Review and Resource Manual

AF800694

Family Nurse Practitioner

6th Edition

Volume 2

Edited by
Courtney Reinisch, DNP, RN, FNP-BC, DCC
Mary Elizabeth Duffy, DNP, RN, FNP-BC, ACNP-BC, DCC

ANA
AMERICAN NURSES ASSOCIATION

The ANA is the only full-service professional organization representing the interests of the nation's 4.2 million registered nurses through its constituent/state nurses associations and its organizational affiliates. The ANA advances the nursing profession by fostering high standards of nursing practice, promoting the rights of nurses in the workplace, projecting a positive and realistic view of nursing, and by lobbying the Congress and regulatory agencies on health care issues affecting nurses and the public.

American Nurses Association
8403 Colesville Road,
Silver Spring, MD 20910

Library of Congress Control Number: 2024940653

ISBNs
Print Volume 1: 978-1-953985-43-9
Print Volume 2: 978-1-953985-44-6
ePDF: 978-1-953985-45-3
ePub: 978-1-953985-46-0
Mobi: 978-1-953985-47-7
SAN: 851-3481

CONTENTS

VOLUME 2

VOLUME 2

CHAPTER 10

RENAL AND UROLOGIC DISORDERS

Heather Marozsan, MSN, FNP

General Approach

- Examination begins with a review of vital signs, with attention to the presence of fever.
- In patients with renal disorders, symptoms and signs may be nonspecific or absent until the disorder is severe.
- Kidney pain is commonly located in the costovertebral angle (CVA).
- A pelvic exam may be necessary in women.
- In men, the penis should be examined for discharge, lesions, and ulcerations when indicated.
- The epididymis and prostate may also need to be evaluated for tenderness, swelling, masses, or nodules.
- Pain associated with infection is typically constant.
- Pain associated with calculi is typically intermittent and immobilizing.
- The normal urinary tract is sterile, and the immunocompetent patient is resistant to bacterial colonization.
- Urinary tract infection (UTI) is the most common bacterial infection in all age groups.
- UTI should be part of differential diagnoses in any febrile infant, child, or older adult.
- UTI is a marker in young children for abnormalities of the urinary tract. Imaging tests should be conducted in all boys of any age with a first UTI, girls younger than 5 years with a first UTI, older girls with recurrent UTIs, and any child with pyelonephritis to identify abnormalities that may lead to renal damage (e.g., vesicoureteral reflux [VUR]).
- Limit antibiotics to category B if the patient is pregnant or lactating; most antibiotics enter breast milk.
- Consult or refer unusual presentations of disease, persons with recurrent UTIs (especially men), and those who do not respond to standard treatment to a urologist.

RED FLAGS

- Wilms' tumor: Embryonal malignant renal tumor. Two-thirds of cases of Wilms' tumor are diagnosed before 5 years of age and 95% before 10 years of age. Patients are typically asymptomatic and present with a smooth, nontender abdominal mass that does not cross the midline. *If tumor is suspected, abdominal exam should be performed carefully.* Referral to appropriate specialist.
- Patients with signs of UTI who are hemodynamically unstable, severely dehydrated, or unable to take oral medications require hospitalization.
- Gross hematuria without evidence of acute UTI should be considered an indication of malignancy until proven otherwise.
- Oliguria or anuria may be evidence of renal insufficiency or mechanical obstruction.
- A palpable bladder on exam may be a sign of complete or incomplete emptying and blockage and if not addressed can lead to autonomic manifestations including bradycardia, hypotension, and even cardiac arrhythmia.

Common Urologic Disorders

ASYMPTOMATIC BACTERIURIA (ASB)

Description

- ASB is the presence of a colony count of at least 100,000/mL in the absence of symptoms of a urinary tract infection. It is more common in women and increases in both sexes with advancing age, pregnancy, structural abnormalities, prostatic hypertrophy, and asymptomatic calculi, and in patients with an indwelling urinary catheter. ASB in asymptomatic women is defined as two positive clean-catch specimens collected within a 2-week time frame to confirm growth of the same organism. In asymptomatic men and catheterized patients, it is defined as a single clean-catch specimen with isolation of a single organism.

Etiology

- Most commonly caused by gram-negative bacteria such as *Escherichia coli*

Incidence and Demographics

- The prevalence of ASB among healthy women increases with advancing age, from about 1% in the general population to greater than 20% among women 80 years and older residing in the community, with higher incidence correlating to sexual activity
- Prevalence among diabetic women is 8% to 14% and is usually correlated with duration and presence of long-term complications of diabetes.
- ASB is rare among healthy young men and occurs in low numbers in men 75 years and older residing in the community, ranging from 6% to 15%.

Risk Factors

- Indwelling catheter use
- Sexual activity
- Age
- Pregnancy
- Diabetes mellitus
- Spinal cord injury
- Nephrolithiasis
- Kidney transplant
- VUR in children

Prevention and Screening

- Screen, culture, and treat ASB in pregnant women, kidney transplant recipients (up to 3 months post-operatively), children with VUR, and persons who will have or have recently had urologic surgery.
- There is no role for routine screening for or treating asymptomatic bacteriuria in the general, nonpregnant population or in health care facilities.

Assessment

History

- ASB causes no symptoms.

Physical Exam

- Benign

Diagnostic Studies

- Urinalysis reveals bacteria, white blood cells (WBCs)
- Urine culture

Differential Diagnosis

- Cystitis
- Urethritis
- Vaginitis
- Acute pyelonephritis

Considerations

- The U.S. Preventive Services Task Force recommends screening for ASB with urine culture for pregnant women at 12 to 15 weeks of gestation because 20% to 35% of women with ASB in pregnancy will develop overt UTIs.
- There is no evidence that treatment of ASB in older adult women and those with diabetes mellitus reduces long-term renal problems.
- Antibiotic therapy is controversial except in patients who are immunocompromised, have malignancy, with spinal cord injuries, or who are pregnant.

Management

Nonpharmacologic Treatment

- Increase fluids
- Empty bladder fully and frequently to avoid stasis
- Review toileting hygiene

Pharmacologic Treatment

- Antibiotic treatment is tailored to the susceptibility pattern of the isolated organism.
  - Pregnancy:
    - Nitrofurantoin (Macrobid) 100 mg orally twice a day for 5–7 days; avoid use in first trimester if possible
    - Cephalosporin 500 mg orally four times a day for 7 days
    - Fosfomycin 3 g orally as a single dose
    - Trimethoprim-sulfamethoxazole (Bactrim DS) 800/160 mg orally twice a day for 3 days; avoid use in first trimester and at term
- Consider decreased length of treatment to reduce fetal exposure to antibiotics unless infection is recurrent or patient has a history of pyelonephritis.
- Therapeutic levels in renal tissue not achieved with nitrofurantoin and fosfomycin—avoid if pyelonephritis is suspected.
- Consider prophylactic nitrofurantoin (Macrobid) following pyelonephritis in pregnancy
- Nonpregnant patients are typically NOT treated for ASB; however, if treatment is needed they should be treated with antibiotics appropriate to their conditions.

When to Consult, Refer, Hospitalize

- Consult a urologist for frequent recurrence or if nonresponsive to treatment.
- Hospitalization for urinary sepsis may be necessary in older patients.

Follow-Up

Expected Outcomes

- If treated with antibiotics, follow-up 1 to 2 weeks after completion of course with repeat urinalysis and culture, also known as a test of cure. Test of cure is appropriate ONLY in pregnant persons.

Complications

- Pyelonephritis, urinary sepsis

HEMATURIA

Description

- The presence of red blood cells (RBCs) in the urine; microscopic (more than3 RBCs/high-power field [hpf]) or macroscopic/gross (visible to naked eye)

Etiology

Nonglomerular

- Infection (cystitis, urethritis, pyelonephritis, prostatitis)—bacterial, fungal, or viral
- Neoplasm of the bladder (increased with environmental exposure), ureter, prostate, or kidney
- Renal or bladder calculi
- Polycystic kidney disease
- Schistosomiasis
- Trauma—recent instrumentation/procedure (catheterization, lithotripsy, transurethral resection of the prostate [TURP])
- Benign prostatic hypertrophy (BPH) and polyps
- Bleeding diathesis
- Strenuous exercise—benign, short-term, seen in 30% of long-distance runners
- Endometriosis
- Nutcracker phenomenon—left renal vein compression causing increased venous pressure

Glomerular

- Benign renal mass (angiomyolipoma, oncocytoma, abscess)
- Malignant renal mass (renal cell carcinoma, transitional cell carcinoma)
- Structural disease
    - Polycystic kidney disease
    - Medullary sponge kidney
- Lupus nephritis

- Papillary necrosis (sickle-cell disease)
- Malignant hypertension
- Hydronephrosis
- Schistosomiasis
- Interstitial nephritis (71% drug-induced, 15% infection, 14% autoimmune)
- Pyelonephritis
- Hypercalciuria/hyperuricosuria
- AV malformations, fistulas
- Renal infarction secondary to emboli (consider in atrial fibrillation and coronary artery disease [CAD])
- Familial nephritis (Alport syndrome—X-linked disorder causing chronic glomerular nephritis)

Mimics of Hematuria

- Menstruation
- Drugs (Phenazopyridine, phenytoin, rifampin, nitrofurantoin)
- Pigmenturia
- Beeturia

Incidence and Demographics

- Four per 1000 patients per year and represents about 6% of new patients seen by urologists.
- Higher risk in older adult men who are at high risk for obstructive and other urologic diseases
- Gross hematuria in older men is correlated with rates of malignancy up to 20%

Risk Factors

- UTI
- Renal calculi

- Smoking increases risk of bladder cancer, which may present as hematuria
- Environmental exposure to elements that can cause bladder cancer

Prevention and Screening

- U.S. Preventive ServicesTask Force on the Periodic Health Examination does *not* recommend routine screening for hematuria.

Assessment

History

- Concurrent symptoms of dysuria, frequency, and urgency are classically symptomatic of an infectious process.
- Unilateral flank pain with radiation to the groin is typically obstructive in nature (calculi, clot, stricture, or tumor).
- Unilateral flank pain without radiation but with fever, dysuria, and frequency/urgency is consistent with pyelonephritis.
- Urinary hesitancy or dribbling may indicate prostatic involvement (BPH or cancer).
- Systemic symptoms such as weight gain, edema, facial swelling, anuria, or oliguria may suggest a glomerular cause.
- With recent upper respiratory infection (URI) and sore throat, consider poststreptococcal glomerulonephritis.
- Intermittent, painless, gross hematuria is the most common presenting symptom for bladder cancer.
- Assess for recent trauma.

Physical Exam

- Fever often indicates infectious or inflammatory cause.
- Assess for edema or recent weight gain.
- Examine abdomen for discomfort or masses.
- CVA tenderness—pyelonephritis or nephrolithiasis

- Digital rectal exam (DRE)—rule out prostatitis, BPH
- Examination of external genitalia to rule out trauma

Diagnostic Studies

Laboratory

- Urinalysis, microscopic examination of urinary sediment, urine culture
  - Red cell casts and/or marked proteinuria indicate glomerular origin probable.
  - Crystals may be present with nephrolithiasis.
- Urine culture
- Urine cytology to rule out malignancy (uncommon)
- Renal function (blood urea nitrogen [BUN], creatinine [CRE]), electrolytes (comprehensive metabolic panel [CMP]), CBC, coagulants, hemoglobin electrophoresis to rule out sickle-cell trait, erythrocyte sedimentation rate (ESR), anti-nuclear antibody (ANA), and sexually transmitted disease (STD) testing

Imaging

- Intravenous pyelography or computerized tomography (CT) urography (intravenous pyelogram [IVP]) to r/o malignancy
- Renal ultrasound (low cost, no radiation)—exclude cysts, hydronephrosis, hydroureter
- CT scan—noncontrast stone study or with/without if trauma is suspected
  - KUB (kidneys, ureters, bladder)—detect radiopaque stones
- Cystoscopy
- Renal biopsy

Differential Diagnosis

- UTI
- STD
- Tuberculosis
- Hemorrhagic cystitis
- Renal carcinoma (risk factors: smoking, obesity, male sex, family history)

- Bladder cancer (predominantly men 60 years of age and older)
- Vesicoureteral Reflux (VUR)
- Ingestion of dyes and pigments
- Glomerulopathy
- Pyelonephritis
- Renal calculi
- Pelvic inflammatory disease

Management

Nonpharmacologic Treatment

- Infection—see Urinary Tract Infection (UTI, cystitis)
- Nephrolithiasis/urolithiasis—see Urolithiasis/Nephrolithiasis

Pharmacologic Treatment

- Infection—see Urinary Tract Infection (UTI, cystitis)
- Nephrolithiasis/urolithiasis—see Urolithiasis/Nephrolithiasis

Special Considerations

- People who ingest large amounts of beets and foods containing red dye may have pseudohematuria.

When to Consult, Refer, Hospitalize

- Refer for persistent, unexplained hematuria; no resolution with treatment of infection; need for invasive testing or treatment. Gross hematuria always warrants referral for further evaluation due to strong evidence associating it with urologic malignancies.
- Hospitalize for uncontrolled pain, uncontrolled bleeding, or unstable vital signs.

Follow-Up

Expected Outcomes

- A cause for hematuria is often not identified. A negative evaluation for hematuria warrants annual urinalysis and blood pressure monitoring. In some high-risk patients, repeat imaging and cystoscopy is appropriate for persistent hematuria.

Complications

- Infection—UTI—> urosepsis
- Urinary obstruction
- Hydronephrosis
- Renal failure—> anemia

PROTEINURIA

Description

- Total urinary protein excretion greater than 150 mg/day; persistent proteinuria is a hallmark of renal disease

Etiology

Types of Proteinuria

- **Transient**
  - Exercise, fever induced
- **Persistent**
  - Orthostatic: uncommon over age 30, occurs in 2%–5% adolescents
  - Glomerular: due to increased filtration of macromolecules (such as albumin) across the glomerular capillary wall.
- Diabetic neuropathy, hypertensive nephrosclerosis, sickle cell disease, radiation nephritis
  - Tubular: increased secretion due to renal tubular dysfunction.

- Heavy metal poisoning, autoimmune disease, allergic interstitial inflammation, medication induced (nonsteroidal anti-inflammatory drugs [NSAIDs], lithium, etc.)
  - Overflow: increased excretion of low-molecular-weight proteins due to overproduction of protein, leading to increased glomerular filtration and excretion.
- Myeloma, hemolysis, rhabdomyolysis
  - Postrenal: due to inflammation in the urinary tract
- Infection, nephrolithiasis or mass

Risk Factors

- Advanced age
- Obesity
- People of African American, Native American, and Pacific Island descent

Prevention and Screening

- Annual screening for proteinuria is not cost effective in the general population of healthy people under age 60 years; however, early detection of proteinuria is useful in patients 60 years of age or older and patients with diabetes and hypertension.
- Proteinuria in pregnant women: fewer than 24 weeks can indicate glomerulonephritis; 24 weeks and over can indicate preeclampsia

Assessment

History

- Recent acute or chronic illness
- Surgery or procedure requiring contrast media
- UTI signs and symptoms, risk factors for HIV
- Family history of renal disease or diabetes

Physical Exam

- Thorough physical examination with fundoscopic examination/referral to ophthalmology to exclude diabetic retinopathy
- Consider diabetic foot examination

Diagnostic Studies

Laboratory

- Urinanylasis (U/A), Bence-Jones proteins to evaluate for multiple myeloma
- Sulfosalicylic acid test and 24-hour collection in children
- CBC, CMP, albumin, calcium, phosphorus; lipids, ESR, ANA

Imaging

- Renal ultrasound
- IVP

Differential Diagnosis

- Transient proteinuria (temporary, self-limiting)
- Persistent proteinuria (two or more incidences over a 3-month period)
- Orthostatic/nonorthostatic proteinuria (increased urinary protein after prolonged sitting)
- Glomerulonephritis
- Diabetic neuropathy
- Vasculitis
- Medication-induced

Management

- Aggressively treat underlying cause

Nonpharmacologic Treatment

- Sodium and protein-restricted diet

Pharmacologic Treatment

- Renal protection with angiotensin-converting enzyme inhibitors (ACEIs) and angiotensin receptor blockers (ARBs)

When to Consult, Refer, Hospitalize

- All renal patients should be referred to a specialist for consultation and management guidance.

LOWER URINARY TRACT INFECTION (CYSTITIS)

Description

- Cystitis or an acute UTI is presumed to be confined to the bladder. Such infections lack signs or symptoms that suggest an infection extending beyond the bladder (see Pyelonephritis).

Etiology

- Uncomplicated, lower UTI is most commonly caused by *E. coli* (80% to 90%) or other gram-negative bacteria from gastrointestinal tract (*Proteus mirabilis, Klebsiella pneumoniae, Enterobacter* spp.).
- Gram-positive organism (*Staphylococcus saprophyticus*) is common in sexually active young women but uncommon cause of infection in men.
- Symptomatic women with pyuria but without significant bacteriuria ("sterile pyuria") may have infection with *Chlamydia trachomatis*.
- Viruses may be associated with hemorrhagic cystitis.
- Most UTIs (more than 95%) are caused by ascending infections from urethra.

Incidence and Demographics

- Most common bacterial infections in women
- In first 2 months of life, incidence higher in males
- May be associated with bacteremia in the first 3 months of life
- After 1 to 2 years of age, females 10 to 20 times more likely to experience UTI than males secondary to shorter urethra, closer proximity to perirectal area
- Reoccurrence in 50% to 75% of females
- VUR found in approximately 20% of females after first UTI and 40% to 45% of those with recurrent UTIs

Risk Factors

- Female gender; sexual intercourse; anal intercourse; failure to void after coitus; fecal contamination; dehydration; history of prior UTI; diabetes mellitus or other immunocompromised state; pregnancy; obesity; use of spermicides, diaphragm, or oral contraceptives; menopause; vaginal pH higher than 4.5
- Structural urinary tract abnormalities (strictures, stones, tumors, neuropathic bladder)
- Procedures such as catheterization or recent urologic surgery
- Aging: relaxation of pelvic-supporting structures; hypoestrogenic state and vaginal atrophy; BPH or prostatitis; incontinence of urine/stool
- Dysfunctional voiding pattern or infrequent voiding, including neurogenic bladder
- Chronic constipation in children

Prevention and Screening

- Frequent bladder emptying; postcoital voiding within 10 to 15 minutes of intercourse
- Urine acidification with cranberry juice (more than 300 mL daily)
- Education of parents and children regarding hygiene, tips on toilet training; education of adolescents regarding sexual intercourse
- In postmenopausal women, systemic or topical estrogen therapy markedly reduces the incidence of recurrent UTI.

- Women with one to two uncomplicated UTIs per year may require postcoital, single-dose antibiotic treatment or appropriate short-course treatment. Women who experience more than three UTIs per year or two in 6 months may warrant low-dose oral antimicrobial prophylaxis.

Assessment

History

- Symptoms: dysuria, urgency, frequency, nocturia, hematuria, suprapubic discomfort
- Rectal pain, change in urine flow or stream
- Low-grade fever and enuresis in children
- Lower abdominal or back pain, fever, chills, and lassitude (may indicate pyelonephritis)
- Presence of vaginal or urethral discharge or odor, pruritus, dyspareunia, or external dysuria without frequency may indicate vaginitis or urethritis
- Perianal itching (may indicate pinworms)
- Mental status change in older adults may be the only symptom of UTI
- History of UTI, pelvic inflammatory disease, cervicitis
- Inquire about last menstrual period

Physical Exam

- Fever
- Suprapubic tenderness to palpation
- CVA tenderness
- Assess signs of hydration status—mucous membranes, skin turgor
- Inspection of genitalia in children for trauma, anomalies, meatal stenosis, phimosis
- Pelvic examination recommended in adolescents and adults to rule out vaginitis if indicated. Assess for discharge, excoriations, tenderness, and ulcerations.
- Male patients should be examined for penile discharge, lesions, ulcerations, and swelling. Prostate exam to evaluate for prostate enlargement or infection, if indicated
- In older adults, mental status changes or new onset of falls may be the only signs of infection.

Diagnostic Studies

Laboratory

- Clean-catch urinalysis. Children: Always obtain culture from midstream; may need to obtain urine by catheterization or SPA (suprapubic bladder aspiration) in infants and children.
- Urine culture and sensitivity
- Cultures for STDs

Imaging

- Radiographic follow-up with a renal and bladder ultrasound and a voiding cystourethrogram (VCUG) should be obtained for all children under 5 years with a documented UTI, all males with a UTI, and all females with febrile UTIs to evaluate for VUR and structural abnormalities. The VCUG should be done after 3 to 4 weeks because mucosal changes (edema) during an infection may result in a transient reflux.
- Renal ultrasound—consider for recurrent UTI or treatment failure
- IVP
- CT or magnetic resonance imaging (MRI)
- Dimercaptosuccinic acid (DMSA) scan may be recommended for patients with pyelonephritis to detect renal scarring.
- VCUG is a dynamic test for stricture/reflux; a normal renal ultrasound does not exclude VUR.

Differential Diagnosis

- Urethritis
- Diabetes insipidus
- Cervicitis
- Pelvic inflammatory disease
- Herpes simplex virus (HSV)
- Interstitial cystitis
- Pyelonephritis

- Renal calculi
- Vaginitis
- Encopresis
- Female urethral syndrome
- Chemical vaginitis
- Prostatitis
- Meatal stenosis
- Dysfunctional voiding
- STDs
- Balanitis
- Sexual abuse
- Psychogenic dysuria (a component of somatization disorder, depression, chronic pain, or sexual abuse)
- Foreign body
- Pinworms
- Diaper dermatitis

Management

Nonpharmacologic Treatment

- Hygiene measures (front-to-back wiping, care of uncircumcised penis)
- More frequent and complete voiding, voiding pre- and post-coitus
- Hydration, cranberry juice (some studies show prevents *E. coli* from adhering to bladder)
  - Avoid carbonated beverages

Pharmacologic Treatment

- It is important to know the antimicrobial susceptibility profile of uropathogens causing uncomplicated UTIs in the community to guide therapeutic decisions—verify susceptibility with urine culture and sensitivity (C&S).

- Adolescents and adults
  - See Tables 10–1 and 10–2 for antibiotic regimens.
- Nitrofurantoin (Macrobid) for 5 days. If no resistance in community, short course of treatment with trimethoprim-sulfamethoxazole or a fluoroquinolone is superior to beta-lactams (e.g., Augmentin).
- For pain relief, consider use of urinary analgesic phenazopyridine (Pyridium); inform patient that medication will turn urine orange and possibly affect contact lenses; not recommended for children or patients with known or suspected glucose-6-phosphate dehydrogenase (G6PD) deficiency.

TABLE 10–1.
UTI TREATMENT IN ADULTS (PREFERRED FIRST LINE)—NO RENAL INVOLVEMENT SUSPECTED

DRUG	DOSAGE
Nitrofurantoin monohydrate	100 mg orally q12h
Trimethoprim-sulfamethoxazole DS	160/800 mg orally q12h
Fosfomycin	3 g single dose

TABLE 10–2.
UTI TREATMENT IN ADULTS (ALTERNATIVES)—NO RENAL INVOLVEMENT SUSPECTED

DRUG	DOSAGE
Amoxicillin-clavulanate	500 mg orally q12h
Cefpodoxime	100 mg orally q12h
Cefdinir	300 mg orally q12h
Cefadroxil	500 mg orally q12h
Ciprofloxacin	250 mg orally q12h
Levofloxacin	250 mg orally daily

In general, beta-lactams are second-line agents because they are less effective and have more potential adverse effects than other UTI antimicrobials.

*****If beta-lactams cannot be used (e.g., because of severe allergy), ciprofloxacin (250 mg twice daily or 500 mg extended release daily), and levofloxacin (250 mg daily), each for 3 days, are reasonable alternative agents.***

- Infants and children
  - See Table 10–3 for antibiotic regimens.
- Fluoroquinolones are not recommended in children (<18 years) because of possible adverse effects on developing cartilage.
- Prophylaxis of UTIs in infants and young children with VUR with low-dose antibiotic

Length of Treatment

- In healthy young women, a 3-day course of therapy is superior to a single dose because early recurrence is more common after single-dose therapy. Nitrofurantoin requires 5-day course; amoxicillin and Augmentin require 7 to 10 days.
- Pregnant women should be treated for 7 days. Do not prescribe sulfonamides in the third trimester.
- Short-course therapy is not recommended if symptoms have been present for more than 7 days, if there is a high probability of deep-tissue infection, for any male person with UTI, in the presence of underlying structural or functional defect of the urinary tract, for immunosuppressed persons, or for patients with indwelling catheters.

TABLE 10–3.
UTI TREATMENT IN INFANTS AND CHILDREN—NO RENAL INVOLVEMENT SUSPECTED

DRUG	DOSAGE	RECOMMENDATIONS & COMMENTS
Cefixime	8 mg/kg orally once daily	Cephalosporins are the first-line oral agent
Cefdinir	14 mg/kg orally once daily	Cephalosporins are the first-line oral agent
Ceftibuten	9 mg/kg orally once daily	Cephalosporins are the first-line oral agent
Fluoroquinolones	Ciprofloxacin 10–20 mg/kg orally q12h	American Academy of Pediatrics (AAP) recommends that the use of ciprofloxacin for UTI in children be limited to those infections caused by *Pseudomonas aeruginosa* or other multidrug-resistant, gram-negative bacteria

Amoxicillin and ampicillin are not routinely recommended for empiric therapy because of the high rate of resistance of E. coli. Similarly, amoxicillin-clavulanate and trimethoprim-sulfamethoxazole should be used with caution.

Special Considerations

- In cases of recurrent infection, assume patient has covert renal infection and retreat for a minimum of 14 days.
- Males younger than 50 years with the following risk factors usually receive a 10- to 14-day course: men who have sex with men also having intercourse with women colonized with uropathogens, or AIDS patients with CD4+ lymphocyte count less than 200/mm^3.
- Males 50 years of age or older may require 4 to 6 weeks and up to 12 weeks of treatment to sterilize the urinary tract if the prostate is the source of infection.
- Infants and children: Treat for 10 days or until imaging studies are completed and assessed.
- Geriatric patients (age 65 and older): Mental status change may be the only symptom.
- Pregnancy/lactation: It is generally accepted that penicillin (with or without beta-lactamase inhibitors), cephalosporins, and aztreonam are safe in pregnancy.

When to Consult, Refer, Hospitalize

- Consult or refer to adult/pediatric urologist for recurrent infections if anatomic abnormality is suspected.
- Hemodynamically unstable patients, or patients in whom urosepsis is a potential concern, may require hospitalization or intravenous antibiotics.
- Hospitalize if signs of pyelonephritis in children or pregnant woman for IV antibiotics.

Follow-Up

- Repeat urine culture 3 to 4 days after completion of therapy in children and pregnant women if infection is recurrent.
- Radiographic follow-up with a renal and bladder ultrasound and a VCUG should be obtained for:
  - Children under 5 years with a documented UTI
  - Males of any age with a UTI
  - Females with a febrile UTI to evaluate for VUR.

Expected Course

- If using correct antibiotic (per culture and sensitivity), signs and symptoms should resolve within 48 to 72 hours.
- Note: A test of cure can help to differentiate inadequately treated infection from recurrence, although not routinely recommended

Complications

- Pyelonephritis, recurrent or relapse of infection, urosepsis (especially in older adults), renal abscess
- VUR can result in renal scarring and loss of renal function.

ACUTE PYELONEPHRITIS

Description

- Acute bacterial infection of the soft tissue of the renal parenchyma and pelvis or other portion of the upper urinary tract, typically producing signs and symptoms of systemic toxicity

Etiology

- 75% due to *E. coli*
- 10% to 15% due to other gram-negative organisms (*P. mirabilis, K. pneumoniae, Enterobacter*)
- 10% to 15% due to *S. aureus* or *S. saprophyticus*
- Most common route of infection: ascension from bladder

Incidence and Demographics

- There are 15 to 17 cases per 10,000 females and 3 to 4 cases per 10,000 males annually. More frequent in sexually active females.

Risk Factors

- Urinary tract abnormalities or instrumentation, stones, catheters, diabetes or other immunocompromised states, recent pyelonephritis, BPH, pregnancy, fecal incontinence
- Recent lower UTI

Prevention and Screening

- Hygiene, hydration, voiding after coitus
- Prophylactic antibiotics if infected recurrently or frequently
- Screening pregnant women for asymptomatic bacteriuria

Assessment

History

- Fever (often temperature above 102°F), shaking chills, flank pain, myalgias, abdominal pain
- Hematuria, dysuria, frequency, urgency
- Nausea and vomiting
- Perineal pain in men

Physical Exam

- Fever
- Suprapubic pain, CVA tenderness
- Tachycardia
- General malaise

Diagnostic Studies

Laboratory

- Urinalysis: bacteria and WBCs visible on microscopy, may also see casts; + leukocyte esterase and nitrites on dipstick, possible proteinuria

- CBC: may have elevated WBCs
- Urine culture and sensitivity should be performed on all patients.

Imaging

- Voiding cystourethrogram, IVP, renal scan, and cystoscopy may be indicated if structural abnormality is suspected. If renal abscess suspected, order abdominal/pelvic CT.
- Renal ultrasound preferred for pediatric patients

Differential Diagnosis

- Nephrolithiasis
- Prostatitis
- TB of the kidney
- Acute low back pain
- Tumors

Management

Nonpharmacologic Treatment

- Increase clear fluids
- Avoid caffeinated beverages

Pharmacologic Treatment:

- In an otherwise healthy patient with mild disease, outpatient treatment with oral antimicrobials is possible if patient has no nausea or vomiting, no signs of volume depletion, no evidence of septicemia, and is reliable in following medical advice.
- See Table 10–4 and 10–5 for oral doses of antibiotic therapy. Urine culture and susceptibility testing should be performed in all patients, and the initial empiric regimen should be tailored appropriately to the susceptibility profile of the infecting pathogen, once known.
- Parenteral antibiotics may be indicated for gram-positive cocci, complicated histories, previous episodes of pyelonephritis, or recent urinary tract manipulations.

TABLE 10–4. TREATMENT FOR ACUTE PYELONEPHRITIS FOR ADULTS IN THE OUTPATIENT SETTING

DRUG	DOSAGE
Ciprofloxacin	500 mg twice a day or 1 g extended release (XR) daily for 1 week
Levofloxacin	750 mg daily for 5–7 days
For patients for whom fluoroquinolones are contraindicated	
Ceftriaxone	1 g IM in office
Followed by ONE of the following:	
Trimethoprim-sulfamethoxazole DS	160/800 mg q12h for 7–10 days
Amoxicillin-clavulanate	875 mg orally twice daily for 7–10 days
Cefpodoxime	200 mg orally twice daily for 7–10 days
Cefdinir	300 mg orally twice daily for 7–10 days

TABLE 10–5. TREATMENT FOR ACUTE PYELONEPHRITIS FOR CHILDREN

DRUG	DOSAGE
Cefuroxime	30 mg/kg/day orally in two divided doses
Cefixime	8 mg/kg/day orally once daily
Cefdinir	14 mg/kg/day orally once daily
Ceftibuten	9 mg/kg/day orally once daily

Length of Treatment:

- Total duration of antimicrobial therapy generally ranges from 5 to 10 days for adults, depending on clinical response and the antimicrobial chosen to complete the course.
- Total duration for children ranges from 3 to 5 days if immunocompetent, afebrile and 10 days in children who are febrile or otherwise immunocompromised.
- Infants, children, pregnant women, and older adults are usually hospitalized for initial therapy with IV antibiotics.
- If **chronic** pyelonephritis develops, therapy may be required for 3 to 6 months.
- Use of nitrofurantoin, fosfomycin, and pivmecillinam should be avoided in the setting of pyelonephritis because they do not achieve adequate renal tissue levels.

Special Considerations

- Older adult patients should be hospitalized and started on an aminoglycoside with dosage adjusted for weight and renal function.
- Pregnancy: sulfa drugs and fluoroquinolones contraindicated; use beta-lactams, aminoglycosides, or both

When to Consult, Refer, Hospitalize

- Inpatient management required if patient appears toxic or is an older adult, hemodynamically unstable, immunocompromised, pregnant, or unable to tolerate oral antibiotic therapy or fluids.
- If fever persists for more than3 days and abscess or obstruction is suspected, refer to a urologist.

Follow-Up

- Recheck patient in office in 24 hours.
- Repeat culture 2 weeks after completion of therapy and again at 12 weeks.
- In children, after completion of treatment course, a prolonged 1- to 3-month course of oral therapy is then instituted with follow-up urine cultures at frequent intervals for the next year.

Expected Course

- Good prognosis: Should resolve within 72 hours of institution of appropriate therapy.

Complications

- Sepsis, preterm labor in pregnancy, chronic renal insufficiency, chronic pyelonephritis, renal abscess, death
- Without demonstrable obstruction or recurrent acute infection, asymptomatic renal bacteriuria has not been clearly established as harmful, and repeated courses of antimicrobials or suppression therapy are not indicated.
- If obstruction cannot be eliminated and recurrent UTI is common, long-term therapy is useful.

URINARY INCONTINENCE (UI)

Description

A general term used to describe involuntary loss of urine; further classified based on causation

Etiology

- *Urge:* Involuntary loss of a large amount of urine preceded by strong, unexpected urge to void; most common cause of incontinence
  - Unrelated to activity or position and indicative of detrusor overactivity (DO)
  - DO is instability of the detrusor muscle during bladder filling as a result of:
- *Idiopathic causes*: Theories include $alpha_1$-receptors in the bladder, disruptions of somatic and autonomic nervous systems, efferent/afferent pathways, and increased activation of muscarinic receptors in the bladder.
- *Neurogenic causes*: Spinal cord injuries below T11 to L1-2, multiple sclerosis, diabetes mellitus, spina bifida.
- *Stress:* Involuntary loss of small amounts of urine
  - Associated with activities that increase intra-abdominal pressure, including coughing, sneezing, lifting, certain exercises
  - Urine does not leak when patient is lying down
  - May be due to aging, pelvic floor muscle weakness (e.g., cystocele, rectocele), perineal trauma, prostatitis/pelvic surgery, estrogen deficiency in women
- *Overflow:* From chronic urine retention
  - Results from chronically distended bladder receiving additional increment of urine to exceed intravesical pressure and release small amount of urine
  - May be due to prostatic enlargement, anticholinergics, tricyclic antidepressants, diabetic neuropathy, outflow obstruction, or multiple sclerosis
- *Functional*
  - Physical or cognitive disability, sedating medications that make it difficult to use the bathroom
- *Total*
  - Loss of urine at all times in all positions
  - Due to sphincteric inefficiency from surgery, nerve damage, tumor infiltration, or fistula formation

- *Transient*
  - May be due to delirium, infection, atrophic vaginitis, urethritis, or drugs (sedatives, hypnotics, diuretics, opioids, calcium channel blockers, anticholinergics, antidepressants, antihistamines, decongestants, others)
  - Less common: diabetes mellitus or insipidus, restricted mobility, stool impaction, depression
- *Mixed:* Two causes present
  - Stress and urge incontinence
  - Urge and functional

Incidence and Demographics

- Problem for 5% to 15% of older adult patients in community setting and up to 50% of nursing home residents
- Overall affects 12 million adults; females (51.1%) affected more than males (13.9%)

Risk Factors

- Older adult
- Estrogen deficiency
- Prostatic hypertrophy
- Multiparity
- Dementia
- Diabetes
- Parkinson's disease
- Myelodysplasia
- Multiple sclerosis
- Spinal cord injury or lesion
- Stroke
- Immobility
- Pregnancy
- Use of diuretics

Assessment

History

- Urgency, leaking, dribbling, burning, hesitancy, nocturia, irritation
- Constipation and sexual function
- Assess for abdominal discomfort or distention; pelvic organ prolapse
- Double vision, muscle weakness, paralysis, or poor coordination suggest neurologic disorders
- Assess exposure to medications (particularly potassium-sparing diuretics) and other provoking factors (caffeine, alcohol, physical activity, cough, laughing, sounds of water, and hands in water)
- The 3 Incontinence Questions (3 IQ) tools help provider in differentiating stress and urge incontinence. Ask patient:
  - "In past 3 months have you leaked urine?"
  - "How often?"
  - "Which of the above provoking factors caused leakage more often?"

Physical Exam

- Goal is to detect anatomic and neurological abnormalities
- Examine abdomen (with full bladder if possible) for masses, suprapubic tenderness, or fullness.
- Pelvic exam to assess perineal skin, cystocele/rectocele, uterine prolapse, pelvic mass, perivaginal muscle tone, atrophic vaginitis
- Estimate post-voiding residual by abdominal palpation and percussion and/or bimanual exam.
- Rectal exam for perineal sensation, resting and active sphincter tone, rectal mass, and fecal impaction; assess consistency, size, and contour of prostate
- Neurological exam with deep tendon reflex, sensation, gait
- Mental status exam in older adults
- Musculoskeletal exam for secondary causes such as weakness, ambulation problems

Diagnostic Studies Examination

- 24-hour voiding diary: include type of fluid ingested and when, time and volume voided.
- Observe voiding to detect problems with hesitancy, dribbling, or interrupted stream.
- Measure post-void residual urine (less than 50 mL is normal).

Laboratory

- Urinalysis, C&S
- Urine cytology
- Renal function screening

Imaging

- Cystograms may demonstrate fistula sites
- Stress cystograms may show descent of bladder neck on straining
- Pelvic ultrasound may reveal source of obstruction

Differential Diagnosis

- Stress urinary incontinence (SUI)
  - Anatomic
  - Intrinsic sphincter deficiency
- Urge incontinence
  - DO
  - Poor bladder compliance
- Mixed incontinence
- Overflow incontinence
- Functional or transient incontinence
- Lower urinary tract conditions
- Medications

Management

Nonpharmacologic Treatment

- Use a voiding diary for 3 days to provide information about voiding habits as a diagnostic technique.
- General
  - Good personal hygiene
  - Dietary modifications (avoid caffeine, alcohol, and sugar)
  - Weight loss
  - Limit use of diuretics
  - Eliminate constipation
  - Smoking cessation
- Behavioral techniques
  - Pelvic floor therapy
  - Bladder training for urge UI; may also work for SUI
  - Pelvic muscle exercises (Kegel) for SUI
  - Biofeedback for SUI
  - Vaginal weighted cone for SUI
  - Habit training or timed voiding for functional UI
- Surgical
  - Overflow incontinence from anatomic obstruction (e.g., BPH)
  - Stress incontinence from anatomically reversible condition (prolapse, cystocele)
- Other measures
  - Intermittent catheterization; useful in overflow incontinence
  - External collection catheters/moisture-wicking catheters
  - Incontinence pads or garments
  - Pessaries for prolapsed uterus
  - Vaginal laser therapy

Pharmacologic Treatment

- Treat UTI if present; otherwise, see Tables 10–6 and 10–7

TABLE 10–6. PHARMACOLOGIC TREATMENT FOR URGE INCONTINENCE

CLASS	DRUG	DOSAGE
Antimuscarinic/ antispasmodics	Oxybutynin (Ditropan) IR	2.5–5.0 mg, two, three, or four times a day
	Oxybutynin (Ditropan) ER	5 to 10 mg orally once daily, max dose 30 mg
	OxybutyninTransdermal 10% Gel	Apply 1 sachet or 1 pump once daily
	OxybutyninTransdermal Patch	Apply 1 patch twice per week
	Tolterodine (Detrol) IR	1 to 2 mg orally twice daily
	Tolerodine (Detrol) XR	2–4 mg orally once daily
	Darifenacin (Enablex)	7.5–15 mg daily
	Fesoterodine (Toviaz)	4–8 mg orally once daily
	Trospium chloride (Sanctura) IR	20 mg orally twice daily.
	Trospium chloride (Sanctura) XR	60 mg orally once daily
	Solifenacin succinate (VESIcare)	5–10 mg daily
Beta-3 adrenergic agonists	Mirabegron *can be used with Solifenacin*	25–50 mg orally daily
	Vibegron	75 mg orally daily

TABLE 10–7. PHARMACOLOGIC TREATMENT FOR STRESS INCONTINENCE

CLASS	DRUG	DOSAGE
Hormone therapy	Conjugated estrogen (Premarin)	0.5–2 mg orally vaginally daily, then 3x per week, then 2x per week
	Progestin (Medroxyprogesterone)	2.5–10 mg/day either continuously or (if uterus present) intermittently

How Long to Treat

- Indefinitely or until surgical correction

Prevention and Screening

- Kegel exercises, regular pelvic examination to detect pathology early
- Avoid constipation

- Regular screening for BPH
- Discuss and evaluate for UI and identify factors that might contribute to or exacerbate symptoms for early diagnosis and treatment.

Special Considerations

- More central nervous system (CNS) effects with oxybutynin (headaches, cognitive impairment) plus dry mouth, constipation, urinary retention
- Caution patient to avoid alcohol when taking this medication.
- Tolterodine does not cross blood–brain barrier; less constipation, dry mouth
- Pregnancy: Stress incontinence is common in pregnancy. It should be treated with good hygiene, frequent voiding, and Kegel exercises.
- Lactation: Avoid pharmacologic agents that could be transmitted via breast milk.
- Overactive bladder (OAB) without incontinence (OAB-dry) may be part of the urge incontinence continuum.

Treatment

Pharmacologic Treatment

- Prescription medications, both pills and patches, are similar to treatment for urge incontinence
- Surgeries and procedures, such as sacral neuromodulation and botulinum injections
- Behavioral interventions, such as behavior modification programs and bladder training
- Complementary and alternative medicine, such as acupuncture and reflexology

When to Consult, Refer, Hospitalize

- Consult with specialist for patients with stress and urge incontinence whose conditions fail to respond to behavioral therapy and initial drug treatment.
- Refer if any neurologic abnormalities coexist.
- Refer for overflow incontinence evaluation and treatment.
- Refer to urologist for cystoscopy for persistent RBCs on urinalysis.

Follow-Up

- Weekly visits until most symptoms controlled; then as needed

Expected course

- Long-term prognosis depends on patient compliance and follow-up.

Complications

- UTI, renal failure, skin breakdown, falls, hydronephrosis, depression, social isolation, sleep disturbances
- Dehydration secondary to minimizing fluids

ENURESIS (PRIMARY NOCTURNAL URINARY INCONTINENCE)

Description

- Persistent involuntary loss of urine at least twice a week for at least 3 consecutive months in child who is at least 5 years of age
  - ◊ *Primary monosymptomatic:* enuresis without a history of nocturnal continence
  - ◊ *Secondary monosymptomatic:* recurrence of enuresis after at least 6 months of nocturnal continence
  - ◊ *Non-monosymptomatic:* enuresis associated with urinary urgency, frequency, straining, pain, constipation, or encopresis

Etiology

- Usually multifactorial
- Appears to run in families; has been linked to specific genetic markers (e.g., chromosome 8, 12, 13, 22, and *ENUR*1 gene on chromosome 13); 77% risk if both parents had enuresis, 44% for one parent, 15% if neither
- 20% of children with nighttime incontinence also have daytime problems.
- Primary enuresis may be due to food allergies, disorders of the urinary or nervous systems, psychological factors, reduced bladder capacity, or lack of normal increase in nocturnal antidiuretic hormone (ADH) secretion.

- Primary nocturnal enuresis (PNE) is primarily an arousal disorder with failure of the CNS to recognize bladder fullness or contraction and/or failure to inhibit bladder contraction or sphincter relaxation; detrusor instability.
- Secondary enuresis may be due to bacteriuria, UTI, inability to concentrate urine secondary to insufficient ADH or a renal tubular defect, a pelvic mass or spinal cord malformation, meatal stenosis, ectopic ureter, glycosuria as in diabetes mellitus or diabetes insipidus, or a possible sleep disorder.

Incidence and Demographics

- Occurs in approximately 15% of children; by age 18, incidence has decreased to 1%; 80% are monosymptomatic, 5% have an organic cause.
- Multifactorial, although most children outgrowing monosymptomatic nocturnal enuresis (MNE) indicate maturational delay
- Genetic predisposition: both parents have history, child has approximately 77% chance of developing enuresis; one parent, 44% chance; neither parent, 15% chance

Risk Factors

- Males more than females, 3:1
- Family history in at least one parent
- Institutionalized

Prevention and Screening

- Ask patient and parent at each well-child visit.

Assessment

History

- Family history of enuresis
- Evaluate frequency of enuresis and the presence of daytime incontinence

- Evaluate for dysuria, frequency, and urgency
- Evaluate for constipation
- Evaluate for psychological stress
- Family's/child's response to bed-wetting
- "How have you handled the nighttime accident?"

Physical Exam

- Vital signs
  - Blood pressure
- Growth chart patterns
  - Poor growth, elevated blood pressure, or both may suggest renal disease
- Genitourinary exam—evaluate for genital anomalies (hypospadias, meatal stenosis, ectopic ureter)
- Abdominal exam—evaluate for renal or bladder enlargement, fecal masses (encopresis)
- Neurological exam—evaluate reflexes, perineal sensation, rectal tone, gait; examine lower back/spine for sacral dimpling, abnormal gluteal folds

Diagnostic Studies

Laboratory

- Hemoglobin A1c (HbA1c) for diabetes mellitus
- Urinalysis
  - Specific gravity = 1.005 may indicate diabetes insipidus, acute tubular necrosis, or pyelonephritis.
  - Glycosuria may indicate diabetes mellitus or low renal glycemic threshold.
  - Proteinuria may indicate underlying disease.
  - WBCs may indicate UTI.
- Culture and sensitivity

Imaging

- IVP
- Renal, bladder ultrasound
- Voiding cystourethrogram (VCUG) with significant daytime complaints
- MRI for abnormal neurological exam

Differential Diagnosis

- Urinary tract structural abnormalities
- UTI
- Neurologic bladder dysfunction
- Spinal cord malformations (hair tuft, abnormal gluteal folds)
- Malignancy
- Diabetes mellitus or insipidus
- Psychogenic polydipsia
- Sleep apnea
- Sickle-cell disease

Management

Nonpharmacologic Treatment

- Behavioral or motivational therapy
    - Counseling, behavior modification, and anticipatory guidance
    - Conditioning therapy
    - Voiding diaries
    - Avoid fluids 2 hours before bedtime.
    - Improve access to toilet.
    - Encourage toileting before bedtime.
    - Discontinue diapers and pull-ups to allow for sensation of wetness.

- ◊ Nonpunitive involvement of child in morning cleanup
- ◊ Positive reinforcement

- ♦ Bladder stretching and strengthening exercises
    - ◊ Bladder training with a toileting schedule, avoid holding urine
- ♦ Enuresis alarms: requires committed and motivated family and takes 12 to 16 weeks to be effective; 70% success rate

Pharmacologic Treatment

- ♦ Desmopressin (DDAVP) one spray each nostril 10 to 20 µg or 0.2 to 0.6 mg orally at bedtime
    - ◊ DDAVP may be used for a 3-month trial to break the cycle of intermittent wetting and intermittently for camping trips, vacations, sleepovers, etc.—start a few days prior
    - ◊ Initial cure rate is 86%; relapse with discontinuation 94%.
    - ◊ In combination with propiverine, cure rate increases to 97%.
- ♦ Anticholinergics
    - ◊ Imipramine (Tofranil) 25 to 50 mg orally at bedtime in ages 7 to 12 years; may increase to 75 mg in patients more than 12 years old.
    - ◊ 40% to 60% efficacy at 6 months; relapse with discontinuation is 50%
    - ◊ Gradually taper dose after 14 to 28 consecutive dry nights
    - ◊ Oxybutynin (Ditropan)

Special Considerations

- ♦ Enuresis alarms are the most effective intervention.
- ♦ Consider medication side effects before initiation and monitor closely.

When to Consult, Refer, Hospitalize

- ♦ Psychosomatic cause may require referral.
- ♦ Genitourinary dysfunction or neurological symptoms warrant referral for clinical radiographic findings that suggest renal or urologic abnormality or bladder instability.
- ♦ Consult with neurosurgery for evidence of occult spinal dysraphism.

Follow-Up

- Regular follow-up visits are important to address issues or concerns and to encourage patient and family.
- Patients on medication should be seen 2 weeks after initiation of therapy, and then monthly for 3 months.

Expected Course

- Typically, self-limiting

Complications

- Emotional distress, social isolation, depression

UROLITHIASIS/NEPHROLITHIASIS

Description

- Urolithiasis: stones occurring within the urinary tract
- Nephrolithiasis: stones within kidney
- Stones initially form in proximal urinary tract and then pass distally.
- Usually lodged in ureter and cause pain, infection, and obstruction
- Most composed of calcium (80%), uric acid (5%), cystine (2%), or struvite (10%)
- Up to 98% of stones smaller than 0.5 cm in diameter will pass spontaneously, especially in the distal ureter.
- Calcium stones are the most common. When they cause obstruction, it tends to be acute and intermittent, producing no long-term effects on renal function.
- Cystine and struvite stones are more likely to be associated with renal damage.

Etiology

- Supersaturation of urine with stone-forming salts

- In many instances, may be manifestation of systemic disease (e.g., bone diseases, immobilization, hyperthyroidism, primary hyperparathyroidism, hypervitaminosis D, renal tubular acidosis, mild-alkali syndrome, gout, others), but idiopathic hypercalciuria responsible for about 50% in adults
- Struvite stones form in alkaline urine; may be seen with chronic *Proteus* spp. infections

Incidence and Demographics

- 1% to 3% of population present with urolithiasis at some point during lifetime
- Most occur at age 30 to 50 years
- Male-to-female ratio 3:1 (calcium stones; struvite stones are more common in females)

Risk Factors

- Cystinuria, genetic defects, renal tubular acidosis, low water intake, high-protein diet, excessive oxalate intake, sedentary lifestyle
- Middle age, white, family history, obesity, diabetes mellitus, chronic diarrhea, malabsorption, history of bowel or bariatric surgery, pathologic skeletal fractures, gout, Paget's disease
- Certain medications: vitamins A, C, and D; loop diuretics; ammonium chloride; acetazolamide; alkali; antacids

Prevention and Screening

- Adequate fluid intake
- If prone to calcium stones, restrict protein, sodium, dairy products, alcohol, and other oxalate-rich foods
- If prone to uric acid stones, alkalinization of urine may prevent formation

Assessment

History

- May be asymptomatic even with severe obstruction, or present with acute back and flank pain that comes and goes.

- Obstruction of the ureter: acute, colicky flank pain that may be episodic in nature; anterior radiation of pain; nausea and vomiting; diaphoresis; patient constantly moving to relieve pain
- Progression of stone: pain referred to ipsilateral testis or labia; urinary urgency or hesitancy
- Ingestion of large amounts of fluids or diuretic use may precipitate attack
- May be associated with dysuria, frequency, hematuria, diaphoresis, restlessness, chills and fever, nausea, and/or vomiting

Physical Exam

- Acute obvious discomfort, pacing, grimacing, unable to get comfortable
- Fever, tachycardia, tachypnea, diaphoresis, restlessness, CVA tenderness
- Be alert to signs of systemic disease (e.g., lymphadenopathy, organomegaly, adenopathy)

Diagnostic Studies

Laboratory

- Urinalysis, culture, CBC, BUN, creatinine
- Urinalysis that shows hematuria with or without proteinuria may suggest calculus or tumor

Imaging

- Plain film of the abdomen (KUB) will show calculi (85% to 90% of which are radiopaque) in the renal pelvis, along the course of the ureter, or in the bladder. Limitations: Overlying bowel gas and rib cartilage calcification may make interpretation difficult.
- Ultrasound is the preferred screening modality when obstruction is suspected (high sensitivity for hydronephrosis) and in pregnancy to assess renal colic. However, it can only suggest (not reveal) the presence of obstruction.
- Noncontrast CT of the abdomen and pelvis is now preferred over imaging; visualizes both radiopaque and radiolucent stones

Differential Diagnosis

- Acute pyelonephritis
- Lower UTI
- Pulmonary (pneumonia, pneumothorax)
- Musculoskeletal (costochondritis, back pain, rib fracture, muscle strain)
- Abdominal pain

Management

Nonpharmacologic Treatment

- For small stones (less than 0.5 cm), observe, and treat pain.
- Strain urine by pouring through strainer, gauze, or coffee filter to collect stones or sediment as they pass; stone analysis is required.
- For larger stones, may refer for extracorporeal shock wave lithotripsy, ureteroscopy, percutaneous nephrolithotomy, or open surgery for removal of stone
- Difficulties in tolerating pain or other factors may mandate treatment with shock wave lithotripsy or ureteroscopy in a patient who otherwise might be expected to pass the stone
- Increase fluid intake to maintain urinary output at 2 to 3 L/day; increase fiber in diet
- Decrease animal fat in diet

Pharmacologic Treatment

- Pain management with NSAIDS and opioids as required
- Antiemetics as needed

Special Considerations

- For prevention of recurrence of all types of stones, stress importance of adequate hydration: 2–3 L per day, dividing intake evenly to produce dilute urine at all times.
    - Avoid apple and grapefruit juices.
    - Avoid long periods of immobilization.

- To prevent recurrence of calcium stones, limit protein, oxalate, and sodium intake; hydrochlorothiazide 50 mg once a day (rule out hyperparathyroidism before prescribing).
- To prevent recurrence of oxalate stones, restrict dietary oxalate (tea, rhubarb, leafy green vegetables, and peanuts).
- To prevent recurrence of uric acid stones, restrict protein, consider allopurinol if serum uric acid is elevated, and take sodium bicarbonate.

When to Consult, Refer, Hospitalize

- Refer to urologist if obstruction is suspected or if symptoms persist over 3 to 4 days.
- Hospitalize if infection is present, stone is larger than 6 mm in diameter, or patient has excessive nausea and vomiting, intractable pain, or gross hematuria.

Follow-Up

- Plain films of abdomen at 1 to 2 week intervals to monitor progress of stone in ureter
- Continue to strain urine until stone has passed. Monitor potassium and blood pressure in patients taking hydrochlorothiazide.

Expected Course

- 98% pass spontaneously
- Usually resolves within 4 weeks
- Recurrences within 5 years common in up to 50% of patients

Complications

- Complete urinary obstruction, hydronephrosis, renal failure, infection

Common Renal Disorders

ACUTE GLOMERULONEPHRITIS

Description

- Glomerulonephritis is a group of kidney diseases characterized by inflammation of the glomeruli causing hematuria and proteinuria. Left untreated, chronic inflammation can lead to scarring, loss of kidney function, high blood pressure, and kidney failure requiring dialysis or transplantation.

Etiology

Infectious

- Bacterial infections (for example, with *Streptococcus, Staphylococcus*)
- Fungal infections
- Parasitic infections (for example, malaria)
- Viral infections (hepatitis B and C or HIV infections)

Vasculitis

- Cryoglobulinemia
- Eosinophilic granulomatosis with polyangiitis (formerly Churg-Strauss syndrome)
- Granulomatosis with polyangiitis (formerly Wegener's granulomatosis)
- Microscopic polyangiitis

Immune

- Goodpasture syndrome
- Systemic lupus erythematosus

Other Causes

- Hereditary nephritis
- Drugs (for example, quinine, gemcitabine, or mitomycin C)

Incidence and Demographics

- Represents 10% to 15% of glomerular diseases and 25% to 30% of all cases of end-stage renal disease (ESRD)
- Postinfectious glomerulonephritis primarily in ages 5 to 15 years; only 10% occurs in patients 40 years and older.
- Acute nephritis may occur at any age, including infancy.
- Acute glomerulonephritis predominantly affects males (2:1 male-to-female ratio).
- A higher incidence (related to poor hygiene) may be observed in some socioeconomic groups.

Prevention and Screening

- Early and aggressive treatment of source/etiology

Assessment

History

- Edema, particularly of face, hands, and feet; malaise; fever; abdominal or flank pain
- Cutaneous or pharyngeal streptococcal infection within preceding 2 to 3 weeks; often cannot identify exact cause
- Abrupt onset of hematuria, oliguria, or anuria

Physical Exam

- Edema (90%), hypertension (75%), fever, abdominal tenderness

Diagnostic Studies

Laboratory

- Urinalysis
- CBC
- BUN, serum creatinine, and serum electrolytes
- ESR
- Complement levels (C3, C4, CH50)
- Streptozyme testing—antistreptolysin O (ASO) titer is increased in 60% to 80% of patients.

Differential Diagnosis

- Systemic lupus
- Anaphylactoid purpura
- Subacute bacterial endocarditis
- Congestive heart failure

Management

Nonpharmacologic Treatment

- Treat as inpatient until edema and hypertension are under control
- Restrict fluid to replacement of insensible losses plus two-thirds of the urine output until diuresis; use no-salt-added diet.
- Restrict protein in presence of azotemia and metabolic acidosis.
- Avoid high-potassium foods.
- May need dialysis

Pharmacologic Treatment

- Streptococcal infection: Penicillin VK if no allergy
  - May prevent the development of glomerulonephritis if given within the first 36 hours
  - Treatment of close contacts may help prevent development.

- Treatment of hypertension and edema secondary to glomerulonephritis
  - Loop diuretics may be required in patients who are edematous and hypertensive to remove excess fluid and to correct hypertension.
  - Vasodilator drugs (e.g., nitroprusside, nifedipine, hydralazine, diazoxide) may be used if severe hypertension or encephalopathy is present.
  - Glucocorticoids if secondary to autoimmune disorder
  - Antimalarial drugs if secondary to malaria

How Long to Treat

- Spontaneous diuresis typically occurs within 7 to 10 days after onset of illness; then supportive care is no longer required.

Special Considerations

- Caution in older adults as frank heart failure occurs in 40%

When to Consult, Refer, Hospitalize

- Consult with physician for inpatient management in acute stage or with significant edema/hypertension.

Follow-Up

- Several times per week until resolution of infection

Expected Course

- Most cases are self-limited and resolve in 2 to 3 weeks; second episodes are rare.
- 95% of patients recover fully.
- There is more morbidity in patients with preexisting renal disease.
- Proteinuria may persist for up to 2 years.

Complications

- Most common long-term sequelae: mild hypertension
- Hypertensive encephalopathy or retinopathy
- Rapidly progressive glomerulonephritis, acute renal failure, nephrotic syndrome, chronic heart failure (CHF)

CHRONIC KIDNEY DISEASE (CKD)

Description

- CKD is diminished renal reserve, renal insufficiency, or renal failure (end-stage renal disease). Initially, as renal tissue loses function, there are few abnormalities because the remaining tissue increases its performance (renal functional adaptation); a loss of 75% of renal tissue causes a fall in glomerular filtration rate (GFR) to only 50% of normal.
- Compromise of renal function as evidenced by a decrease in GFR.
- Characterized by elevated BUN and creatinine and greatly diminished capacity for dealing with water solute fluctuations, but otherwise can maintain homeostasis
- First finding often abnormal urinalysis (proteinuria, hematuria, pyuria, casts)
- Patients may be asymptomatic but may have extra-renal symptoms of edema, hypertension, or signs of uremia.
- Patients may remain asymptomatic until GFR is less than 10% of normal.
- Chronic renal failure (CRF): reduction in GFR for at least 2 to 3 months
    - Chronic renal insufficiency: serum creatinine 1.5 to 3.0 mg/dL
    - Chronic renal failure: serum creatinine higher than 3.0 mg/dL
- Acute renal failure (ARF): an increase in serum creatinine of 0.5 mg/dL or more within 24 hours

Etiology

- Metabolic syndrome, which includes diabetes (44.8%) and hypertension (27.1%)
- Glomerulonephritis (8.5%), polycystic renal disease (3.5%), obstructive uropathy, amyloidosis
- Congenital anomalies, infection, collagen vascular disease, nephrotoxins, ischemia, ARF
- Deterioration may continue after initial insult resolves.

Incidence and Demographics

- 2.8 per 100,000 people in the United States with renal insufficiency or failure
- Males more than females, increased incidence in people of color

Risk Factors

- Poorly controlled chronic conditions including diabetes, hypertension, and others indicated in etiology section
- Chronic NSAID use, especially in patients with hypertension
- Aging

Prevention and Screening

- Preventive health maintenance to screen, diagnose, and treat metabolic syndrome and other conditions
- ACEIs have been demonstrated to decrease progression to renal failure in both diabetic and nondiabetic patients.
- Protein restriction may reduce progression of chronic renal disease.
- Blood pressure in control is crucial.

Assessment

History

- Many patients are asymptomatic.
- Early manifestations may include nocturia because of inability to concentrate urine.
- Later patients may complain of anorexia, fatigue, weakness, edema, pruritus, nausea, vomiting, constipation or diarrhea, shortness of breath, hiccups, lethargy, insomnia, or stocking-glove paresthesia.

Physical Exam

- Vital signs including bilateral and orthostatic blood pressures
- Funduscopic exam to evaluate for arteriovenous (AV) nicking, retinopathy, and papilledema

- Evaluate for volume overload
  - Lung and heart sounds
  - Jugular venous distension
  - Edema
- Abdominal exam: auscultate for renal artery bruits
- Skin: ecchymosis, rashes, pallor, uremic frost
- Neuro: deep tendon reflexes, Mini-Mental State Examination

Diagnostic Studies

Laboratory

- Urinalysis, osmolality
- Urine for microalbumin
- Elevated 24-hour urine for volume, protein, creatinine clearance
- Elevated serum BUN, creatinine, potassium, phosphate, uric acid, and sodium
- Decreased serum calcium (ionized) and hemoglobin/hematocrit
- Prolonged bleeding time due to platelet dysfunction
- Hepatitis B, HIV
- ANA, rheumatoid factor, antistreptococcal antibody

Classification

- Stage 1: normal eGFR (greater than or equal to 90 mL/min/1.73 m^2) plus either persistent albuminuria or known structural or hereditary renal disease
- Stage 2: GFR 60 to 89 mL/min/1.73 m^2
- Stage 3: GFR 30 to 59 mL/min/1.73 m^2
- Stage 4: GFR 15 to 29 mL/min/1.73 m^2
- Stage 5: GFR less than 15 mL/min/1.73 m^2

Imaging

- Renal ultrasound to rule out cysts or obstruction and document kidney size
- Electrocardiography (ECG)

Differential Diagnosis

- Acute renal failure
- Chronic renal failure
- Prerenal failure
- Intrarenal failure
- Postrenal failure

Management

The goal is to delay or halt the progression of CKD:

- Treatment of the underlying condition if possible
- Treatment is guided by staging:
  - Stage 1 and 2: diagnosis and treatment, treatment of comorbid conditions, interventions to slow disease progression, reduction of risk factors for cardiovascular disease
  - Stage 3: evaluation and treatment of disease complications
  - Stage 4: preparation for kidney replacement therapy (dialysis, transplantation)
  - Stage 5: kidney replacement therapy if uremia is present
- Aggressive blood pressure control to target values per current guidelines
- Treatment of hyperlipidemia to target levels per current guidelines
- Aggressive glycemic control per the American Diabetes Association (ADA) recommendations (target HbA1c <7%)
- Avoidance of nephrotoxins, including IV radiocontrast media, NSAIDs, and aminoglycosides
- Use of renin-angiotensin system (RAS) blockers among patients with diabetic kidney disease (DKD) and proteinuria
- Use of ACEIs or ARBs in patients with proteinuria

- Patients with CKD should be referred to a nephrologist for consultation and co-management if a clinical action plan cannot be prepared, the appropriate evaluation cannot be performed, or the recommended treatment cannot be implemented. In most cases, patients with a GFR below 30 mL/min/1.73 m^2 should be referred to a nephrologist.

Nonpharmacologic Treatment

- Nutritional modifications
  - Maintain calorie intake at 35 to 50 kcal/kg daily.
  - Protein restricted to 0.8 g/kg/day of balanced amino acids; may reduce acidosis and symptoms from elevated BUN and may slow disease progression
- Closely monitor the patient's nutritional status. Pre-dialysis low serum albumin is associated with a poor outcome among dialysis patients. Protein restriction is not recommended in pediatric patients with CKD.
  - Potassium restriction to 2 g/day may be required if K is elevated or urine output is less than 1 L/day.
  - Fluid restriction if sodium concentration is less than 135 mmol/L
  - Phosphorus, 8 to 15 mg/kg/day
  - Calcium, 1.2 to 1.6 g/day
  - Sodium, 1 to 3 g/day
- Monitor for both hypokalemia and hyperkalemia and avoid potassium-sparing diuretics. Treat hyperkalemia higher than 6 mEq/L and watch for ECG changes, especially above 6.5 mEq/L.
- Monitor serum phosphate and calcium levels.

Pharmacologic Treatment

- Anemia: When the hemoglobin level is below 10 g/dL, treat with an erythropoiesis-stimulating agent (ESA) such as epoetin alfa or darbepoetin alfa; caution should be exercised in patients with malignancy. Severe anemia (e.g., with angina, high output failure) may require transfusion.
- Bleeding can be treated with fresh frozen plasma (FFP) or cryoprecipitate.
- Hyperphosphatemia: Treat with dietary phosphate binders and dietary phosphate restriction.

- Use vitamin D supplementation to prevent secondary hyperparathyroidism.
- Hypocalcemia: treat with calcium supplements with or without calcitriol.
- Hyperparathyroidism: treat with calcitriol, vitamin D analogues, or calcium mimetics.
- Volume overload: treat with loop diuretics or ultrafiltration.
- Metabolic acidosis: treat with oral alkali supplementation.
- Uremic manifestations: treat with long-term renal replacement therapy (hemodialysis, peritoneal dialysis, or renal transplantation).
- Cardiovascular complications: treat as appropriate.
- Growth failure in children: treat with growth hormone.

How Long to Treat

- May require indefinite treatment

Special Considerations

- Geriatric patients (age 65 and older): highest incidence, highest morbidity and mortality, exacerbated by many age-related conditions

When to Consult, Refer, Hospitalize

- Consult for chronic renal insufficiency/abnormal laboratory tests beyond baseline (creatinine, serum albumin, creatinine clearance, electrolytes, calcium, phosphate, CBC, platelets)
- Refer to nephrologist for dialysis and/or transplantation when indicated
- Refer to nutritionist/dietician for dietary modifications

Follow-Up

- Monthly

Expected Course

- Progression of CKD is predicted in most cases by the degree of proteinuria. Patients with nephrotic-range proteinuria (more than 3 g/24 hours or urine protein/creatinine higher than 3) usually have a poorer prognosis and progress to renal failure more rapidly. The leading cause of death in patients with CKD is cardiovascular disease, regardless of whether there is progression to stage 5.

Complications

- Anemia, congestive heart failure, pericardial tamponade, electrolyte imbalance, acidosis, death.

CASE STUDIES

CASE 1

A 62-year-old man presents to your office for evaluation of blood in his urine after having a routine work physical and UA that showed 2+ blood on dipstick. The remainder of the UA and microscopic examination was normal.

Past Medical History: Hypertension, hyperlipidemia

1. What additional history will you need?

   Exam: Vital signs stable, afebrile, no acute distress, positive left-sided CVA tenderness.

   Consider a prostate exam if not done recently and with complaints of changes in urine flow, incontinence, or testicular pain (rule out BPH, prostatitis, cancer).

2. What are the differential diagnoses?
3. What diagnostic studies will you consider?

   Results: Repeat urinalysis shows 2+ blood with 1+ proteinuria, negative leukocytes, negative nitrates. A KUB was ordered and demonstrated a small stone in the distal ureter (4 mm).

4. What treatment will you consider?

CASE 2

A 25-year-old woman, recently married, comes in complaining of painful urination for 2 days. She has no fever. She uses a diaphragm for birth control.

History of Present Illness: No medications. Reports burning, frequency, hematuria, urgency. PMH is significant for one urinary tract infection at age 19. Otherwise in good health.

1. What are the differential diagnoses?

   Exam: Vital signs are stable, afebrile, mild suprapubic tenderness. Normal pelvic exam.

2. What diagnostic studies will you order?
3. What risk factors can you identify?

   Results: Urinalysis shows trace blood, large leukocytes, and positive nitrates.

4. What treatment measures will you prescribe?
5. What follow-up is necessary?
6. What will you do if this patient follows up 2 weeks later with another UTI?

CASE 3

A 10-year-old boy comes in with his parents to discuss bedwetting. He has daytime continence but has always had nocturnal enuresis once or twice a week. He has been diagnosed with attention-deficit/hyperactivity disorder but is not receiving any drug treatment; however, he has recently been placed in a special education class in school. Episodes of enuresis are now occurring almost nightly.

History of Present Illness: Normal gestation, normal labor and delivery. No serious childhood illnesses. No history of UTI. No medications or allergies.

1. What additional history would you like?

   Exam: Physical exam and neurological exam are normal (i.e., no anatomic abnormalities, normal gait and reflexes).

2. What are the differential diagnoses?
3. What diagnostic studies will you order?
4. What treatment would you consider?

CASE STUDIES DISCUSSION

CASE 1

1. What additional history will you need? Any fevers, chills, or muscle aches?

   Any change in urine flow, initiation of urine flow, or incontinence?

   Any personal or family history of renal stones or bladder or prostate cancer?

2. What are the differential diagnoses? Nephrolithiasis, UTI

3. What diagnostic studies will you consider?

   Repeat UA (microscopic exam may show indication of stones) and culture and sensitivity KUB vs. CT of the abdomen and pelvis without contrast

4. What treatment will you consider? Encourage patients to increase fluids.

   Consider treatment with tamsulosin (Flomax) HCl 0.4 mg.

   Treat for infectious lithiasis with indications of infection—fevers, chills, leukocytes *or* in high-risk patients, including men.

   Strain urine; all available stones should be analyzed to determine their crystalline composition.

   Discuss dietary modifications and drug therapies that can reduce the likelihood of recurrence of calcium oxalate stones.

   For recurrent stones: Consider checking serum electrolyte levels and a chemistry panel because doing so may help identify certain disorders—such as primary hyperparathyroidism, hyperuricemia, and distal renal tubular acidosis—that are associated with nephrolithiasis.

CASE 2

1. What are the differential diagnoses? UTI, vaginitis (bacterial vaginitis vs. *Candida*), STD
2. What risk factors can you identify? Sexual activity, diaphragm use
3. What diagnostic studies will you order? Uncomplicated/low risk/nonrecurrent—UA Complicated/recurrent infection—UA and C&S Vaginal swab—KOH and wet prep

   If concern for STD—urine or vaginal swab for gonorrhea (GC), *Chlamydia*, and trichomoniasis
4. What treatment measures will you prescribe? Antibiotic treatment for UTI—see Table 10-1—Increased fluids; empty bladder regularly; postcoital voiding
5. What follow-up is necessary?

   Follow-up not necessary for uncomplicated UTI unless symptoms persist or recur.
6. What will you do if this patient follows up 2 weeks later with another UTI? Send UA and C&S Treatment with different class of antibiotic, test of cure. Consider further evaluation for more than three UTIs in 1 year.

CASE 3

1. What additional history would you like? Evaluate for dysuria, frequency, and urgency; evaluate for constipation. Evaluate for psychological stress; family history of enuresis or diabetes.
2. What are the differential diagnoses? UTI, constipation, neurologic bladder dysfunction, diabetes mellitus or insipidus, psychogenic polydipsia
3. What diagnostic studies will you order? UA with specific gravity and C&S; Consider further imaging for persistent symptoms (see Enuresis [Primary Nocturnal Urinary Incontinence])
4. What treatment would you consider? Start with behavior or motivational therapy. Consider pharmacologic therapy for persistent symptoms.

REFERENCES

American Academy of Pediatrics. (2021). Red Book: *2021–2024 Report of the Committee on Infectious Diseases*, (32nd ed.). American Academy of Pediatrics.

Baldor, R. A., Berry, K., Domino, F. J., Golding, J., & Stephens, M. B. (2020). *The 5-minute clinical consult 2021* (29th edition). Lippincott Williams & Wilkins.

Buttaro, T. M., Polgar-Bailey, P., Sandberg-Cook, J., Trybulski, J. A., & Distler, J. (2021). *Primary care: Interprofessional collaborative practice*. Elsevier.

Center for Drug Evaluation and Research. (n.d.). FDA advises restricting use of fluoroquinolones for certain infections. U.S. Food and Drug Administration. http://www.fda.gov/Drugs/DrugSafety/ucm500143.htm

Culbertson, S., & Davis, A. M. (2017). Nonsurgical management of urinary incontinence in women. *Journal of the American Medical Association, 317*(1), 79. https://doi.org/10.1001/jama.2016.18433

Elsevier. (n.d.). Brenner and Rector's the Kidney, 2-Volume Set (11th ed.) https://www.elsevier.com/books/brenner-and-rectors-the-kidney-2-volume-set/yu/978-0-323-53265-5

Gharbi, M., Drysdale, J. H., Lishman, H., Goudie, R., Molokhia, M., Johnson, A. P., Holmes, A. H., & Aylin, P. (2019). Antibiotic management of urinary tract infection in elderly patients in primary care and its association with bloodstream infections and all-cause mortality: Population based cohort study. *British Medical Journal*, l525. https://doi.org/10.1136/bmj.l525

Gilbert, D. N., Chambers, H. F., Schwartz, B. S., Kami, K., Freedman, D. O., Boucher, H., Pavia, A. T., & Saag, M. S. (Eds.). (2022). *The Sanford guide to antimicrobial therapy* (52nd ed.). Antimicrobial Therapy, Inc.

Grantham, E. C. (2022). Enuresis. *BMJ Best Practice*. https://bestpractice.bmj.com/topics/en-us/690.

Hanretty, A. M., & Gallagher, J. C. (2018). Shortened courses of antibiotics for bacterial infections: A systematic review of randomized controlled trials. *Pharmacotherapy: The Journal of Human Pharmacology and Drug Therapy, 38*(6), 674–687. https://doi.org/10.1002/phar.2118

Kronenberg, A., Bütikofer, L., Odutayo, A., Mühlemann, K., da Costa, B. R., Battaglia, M., Meli, D. N., Frey, P., Limacher, A., Reichenbach, S., & Jüni, P. (2017). Symptomatic treatment of uncomplicated lower urinary tract infections in the ambulatory setting: Randomised, double blind trial. *British Medical Journal*. https://doi.org/10.1136/bmj.j4784

Papadakis, M. A., McPhee, S. J., & Rabow, M. W. (2021). *Current medical diagnosis & treatment*. McGraw-Hill Education.

Romero, C., & Uyeda, J. W. (2019). Patient-friendly summary of the ACR appropriateness criteria: Acute pyelonephritis. *Journal of the American College of Radiology, 16*(10). https://doi.org/10.1016/j.jacr.2019.06.015

Smith, M. S., Shimp, L. A., & Schrager, S. (2017). Urological care. In *Family medicine: Ambulatory care & prevention* (6th ed.). McGraw Hill Medical.

U.S. Preventive Services Taskforce. (2019a). Asymptomatic bacteriuria in adults: Screening. Home page. https://www.uspreventiveservicestaskforce.org/uspstf/document/evidence-summary/asymptomatic-bacteriuria-in-adults-screening

U.S. Preventive Services Taskforce. (2019b). Asymptomatic bacteriuria in adults: Screening. United States Preventive Services Taskforce. https://www.uspreventiveservicestaskforce.org/uspstf/recommendation/asymptomatic-bacteriuria-in-adults-screening

Walker, E., Lyman, A., Gupta, K., Mahoney, M. V., Snyder, G. M., & Hirsch, E. B. (2016). Clinical management of an increasing threat: Outpatient urinary tract infections due to multidrug-resistant uropathogens: Table 1. *Clinical Infectious Diseases, 63*(7), 960–965. https://doi.org/10.1093/cid/ciw396

Welk, B., & Baverstock, R. J. (2017). The management of mixed urinary incontinence in women. *Canadian Urological Association Journal, 11*(6S2), 121. https://doi.org/10.5489/cuaj.4584

CHAPTER 11

FEMALE REPRODUCTIVE SYSTEM DISORDERS

Rosita Rodriguez, DNP, PMHNP-BC, AGPCNP-BC, FNP-BC, WHNP-BC, CDCES, CNE

General Approach

DESCRIPTION

- Because of the high number of women who seek health care, the primary care clinician must be prepared to handle a broad variety of women's health concerns.
- The clinician may view women's health concerns in terms of common groupings: menstrual cycle, normal changes (menopause), variations (premenstrual syndrome [PMS]), abnormalities of that cycle (abnormal bleeding), and fertility issues.

Red Flags

OVARIAN CANCER

- The second (developed countries) or third (developing countries) most common type of gynecological cancer, worldwide
- High-risk women: familial cancer syndromes; history of breast, colon, or uterine cancer; two first-degree relatives with ovarian cancer; smokers
- Presentation with ovarian cancer is vague: mild, nonspecific gastrointestinal symptoms; dyspareunia; abdominal pain; bloating; urinary symptoms; dyspepsia; abdominal fullness; increasing abdominal girth; cramping; irregular vaginal bleeding; fatigue; or pelvic pressure; most present with advanced disease
- Persons with ovarian cancer presented prior to diagnosis with the following symptoms: abdominal (77%), gastrointestinal (70%), pain (58%), constitutional (50%), urinary (34%), and pelvic (26%).

- Weight loss and anorexia are poor prognostic signs.
- Physical exam findings occur late in disease: palpable adnexal mass; ascites (poor prognostic sign).
- If suspicious, obtain transvaginal ultrasound. May consider obtaining CA-125 and refer to gynecologic oncology specialist
- Refer women in high-risk groups to gynecologic oncologist—premenarchal or postmenopausal females with a palpable ovary, persistent ovarian cyst ≥5 cm (beyond 6 weeks) among reproductive-age women

ENDOMETRIAL CANCER

- Risks include any condition leading to unopposed estrogen, prolonged anovulation, oligomenorrhea, nulliparity, obesity, diabetes, early menarche/late menopause, endometrial hyperplasia, hormone replacement therapy (HRT) with estrogen alone, smokers, polycystic ovary syndrome (PCOS), tamoxifen therapy; if diagnosed in early stages, 5-year survival is 80%–90%.
- About 75% to 90% present with painless abnormal bleeding pattern as cardinal sign, but may also present with watery vaginal discharge.
- Pelvic pain, pressure, or mass present late in disease (entire uterus may be boggy, enlarged).
- Refer if Papanicolaou (Pap) test reports atypical glandular cells of undetermined significance (AGCUS) or if transvaginal ultrasound reports endometrial stripe ≥10 mm among postmenopausal women.
- Any postmenopausal vaginal bleeding merits a referral to gynecology for further workup; women older than 35 or with risk factors should have a pelvic ultrasound, an endometrial biopsy, or both. Younger women with vaginal bleeding unresponsive to therapies also merit pelvic ultrasound, endometrial biopsy, or both.

VULVAR CANCER

- Pruritus is the most common symptom, followed by burning or dysuria, bleeding, pain, or discharge.
- Common areas for lesions include labia majora, clitoris, and periurethral areas, but may occur anywhere on vulva.
- Suspicious findings include changes in pigmentation or tissue that is thickened, reddened, ulcerated, nodular, fissured, or with abnormal raised areas.

- Refer any lesions that fail to spontaneously resolve in several weeks or with therapy; promptly refer new lesions in women ≥60 years of age.

VAGINAL CANCER

- Frequently secondary to cervical or endometrial cancer, diethylstilbestrol (DES) exposure
- Signs and symptoms include bleeding from vaginal wall, chronic pruritus, and vaginal or pelvic pain
- Usually found in proximal third of posterior vagina; most lesions raised, granular, friable; lesions may be palpable, but not visible
- Refer all lesions for biopsy.
- Refer all women with a history of DES exposure.

ECTOPIC PREGNANCY

- Represents 1%–2% of pregnancies but accounts for 13% of maternal deaths
- Most ectopic pregnancies implant in fallopian tubes (97%).
- Most common time for rupture is during the first 8–12 weeks.
- Approximately 50%–80% of women with a history of an ectopic pregnancy will go on to have an intrauterine gestation; 10%–25% will have a repeat ectopic pregnancy.

Risk Factors

- History of sexually transmitted diseases (STDs; especially multiple episodes), pelvic inflammatory disease (PID), adhesions, intrauterine device (IUD) use, tubal ligation failure, pelvic or abdominal surgery, prior ectopic gestation, inconsistent or nonuse of birth control methods, infertility therapy
- Classic symptoms: amenorrhea, abdominal pain, abnormal bleeding
- Late menses that is lighter than normal or amenorrhea of 4–6 weeks' duration followed by erratic vaginal bleeding (75%) is commonly seen.
- Abdominal tenderness (95%); adnexal tenderness (87%–99%); adnexal mass (33%–53%); cervical motion tenderness in almost all cases
- Peritoneal signs: involuntary guarding, rigidity (75%)

- Late and more ominous signs indicating potential rupture: syncope or orthostatic blood pressure changes (shock, 2%–17%), shoulder pain similar to cholecystitis (10%), increase in vaginal bleeding (dark red or bright red), and significant worsening of abdominal pain
- If urine human chorionic gonadotropin (hCG) or serum beta-hCG is positive, obtain a series of quantitative serum hCG (low and not doubling every 24–48 hours indicates ectopic); if urine hCG is negative, obtain a serum beta-hCG. A negative serum beta-hCG rules out pregnancy and thus presence of an ectopic pregnancy.
- Transvaginal ultrasound may be done to exclude intrauterine pregnancy more than 6 weeks from last menstrual period (LMP).
- If condition is stable, refer to gynecologist for possible medical treatment with methotrexate, laparoscopy, or laparotomy.
- Transfer to emergency facility immediately for signs of rupture.
- Rho(D) immune globulin (RhoGAM) 300 µg will need to be administered to any Rh-negative woman.

TOXIC SHOCK SYNDROME (TSS)

- Caused by strain of *Staphylococcus aureus*; risk factors include menstruation (especially with tampon use), skin and respiratory infections, post-surgery, postpartum
- Signs and symptoms: 2- to 3-day prodrome including but not limited to malaise, myalgia, fever (temperature higher than102°F), erythematous rash (particularly palms and soles), vomiting, watery diarrhea, or abdominal pain followed by signs of shock and organ failure
- Consult with physician promptly for hospitalization or immediate transfer to emergency facility.

Contraception

DESCRIPTION

- Voluntary control of childbearing
- About 45% of pregnancies in the United States are unintentional.
- Most popular methods in the United States are oral contraceptives, female sterilization, condoms, and male sterilization. Many forms of contraception do not decrease the risk of STDs.

- Abstinence is the only method with 100% safety and efficacy for preventing pregnancy and STDs.
- Surgical sterilization via tubal ligation has efficacy greater than 99% and is considered to be irreversible.
- Choice of contraceptive method is based on lifestyle, developmental level, efficacy, safety, and characteristics of sexual relationships. Adolescents are typically sexually active 6 months before seeking counseling and information regarding contraception; contraception failure rates are highest among adolescents.
- By high school graduation, approximately 57% of all adolescents are sexually active; providers must know state regulations regarding adolescent confidentiality when they are seeking contraception.

SPERMICIDES

- Spermicides (gels, creams, suppositories, vaginal film, foam) usually contain Nonoxynol-9 (N-9), are sold over the counter with specific instructions for each type, and are hormone free. N-9 or octoxynol-9, the active ingredient, are detergents that damage membranes and inhibit or kill sperm. The spermicide must be present in the vagina before intercourse to be effective.
- Spermicidal products sold separately in the United States are intended for use alone, with condoms, or with vaginal or cervical barrier devices.
- Products intended for use alone or with condoms contain 4% N-9 and are free of petroleum products.
- Products designed for use with cervicovaginal barriers contain 2% N-9 or octoxynol-9.
- For optimal effectiveness, spermicides must be placed in the vagina before each coital act (5–15 minutes up to 1 hour, or according to package labeling) and retained in the vagina for 6 hours afterward. If spermicide is used alone, it should be reapplied before each ejaculation.
- Spermicides may be combined with periodic abstinence or withdrawal to improve efficacy.
- Users should avoid douching after placement of spermicide until 6 hours after the last ejaculation.
- Can be effective if used consistently, but first-year failure rate of typical users is 21%.
- More effective when combined with barrier method
- Spermicides with a petroleum base should not be used with latex condoms because they may damage or weaken the latex.

- Spermicides may irritate vagina or urinary tract; they alter normal vaginal flora or may alter normal vaginal barriers (mucus, flora, pH) that protect from infection.
- No major contraindications, except women with allergy to N-9, octoxynol-9, or the additives commonly found in N-9 should avoid exposure; common product additives are methylparaben, sorbic acid, cellulose gum, lactic acid, povidone, propylene glycol, and sorbitol.
- No systemic side effects; safe in postpartum or breastfeeding women.
- Appropriate for women with infrequent coitus or those using contraceptives to space their children and who accept a moderate risk of contraceptive failure.
- *Warning:* The Centers for Disease Control and Prevention (CDC) has indicated that vaginal spermicides that contain N-9 are not effective in the prevention of STDs and HIV. Furthermore, frequent use of spermicides containing N-9 has been associated with disruption of the genital epithelium, which might be associated with an increased risk for HIV transmission with exposure to the virus. Therefore, N-9 is not recommended for STD/HIV prevention or use in the rectum.
- If contraception is used improperly or not used at all, emergency contraception as a backup method should be recommended to decrease the risk of unplanned pregnancy.

NONPRESCRIPTION BARRIER METHODS

- **Over-the-counter barriers**: female or male condoms—prevent sperm from physically entering the woman
  - Up to 97% effective if perfect use (99% if combined with spermicide)
  - Screen for latex allergy (non-latex products may offer less STD/HIV protection)
  - Latex condoms are a good choice for protection from STDs and HIV when used appropriately; require partner cooperation support
- **Female condom**: Single-use, polyurethane sheath with 8 hours of maximal wear time

Contraceptive Sponge

- Nonprescription barrier method of reversible birth control; inserted deep into the vagina before intercourse; made of solid polyurethane foam containing 1 g N-9 spermicide; soft, round, pillow-shaped, and about 2 inches in diameter; has a nylon loop attached to the bottom for removal
- Covers the cervix and blocks sperm from entering the uterus; continuously releases spermicide that immobilizes sperm; cannot reduce the risk of STDs

- Advantages
  - No prescription or fitting needed
  - Can be used during breastfeeding
  - Portable
  - Does not affect a woman's natural hormones
  - Does not interrupt sex play
- Method of use: Before inserting the sponge, wet it with at least two tablespoons of clean water. Gently squeeze the sponge. The spermicide will become active when the sponge is thoroughly wet. Fold the sides of the sponge upward and away from the loop on the bottom to make it look long and narrow. Slide the sponge as far back into the vagina as fingers will reach. The sponge will unfold and cover the cervix once released. To make sure the cervix is covered, slide a finger around the edge of the sponge and check its position. The nylon loop on the bottom of the sponge should also be felt.
- Can be inserted up to 24 hours before intercourse; must be left in place for at least 6 hours after the last act of intercourse; during that time, intercourse may be repeated without additional preparation during the first 24 hours. It should not be worn for more than 30 hours in a row. Use sponge only once, then discard.
- To remove the sponge, insert a finger inside the vagina and through the loop. Pull the sponge out slowly and gently.
- Contraindications to use: allergy to polyurethane, spermicide, or sulfa drugs; current menstruation; current reproductive tract infection; difficulty with insertion; discomfort with touching one's genitals; history of TSS; recent abortion, childbirth, or miscarriage; vaginal obstructions; any kind of vaginal bleeding, including menstruation.
- Disadvantages: Few side effects reported. Sponge may be difficult to remove. If the sponge cannot be removed, or if it breaks into pieces that cannot be completely removed, instruct patient to be seen by her health care provider immediately. Some women may notice vaginal irritation. Sponge users may be at slightly increased risk of TSS, which is also associated with the prolonged use of highly absorbent tampons.

EMERGENCY CONTRACEPTION

- Emergency contraception (EC) is used within a short interval after a coital event to reduce the chance of pregnancy.
- May be used within 72 hours and up to 120 hours after unprotected vaginal intercourse to prevent pregnancy; however, it is most effective when used as soon as possible after having unprotected sex.

- Available over the counter in the United States to men and women without age restrictions
- Mechanism of action: depends on where the woman is in her menstrual cycle; inhibition or delay in ovarian follicular development or maturation; typically prevents luteinizing hormone (LH) surge and thus ovulation; alters endometrium to prevent implantation; promotes thickening of cervical mucus, impeding sperm transport; or alteration of fallopian tube transport of sperm, egg, or fertilized ovum. The copper T IUD prevents fertilization of the ovum and may prevent implantation of a fertilized egg.
- Use of EC could prevent as many as 1.5 million unintended pregnancies annually; 90% of pregnancies following rape could be prevented if all women had access to EC after a sexual assault; an estimated 51,000 abortions were avoided through EC use in 2000; most women seeking EC use a regular form of contraception, usually condoms; up to 50% of clients request EC after condom failure.
- Options for EC in the United States are ulipristal acetate (UPA) progesterone receptor modulator (prescription only); combined estrogen and progestin; progestin-only (levonorgestrel tablets under the names Plan B One-Step, Next Choice, Next Choice One Dose); and copper T IUD.
- Combined estrogen and progestin pills (Yuzpe method) which utilizes pills already formulated for use as birth control pills:
- Take 2 doses of pills orally 12 hours apart as soon as possible up to 120 hours after unprotected intercourse; each dose contains 100–120 mg ethinyl estradiol and 0.50–0.60 mg levonorgestrel; the regimen is one dose followed by a second dose 12 hours later, where each dose consists of 1, 2, 4, 5, or 6 pills, depending on the brand used; approximately 75% effective; may cause nausea and vomiting.
- Plan B One-Step (which has replaced the two-pill predecessor Plan B) and Next Choice One Dose (a generic form of Plan B One-Step) one-pill system: take 1 tablet orally single dose as soon as possible up to 120 hours after unprotected intercourse; the dose contains 1.5 mg levonorgestrel; much less nausea and vomiting are reported than with combined estrogen and progestin pills use; 89% effective.
- Next Choice and levonorgestrel tablets (generic forms of the original two-pill version of Plan B): take 2 tablets orally together or 1 tablet orally 12 hours apart as soon as possible up to 120 hours after unprotected intercourse; each dose contains 0.75 mg levonorgestrel.
- Ulipristal acetate progesterone, a receptor modulator anti-progestin pill (prescription only; brand name Ella): take one pill orally single dose as soon as possible up to 120 hours after unprotected intercourse; the dose contains 30 mg ulipristal acetate; ulipristal binds to the human progesterone receptor, thereby preventing the binding of progesterone; contraindicated in pregnancy; unlike other hormonal ECs, existing pregnancy must be ruled out before prescribing ulipristal, because of the risk of fetal loss if used in the first trimester of pregnancy; obtain urine hCG (or serum beta-hCG, if

indicated) before administering; patient must return if menses does not occur after taking ulipristal to assess for pregnancy and to rule out ectopic pregnancy if severe abdominal pain occurs 3–5 weeks after the dose.

- CopperT IUD: may be inserted within 5 days (120 hours) after unprotected intercourse to reduce the risk of pregnancy by 99.9%; prevents fertilization of ovum and may prevent implantation of a fertilized egg
- Provide thorough education regarding correct use of emergency contraceptive regimen selected.
- EC must be initiated within 120 hours of need, preferably as soon as possible after unprotected intercourse.
- Nausea (30%–50%) and vomiting (15%–20%) are the most common complaints associated with EC with combination pills; the woman should take the pills with food, not on an empty stomach.
- Advise the patient to return for a pregnancy test if there is no menses in the next 3–4 weeks.
- Medications that reduce the efficacy of EC are rifampin, griseofulvin, phenytoin, St. John's wort, and some antiretroviral agents.
- Emergency follow-up is recommended if patient experiences severe abdominal pain or other severe side effects possibly related to the treatment, possible ectopic gestation, or miscarriage.
- Obtain date of LMP and whether it was normal; determine date and time of first episode and most recent episode of unprotected intercourse.
- Physical exam is not necessary before EC use when otherwise asymptomatic; before IUD insertion, perform a pelvic exam to assess uterine size and position and rule out pelvic infection.
- Plan for future use of a reliable contraceptive method.
- Note: EC is different from mifepristone (RU-486) and does not cause an abortion. EC is not effective if a woman is already pregnant and will not adversely affect an established pregnancy.

NATURAL FAMILY PLANNING

- Efficacy is variable but can be high if the couple is very dedicated.
- Several visits or specialized classes are recommended to provide instructions for using one or more of the natural family planning methods, practicing the record keeping, and learning to observe the signs correctly; instructor should be specially trained.

- The calendar rhythm method uses calendar charting to calculate a woman's fertile period, averaging the longest and shortest cycles and identifying times of likely ovulation.
- Basal body temperature (BBT) method: Daily a.m. basal body temperatures are monitored for a sustained rise (0.4°F—0.8°F degrees) at ovulation that continues until next menses.
- Ovulation or "Billings" method*:* Daily changes in cervical mucus are observed for characteristics at ovulation (sticky and pasty mucus precedes ovulation, silky and stretchy mucus occurs at ovulation).
- A variety of factors may interfere with the characteristics of cervical mucus: douching, spermicides, vaginal infections, lubricants, semen, vaginal medications, and normal lubrication of sexual arousal.
- Symptothermal method: combines changes in cervical mucous and recognition of ovulation symptoms with BBT; charted daily and used to assess fertile times
- Cooperation between partners and agreement about any backup methods are needed. Typically, the ovum is viable for 24 hours and sperm up to 72 hours; however, ova can survive up to 72 hours and sperm can survive 72 or more hours, so couples must factor this knowledge into fertile interval planning; this method requires a woman to have regular cycles to be most successful.

PRESCRIPTION BARRIER METHODS

- Diaphragms, caps, and shields are soft latex or silicone barrier devices that cover the entire cervix, blocking the opening to the uterus to prevent sperm from physically entering the cervix; used with spermicidal jelly or cream to enhance contraceptive effect.
- A diaphragm is a shallow, dome-shaped cup with a flexible spring rim. There are several types of diaphragms as determined by the spring rim: coil, flat, or arcing. Coil-spring and flat-spring diaphragms become a flat oval when compressed for insertion. Arcing diaphragms form an arc or half-moon when compressed and are the easiest to insert. Efficacy may reach 96% if used properly; use with 1 teaspoon of spermicidal jelly; insert to back of vagina and tuck behind the pubic bone, ensuring the cervix is covered; must stay in place 6 hours after last act of intercourse; if intercourse is repeated or occurs more than 6 hours after insertion, leave the diaphragm in place and apply more spermicide; do not leave the diaphragm in place for more than 24 hours.
- FemCap is a silicone rubber cup-shaped device that fits securely in the vagina to cover the cervix; efficacy may reach 94% if used properly. Cap must stay in place for 8 hours after intercourse; do not leave cap in place for more than 48 hours; cannot use cervical cap if woman has short or irregular cervix, is post-cervical conization, or has abnormal Pap test. Use with spermicidal jelly; insert cap into the vagina and onto the cervix,

ensuring that the cervix is completely covered; with each act of intercourse, check that cap is still covering the cervix; apply more spermicide if needed.

- Fitting or sizing is performed by a clinician to determine the correct size needed for the diaphragm or cap.
- There are generally no systemic side effects with barrier methods; increased urinary tract infections (UTIs) may occur in some women; ask about allergy to latex and N-9, as well as history of toxic shock syndrome (TSS).
- Protection may be increased by ensuring that the cervix is covered before each act of intercourse; using spermicide as recommended; or using a latex condom.
- Diaphragm and cap offer no protection against STDs. Use a latex condom to reduce the risk of infection.
- Diaphragms are available in many sizes and designs. A new size may be needed after any of the following: full-term pregnancy; abdominal or pelvic surgery; miscarriage; abortion after 14 weeks of pregnancy; or 20% change in weight.
- FemCap is available in three sizes: small, for women who have never been pregnant; medium, for women who have had an abortion or a cesarean delivery; large, for women who have given birth vaginally.

Warning Signs

- Toxic shock syndrome (TSS): rare cases of TSS have been reported with diaphragm, sponge, and other cervical barrier method use. Symptoms include a sunburn-type rash; diarrhea; dizziness, faintness, weakness; sore throat; aching muscles and joints; sudden high fever; and vomiting.

Contraindications

- Allergy to latex, silicone, or spermicide; childbirth in the previous 6 weeks (10 weeks for FemCap); difficulty with insertion; discomfort with touching one's genitals; history of TSS; recent cervical surgery; recent abortion after the first trimester (after any recent abortion for FemCap); uterine prolapse; vaginal obstructions
- Inability to use a diaphragm if woman has frequent UTIs, poor vaginal muscle tone
- Inability to use FemCap if there are breaks in the vaginal or cervical tissue; cancer of the uterus, vagina, or vulva; reproductive tract infection; poor vaginal muscle tone
- Diaphragm and cap should never be used during any kind of vaginal bleeding, including menstruation.

Advantages

- Can be used during breastfeeding; portable; usually cannot be felt by the woman or her partner; immediately effective and reversible; no effect on a woman's natural hormones; no interruption of sex play; can be inserted hours ahead of time

Disadvantages

- Cannot be used during menstruation; may be difficult for some women to insert; may be pushed out of place by some sexual positions; must be in place every time a woman has vaginal intercourse; diaphragms and caps may require refitting
- Use of spermicide N-9 many times a day by people at risk for HIV may irritate tissue and increase risk of HIV and other STDs
- Care of diaphragm and cap: diaphragm and cap may last 2 years; wash with warm soapy water and air dry; do not use powders; never use oil-based lubricants such as petroleum jelly (Vaseline), creams, or lotions because they will damage latex; examine devices for small holes or fill the cup of the diaphragm or cap with water and look for leaks; diaphragm and cap can still be used if the rubber becomes discolored. However, if the rubber puckers, especially near the rim, it has become too thin.

INTRAUTERINE CONTRACEPTIVE DEVICES (IUDS)

- IUDs are small, T-shaped contraceptive devices made of flexible plastic; can be embedded with progestin or wrapped with copper; sit in the uterine cavity and prevent implantation of fertilized ovum; are greater than 99% effective, with no user error.
- There are five U.S. Food and Drug Administration (FDA)–approved brands of IUDs available in the United States: ParaGard, Kyleena, Liletta, Mirena, and Skyla. All IUDs are considered as long-acting reversible contraceptives (LARCs).
- Two types of IUDs available in the United States are:
  - Non-Hormonal ParaGard (CopperT 380A) contains copper and can be left in place for 10 years but can be effective for up to 12 years; causes increased copper in the form of ions, enzymes, and prostaglandins that enhance inflammatory response and impede sperm transport, fertilization, and implantation.
  - Hormonal-Containing Levonorgestrel—Mirena, Skyla, Liletta, and Kyleena are all levonorgestrel-containing intrauterine devices (LNG-IUDs) that continuously release a small amount of the hormone progestin.
  - Each brand is recommended for a specified time period ranging from 3 to 8 years and must be removed or replaced at that time.

- Both devices contain barium sulfate for detection by radiograph.
  - Mirena 52 mg initially releases 20 µg of levonorgestrel per day and is FDA-approved for up to 8 years of use; decreases bleeding and cramping; 20% of users become amenorrhoeic; device must be inserted by a trained clinician; irregular bleeding/spotting first 3 months; abdominal pain, back pain, breast pain, mood changes, acne, headaches, and nausea may occur; user must be comfortable checking string monthly.
- Liletta 52 mg initially releases approximately 20 µg per day of levonorgestrel and is FDA-approved for 6 years of use.
- Kyleena 19.5 mg initially releases 17.5 µg of levonorgestrel per day and is FDA-approved for 5 years of use.
- Skyla 13.5 mg initially releases 14 µg of levonorgestrel per day and is FDA-approved for 3 years of use.
- Hormonal IUD thickens cervical mucus, disrupts the pattern of ovulation, and impairs uterine and tubal motility.
- LNG-IUDs decrease bleeding and cramping; up to 20% of users become amenorrhoeic; device must be inserted by a trained clinician; irregular bleeding/spotting first 3 months; abdominal pain, back pain, breast pain, mood changes, acne, headaches, and nausea may occur; user must be comfortable checking string monthly.
- May be inserted at any time in woman's cycle if negative hCG pregnancy test, mid-cycle, and no unprotected coitus since LMP; may insert immediately after an uncomplicated abortion, 4–6 weeks after delivery, or a second-trimester abortion.
- LNG-IUDs are effective immediately if inserted within 7 days of LMP. If an LNG-IUD is inserted at any other time of the menstrual cycle, the patient will need to use another method of birth control if vaginal intercourse occurs during the first week after insertion. Protection begins after 7 days. The copper IUD begins to work immediately; therefore, no back up method is required.
  - Choose candidates based on careful assessment of risk factors (PID risk related to multiple partners; history of heavy menses; dysmenorrhea); clinicians require specialized training for insertion.
  - Nulliparous women can safely use IUDs.
  - IUDs are not abortifacients.
  - May be inserted at any time in woman's cycle if negative hCG, midcycle, and no unprotected coitus since LMP; may insert immediately after an uncomplicated abortion or delivery.

Common Complaints

- Dysmenorrhea and increased blood flow
- Consider IUD removal in addition to antibiotic therapy when treating endometritis, STD, PID; IUD should be removed at the time pregnancy is diagnosed if strings are visible, regardless of patient's plan for the pregnancy; 40%–50% risk of spontaneous abortion if IUD is left in place and 30% risk of spontaneous abortion after IUD is removed.

Risk Factors

- Highest risk of perforation is at time of insertion; early perforation warning signs are:
  - **P:** Period late, abnormal spotting, bleeding
  - **A:** Abdominal pain, or pain with intercourse
  - **I:** Infection exposure (STDs), abnormal discharge, itching, pain
  - **N:** Not feeling well, fever, chills, fatigue
  - **S:** String missing, shorter, or longer (check monthly)

HORMONAL CONTRACEPTION

The first question to be decided is whether the presence of estrogen is medically acceptable and not contraindicated for the woman.

Oral, Transdermal, Vaginal, Injectable Progestin, and Progestin Implants

- Hormonal methods interfere with negative feedback loop with steady hormonal doses, inhibiting ovulation, decreasing endometrial lining (less flow, less area to implant in), and altering cervical mucus.
- Estrogen effects: follicle-stimulating hormones (FSH) and LH are suppressed, ovary is not stimulated, and secretions and cellular structure of endometrium are altered.
- Progestin effects: inhibits FSH and LH, which suppresses ovulation, thickens cervical mucus so sperm transport is inhibited; decidualized endometrial bed inhibits implantation.

Contraindications

- Thrombophlebitis; thromboembolic disease; cerebrovascular accident (CVA); coagulopathies; uncontrolled hypertension (progestin-only pills may be used); vascular disease (coronary artery disease (CAD), peripheral vascular disease [PVD]); breast cancer; estrogen-dependent neoplasia; hepatic adenoma/cancer; pregnancy; impaired renal function/hepatitis; diabetes with nephropathy, neuropathy, retinopathy, or other vascular disease; lactation fewer than 6 weeks postpartum; major surgery with immobilization; hypertension (160+/100+ mmHg); smoking (age older than 35 smoking more than 20 cigarettes/day); migraines with focal neurological symptoms that worsen with any hormonal contraceptive use; usually not given to smokers
- Relative contraindications, exercise caution: undiagnosed vaginal bleeding, active gallbladder disease, family history of hyperlipidemia/myocardial infarction (MI) younger than age 50, smoking (age older than 35 and smoking more than 15 cigarettes/day)
- No significant adverse fetal effects have been documented regarding exposure before and early in pregnancy.
- Highly effective (higher than98%) when used correctly; reversible, widely studied for years, menstrual benefits (especially with endometriosis)
- No STD protection is provided.

Side Effects

- Acne (with high-androgenic-activity pills), light/no menses (clinician should always be sure to rule out pregnancy), breakthrough bleeding or spotting between periods, breast pain (mastalgia), depression, headaches, libido changes, nausea, weight changes
- Serious: stroke, pulmonary embolus, thrombophlebitis, hepatitis; stroke risk increased in smokers
- Some drugs reduce oral contraceptive levels such as (carbamazepine [Tegretol], phenytoin [Dilantin], Rifampin [Refadin])
- Antibiotics *do not* decrease oral contraceptive steroid levels: ampicillin, clarithromycin (Biaxin), metronidazole (Flagyl), quinolone antibiotics (ciprofloxacin, ofloxacin), doxycycline, tetracycline, fluconazole (Diflucan)

Oral Contraceptives (OCs)

- Multiple dosage arrangements are available combining estrogens and progestins in fixed amounts during 21 days of the cycle, or varying amounts of progestin and sometimes estrogen. Side effects (breakthrough bleeding) and beneficial effects (acne reduction) based on the estrogenic, progestational, androgenic, endometrial, and lipid biological activity of each type

- Ocs act on the pituitary and hypothalamus to inhibit gonadotropin secretion, thereby preventing ovulation; progestin suppresses LH secretion, eliminating the LH surge; estrogen suppresses FSH secretion, decreasing follicular maturation.
- Progestational agent also thickens cervical mucus, decreases peristalsis in the fallopian tube, and makes the endometrium unreceptive to implantation; estrogen stabilizes the endometrium to prevent irregular bleeding.
- Perfect use failure rate is 0.1%; typical use failure rate is 7.6%
- Extended or continuous cycles:
  - Good options for women who do not want monthly menses or have medical issues during the menses. Seasonique and Seasonale are both extended uses combined Ocs using a 13-week (91-day) cycle and four withdrawal bleeds per year. Formulation consists of 84 active hormonal pills containing levonorgestrel 0.15 mg and ethinyl estradiol 30 µg and 7 days of inert placebo pills.
  - Amethyst is a continuous-cycle combined OC where the next 28-day pill pack is taken without in-between placebo pills. Like its now-discontinued, continuous combined OC predecessor Lybrel, Amethyst contains levonorgestrel 90 µg and ethinyl estradiol 20 µg.
- Low-dose estrogen Ocs (20–25 µg) decrease estrogen side effects; possible increased breakthrough bleeding; decreased suppression of cyst formation/reduction; decreased margin of error for noncompliance, late or missed dosing; variety of cycle regimens are available: 21/7 (hormonally active/placebo), 21/2/5 (hormonally active/ placebo/ ethinyl estradiol(EE)), 24/4 (hormonally active/placebo); monophasic pills contain the same dose of EE and progestin for all hormonally active days; multiphasic preparations use varying levels of EE or progestin.
- Progestin-only OCs—"mini-pill": contain only progestin, not estrogen; norethindrone 0.35 mg is available in the United States; 28 pills per month; all pills contain active hormone dose, no placebos; failure rate is 5 times that of combination OCs; taken continuously with no placebos; breakthrough bleeding more common, especially if pills are missed or taken late; need backup method for missed or late pills.

Warning Signs

- **A**bdominal pain (severe)
- **C**hest pain (severe, cough, short of breath, sharp pain on breathing in)
- **H**eadache (severe), dizziness, weakness, numbness, especially if one-sided

- **E**ye (visual blurring, visual loss), speech problem
- **S**evere leg pain (calf or thigh)

OC Initiation

- Screen patient for personal or family history of venous thromboembolism, complicated valvular heart disease, or history of an estrogen-dependent tumor or known or suspected breast cancer.
- Use the pill with the fewest bleeding side effects, better lipid profile, fewer estrogenic effects
- Can be initiated on any day of the menstrual cycle; pregnancy test is not necessary for the first cycle because the pill is easily withdrawn and has an excellent safety record in early pregnancy over the past 40 years.
- Patients are instructed to return if no withdrawal bleeding occurs on inert pills of the first pack to evaluate for pregnancy.
- "Quick start" method: initiation of the pill on the day patient is given the prescription improves compliance and does not increase breakthrough bleeding; must use a backup method for 7–10 days.
- With the "Quick start" method, clinicians typically perform a pregnancy test on the day the pill is prescribed if the patient is not already actively menstruating. If the pregnancy test is negative, the patient is asked to return in 1 week for a repeat pregnancy test and to use condoms consistently during the first 7–10 days of pill use. Patients should be instructed to return if no withdrawal bleeding occurs on the inert pills of the first pack.
- Use alternative contraceptives (such as the condom, the sponge, contraceptive foam or gels) in addition to OCs during first 7–10 days of starting pill; also use alternative contraceptive if pills are missed, taken late, or used with certain drugs such as carbamazepine [Tegretol], phenytoin [Dilantin], rifampin [Rifadin]), which can reduce steroid contraceptive levels and lower the efficacy of OCs.
- With combination forms of OCs: if one pill is missed, take it immediately or two pills together the next day; if 2 days of pills are missed, take two pills immediately and two pills the following day; avoid intercourse on days when pills are missed or use condoms for 7 days. If more than 2 days of pills are missed in a row, discard the pack, use another form of birth control such as condoms, and start a new pack within 7 days of the onset of the next menses.
- With progestin-only forms: If the mini-pill is taken even 2–3 hours late, use a backup method. Report severe headache or severe lower abdominal pain that may indicate pregnancy or ruptured cyst.

- In the first 6 weeks postpartum, avoid combination OCs because of clotting risk; progestin-only pill may be used; OCs pose no apparent harm to the breastfeeding neonate but lactation may be impaired.
- Thorough history and physical examination with attention to the breasts, blood pressure, abdomen, pelvic organs, and cervical cytology should be done on initiation of the pill and at least yearly.

Transdermal Patch

- The Ortho Evra transdermal contraceptive patch contains norelgestromin 150 µg and ethinyl estradiol 20 µg, which both release continuously. The patch is applied to abdomen, buttock, upper outer arm, or upper torso (except breasts) weekly for 3 weeks, followed by a patch-free week, causing withdrawal bleeding/menses to occur. A backup method should be used the first week after starting the patch.
- Start first patch cycle on day 1 of menses or the first Sunday after the first day of menses.
- Same indications, risk factors, mechanisms, and side effects as for OCs
- May be less effective in women who weigh more than 198 pounds
- About 2%–4.7% of patches have to be replaced because of detachment.
- No powder, lotion, or other products should be applied around the site of the patch.
- The user may bathe, exercise, and swim.
- There is a 3% discontinuation rate because of application-site reaction.
- Increased breakthrough bleeding in the first one to two cycles
- Antibiotics do not affect contraceptive efficacy of the patch; however, drugs such as carbamazepine [Tegretol], phenytoin [Dilantin], and rifampin [Rifadin] alter steroid contraceptive levels and lower contraceptive efficacy.

Warning Signs

- The FDA issued a warning regarding a higher risk of venous thromboembolisms with use of the transdermal patch as compared with standard combined OCs. The FDA recommends that an alternative contraceptive be used in women at higher risk of blood clot formation, including those older than 35 years, obese, smokers, or having a personal or family history of venous thrombosis.

Vaginal Ring Contraceptive

- NuvaRing: etonogestrel 120 µg and ethinyl estradiol 15 µg, delivers a daily dose of etonogestrel 120 µg and 15 µg of ethinyl estradiol both amounts released each day; 21 days on/7 days off; device is a 5.4 cm in diameter and 4-mm thick, flexible donut-shaped ring (2 inches); ethylene vinyl acetate copolymer (not latex)
  - Insert 1 ring vaginally on day 1–5 of menstrual cycle. Leave in place for 3 weeks, and then remove and discard for 1 week, allowing menses to occur; insert new ring following menses and repeat 3-weeks-in/1-week-out pattern; backup method recommended during initial week.
- If ring falls out for less than 3 hours, it may be reinserted.
- Annovera: segesterone acetate and ethinyl estradiol, a combined hormonal contraceptive for women of reproductive age used to prevent pregnancy. It is the first vaginal ring contraceptive that can be used for an entire year. The vaginal ring system releases an approximate average 0.15 mg/day of segesterone acetate and 0.013 mg/day of ethinyl estradiol over the 21 day in-use period of each cycle for up to 13 cycles (total of 273 days). Annovera is a reusable donut-shaped (ring), nonbiodegradable, flexible vaginal system that is placed in the vagina for 3 weeks followed by 1 week out of the vagina, at which time women may experience a period (a withdrawal bleed). This schedule is repeated every 4 weeks for 1 year (thirteen 28-day menstrual cycles).
- Same indications, risk factors, mechanisms, and side effects as for OCs; may cause some irregular bleeding, leukorrhea, vaginitis, foreign body sensation, coital problems, and expulsion
- Antibiotics do not affect contraceptive efficacy of the ring; however, drugs such as carbamazepine [Tegretol], phenytoin [Dilantin], and rifampin [Rifadin]) alter steroid contraceptive levels and lower contraceptive efficacy.

Warning Signs

- Cautious use in women with vaginal abnormalities (rectoceles, stenosis, cervical prolapse)
- The FDA issued a warning regarding a higher risk of venous thromboembolisms with use of the vaginal ring as compared with standard combined oral contraceptives. It recommends that an alternative contraceptive be used in women at higher risk of blood clot formation, including those older than 35 years, obese, smokers, or having a personal or family history of venous thrombosis.

Depot Medroxyprogesterone Acetate (DMPA; Depo-Provera)

- Depo-Provera: progesterone only, 150 mg IM injection every 12–13 weeks (not later than 14 weeks); may use deltoid or gluteal muscles; do not rub site after injection; given within first 5 days of menses; cannot be immediately reversed, may take 6–18 months for return of fertility; recommend a urine hCG before administering the first two DMPA injections to rule out pregnancy
- Also available as depo-subQ provera 104, administered subcutaneously (SC) 104 mg every 12 weeks. The IM and SC formulations provide the same duration of effect.
- Amenorrhea, spotting, and irregular bleeding are most common in the first 3 months.
- May be started at 30 days postpartum

Complications

- Frequently causes weight gain, headaches, mood changes, menstrual irregularities (amenorrhea in 60%–70%), hair loss/thinning, lowering of high-density lipoprotein (HDL) cholesterol level, decreased bone density

Contraindications

- Absolute: pregnancy and unexplained vaginal bleeding
- Relative: weight gain issues, headaches, and liver or gallbladder disease
- May take as long as 18–22 months for fertility to return after stopping DMPA; therefore, another contraceptive method may be more appropriate for women considering a pregnancy within the following year
- Bone mineral density (BMD) fully recovers in teens and adult women following DMPA discontinuation and should not be withheld because of skeletal health concerns.

Nexplanon

- Nexplanon contains the same hormone for birth control as its predecessor Implanon; however, the new and improved implant Nexplanon is quicker and easier to insert and is radiopaque. Therefore, Nexplanon can be seen on an X-ray, computerized tomography (CT scan), ultrasound scanning, and magnetic resonance imaging (MRI) to confirm proper placement or assist with removal.

- Single rod, progestin-only subdermal implant containing etonogestrel implant 68 mg; LARC effective for up to 3 years
- Packaged as a sterile, disposable, preloaded applicator; prevents insertion errors from occurring, such as the device being inserted too deeply into the arm; clinicians are qualified insert/remove device after completing a sponsored training program.
- Solid core contains etonogestrel 68 mg; initial release is 60–70 µg/day; after a few weeks releases 40–50 µg/day; the at end of the third year it releases 25–30 µg/day; after the third year, not enough hormone is present to prevent pregnancy; may cause irregular bleeding.
- Inhibits ovulation, increases viscosity of cervical mucus; drug below detectable levels within 1 week of removal, more than90% women ovulated well within 3 months after removal.

Contraindications

- Pregnancy, current or past history of thrombotic disease, undiagnosed vaginal bleeding, history of breast cancer, hypersensitivity to any of the components; not recommended with hepatic enzyme–inducer drugs; women desiring to use implantable birth control are advised to quit before beginning this form of birth control.
- Immediately after insertion, the clinician and patient have to check the rod for placement in the arm. If the rod cannot be felt, a nonhormonal backup birth control method such as condoms has to be used until placement is confirmed.
- No STD protection is provided by this method.

Essure Permanent Birth Control System

- Essure is no longer sold or distributed in the United States, effective December 31, 2018, a decision made by the manufacturer, Bayer.
- Women who have been using Essure successfully to prevent pregnancy can continue to do so. Those with Essure who suspect they may be having symptoms related to the device, such as persistent pain, should consult with their physician on what steps may be appropriate for them to take.

Conditions of the Menstrual Cycle

NORMAL MENSTRUAL CYCLE

Description

- Complex rhythmic hormonal interchange among the hypothalamus, pituitary gland (the hypothalamic-pituitary axis), ovaries, and uterine endometrium
- Cycle requires intact hormonal feedback, functional organs, and open cervical and vaginal orifices
- Cycle divided into two phases: follicular phase starts with day 1 of menses and ends with LH surge; luteal phase begins with preovulatory LH surge and ends with menses
- Low estrogen level causes the hypothalamus to produce pulsatile waves of gonadotropin-releasing hormone (GnRH).
- GnRH causes the anterior pituitary to produce follicle-stimulating hormone (FSH) and LH.
- The ovary responds to FSH production and the higher level of estrogen (estradiol) with follicle stimulation to prepare the ovum. Estrogen also produces proliferation of the endometrial lining.
- Rising estrogen provides feedback to the pituitary; LH surges and stimulates release of the egg follicular material (ovulation).
- Estradiol continues to rise and progesterone starts increasing.
- Progesterone thickens and stabilizes the endometrial lining. (If the zygote needs to implant, the endometrium is ready.) Time from LH surge to endometrial shedding (menses) is approximately 14 days for most women.
- A negative feedback cycle occurs as rising estrogen and progesterone levels "switch off" the stimulating hormones from the pituitary/hypothalamus.
- The corpus luteum begins to shut down, estrogen and progesterone production falls, and the endometrial tissue loses hormonal support.
- Ischemia and vasoconstriction ensue 4–24 hours before menstruation and cause degeneration of the endometrium, which eventually sloughs away.
- The average age of menarche is 12 years; range 10–16 years
- Average duration of menses is 2–7 days and average interval between menstrual periods is 28 days ±7 days. The normal amount of blood loss per menstrual period is approximately 5–80 mL.

- If a conceptus implants in the endometrial lining, the beta-hCG produced will help the ovary maintain the corpus luteum, which helps maintain the progesterone levels, which in turn maintains the protective endometrial lining and supports gestation. This process short-circuits the "negative feedback loop."

PREMENSTRUAL SYNDROMES (PMS)

Description

- Clusters of mood and behavioral symptoms (somatic, affective, or both) occurring or worsening cyclically during the luteal phase (between ovulation and onset of menstruation), followed by resolution after menses
- Has some negative impact on one or more aspects of the patient's life (work, social, lifestyle, interpersonal relationships)
- Premenstrual symptom clusters occur within a continuum.
  - Premenstrual syndrome (PMS), a mild to moderate form
  - Premenstrual dysphoric disorder (PMDD), a subset of PMS; more severe with major impairment
- Diagnosis of exclusion (see differential diagnosis list)

Etiology

- Precise pathogenesis unknown; presumed to relate to hormonal fluctuations preceding menses
- Psychophysiologic disorder tied to menses by unknown biological link
- May be caused by increased sensitivity of one or more neurotransmitters to the cyclic fluctuation of ovarian hormones, particularly for PMDD; theorized to be due to neurotransmitter dysregulation
- Serotonin deficit may play a role.

Incidence and Demographics

- 90% of all women report at least one premenstrual symptom.
- 10% of these women report adverse lifestyle impact of symptoms and have severe PMS or PMDD.

- These syndromes most frequently affect women in childbearing years ages 25 to 45.
- Symptom onset often occurs in adolescence; affects approximately one-third of premenopausal women.

Risk Factors

- Strongly associated with a past personal or family history of mood disorders (including depression and anxiety) and psychiatric disorders; history of sexual abuse or domestic violence; stress may precipitate the condition.
- Familial trend in female relatives

Prevention and Screening

- Balanced diet; regular exercise; decreased alcohol intake; elimination of caffeine, sodium to reduce symptoms; smoking cessation; adequate sleep

Assessment

History

- PMS and PMDD are diagnoses of exclusion.
- Symptoms often begin 7–10 days before menses after ovulation has occurred.
- Fatigue/lack of energy, sleep changes
- Depression, affective lability, panic attacks, anxiety, lethargy, persistent marked anger or irritability, changes in libido, difficulty concentrating, feelings of being overwhelmed or out of control
- Breast tenderness
- Abdominal bloating, thirst, and appetite changes
- Other: headaches, edema, joint or muscle pain, weight gain
- Anxiety may peak 1–2 days before menses.
- Severe emotional symptoms predominate for PMDD; symptoms also tend to become more severe and of greater duration with time. In mild or moderate PMS, symptoms do not cause functional impairment; neither the affective nor somatic symptoms predominate.

Physical Exam

- Affect, speech, mood, mental status, depression scale to evaluate for other mood disorder
- General appearance, skin, thyroid exam to look for signs of adrenal or thyroid disorder
- Cardiac exam for changes with thyroid disorder, substance abuse
- Musculoskeletal exam for trigger points of fibromyalgia
- Complete pelvic examination screening for focal pain, masses
- Complete neurologic exam to evaluate headache, mood changes

Diagnostic Studies

- Thyroid-stimulating hormone (TSH), cortisol level as indicated to rule out thyroid adrenal disorders; prolactin if headache severe
- Consider complete blood count (CBC), glucose and serum chemistries, liver function tests (LFTs), renal function to evaluate lethargy
- If perimenopause or premature menopause is suspected: FSH, estradiol, progesterone, testosterone, and dehydroepiandrosterone-sulfate (DHEA-S) hormone testing may be indicated.
- Patient can do Self-Rating Scale for PMS (Steiner, Haskett, & Carroll, 1980) or calendar of symptoms; must have a minimum of 2 months of charting of symptoms
- To differentiate PMDD from PMS, see Table 11–1.

Differential Diagnosis

- Thyroid disorders
- Substance abuse
- Adrenal disorders (Cushing's syndrome)
- Depression (often with suicide ideation)
- Anxiety disorders
- Bipolar disorder
- Fibromyalgia

TABLE 11–1. DSM-5-TR CRITERIA FOR PREMENSTRUAL DYSPHORIA DISEASE (PMDD)

Patients must have 5 or more of the following symptoms, and 1 of them must be from column 1. None of the symptoms can be an exacerbation of another disorder. The symptoms interfere with work or usual activities, or relationships.

COLUMN 1	COLUMN 2
Feeling sad, hopeless, or self-deprecating	Decreased interest in usual activities, which may be associated with withdrawal from social relationships
Feeling tense, anxious, or "on edge"	Difficulty concentrating
Marked lability of mood interspersed with frequent fearfulness	Feeling fatigue, lethargic, or lacking in energy
Persistent irritability, anger, and increased interpersonal conflicts	Marked changes in appetite, which may be associated with binge eating or craving certain foods Hypersomnia or insomnia A subjective feeling of being overwhelmed or out of control Physical symptoms such as breast tenderness or swelling; headaches, joint, or muscle pain; sensations of bloating or weight gain with tightness of fit of clothing, shoes, or rings

- Chronic fatigue syndrome
- Irritable bowel syndrome
- Personality disorders
- PCOS
- Sleep disorders
- Chronic pelvic pain syndromes; endometriosis
- Dysmenorrhea
- Perimenopause
- Menopause
- Drug and alcohol abuse

Management

- Focus therapeutic management on self-care approaches and lifestyle modification. No treatment of PMS has been validated by evidence-based studies. However, the following lifestyle changes are reported effective for some patients with PMS:

Nonpharmacologic Treatment

- During evaluation, consider discontinuing all self-remedies such as vitamins and supplements.
- Menstrual charting for symptom assessment during management
- Aerobic exercise 3–4x weekly, especially during luteal phase
- Stress reduction
- Reduction of alcohol, caffeine, sugar, sodium during most-symptomatic times
- Balanced diet; increase consumption of dairy and complex carbohydrates
- Adequate sleep
- Smoking cessation

Pharmacologic Treatment

- Calcium carbonate 1,200 mg daily
- Dietary supplements: vitamin B6 100 mg/day, vitamin E 400 IU/day, and magnesium 200–400 mg/day
- Selective serotonin reuptake inhibitors (SSRIs), tricyclic antidepressants, benzodiazepines helpful in clinical trials; SSRIs are the drug of choice for PMDD
- NSAIDs taken with food are effective for pain and cramping components.
- Evening primrose oil, OCs, progesterone, monoamine oxidase (MAO) inhibitors, bromocriptine, vitamins, lithium, and spironolactone not demonstrated in clinical trials to reduce PMS symptoms.
- To reduce symptoms by minimizing the number of menstrual cycles a patient with PMS/PMDD experiences (4 per year instead of 12) the use of continuous monophasic OCs may be prescribed (called "tricycling"):
  - Patient is instructed to take 3 months of 21-day OC packets sequentially with no placebo pills provided at the end of packs #1 & #2. After completing pack #3,

patient takes inert pills × 1 week and has withdrawal bleeding. A new three-pack cycle of OCs is started the first Sunday after withdrawal bleeding occurs.

◇ "Tricycling" typically reduces menses to 4 times per year, and may thereby improve PMS symptoms; however, recurrence is common with discontinuation of OCs.

- Psychological support is helpful to patients experiencing severe manifestations of PMS/PMDD symptoms

How Long to Treat

- Therapy is based on patient response; expect long intervals of treatment.

Special Considerations

- Accurate identification of PMS or PMDD requires excluding other disorders and careful evaluation of menstrual charts and symptom diaries for at least 3 months.
- Placebo effect is very potent; confidence in the clinician and improved understanding of the condition can eliminate some fears, provide some hope, and improve self-control.
- More research evidence substantiating the efficacy of complementary therapies in the treatment of PMS/PMDD is needed. However, patients who report benefits from using complementary therapies to manage their PMS/PMDD symptoms should be supported providing that no adverse reactions are experienced by the patient.

When to Consult, Refer, Hospitalize

- Psychological counseling may be indicated.

Follow-Up

- After charting symptoms for two to three cycles; follow-up every 3–4 months to assess or evaluate the effectiveness of therapy.

Expected Course

- In the absence of treatment, signs and symptoms are expected to persist as long as the woman has ovulatory menstrual cycles; spontaneous remission occurs with menopause and otherwise anovulatory cycles.

Complications

- None

AMENORRHEA

Description

- Absence of menses
- Physiologic amenorrhea occurs with pregnancy, lactation, and menopause.
- Primary amenorrhea is lack of menarche by 14 years of age with absence of secondary sex characteristics, or lack of menarche by age 16, regardless of the presence of secondary sex characteristics, or absence of menses more than5 years after thelarche.
- Secondary amenorrhea is the absence of menses for a minimum of 90 days or three missed cycles to 6 months' cessation of menses after menarche has been previously established.

Etiology

For Primary Amenorrhea

- Constitutional delay of puberty
- Müllerian agenesis (second most common cause of primary amenorrhea) is caused by underdevelopment of the Müllerian duct resulting in absence or abnormal narrowing of the vagina, uterus, or both
- Mayer-Rokitansky-Küster-Hauser syndrome: 46 XX; absent vagina and uterus, but ovaries and sexual hair normal
- Androgen sensitivity syndrome (testicular feminization): 46 XY; X-linked recessive defect; uterus and adnexa absent with testes and blind-pouched vagina; breasts well developed but scant sexual hair; elevated testosterone
- Müllerian fusion anomalies: Müllerian duct fails to fuse with urogenital sinus, resulting in transverse septum of vagina, usually located in middle or upper vagina; normal uterine development
- Turner syndrome: 45 XO; ovarian dysgenesis; most common chromosomal abnormality causing gonadal failure and primary amenorrhea
- Gonadal dysgenesis: lack of mature breast/pubic hair development, but some initial stages of development may be present

- Approximately 30% of patients with primary amenorrhea have an associated genetic abnormality.
- Congenital defects in steroid synthesis
- Late-onset congenital adrenal hyperplasia
- Depending on onset, some disorders classified under secondary amenorrhea may present as primary amenorrhea.

For Secondary Amenorrhea

- Pregnancy is the most common cause of secondary amenorrhea. The next five most common causes are PCOS, hypothalamic amenorrhea, thyroid dysfunction, hyperprolactinemia, and ovarian failure.
- Hormonal contraception such as depo medroxyprogesterone, combined OCs
- Hypothalamic dysfunction, as seen in cases of excessive exercise, severe drop in body fat (less than 22%) associated with anorexia nervosa, severe malnutrition, severe systemic illness, and stress
- Pituitary dysfunction (adenoma, idiopathic hyperprolactinemia)
- Other endocrine causes: severe hypothyroidism or hyperthyroidism, adrenal disorders, diabetes
- Ovarian dysfunction: premature ovarian failure; PCOS (characterized by amenorrhea, obesity, infertility, and hirsutism)
- Other medications: phenothiazine antipsychotics, antidepressants, antihypertensives, complication of chemotherapy or radiation therapy, systemic steroids, GnRH agonists
- Surgical: oophorectomy, hysterectomy
- Outflow tract obstruction: severe cervical stenosis, severe endometrial scarring and obliteration of endometrium, vaginal scarring, labial fusion

Incidence and Demographics

- Incidence for primary amenorrhea is 0.3%
- Incidence for secondary amenorrhea is 3.3%

Risk Factors

- Vary according to underlying etiology
- Endocrine disorders, stressful life events, and a variety of medications may produce amenorrhea: phenothiazines, antidepressants, antihypertensives, chemotherapy, systemic steroids, GnRH agonists
- Obesity, weight loss, excessive exercise, and chronic disease

Assessment

History

- Assess first for pregnancy and then galactorrhea (in addition to amenorrhea).
- Gynecologic history: infertility, PID, STDs, surgical procedures such as dilation and curettage (D&C), cryotherapy, ovarian wedge resection (for PCOS), myomectomy, hysterectomy
- Pubertal development history
- Menstrual history with attention to past episodes of erratic bleeding or absence of bleeding
- Update obstetrical history; update contraceptive history.
- Endocrine: thyroid, diabetes signs and symptoms
- Headaches, visual changes
- Acne, hirsutism (include adolescent as well as family history)
- Emotional stress: recent major life events such as divorce, death of a loved one
- Depression or other psychological symptoms
- Nutritional patterns, weight changes, history of eating disorder
- Family history of genetic anomalies
- Athletes who exercise excessively

Physical Exam

- Weight changes since last visit, body habitus/height
- Observe for common anomalies associated with gonadal dysgenesis, such as neck folds and low-set ears

- Secondary sexual characteristics and Tanner staging: pubic and axillary hair patterns, breast development, genital appearance
- Eyes: impaired visual fields, ptosis, nystagmus, papilledema
- Skin: hirsutism, acne, hyperpigmentation, vitiligo, fat distribution
- Thyroid: tenderness, nodules, enlargement
- Breasts: galactorrhea, engorgement
- Pelvic: assess for presence/absence of normal structures; clitoromegaly, vulvar or vaginal atrophy, imperforate hymen, uterine enlargement (pregnancy), cervical stenosis, tenderness, adnexal masses, ovary greater than 5 cm, masses

Diagnostic Studies

- First rule out pregnancy with a urine hCG or serum beta-hCG test.
- Workup for primary amenorrhea
- If secondary sex characteristics are absent or poorly developed, obtain karyotype to rule out genetic etiology.
- If breast tissue is absent or poorly developed and uterus present, obtain serum FSH.
  - If elevated, suggests ovarian failure; obtain karyotype to rule out ovarian dysgenesis
  - If low, suggests pituitary or hypothalamic dysfunction
- If breast development is present but uterus is absent, obtain serum testosterone.
  - If results are appropriate for males, obtain karyotype to rule out testicular feminization.
- If breast tissue and uterus are present, obtain serum prolactin.
  - If elevated, include pituitary tumor in differential diagnosis.
  - If normal, begin progesterone challenge test (see below).
- If workup is negative, proceed to workup for secondary amenorrhea.
- Workup for secondary amenorrhea (obtain serum prolactin at start of challenge): CBC, erythrocyte sedimentation rate (ESR), TSH levels, bone age, FSH and LH levels, estradiol, LFTs, blood urea nitrogen (BUN), creatinine levels, urinalysis (UA), urine hCG, karyotyping, DHEA-S levels, androstenedione levels, testosterone levels, adrenal suppression test for 17-hydroxyprogesterone, magnetic resonance imaging (MRI) of brain to rule out pituitary tumor (prolactinoma)

- Progesterone challenge: prescribe oral Provera (medroxyprogesterone acetate [MPA]) 10 mg daily for 5 days.
  - Positive: withdrawal bleeding (or spotting) within 7 days of last MPA pill; suggests adequate endogenous estrogen present to prime endometrium; suggests anovulation, meaning presence of intact outflow tract; intact functioning of endometrium, ovary, pituitary, central nervous system (CNS). If prolactin is normal and there is no galactorrhea, no further workup is needed.
  - Positive: withdrawal bleeding/spotting within 14 days; no outflow tract problem (uterus, cervix, or vagina) but estrogen deficiency
  - Negative: no withdrawal bleeding or spotting; suggests either inadequate estrogen levels to prime uterus or absent endometrial cavity (in case of primary amenorrhea). No withdrawal bleeding suggests end-organ failure possibly due to congenital malformation or distortion (e.g., intrauterine adhesions) of the uterus, vagina; need to repeat estrogen/MPA trial to confirm
  - If negative progesterone challenge, wait 2 weeks and then prescribe conjugated estrogen 1.25 mg daily for 21 days or 2 mg estradiol orally once a day. for 21 days, with MPA 10 mg orally for the last 5 days of the estrogen, or combination oral contraceptives (monophasic) 1 tab orally for 21 days
- If negative, obtain serum TSH/thyroid panel, FSH, LH, and LH/FSH ratio.
- Elevated TSH suggests hypothyroidism.
- Low or undetectable TSH suggests hyperthyroidism.
- If LH is elevated or LH/FSH ratio is higher than 3 (especially with signs of androgen excess), include PCOS in differential.
- If LH is normal or low, include hypothalamic/pituitary regulation defect in differential.
- Low LH plus low FSH suggests hypothalamic etiology—e.g., stress, excessive exercise, anorexia, or pituitary malfunction.
- High LH plus high FSH suggests ovarian failure/menopause secondary to radiation, chemotherapy, autoimmune disease, or chromosomal abnormalities.
- If Cushing's syndrome is suspected, check adrenocorticotropic hormone (ACTH), DHEA-S, urinary free cortisol.
- Transvaginal and pelvic ultrasounds if any abnormality found on physical exam (masses, absent organs, enlarged organs) or if PCOS suspected
- If galactorrhea is present or prolactin is elevated, must get an MRI of the sella turcica to assess for adenoma or necrosis/ischemia (Sheehan's syndrome); coned down
- X-ray of sella turcica is also appropriate.

Differential Diagnosis

- Pregnancy
- Chromosomal abnormality
- Secondary causes

Management

- Treat any underlying conditions or abnormality identified and assess in 3–6 months for spontaneous return of menses

Nonpharmacologic Treatment

- Pituitary adenoma: may need surgical treatment
- Increase caloric intake if underweight, encourage adequate calcium intake, reduce exercise if excessive, help patient cope with stress, refer to eating disorder center as needed, and maintain appropriate body weight.

Pharmacologic Treatment

- If positive MPA challenge, give MPA monthly 10 mg once a day. for a minimum of 10 days or progesterone (Prometrium) 100–200 mg orally once a day (day 14–16 until menses onset) for 3–6 cycles *or* can treat with combined OCs for minimum of 3–6 cycles.
- Start hormonal therapy with oral contraceptives *or* HRT regimen if no menstruation occurs for more than 6 months (or sooner if estradiol levels lower than 20, FSH levels above 20).
- Suggest *not* using progestin-only contraception until regular cycles recur.
- If no withdrawal bleed occurs, further exploration is needed.
- For pituitary adenoma, referral to an endocrinologist for bromocriptine (Parlodel) treatment.

Special Considerations

- Endometrial biopsy is recommended for women experiencing a prolonged duration of unopposed estrogen (e.g., erratic, variable episodes of bleeding without premenstrual prodrome), amenorrhea for more than 12 months, or more than 3-month history of undiagnosed abnormal vaginal bleeding

When to Consult, Refer, Hospitalize

- Consult with an endocrinologist for pituitary adenoma or PCOS.
- Refer to a gynecologist if no withdrawal bleeding occurs; for patients who do not respond to therapy; if prolonged amenorrhea recurs; or for infertility management or HRT.

Follow-Up

- As appropriate for cause

Complications

- Endometrial cancer is a complication of unopposed estrogen.
- Reduced bone mass with prolonged amenorrhea

DYSMENORRHEA

Description

- Painful menstruation associated with the menstrual cycle may be primary (absence of pelvic pathology) or secondary (organic cause of pain may be identified).

Etiology

- Typically, worse in early years of menses and lessens after early 20s
- Not common in the first 2–3 years after menarche, when most menstrual cycles are anovulatory
- Incidence of primary dysmenorrhea decreases with age, parity, and the use of hormonal contraceptives.
- Considered to be chiefly mediated by prostaglandins (E and F) produced within the endometrial tissue by influence of progesterone and secretory phase of cycle

- Diagnosed by history and excluding other causes, especially pregnancy and PID
- Presents as crampy middle to lower abdominal pain, occurs with menses, and is worst the first 1–2 days; may radiate to the lower back, thighs
- Secondary dysmenorrhea is painful menstruation due to an identifiable organic cause.
  - Occurs chiefly in women years after menarche and into fourth decade; incidence increases with age
  - Associated with pain frequently but not limited to the menstrual phase; the pattern of pain may become more severe over time.
  - Symptoms suggest a specific etiology, such as endometriosis, tumors, adhesions, adenomyosis, leiomyomas, polyps, or infection.

Incidence and Demographics

- Affects 50%–75% of menstruating women; approximately 10% have severe symptoms
- High incidence in adolescents, 60%–92%

Risk Factors

- Primary dysmenorrhea: adolescent age, nulliparity, heavy menstrual flow, cigarette smoking, low fish intake; depression/anxiety/sexual abuse and poor school/work performance are weaker factors
- Secondary dysmenorrhea: varies with etiology, usually older than 30 years, PID/STDs, endometriosis, family history of endometriosis, non-medicated IUD use, uterine fibroids

Assessment

History

- History should direct the clinician to a likely etiology; emphasis on menstrual history, descriptors of pain relative to menses
- Low midline "cramping" pain, occurs in waves, may radiate to back or thighs, lasts one or more days with headache, diarrhea, vasomotor flushing, nausea
- Associated symptoms indicating underlying problem include fever, unilateral pain, dizziness, unusual bleeding, increased pain with coitus

- Symptoms associated with primary dysmenorrhea include fatigue, nervousness, irritability dizziness, syncope, bloating, headache, mood changes, nausea, vomiting, constipation, diarrhea.
- Important to ask patient about onset of menstrual pain. Primary dysmenorrhea rarely occurs in the first 1–2 years of menarche. Typically, in the absence of pathology, menstrual pain begins 2–3 years after menarche once a regular ovarian cycle is established.
- Review past medical history, surgeries, complications of pregnancy (infection), fibroids, STDs, bowel disorders

Physical Exam

- Assess for fever or signs of shock (e.g., low blood pressure, rapid pulse).
- Abdominal masses, abdominal tenderness, guarding, or rebounding; focal abdominal pain can identify source (e.g., lower left quadrant pain suggests bowel, ureter, fallopian tube, ovary).
- Vaginal discharge, odor
- Cervical erythema, purulent mucus, friability, cervical motion tenderness
- Uterine enlargement or tenderness, masses, immobility, firmness
- Adnexal or ovarian masses, or adnexal tenderness
- Exam and diagnostic studies will be normal in primary dysmenorrhea.

Diagnostic Studies

- Vaginal/cervical smear and wet mount to rule out STD—increased white blood cells (WBCs) indicating STDs or PID
- Chlamydia/gonorrhea testing
- Pregnancy test
- Pap screen may be deferred if obvious vaginal or cervical infection exists; obtain later
- Ultrasound if ectopic or intrauterine pregnancy, ovarian masses, or fibroids are suspected

Differential Diagnosis

- Pregnancy
- Ectopic gestation

- Endometriosis
- STDs
- PID
- Leiomyoma (fibroids)
- Chronic pelvic pain syndromes
- Irritable bowel syndrome (IBS) or another bowel disorder
- Fibroids
- Urinary tract disorder (calculi, UTI)
- Must always consider carcinoma

Management

Nonpharmacologic Treatment

- Treat causes of secondary dysmenorrhea as indicated.
- For primary dysmenorrhea, evidence of interference in activities of daily living and severity of complaints determines management protocols.
- Grade 1 (mild dysmenorrhea): little or no interference in activities of daily living, mild somatic complaints
- Grade 2 (moderate–severe dysmenorrhea): complaints of significant interference in daily living, positive systemic somatic complaints
- Grade 3 (severe dysmenorrhea): severely restricted activities, large degree of systemic somatic complaints
- Supportive treatment of primary dysmenorrhea: eating regularly, using dry or moist heat to abdomen to hasten pain relief, high intake of fish rich in omega-3 fatty acids, aerobic exercise helpful for some women
- Transcutaneous electrical nerve stimulator (TENS) appliance may be helpful.

Pharmacologic Treatment

- NSAIDs are the treatment of choice for primary dysmenorrhea; work most effectively when taken before pain becomes severe. Take with food.
- NSAIDs should be taken 2 days or more (up to 1 week) before onset of menses, at regular intervals around the clock; with food to avoid GI upset.

- Be aware of Black Box Warnings for NSAIDS concerning GI and cardiovascular risk when prescribing.
- If inadequate response, increase dose or switch to other product; allow minimum of 2–3 cycles to evaluate before switching
- Various pharmacologic agents are available for pain management such as, but not limited to the following commonly prescribed prostaglandin inhibitors:
  - Mefenamic acid (Ponstel) 500-mg orally loading dose, then 250–500 mg orally every6 hours as needed.
  - Naproxen (Anaprox, Naprosyn), 500-mg orally loading dose, then 250 mg orally every6–8 hours as needed. (Maximum 24-hour dose is 1,250 mg)
  - Ibuprofen (Motrin), 400–800 mg orally three to four times a day as needed.
  - Naproxen sodium extended release (Anaprox DS) 550 mg 1 tablet orally twice a day, as needed.
  - Naproxen sodium (Naprelan) 500 mg, 2 tablets orally once daily.
  - Indomethacin (Indocin) 50 mg loading dose, followed by 25 mg twice a day
  - Diclofenac potassium (Voltaren) 50 mg loading dose, followed by 50 mg twice a day
  - Ketoprofen extended-release (Oruvail) 200-mg caplet orally daily (single dose)
  - Another class of NSAIDs that has been shown to work for treatment of primary dysmenorrhea is the cyclooxygenase-2 (COX-2) inhibitors; celecoxib (Celebrex) is approved for this indication.
- Controlling menses with oral contraception can also be beneficial. Options include the following:
  - Combined OCs may be considered for first line of therapy in a sexually active female with 21/7 or extended cycling.
  - Tricycling (take active contraceptive pills for three cycles without allowing withdrawal bleeding) is especially beneficial.
  - Use the first day start system.
  - After two to six cycles, some patients can discontinue OCs and will respond to NSAIDs.
  - Consider DMPA or the levonorgestrel intrauterine system (Mirena).
  - Vitamin B1 100 mg orally daily
  - Magnesium (limited evidence, optimal regimen unknown)

Special Considerations

- Aspirin, a mild prostaglandin inhibitor, tends to increase menstrual flow, whereas ibuprofen, a potent prostaglandin inhibitor, lessens flow and controls cramping more effectively.

When to Consult, Refer, Hospitalize

- Refer to gynecologist if the patient responds poorly to NSAID therapy or needs evaluation and management of secondary dysmenorrhea.

Follow-Up

- Every 2–3 months as necessary to evaluate efficacy of therapy or as appropriate for underlying cause
- *Expected Course*
- Primary dysmenorrhea: tends to improve with age and pregnancy
- Symptoms resolve with NSAIDs or OCs within three cycles
- For Grade 1, use medication for 24–72 hours; Grade 2, treat with NSAIDs for 3–4 cycles or continuous NSAIDs for 3–4 months; Grade 3, try NSAIDs, then use OCs for 2–6 months then stop; retry NSAIDs.
- Secondary dysmenorrhea: depends on cause

Complications

- Primary dysmenorrhea: none
- Secondary dysmenorrhea: depends on cause

ABNORMAL UTERINE BLEEDING (AUB)

Description

- Any vaginal bleeding that is not attributed to normal menstrual flow. It is classified as premenopausal or postmenopausal, bleeding at inappropriate times, amount, or duration. It is a symptom, not a diagnosis.
- Dysfunctional uterine bleeding (DUB) is a diagnosis of exclusion defined as painless, irregular bleeding because of anovulation.
- Blood loss during normal menses averages 30 mL ranging from 5 to 80 mL over a maximum of 7 days

- AUB can be classified as:
  - Menorrhagia: menstrual periods occurring at regular intervals but of excessive duration and flow. Total blood loss of more than 80 mL and duration more than 7 days
  - Metrorrhagia: menstrual periods occurring at irregular intervals of varying flow and duration
  - Oligomenorrhea: menstrual periods occurring irregularly at intervals of greater than 40 days, but less than 6 months
  - Hypomenorrhea: regular menstrual periods but with reduced amount or duration, lesser than 30 mL
  - Menometrorrhagia: irregular menstrual periods of increased amount or duration
  - Polymenorrhea: regular menstrual periods but at intervals of less than 21 days
  - A single spot of blood with ovulation is common and benign.

Etiology

- Women younger than 20 years old: anovulation because of immature pituitary-hypothalamic-ovarian axis
  - Over 90% of AUB is anovulatory in this age range.
  - Estimates suggest 55% of teens have anovulatory cycles the first year after menarche.
  - Less-frequent cycles and erratic ovulation may lead to AUB (mostly anovulatory), intervals of amenorrhea, and reduced fertility.
- Women age 20–40 years
  - Usually ovulatory (less than 20% of cases are due to anovulatory problems)
  - Pregnancy, PID, OCs, DMPA, other drugs, IUCs, severe stress, thyroid disease, endometriosis, polyps, fibroids, and neoplasm
- Women age 40 years or older
  - Anovulation due to perimenopause, aging, polyps, fibroids, uterine atrophy or thickening (hyperplasia), uterine cancer
  - 40% of all DUB cases occur in women over age 40—more likely to have disruptions in ovarian function
  - Perimenopausal women have menstrual changes, including altered intermenstrual intervals (shorter, longer, or variable) and altered menstrual flow (heavier, lighter, longer, or shorter patterns).

Incidence and Demographics

- Approximately 10 to 30% of women are affected by AUB
- Yearly about 5% of women visit medical treatment for AUB

Risk Factors

- Adolescents and perimenopausal women; copper IUD, disorders of systemic hemostasis

Assessment

History

- Complete menstrual history and patterns; STD; nipple or vaginal discharge; contraceptive patterns; abdominal pain; dyspareunia; heat/cold intolerance; bleeding or bruising; weight changes; headaches; visual problems; male pattern hair growth; drugs and medication, use including oral and long-acting contraceptive use
- Abnormal bleeding is the primary symptom

Physical Exam

- Perform a thorough pelvic exam to rule out structural abnormality of the uterus and pelvic organs.
- Thyroid nodules, enlargement, tenderness
- Visual field defects
- Galactorrhea: often present with hyperprolactinemia
- Abdominal pain, guarding, rebound
- Pelvic: polyps, lesions, cervical motion tenderness, cervicitis, cervical discharge or blood, enlarged uterus, adnexal pain or masses, infection, pregnancy
- Moon facies, truncal obesity, abdominal striae, elevated blood pressure: include Cushing's syndrome in differential
- Check for hirsutism.

Diagnostic Studies

- Urine or serum hCG, CBC, TSH, Pap test, prolactin, chlamydia/gonorrhea testing
- If indicated by history or physical exam, evaluate glucose, renal function, hepatic function, bleeding studies (platelet count, prothrombin time [PT], partial thromboplastin time [PTT], bleeding time); adolescents with heavy menstrual bleeding should be evaluated for underlying systemic disorder such as von Willebrand factor or other inherited disorders of hemostasis
- Endometrial biopsy or hysteroscopy: need determined by history but generally more than 3–6 months of unexplained AUB despite therapies
- Pelvic or transvaginal ultrasound: rule out pregnancy or its related complications, assess endometrial stripe to rule out endometrial hyperplasia, other masses (e.g., fibroids)
- Dexamethasone test, ACTH, serum cortisol, and urine cortisol
- FSH, LH, LH/FSH ratio
- MRI of sella turcica

Differential Diagnosis

- Pregnancy
- Spontaneous abortion
- Ectopic pregnancy
- Polyps
- Hyper/hypothyroidism
- PCOS
- Infection
- Gynecologic cancer (usually endometrial)
- Salpingitis (especially chronic)
- Endometritis
- Fibroids
- Adenomyosis
- Copper IUD
- Thrombocytopenia

- Coagulopathy
- Blood dyscrasia
- Hyperprolactinemia (rule out pituitary adenoma, medications)

Management

- The main goal of management is to determine which patients require intervention and which patients require close surveillance.
- In adolescents, advise that the problem is often self-limiting and should resolve within a year or two of menarche.
- Treat any causes identified as indicated.
- DUB is the working diagnosis if other causes are ruled out.

Pharmacologic Treatment

- Oral contraceptives or HRT for several cycles
- Monophasic combination OC with 30–35 μg estrogen may be given 1 tab orally two to three times a day. for 7–10 days until bleeding is controlled.
- If bleeding stops within the treatment period, advise one OC once a day, uninterrupted without a withdrawal bleed for another 21 days.
- Stopping withdrawal bleeding for 6–12 weeks allows for minimal endometrial growth and thereby gradual thinning of the endometrium resulting in a lighter withdrawal bleed.
- Another treatment is 1.25 mg conjugated estrogens orally or 2 mg estradiol orally every 4 hours for 24 hours, then a daily dose for 7–10 days
- Follow with progestin coverage allowing withdrawal bleed; treatment after this is OC cycles × 3.
- Consider continuous/extended OC cycle therapy.
- Medroxyprogesterone acetate (MAP, Provera)
    - May be given 10 mg orally for 10–14 days every month.
    - The first withdrawal bleed will be heavy but the woman should cycle after that.
    - MPA may be used monthly.
- Depot medroxyprogesterone acetate (DMPA, Depo-Provera)
    - Give DMPA 150 mg IM every 12 weeks

- Levonorgestrel intrauterine system (IUS): progestin-impregnated IUD
    - Reduces blood loss by up to 94% in the first 3 months of use
    - Amenorrhea in 20%–40% at 1 year
- Supportive therapy
    - Iron replacement therapy if needed for anemia
    - NSAIDs (which act as prostaglandin synthetase inhibitors): a 20%–30% reduction in bleeding may occur. Start NSAIDs the first day of menses and continue through the heavy flow days.
    - Mefenamic acid 500 mg orally three times a day for 3 days
    - Naproxen 500 mg orally twice a day
    - Ibuprofen 400 mg every 6 hours

Surgical Treatment

- Surgical interventions for idiopathic heavy menstrual bleeding are usually reserved for those patients who have failed to response or are intolerant of medical therapy and who are willing to forgo fertility; surgical interventions may include but are not limited to endometrial ablation and hysterectomy.

Special Considerations

- With postmenopausal women, any bleeding/spotting is presumed to be of malignant origin until proven otherwise.

When to Consult, Refer, Hospitalize

- Refer to gynecologist for acute menorrhagia if the bleeding is sufficiently severe to cause volume depletion, shortness of breath, fatigue, palpitations, and other related symptoms. This level of anemia necessitates hospitalization for intravenous fluids and possible transfusion, as well as possible intravenous estrogen therapy. Patients who do not respond to medical therapy may require surgical intervention to control the menorrhagia.

Follow-Up

- Varies according to etiology

Expected Course

- Varies with etiology

Complications

- Varies with etiology

ENDOMETRIOSIS

Description

- Endometrial glands and stroma outside of uterine endometrial cavity—sometimes well outside pelvic cavity
- Common cause of secondary dysmenorrhea, abnormal bleeding patterns, altered fertility, dyspareunia
- Staging: based on the site(s) and severity of involvement at the time of surgery
  - Stage I (minimal): isolated implants, no significant adhesions
  - Stage II (mild): superficial implants with smaller than 5 cm of total disease, no significant adhesions
  - Stage III (moderate): multiple superficial and deep implants, with or without peritubal and periovarian adhesions
  - Stage IV (severe): multiple superficial and deep implants, large ovarian endometrioma(s), with presence of adhesions

Etiology

- Pathogenesis poorly understood; theories include retrograde menstruation, abnormal cellular process from embryogenesis, lymphatic or vascular transplantation, autoimmune disorders

Risk Factors

- Increased risk with affected first-degree female relatives
- History of uninterrupted, prolonged menstrual cycles

- Delayed childbearing/parity
- Increased incidence in women with uterine anomalies leading to outflow obstruction, such as transverse vaginal septum

Incidence and Demographics

- Six percent to 10% prevalence in fertile women and 20%–50% in infertile women
- Commonly seen with chronic pelvic pain in about 71% to 81% of cases

Assessment

History

- Gradual onset of constant, achy pain starting on or near menses, with increasing severity for few days and relenting only when menses starts to abate
- History of pain-free cycles then gradual pain, with recurrences for months or years with increasing intensity over time, will help rule out most acute abdominal conditions.
- History of large doses of NSAID analgesics with or without narcotics can be a tip toward assessing pain severity.
- Severity of symptoms may not correlate with extent of disease.
- Symptoms include pain, infertility, dysmenorrhea, nonmenstrual pelvic pain, dyspareunia, low back pain, bladder pain, frequent urination and dysuria, irregular vaginal bleeding, partial bowel obstruction, irritable bowel syndrome, perimenstrual chest and shoulder pain, abdominal wall pain, and nonpelvic pain.

Physical Exam

- Physical examination at the time of menses may identify typical patches of enlarged tissue palpable at points of pain (some only identifiable at time of laparoscopic examination).
- There may be fixed uterine position, adnexal enlargement, cervical motion tenderness, or tenderness in vaginal cul-de-sac.

Diagnostic Studies

- Diagnosis is suggested by history and physical, and tests to exclude other sources.
- Lab test to rule out other causes of pain: STDs screens, urinalysis, fecal occult blood testing, Pap testing
- Vaginal/abdominal ultrasound may show complex fluid-filled masses or diagnose endometrioma.
- Abdominal CT or MRI may show masses but not small implants; may help in mapping extent of disease.
- Confirmation of diagnosis by direct visualization can be made only by laparoscopy or surgical exploration with biopsy.

Differential Diagnosis

- Leiomyomas
- STDs or PID
- Irritable bowel other GI disorders
- Adenomyosis
- Ectopic pregnancy
- Urinary tract disorders
- Chronic pelvic pain
- Nerve pain syndromes
- Musculoskeletal pain disorders
- Ruptured ovarian cyst
- Neoplasms
- Pelvic adhesions

Management

Nonpharmacologic Treatment

- Surgical management may involve excision of implants, lysis of adhesions, reduction of ovarian tissue, or total abdominal hysterectomy with bilateral salpingo-oophorectomy (TAH-BSO).

Pharmacologic Treatment

- Treatment goals are pain relief, control of endometrial patch growth, preservation of fertility
- These first-line therapies should be combined with NSAIDs; additional analgesics may be necessary when menses occurs.
- Hormonal contraception may be used (omitting the withdrawal bleed interval) for 6–12 months (continuous use OCs daily without placebo pills or break; DMPA injections on accelerated schedule). Continuous OCs may be associated with breakthrough bleeding if taken for more than 3 months continuously. Patient must be informed about this possibility.
- LNG-IUD: Not FDA approved to treat endometriosis but may decrease recurrence of painful period.
- Second-line treatments are gonadotropin-releasing hormone (GnRH) agonist; third-line treatment are GnRH analogues

How Long to Treat

- Until pain relief, pregnancy, or menopause (biologic or surgical)

Surgical Treatment

- Laparoscopy with destruction of identifiable lesions via excision, laser vaporization, electrocautery, or endocoagulation

Special Considerations

- Calcium supplementation is advised during therapy.
- After TAH-BSO, HRT is needed (both estrogen and progesterone, to reduce endometrial cancer risk from residual implants), as well as calcium supplementation

When to Consult, Refer, Hospitalize

- Refer to gynecologist if the condition responds poorly to medical therapy or if the patient desires fertility assistance.

- Refer for other hormonal suppression with GnRH analogs such as leuprolide (Lupron), or androgens such as danazol, significant side-effect profile and expense

Follow-Up

- Gynecologist should be managing any follow-up required if the patient is receiving GnRH agonists or danazol, to assess side effects and evaluate efficacy

Expected Course

- After surgery or suppressive drug therapies (e.g., GnRH agonists or danazol), women may have 18–24 months of pain relief.

Complications

- Infertility

PERIMENOPAUSE/MENOPAUSE

Description

- Age-related reduction in ovarian function with end of fertility and menstrual cycle
- Biological menopause is natural failure of ovaries after age 40–45, resulting in absence of fertility and ≥12 months without menses.

Etiology

- The actual cause of natural menopause is unknown.
- The ovary becomes less responsive to FSH; therefore, the pituitary increases production of FSH in an attempt to stimulate the ovary. During the perimenopausal period, estrogen levels remain normal or slightly elevated, and monthly ovulation becomes more inconsistent until menstruation ceases.
- Fluctuation in estrogen levels creates menstrual cycle changes, hot flashes and sweats (vasomotor instability), sleep disturbances, fatigue, irritability, PMS, mood changes, vaginal dryness, and urinary complaints.

- Perimenopause is suggested when FSH levels are greater than 20 IU/mL despite continued menstrual bleeding.
- Adverse postmenopausal body changes include:
  - Increased bone reabsorption and decreased bone formation, leading to decreased bone density (osteoporosis)
  - Rise in total cholesterol, low-density lipoprotein (LDL), and very low-density lipoprotein (VLDL); high-density lipoprotein (HDL) declines and triglycerides show no change
  - Diminished bladder control (may occur months to years later)
- Positive postmenopausal changes include:
  - FSH levels greater than 30 IU/mL
  - Reduction in leiomyomata, endometriosis, adenomyosis
  - Gradual decrease in PMS-type symptoms is common: less mastodynia, bloating, edema, headache, and cyclical mood swings
  - Women can enjoy sexual intercourse without the need to use contraceptives to prevent unplanned pregnancy.

Incidence and Demographics

- Each year in the U.S. about 1.3 million women reach menopause, 5% between 40 and 45 years of age; 5% after 55 years of age.
- Average age at perimenopause is 47.5 years.
- Duration of the perimenopausal period is approximately 4 years.
- Average age of biological menopause is 51.4 years.
- About 10% of women have abrupt cessation of menses and 90% of women have menstrual changes before menstrual cessation.
- About 0.9% of women experience menopause before age 40 (premature menopause).
- Artificial menopause can occur at any time the ovaries are removed or irradiated before biologic failure occurs.

Risk Factors (for Premature Menopause)

- Turner syndrome (mosaic variant)
- Autoimmune endocrinopathy

- Severe systemic illness
- Chemotherapy and radiation
- Possible familial component

Prevention and Screening

- All women should be asked about menstrual history and onset of menopausal symptoms after age 40.
- Assess risk for coronary heart disease (CHD), osteoporosis, and breast and endometrial cancer.

Assessment

History

- Obtain complete medical, gynecological, and menstrual history; contraceptive use, and medication use; and family history of menopause.
- Associated symptoms: mood and sleep changes, hot flashes, vaginal dryness, and vaginal bleeding not related to menses

Physical Exam

- Complete physical exam, including breast and pelvic exam; uterus and ovaries become smaller after menopause
- Rectovaginal exam, stool for occult blood in women over 50 years old

Diagnostic Studies

- Some experts suggest diagnosis should be based on clinical symptoms, not laboratory criteria (e.g., cessation of menses, age, vasomotor symptomatology).
- Pregnancy test—always rule out possibility of pregnancy during the perimenopausal period; obtain thyroid studies such as TSH, T3, and T4 if thyroid problems are suspected.
  - Obtain baseline and periodic FSH and LH levels; fluctuation in FSH, LH, and estradiol levels are common until menopause.

- Within 1 full year after cessation of menses, there is an expected three- to fourfold increase in FSH levels, a threefold increase in LH levels, and estradiol levels typically fall below 20 pg/mL. Such diagnostic results are strong indicators used to confirm ovarian failure:
  - Predominance of immature epithelial cells on vaginal wet mount (simple, inexpensive)
  - CBC, thyroid function tests, Pap testing, mammogram, dual-energy X-ray absorptiometry (DEXA) scan, STD testing if indicated, fecal occult blood/sigmoidoscopy. Follow guidelines for periodic health screening and evaluation for adults as recommended by the U.S. Preventive Services Task Force (USPSTF, 2021).

Differential Diagnosis

- Pregnancy
- Depression
- Thyroid and other endocrine disorders
- PMS
- Hot flashes
- Pheochromocytoma
- Cancer
- Leukemia
- Thyroid tumors
- Pancreatic tumors

Management

- The American Association of Clinical Endocrinologists (AACE) has published an extensive menopause management guideline for clinician's use (Goodman et al., 2011): https://www.endocrinepractice.org/article/S1530-891X(20)43378-6/fulltext
- The FDA and the American College of Obstetricians and Gynecologists (ACOG) recommend the following guideline when hormone therapy is required to treat menopausal symptoms: treatment should be at the lowest dose and for the shortest possible time, and only during the first few years after the final menstrual period (https://www.acog.org/womens-health/faqs/hormone-therapy-for-menopause).

- The North American Menopause Society (NAMS) is an excellent resource on menopause management available online via this link https://www.menopause.org/ and this society also sponsors the free app MenoPro app for provider point of care use or patient usage.

Nonpharmacologic Treatment

- Exercise and weight management
- Smoking cessation: reduces heart disease and osteoporosis, may relieve hot flashes, may avoid early menopause
- Healthy nutritional and dietary practices, including a well-balanced diet consisting of fresh fruits and vegetables, whole grains, lean proteins, low saturated fats; daily multivitamin, daily recommended dosage of calcium (1,500 mg/day), and vitamin D (800 IU per day for individuals at risk of deficiency). See Chapter 14 for osteoporosis prevention; avoid hot flash triggers such as spicy foods, face heat, hot baths, and tanning booths.
- Limit alcohol to one drink/day or less; limit caffeine.
- Kegel exercises for coitus and urinary incontinence; weight-bearing exercise
- Vaginal lubricants for coitus
- More research evidence substantiating the efficacy of herbal remedies and vitamin supplementation in the treatment of perimenopausal symptoms is needed. However, patients who report obtaining benefits from using these products to manage their symptoms should be supported providing no adverse reactions are experienced and there are no contraindications or drug to drug interactions.

Pharmacologic Treatment

- Research data obtained from the Women's Health Initiative study has effected change in medical opinion and practice concerning HRT:
  - Data suggest that long-term use of estrogen and estrogen plus progestin may increase the risk of breast cancer in some women.
  - HRT has no beneficial effect on CHD.
  - HRT may increase the risk of CHD among generally healthy postmenopausal women, especially during the first year after the initiation of hormone use.
  - HRT increases the risk of thromboembolic events and stroke.
- Other research suggests that long-term HRT may increase the chance of dementia and breast cancer.

- Some women will still require HRT; the regimen should be individualized and based on the specific diagnosis.
- HRT relieves vasomotor flushing and may prevent osteoporosis; is available in oral forms or transdermal patch; offered as progestin only for those who cannot take estrogen; progestin must be included for women with an intact uterus to protect against endometrial hyperplasia or cancer.
    - Absolute contraindications: pregnancy, thromboembolus, unexplained genital bleeding, endometrial cancer, undiagnosed breast mass, active liver disease
    - Relative contraindications: seizure disorder, hypertension, familial hyperlipidemia, migraines, gallbladder disease, past history of thrombosis
    - Vaginal creams for atrophic vaginitis (stop after 3–6 months; reassess)
        - Estradiol (Estrace) 0.01% cream 1 g twice weekly for 3 weeks/off for 1 week
        - Estropipate (Ogen) 1.5 mg/g cream 2–4 g daily for 3 weeks/off for 1 week
        - Conjugated estrogens (Premarin) 0.625 mg/g cream 0.5–2 g daily for 3 weeks/ off for 1 week
    - Vaginal ring
        - Estring vaginal ring releases 7.5 µg/24 hours; is inserted deeply into upper one-third of vaginal vault by patient; removed and replaced after 90 days; reassess at 3–6 month intervals
- Treatment of DUB: The goal is to restore the stabilizing effect of luteal progesterone and prevent hyperplasia.
    - Low-dose monophasic OCs; extended-cycle OCs
    - Oral progestin 10–14 days every1–2 months; does not provide contraceptive benefit; MPA 10 mg daily, or progesterone 200 mg daily or norethindrone (Aygestin) 2.5–10 mg daily
    - LNG-IUS (Mirena) for 80% reduction in bleeding after 3 months and provides contraception protection
    - NSAIDs
- Preparation for hot flashes
    - Hormone therapy: gold standard for relief of hot flashes; contraindicated in women with hormonally mediated cancers, undiagnosed vaginal bleeding, active liver disease, increased risk clotting, and coronary artery disease
    - Estrogen therapy (ET) for women without a uterus and estrogen/progestin therapy (EPT) for women with a uterus; unopposed estrogen increases risk of endometrial cancer; progestin therapy reduces risk back to baseline
    - Goal is to use the lowest dose for the shortest amount of time

- The FDA has approved the following drugs specifically to treat hot flashes; however, they are approved for treating other conditions as well. Information is available on the FDA website at www.fda.gov.
  - **Antidepressants**. Low doses of certain antidepressants may decrease hot flashes. Antidepressants from classes of medications known as selective serotonin reuptake inhibitors (SSRIs) and serotonin and norepinephrine reuptake inhibitors (SNRIs)—including venlafaxine (Effexor), paroxetine (Paxil), fluoxetine (Prozac), citalopram (Celexa), and others—have been found to relieve hot flashes in some clinical trials. Many clinicians now consider these antidepressants the treatment of choice for moderate to severe hot flashes for patients who refuse or are not candidates for HRT. However, these medications are not as effective as hormone therapy for severe hot flashes and may cause unwanted side effects, such as nausea, dizziness, weight gain, and sexual dysfunction.
  - **Gabapentin (Neurontin)**. Approved for treating seizures or pain associated with shingles. Some studies have found that gabapentin is moderately effective in reducing hot flashes. Side effects can include drowsiness, dizziness, nausea, imbalance when walking, and swelling.
  - **Clonidine (Catapres)**. A pill or patch typically used to treat high blood pressure; may provide some relief from hot flashes. Side effects such as dizziness, drowsiness, dry mouth, and constipation are common, sometimes limiting the medication's usefulness for treating hot flashes.
  - MPA 10–20 mg once a day or depo medroxyprogesterone 150 mg IM every 3 months
    - Megestrol acetate (Megace) 20 mg twice a day
    - Progesterone 100 mg once a day (or 200 mg 12 days a month)
    - Transdermal clonidine 0.1 mg/day, apply weekly (side effects: hypotension, dizziness, nausea, mood swings)
    - Clonidine 0.1 mg daily (orally or transdermally) is another option to treat vasomotor flushing
- Prevention and treatment of osteoporosis
  - Oral bisphosphonates (alendronate [Fosamax], risedronate [Actonel], ibandronate [Boniva]) for prevention and treatment
  - Raloxifene (Evista). Another drug used in the treatment of osteoporosis and prevention of breast cancer in women at high risk for invasive breast cancer recurrence. Raloxifene is an estrogen receptor modulator that binds selectively to estrogen receptors, producing an estrogen agonist effect on bone and decreasing bone resorption and turnover. Raloxifene also has an antiestrogen antagonist effect on breast and uterine tissue, inhibiting breast epithelium proliferation and decreasing the risk of endometrial hyperplasia.

How Long to Treat

- Until symptoms resolve or, with HRT use, for no more than 10 years (controversial)

Special Considerations

- Do not start HRT in a woman who is being treated for ovarian or breast cancer or who has a history of either; consult with the oncologist/surgeon.
- Do not use HRT as a birth control method.
- All undiagnosed vaginal bleeding is cancer until proven otherwise.

When to Consult, Refer, Hospitalize

- Consult or refer for all relative contraindications and questionable uses for HRT.
- Consult or refer for endometrial biopsy for episodes of vaginal spotting/bleeding, even though this side effect of HRT is common.

Follow-Up

- Three months after initiating HRT or as often as necessary to evaluate efficacy and side effects
- Review danger signs of HRT: vaginal bleeding not associated with HRT use, calf pain, chest pain, shortness of breath, hemoptysis, severe headache, vision problems, breast changes, abdominal pain, and jaundice
- Annual exams after HRT regimen is established

Complications

- Postmenopausal problems: cardiovascular problems, osteoporosis, vasomotor symptoms, urogenital atrophy and incontinence, atrophic vaginitis, diminished libido

Breast Conditions

BREAST CANCER, BREAST MASSES

Description

- Malignancy of the breast

Etiology

- Precise etiology unknown
- Noninvasive: intraductal tumors, including ductal carcinoma in situ (DCIS) or lobular carcinoma in situ (LCIS)
- Invasive: tumor no longer contained within basement membrane
- Invasive ductal carcinoma is most common; originates from epithelial cells lining the mammary ducts; subtypes include medullary, papillary, tubular, colloid
- Invasive lobular carcinoma arises from mammary lobules

Incidence and Demographics

- Breast cancer is the most commonly diagnosed type of cancer in women; to a lesser extent, men can develop breast cancer.
- In the United States there are about 3.8 million breast cancer survivors.
- Second leading cause of death in women and approximately 2.6% women diagnosed die in the United States related to breast cancer
- Rare in women under 25; 95% of new breast cancer cases occur in women over 40 years old, with a median age of 65 years of age for diagnosis
- The most common site is the upper outer quadrant (49%).

Risk Factors

- Female gender; living in North America, northern Europe, and older age; early menarche (before age 11) or late menarche (after age 14); late menopause (after age 55 or more than 35 years of menses); nulliparity; first pregnancy after age 35; prior breast cancer; obesity (may be linked to hyperinsulinemia or fat cell production of androgens converted to estrogens); android fat distribution; excess alcohol use; tobacco use; never any breastfeeding; use of hormone therapy for more than 4 years, especially combined estrogen plus progestin use

- Significant risk factor for the development of breast cancer is family history; a person's risk increases a fourfold if a mother and sister affected; in women the risk is greater with a single first-degree relative, especially if diagnosed before age 50 years and about 5 times greater if two or more first-degree relatives are affected.
- BRCA (breast cancer recessive autosomal) carriers have risks for breast and ovarian cancers, usually early onset.
- BRCA1 carriers have 57% breast cancer risk and 40% ovarian cancer risk with estrogen receptor negative
- BRCA2 carriers' breast cancer risk is high with estrogen receptor positive

Prevention and Screening

- Protection may be conferred by exercise and weight control, especially in postmenopausal years.
- Raloxifene and tamoxifen as prophylaxis in high-risk women (watch for endometrial abnormalities)
- Aromatase inhibitors have been shown to be more effective than tamoxifen in preventing second breast cancers.
- Breastfeeding may reduce the risk by about 4% per year; this reduction of risk is cumulative per child.
- Women with *BRCA1* mutations who breastfed for more than 1 year are less likely to have breast cancer than those who never breastfed.
- Avoid excessive daily use of methylxanthines (caffeine) which may cause increased breast tissue tenderness in susceptible women.

Screening

- Although some controversy surrounds the breast self-exam (BSE), it is still recommended by many clinicians.
- Age 20–39: monthly BSE and clinical breast examination every 1–3 years
- Baseline digital mammogram at age 40–49 is an individualized decision based on patient's history and risk factors for biennial screening; starting age 50–74 digital

mammogram every 1–2 years; or 10 years earlier than age at onset of a first-degree relative with history of breast cancer

- Age 40–49: monthly BSE, annual clinical breast examination, digital mammography every 2 years per patient's history and risk factors
- Age 50–74: monthly BSE, annual clinical breast examination, digital mammography every 1–2 years (reduces cancer mortality by 30%–50% in women ages 50–69; 70 years of age and older, data are conflicting; no evidence to benefit women over age 75)
- Screening digital mammogram yields a false-negative rate of about 15% and a false-positive rate of 15%–20%
- Clinical breast examination to find changes that may indicate a malignancy soon enough for timely intervention, and to teach or to reinforce BSE
- Yearly digital mammogram for women who have had breast cancer; MRI for women with history of breast cancer for close surveillance
- Sentinel node biopsy is an accurate tool for assessment of axilla in early breast cancer.

Assessment

History

- Assess for risk factors
- Obtain detailed medical/gynecological history, history of breast mass development; document all prior mammogram dates and results, contraceptive and HRT use, prior breast biopsies, and breast surgery
- Painless or tender persistent breast mass; unilateral nipple inversion, discharge, itching; breast cellulitis that fails to respond or resolve; symptoms of systemic disease (bone pain, cough, or shortness of breath, epigastric discomfort or nausea); family history of breast and ovary cancers; ethnicity (Ashkenazi Jewish, Scandinavian)

Physical Exam

- Persistent nipple itching or burning suggests Paget's disease; may present with minimal skin changes, no mass palpable; may have erosion or ulceration.
- Exam shows solitary, nontender, firm-to-hard mass without well-defined margins; often fixed position.
- Ominous signs are enlarged or tender lymph nodes, skin color changes, skin erosion, peau d'orange (edema), dimpling, nipple retraction, pain, breast enlargement.

- Assess for nipple discharge, thickening, scaling, or inversion.
- Lymphadenopathy noted in axilla, neck, or supraclavicular regions

Diagnostic Studies

- Negative test results are not necessarily diagnostic in the presence of a palpable breast mass.
- Diagnostic mammography
- Ultrasound
- CBC, LFTs, chest X-ray, estrogen/progesterone receptor determination (usually ordered after biopsy), bone scan, CT scan, or ultrasound to assess lymph node involvement and metastasis
- Breast MRI if exam is suspicious and mammogram is not definitive
- Cytologic tests of nipple discharge

Differential Diagnosis

- Fibrocystic changes
- Fibroadenoma
- Intraductal papilloma
- Lipoma
- Fat necrosis

Management

- Mastectomy (radical and modified radical) and lumpectomy when combined with radiation appear to have similar cure rates.
- In addition to surgical excision:
    - Premenopausal women with positive lymph nodes often receive cyclophosphamide (Cytoxan) chemotherapy, followed by tamoxifen if estrogen receptor positive.
    - Postmenopausal women with positive lymph nodes and a positive estrogen receptor assay are commonly treated with tamoxifen and are less likely to benefit from chemotherapy.

- ◇ Controversy exists whether women with negative lymph nodes would benefit from chemotherapy (but modest success is shown in postmenopausal women with positive estrogen receptors)
- ◇ High-dose chemotherapy with autologous bone marrow transplant has proven no more effective than standard treatment in many women but is still in clinical trials.

Special Considerations

- Toremifene (Fareston), fulvestrant (Faslodex), raloxifene, or anastrozole (Arimidex) may be given to women at high risk for breast cancer recurrence.

When to Consult, Refer, Hospitalize

- Refer all suspicious breast lumps and abnormal mammograms to surgeon for excision biopsy.
- Additional referrals may be made to a medical radiation oncologist.

Follow-Up

- After diagnosis and therapy for breast cancer, a physical examination is indicated every 3–4 months for the first 5 years and every year thereafter.
- Regular follow-up visits include chest X-rays and LFTs.
- Yearly mammogram and possible MRI for women who have had breast cancer

Expected course

- Highly variable; prognosis is best reflected by stage; stage I treated with the standard of care has up to 95% survival over 10 years

Complications

- Metastatic disease

Noninfectious Breast Disorders

BENIGN BREAST MASSES

Description

- Benign mammary dysplasia is also referred to as fibrocystic changes (FCCs); most cases not at risk for breast cancer.
- Fibroadenomas are the most common benign palpable breast lesions seen in adolescents and young adults to age 25; solid benign masses.

Etiology

- FCCs are the most common benign breast condition; caused by ductal dilation, usually 2 mm or less; 20%–40% enlarge to palpable cysts (usually fluid filled); may increase and decrease with menstrual cycle.
- Fibroadenomas are made of glandular fibrous tissue, often located in the right or left upper, outer quadrants, caused by an inflammatory reaction from ductal irritation, with onset from late teens to early 20s.

Incidence and Demographics

- Fibrocystic breasts: most common in ages 30–50; rare in women younger than 20 years of age
- Cysts and fibroadenomas: most commonly benign breast changes, followed by duct ectasia
- Up to 50% of women are affected with FCCs.
- About 10% of women have a fibroadenoma in their lifetime.

Risk Factors

- Fibrocystic disease: caffeine, chocolate, tea, coffee, smoking, family history

Prevention and Screening

- Monthly breast self-exams are encouraged.
- Avoid methylxanthines, whose side effects are similar to excessive caffeine intake

Assessment

History

- Achy, tender, or painless lumpy breasts
- More tender with menses
- Any nipple discharge; may be seen in galactocele or ductal ectasia, papilloma, or cancer

Physical Exam

- Benign multiple breast masses, size fluctuating with menses (cystic, adenosis, fibrosis, ductal hyperplasia), occasionally with unilateral or bilateral nipple discharge. May feel one or two dominant cysts, usually 1–2 cm
- Fibroadenomas: unilateral mass, often solitary; well-defined, round, rubbery, mobile masses
- Fibrocystic disease: multiple masses, tender with menses, fluctuating size, rare nipple discharge
- Examine axillary, supraclavicular, infraclavicular lymph nodes for enlarged nodes

Diagnostic Studies

- Breast ultrasonography can identify cystic structures vs. solid mass.
- Suspicious masses should be evaluated by ultrasonography or mammogram.
- Cytologic evaluation of nipple discharge

Differential Diagnosis

- Breast cancer
- Fibroadenoma
- Breast abscess
- Galactocele
- Fat necrosis
- Benign cyst
- Prolactinoma

Management

Nonpharmacologic Treatment

- Fibroadenoma: watch, excise, or aspirate
- Fibrocystic disease: reduce caffeine and chocolate in diet, wear a supportive brassiere, take oral contraceptive pills

Pharmacologic Treatment

- Vitamin E supplements 400 IU daily (for 2 weeks then discontinue), vitamin B6 25–50 mg daily, magnesium 200–400 mg/day supplements
- Oral contraceptives may or may not relieve symptoms of fibrocystic disease.
- Over-the-counter analgesics, NSAIDs; take with food

Special Considerations

- Breast pain in postmenopausal women not on HRT should be worked up for cancer.
- Despite limitations (for example, reduced mammographic sensitivity), women with implants should continue to be radiographically screened as appropriate for their age and risk factors.

When to Consult, Refer, Hospitalize

- Refer to a surgeon for fine needle aspiration to confirm that a cyst is fluid filled, for excisional biopsy, or for biopsy of suspicious areas, bloody fluid, persistent mass, or excision as indicated.

Follow-Up

- For fibrocystic disease (with multiple or single small cysts smaller than 1 cm), reevaluate in 1–2 months soon after menses to determine efficacy of therapy, whether further workup required

Complications

- Usually none if benign process

GALACTORRHEA/NIPPLE DISCHARGE

Description

- Milky nipple discharge not associated with lactation

Etiology

- Duct ectasia is a collection of dilated terminal collecting ducts in the breast and is commonly associated with nipple discharge. It is not clear if the discharge causes ectasia or the other way around. The problem commonly presents when the woman is in her 40s.
    - Nipple discharge is most commonly associated with endocrine alterations or medications (e.g., methyldopa, illicit drugs, neuroleptics, phenothiazines, oral contraceptives, tricyclic antidepressants, opiates) affecting hypothalamic inhibition of dopamine.
    - Galactorrhea may be due to a prolactin-secreting pituitary adenoma (prolactinoma); usually prolactinomas less than 10 mm resolve on their own.
    - The likelihood of malignancy increases when the discharge is unilateral, arises from a single duct, is accompanied by a palpable mass, is associated with a positive mammographic finding, shows positive cytologic galatotrophic findings, or when the patient is older than 50 years.
    - Physiologic etiologies for galactorrhea include stress, breast stimulation, exercise, eating, and sleep; bilateral nipple discharge can be expressed in up to 80% of asymptomatic women.

Incidence and Demographics

- Galactorrhea is leading cause of breast complaint reported by women in the United States; about 20% to 25% have galactorrhea or have experienced this in their life
- Mostly occurs in women between the ages 20 to 35 years
- Benign discharge spontaneously resolves in up to 73% of patients within 5 years.
- About 10%–12% of breast cancers are associated with nipple discharge.

Risk Factors

- Nipple discharge often results in FCCs, ductal ectasia, or both.

Prevention and Screening

- During clinical breast exam, gently attempt to express any fluid from the nipple.
- Monthly breast self-exams are encouraged.

Assessment

History

- Changes may be unilateral or bilateral, causing discharge from one or several nipple ducts.
- Color of nipple discharge: clear, white, milky, gray, brown, green, or bloody
- Any association with a lump; tenderness
- Medications
- Provoked by nipple stimulation or spontaneous discharge
- Pregnant or lactating
- Relationship with menstrual cycles; menstrual history
- Vision problems, headaches

Physical Exam

- Nipple discharge can vary in color from white, yellow, green, brown, or black.
- To be clinically significant, nipple discharge must be true, spontaneous, persistent, and non-lactational.
- Surgically significant discharge is clear (watery), serous (clear yellow), or serosanguinous (bloody).
- Nipple discharge is typically green to yellow to black in color if physiologic, coming from multiple ducts vs. spontaneous, unilateral.
- Nipple discharge associated with duct ectasia is often thick and cheesy
- Bloody discharge is more likely to be associated with cancer.
- Check vital signs, perform neurologic exam with visual fields, and perform complete breast exam with patient sitting and lying with hands on hips and above head.

Diagnostic Studies

- Mammogram, ultrasound, and possible MRI of breast
- After negative mammographic findings, galactography or ductography is the procedure of choice. Galactography involves the retrograde injection of water-soluble radiopaque contrast material into a discharging duct with subsequent mammographic imaging.
- Hemoccult tests can be used to assess the nipple discharge fluid to confirm or exclude the presence of occult blood.
- Cytologic tests of nipple discharge or breast tissue fluid may be performed; however, cytologic testing is not necessarily conclusive as this test carries notable false-positive and false-negative rates.
- Prolactin, TSH
- MRI or CT of brain to rule out pituitary adenoma if prolactin level is elevated

Differential Diagnosis

- Breast cancer
- Fibroadenoma
- Breast abscess
- Fat necrosis
- Thyroid disease
- Benign cyst

Management

Nonpharmacologic Treatment

- Avoid nipple stimulation.

Pharmacologic Treatment

- None unless specific for treatment of prolactinoma

When to Consult, Refer, Hospitalize

- As needed for suspicious findings, such as positive occult blood or galactorrhea in a nulliparous woman

Follow-Up

- As indicated by breast specialist or primary care provider

MASTITIS ABSCESS

Description

- Mastitis is inflammation of the breast tissue with possible infection. An abscess (a collection of pus) may develop but is more likely when treatment has been delayed or inadequate.

Etiology

- Occurs as a result of milk stasis
- If infection is present, it is usually due to *S. aureus*, which is generally penicillin resistant.
- Nonpuerperal infection can occur, although less common, and is usually due to *S. aureus, Bacteroides, Peptostreptococcus.*
- A break in the integrity of the nipple or areolar area is a risk factor but is neither adequate nor necessary for the development of infection.

Incidence and Demographics

- Puerperal mastitis: 3%–20% in breastfeeding mothers
- Abscess from puerperal mastitis: approximately 3%

Risk Factors

- Lactation
- During lactation, any event that causes milk stasis, such as inadequate drainage of the breast; rapid weaning; oversupply of milk; pressure on the breast (e.g., from a poor-fitting bra); a blocked duct; or missed, scheduled, infrequent, or timed feeds
- Nipple trauma with skin breakdown
- Possibly also infant illness, maternal fatigue or stress, anemia, poor nutrition, or illness
- Eczema; these are mothers prone to colonization with *S. aureus*

Prevention and Screening

- Maintain adequate breast drainage to avoid engorgement. Teach the mother to properly latch and position her infant to maximize milk removal and minimize nipple trauma.
- Encourage feeding demonstration.
- If weaning is desired, recommend dropping one feeding every 2–3 days, taking 2–3 weeks to complete.
- Recommend avoiding abrupt weaning or binding of the breasts.

Assessment

History

- Painful, tender, warm, red breast area (classic presentation is a red wedge-shaped area)
- Fever (may or may not be present)
- Nipple soreness with or without skin breakdown may be present.
- Assess breastfeeding frequency, milk supply

Physical Exam

- Local edema, erythema, induration
- Axillary lymphadenopathy

- Localized, extremely tender, fluctuant mass may develop
- May be bilateral or unilateral (suspect *Streptococcus* group B if bilateral in the early postpartum)
- Check nipples for increased redness, soreness, skin breakdown.
- Examine skin for eczema.

Diagnostic Studies

- Clinical diagnosis: nipple/breast drainage should be sent for culture and sensitivity to rule out infection/causative organism if treatment with antibiotics is indicated for mastitis or breast abscess.
- Should have mammogram, ultrasound, or both for recurrent symptoms or nonpuerperal
- Ultrasound to evaluate for abscess as needed, or if lump does not disappear in a week with massage and warm compress.

Differential Diagnosis

- Breast trauma, breast engorgement, or plugged duct

Management

Nonpharmacologic Treatment

- Warm compresses, massage to promote drainage; cool compresses to reduce local pain and swelling
- Patient should continue to breastfeed or express milk and increase the frequency to shorten symptom duration. (Bacteria in breast milk is shown not to be pathogenic to the infant.)
- If possible, start on the affected side, or start on the unaffected side and switch after letdown occurs. If direct breastfeeding is not possible, regular pumping instead of breastfeeding should be done with a hospital-grade double electric pump 8–12 times per day for 15–20 minutes. When necessary, pumping or expression can be done after feedings if the infant fails to adequately drain the breast.
- During breastfeeding, pointing the infant's chin toward the affected area may improve the drainage.

- Encourage mother to rest, eat nutritiously, and drink plenty of fluids.
- Suspect abscess if the mastitis does not respond to antibiotics.
- Abscesses: warm compresses. It is a relative contraindication to discontinue breastfeeding with an abscess because engorgement may lead to worsening of the infection (because the fluid/milk backs up into the interstitial tissue) and abrupt weaning may cause the mother to develop fever, malaise, and achiness. Maintain adequate breast milk drainage either by direct breastfeeding or with a hospital-grade double electric pump.

Pharmacologic Treatment

- For infectious mastitis during lactation, mothers with acute pain or toxicity: bacterial colony counts, WBC counts, and culture results consistent with infection; and nipple fissures or severe or classic symptoms (fever; myalgias; chills along with a localized, red, hot, swollen, painful breast) generally should be treated with antibiotics. Mothers without these criteria should be instructed to feed frequently and maintain regular drainage of the breast as described previously. If symptoms have not resolved within 12–24 hours, antibiotic treatment should begin promptly.
- For puerperal *S. aureus* infections: dicloxacillin (Dycill) 500 mg orally four times a day or clindamycin (Cleocin) 300 mg orally four times a day; may need to consider IV therapy if mother is toxic or has extensive cellulitis
- For nonpuerperal infection, amoxicillin/clavulanate (Augmentin) 875/125 mg twice a day or IV therapy
- Analgesics: acetaminophen, NSAIDs. (NSAIDs taken with food may be more effective. Ibuprofen and acetaminophen are compatible with breastfeeding.)

How Long to Treat

- Although there is no standard recommendation for treatment length, a 10–14 day course of treatment is advised.

Special Considerations

- When treatment for non-lactational mastitis is unsuccessful and no breast abscess is identified, need to evaluate for presence of squamous metaplasia.
- Monitor for candidiasis in mother or infant; treat them concurrently if it is present or develops.

- If mother is hospitalized, the infant should be in the room with her to facilitate continued breastfeeding.

When to Consult, Refer, Hospitalize

Refer to physician for abscess, toxic mother with persistent fever despite oral antibiotics, extensive cellulitis, or if patient needs hospitalization for IV medications.

- If abscessed, refer for incision and drainage or ultrasound-guided needle aspiration.
- Consult with a lactation specialist for breastfeeding management issues, including oversupply, latching problems, lowered milk supply, persistent nipple pain, damaged nipples, nipple vasospasm (Raynaud's phenomenon), fussy infant.

Follow-Up

- Examination to assess for resolution or identify other differentials
- Evaluate for an underlying mass if more than two to three episodes occur in the same area.

Expected Course

- Frequent breastfeeding or milk expression successfully resolves puerperal mastitis 96% of the time.
- Any lowering of the milk supply will respond to more frequent breastfeeding within a few days.

Complications

- Development of sinus tracts
- Development of nipple soreness or burning breast pain, which may be a sign of mammary candidiasis, necessitating concurrent treatment of mother and child
- Infant thrush
- Functional mastectomy because of extensive incision and drainage; 10% of women affected by a breast abscess experience compromised lactation that includes a functional mastectomy
- Recurrent infectious mastitis may cause chronic inflammation.
- Temporarily lowered milk supply

Conditions of the Vulva, Vagina, and Cervix

ABNORMAL CERVICAL CYTOLOGY

Description

- Abnormal cervical cytology (most likely via Pap test) may indicate cervical cancer.
- In the United States, cervical cancer is a common gynecological cancer diagnosis and cause of death.
- The most common type of cervical cancer is squamous cell carcinoma.
- The Pap test has changed cervical cancer from a top killer (in the United States in the 1940s) to a preventable disease.

Etiology

- Preinvasive cancer of the intraepithelial layers (carcinoma in situ or cervical intraepithelial neoplasia [CIN]) is a common diagnosis in women of childbearing age.

Incidence and Demographics

- Current lifetime risk for death by cervical cancer in the United States is 0.7%.
- Most cervical cancers are diagnosed between the ages of 35 and 44 years of age; average age of diagnosis in the US is 50 and over 20% are diagnosed in women over 65 years of age.
- In the United States there are about 295,382 women currently living with cervical cancer.
- Precancerous lesions are diagnosed more than invasive cervical cancer.
- Half of women diagnosed with invasive cervical cancer have never been screened, and another 10% have not had a Pap test in 5 years.
- Least likely to be screened: older adults; poor, Black, Hispanic, and uninsured women; Black women and American Indian/Alaskan Native women have the highest mortality rates associated with cervical cancer.
- A progression of cellular abnormalities is often evident in the single-layered cervical epithelium; an area of metaplasia occurs.
- A variety of factors lead to additional cellular abnormalities.
- Squamous cell dysplasia or cancer can occur.

- Self-contained dysplasia may invade the basement membrane and surrounding tissues.
- The degree of dysplasia can vary; no strong predictor as to which types will extend; some remain stable, others regress, some extend.
- All types of dysplasia must be observed serially or treated.

Risk Factors

- Early onset coitus, especially within the first year of menarche
- Three or more lifetime sexual partners (4x risk in sex workers); women who have never had vaginal intercourse almost never get cervical cancer
- Male sexual partner who has had other partners (especially one with cervical cancer)
- More than three STDs
- Long-term OC use increases risk of dysplasia and cancer.
- Smoking: nicotine and other substances bind to cells (cancer cofactor)
- Clinical history of human papillomavirus (HPV): documented warts or positive DNA sampling
- Low socioeconomic status (less likely to be screened regularly)
- Diethylstilbestrol (DES) exposure
- HIV: Prevalence of dysplasia without HIV is 3%; with HIV 36%; with AIDS 64%; cervical cancer is an AIDS-defining illness (immunosuppression increases the risk of dysplasia) (CDC, 2023). Any woman in her mid-20s or younger with advanced carcinoma in situ (CIS) or cervical cancer needs assessment for HIV.
- HPV prevalence accounts for more than 90% of abnormal cytology.
- Herpes simplex virus (HSV), partner circumcision, parity, and OC use have not been shown to affect risk.

Current Recommendations

The U.S. Preventive Services Task Force (USPSTF) and the American College of Obstetricians and Gynecologists (ACOG) cervical cancer screening recommendations apply to women who have a cervix, regardless of sexual history or HPV vaccination status. These recommendations do not apply to women who have received a diagnosis of a high-grade precancerous cervical lesion or cervical cancer, women with an in utero exposure to DES, or women who are immunocompromised (such as those who are HIV positive). Women of any age with this history need to have individualized follow-up. The guidelines recommend:

- Cervical screening for women beginning at age 21 to 65 years with cervical cytology every 3 years or, for women ages 30 to 65 years who want to lengthen the screening interval, screening with a combination of cytology and high-risk HPV (hrHPV) testing every 5 years or hrHPV only
- Against screening for cervical cancer in women younger than age 21 years regardless of sexual history; harm outweighs benefit
- That women between the ages of 21 and 29 should have a Pap test every 3 years. They should not be tested for HPV unless it is needed after an abnormal Pap test result.
- Against screening for cervical cancer in women older than age 65 years who have had adequate prior screening and are not otherwise at high risk for cervical cancer. However, women who have been diagnosed with cervical precancer should continue to be screened.
- Against screening for cervical cancer in women who have had a hysterectomy with removal of the cervix and who do not have a history of CIN 2, CIN 3, or cervical cancer.
- Against screening for cervical cancer using HPV testing, alone or in combination with cytology, in women younger than 30 years.
- That women who have had the HPV vaccine should still follow the screening recommendations for their age group
- That women who are at high risk for cervical cancer may need to be screened more often. Women at high risk might include those with HIV infection, organ transplant, or exposure to DES. Consultation with their health care provider is recommended.
- The American Cancer Society recommends screening between 25 and 65 years old with a primary HPV test every 5 years; if a primary HPV test (solely testing for HPV) is not available, recommendations are as follows:
  - Combination HPV with a Pap test every 5 years or,
  - Pap test alone every 3 years

Prevention and Screening

- Abstinence/safer sex to prevent STDs, which increase risk
- Advise patients to avoid initiation of all forms of tobacco use or to stop use as the HPV virus is known to shed via the cervix; nicotine potentiates viral shedding and viral replication.
- HPV vaccine for both genders at 11 to 12 years old; may begin at 9 years old; catch up vaccine through 26 years old for females and 21 years old for males (up to 26 years in

certain populations); potential for vaccine catch up in those who are 27 to 45 years old through a shared decision process

- The only available U.S. HPV vaccine is the 9-valent (9vHPV, Gardasil 9, Merck).
- For the prevention of cervical cancer, precancerous or dysplastic lesions, and genital warts caused by HPV types 6, 11, 16, 18, 31, 33, 45, 52, and 58; the majority of cancers are caused by the 16 & 18 subtype
- Gardasil-9 should be administered in three separate intramuscular injections in the deltoid region of the upper arm or the higher anterolateral area of the thigh over a 6-month period, with the first dose at an elected date, the second dose 2 months after the first dose, and the third dose 6 months after the first dose.
- Vaccination with Gardasil-9 may not result in protection in all vaccine recipients.
- HPV vaccine will prevent up to 70% of cervical cancer cases.
- Contraindicated in individuals who are hypersensitive to the active substances or any of the excipients of the vaccine
- Does not substitute for routine cervical cancer screening; follow the current USPSTF cervical cancer screening recommendations for cervical cancer
- Not recommended for use in pregnant women
- May be administered while breastfeeding.
- Not intended to be used for treatment of active genital warts, cervical cancer, cervical intraepithelial neoplasia, vulvar intraepithelial neoplasia, or vaginal intraepithelial neoplasia
- Has not been shown to protect against diseases caused by HPV types not covered by the vaccine
- The vaccine-related adverse experiences observed among recipients of Gardasil-9 at a frequency of at least 1.0% and greater than placebo were pain, swelling, erythema, fever, nausea, pruritus, and dizziness. In addition, common post-marketing reports include vomiting and syncope.
- The highest-risk area on the uterine cervix for cancer is the "transformation zone" (TZ), where stratified squamous epithelial tissue intersects with columnar epithelial tissue.
- The TZ appears well outside the external os in very young women and migrates into the canal as the woman ages, or as there is disruption in the cervix (childbirth, invasive procedures, cancer treatment). With hormonal stimulation, the TZ may be more visible (hormonal contraception, pregnancy). In DES-exposed women, the TZ may extend into the vagina.

Assessment

History

- Cervical cellular changes and cervical cancer are diagnosed as a result of performing screening annual Pap tests at age 21 or if there is a clinical indication to do so before that age (e.g., rape, history of sexual abuse, known exposure to partner with HPV, or gynecologic pathology). Unfortunately, there are typically no signs or symptoms of cervical intraepithelial neoplasia.
- Assess the history of cervical cancer screening, management of any abnormalities.
- Note any colposcopy, biopsy, past ablative or surgical therapy.
- Cervical cancer is asymptomatic until well advanced.
- Exposure to DES

Physical Exam

- Most abnormal cytological changes are identified on cytologic screening.
- Vaginal discharge; vaginal cervical lesions; vaginal bleeding (metrorrhagia, postcoital spotting, cervical lesion or ulceration, abnormal uterine bleeding); and malodorous, bloody, nonpruritic vaginal discharge usually are caused by STDs and other conditions, which bring attention to cervical screening.
- If evidence exists of an infectious process, treat condition and defer Pap test for 3–6 months.
- If inflammation is noted on follow-up, obtain cervical cytology; note this on request slip.

Diagnostic Studies

Screening methods for cervical cancer

- Colposcopy
  - Recall that false negatives occur from sampling error (poor specimen collection) and from detection error.
- Thin prep
  - Specimen is obtained from a non-menstruating patient.
  - Specimen should include squamocolumnar junction and endocervix.
  - The cervical specimen is placed directly into a preservative vial.

- ◊ Increases number of cells sampled by removing confounding mucus, blood, and debris
- ◊ Reduces inadequate specimens and sampling errors by 50%

- ♦ Conventional Pap screening
  - ◊ Has a sensitivity of 51% and a specificity of 98%
  - ◊ Most accurate and very specific for carcinoma or invasive cancer and high-grade lesions
  - ◊ Low-grade lesions often over diagnosed: false-negative rate can be 10%–20% (vs. false–positive rate of less than 1%)
- ♦ Auto Pap
  - ◊ Computer-based algorithm classification of standard Pap specimen that reviews the number of abnormal cells per slide
  - ◊ Increased sensitivity (picks up more abnormal results) and specificity (decreases the number of false positives)
- ♦ Bethesda System for grading cervical or vaginal cytologic specimens: most recently revised in 2014; very comprehensive
  - ◊ Specimen adequacy
  - ◊ Satisfactory for evaluation
  - ◊ Presence or absence of endocervical or transformation zone components or other quality indicators such as partially obscuring blood or inflammation
- ♦ Unsatisfactory for evaluation (specify reason)
- ♦ Specimen rejected or not processed (specify reason)
- ♦ Specimen processed and examined, but unsatisfactory for evaluation of epithelial abnormalities (specify reason)
- ♦ General categorization: optional
  - ◊ Negative for intraepithelial lesion or malignancy
  - ◊ Epithelial cell abnormality
  - ◊ Other
- ♦ Interpretation/result
  - ◊ Negative for intraepithelial lesion or malignancy
- ♦ Organisms
  - ◊ *Trichomonas vaginalis*
  - ◊ Fungal organisms morphologically consistent with *Candida* species
  - ◊ Shift in flora suggestive of bacterial vaginosis

- ◊ Bacteria morphologically consistent with *Actinomyces* species
- ◊ Cellular changes consistent with herpes simplex virus

- Other nonneoplastic findings (optional to report)
- Reactive cellular changes associated with:
  - ◊ Inflammation (includes typical repair)
  - ◊ Radiation
    - Intrauterine contraceptive device
- Glandular cells status post hysterectomy
- Atrophy
- Epithelial cell abnormalities
- Squamous cell
- Atypical squamous cells (ASC)
- ASC of undetermined significance (ASC-US)
- ASC; cannot exclude high-grade squamous intraepithelial lesion (ASC-H)
- Low-grade squamous intraepithelial lesion (LSIL) encompassing HPV, mild dysplasia, CIN 1
- High-grade squamous intraepithelial lesion (HSIL) encompassing moderate and severe dysplasia, CIS/CIN 2, and CIN 3 with features suspicious for invasion
- Squamous cell carcinoma
- Atypical glandular cell:
  - ◊ Endocervical, endometrial, or glandular cells (not otherwise specified [NOS] or specify in comments)
  - ◊ Atypical glandular cell (NOS or specify in comments) favor neoplastic
- Endocervical adenocarcinoma in situ (AIS)
- Adenocarcinoma
  - ◊ Endocervical
  - ◊ Endometrial cells in a woman 40 years or older
  - ◊ Extrauterine
  - ◊ NOS
- Other malignant neoplasms (list not comprehensive)
- Automated review and ancillary testing (include if appropriate)
- Educational notes and suggestions (optional)

Management

Nonpharmacologic Treatment

- The American Society for Colposcopy and Cervical Pathology (ASCCP) current 2019 guidelines reccomend an individualized risk-based treatment approach.
- The ASCCP has available for a fee a downloadable app to use at point of care to assist with individualized decision making: https://apps.apple.com/us/app/asccp-management-guidelines/id1498550832
- Treatment options range from surveillance, colposcopy, to treatment.

Special Considerations

- Pap screening has a very poor positive predictive value for abnormal vaginal cytology. Vaginal cancers are only 1%–4% of gynecological malignancies.
- Women who have had a hysterectomy (for other than malignant causes) in which the cervix was removed do not require cytologic screening (less than 10% yield on vaginal cuff smears) but should continue to have vaginal inspection annually.
- Annual cytology is advised if hysterectomy is done to treat cervical dysplasia, cervical cancer, uterine cancer
- A hysterectomy may *not* remove the cervix. It is important to visualize the vagina and assess for the presence of a cervix.
- If a woman presents having two cervices, collect a Pap test from each one and label each test appropriately (e.g., right cervix Pap, left cervix Pap).
- Pregnancy changes mimic dysplasia and are sometimes indistinguishable from true neoplasia. Seventy-five percent of "abnormal" Pap tests may regress within 6 months after the pregnancy ends. Confer with or refer to obstetrician or pregnancy specialist for abnormal cytology management in pregnancy. Be sure to obtain follow-up Pap tests during the postpartum period.
- In women at high risk for endometrial hyperplasia (postmenopausal, chronic anovulation), if endometrial cells are noted on the Pap (even without atypia), refer for endometrial sampling.
    - Clinical tip: Postmenopausal women with one or more unsatisfactory Pap tests due to atrophy should use topical estrogen cream for 4–6 weeks, then repeat the Pap after more than 1 week without treatment.

When to Consult, Refer, Hospitalize

- Refer to gynecologist when signs, symptoms of cervical cancer are present.
- Abnormal bleeding (either metrorrhagia or postcoital spotting)
- Visible ulcer or mass on cervix, regardless of the Pap result
- Late signs: anemia, anorexia, urinary frequency, hematuria, weight loss, pelvic or epigastric pain
- Late complications: vaginal fistulas, urinary and fecal incontinence, back pain, leg edema, ureteral obstruction, eventually renal failure
- Two thirds of deaths from cervical cancer are from the uremia; another 10%–20% die from hemorrhage.
- Refer for colposcopy evaluation in individuals with abnormal Pap test results.

Follow-Up

- After ablative treatment, screening cytology should be repeated at accelerated intervals; commonly every 3–4 months for the first year, then every 6 months for the next year, then annually once a pattern of normal readings has been established.
- Any recurrent abnormal Pap needs colposcopy evaluation, repeat endocervical curettage, and biopsy.

Expected Course

- With appropriate management, future cancer risk is less than 5%. Many clinicians use automated cytology procedures if the patient has had therapy.
- Most treatment failures show up within 1–2 years post procedure.
- If undetected or untreated, 15%–20% of cervical lesions progress while the rest either stay stable or regress; up to 10 years from precancerous changes to invasive disease.

Complications

- After invasion, death usually occurs in 3–5 years without treatment or in unresponsive cancers.
- Invasion moves from the cervix to the uterus, the pelvis, internal lymph nodes, ureters, bladder, and rectum.

ATROPHIC VAGINITIS

Description

- Thinning fragility of vaginal and vulvar epithelium

Etiology

- Estrogen deficiency (estradiol levels less than 20 pg/mL); most common in menopausal and postmenopausal women
- Estrogen, along with glycogen, maintains a healthy pH of the vaginal environment between 3.8 and 4.2; estrogen deficiency causes an increased pH, disrupting the normal ecosystem.
- Estrogen deficiency also causes thinning and dryness of vaginal epithelium with loss of natural folds (rugae) in vaginal wall, predisposing the vagina to overgrowth of colonizing organisms or invasion of pathogens; vagina becomes friable, prone to inflammation

Incidence and Demographics

- Forty percent of postmenopausal women not on HRT
- Premenopausal women with low estrogen levels

Risk Factors

- Menopause, either natural or surgical, leading to a decline in endogenous estrogen
- Antibiotic use and antiestrogenic medications
- Stress and conditions suppressing immune function (e.g., diabetes mellitus and HIV)
- Lactation: prolactin, antiestrogenic effects; women who are breastfeeding may be unaware of the possibility of atrophic vaginitis.

Prevention and Screening

- All perimenopausal and postmenopausal women should be asked about signs and symptoms during their annual exams.

Assessment

History

- Complaints include vaginal itching, thin watery discharge or discomfort with coitus, reduced libido, urinary urgency, dysuria; may be asymptomatic
- Obtain history of menopause, use of HRT, vaginal therapies, coital lubricants, UTI history, diabetes

Physical Exam

- Exam: vagina is lighter pink to pale in color, fewer rugae, smaller labia, dry to little discharge, overall decreased vaginal moisture, loss of elasticity or turgor of skin and vaginal epithelium
- Elevated vaginal pH level higher than 5, ranging pH 5.5–7 (a rise over premenopausal levels of approximately 4.0)

Diagnostic Studies

- Pap, wet prep, maturational index: more parabasal cells and fewer intermediate and superficial cells (changes consistent with reduced estrogen)
- Abnormal number of WBCs (greater than 10 per high power field [HPF]) on wet prep
- Any vaginal specimen with blood should prompt a workup for cervical or uterine bleeding sources; there should be minimal trauma during the examination to create vaginal bleeding (except the use of a cytobrush, which often causes slight spotting).
- Urinalysis negative

Differential Diagnosis

- Infectious vaginitis (trichomoniasis, candidiasis)
- Bacterial vaginosis
- Vulvar or vaginal cancer
- Diabetes mellitus
- Trauma or foreign body
- Contact irritation

Management

Nonpharmacologic Treatment

- Use of vaginal water-based lubricants and moisturizers for coitus and general comfort

Pharmacologic Treatment

- Estrogen replacement therapy unless otherwise contraindicated: transvaginal administration of estrogen via intravaginal creams, pessaries, estradiol vaginal tablets (Vagifem); 25 μg oral estradiol twice a week; or a hormone-releasing ring (Estring), an estradiol-impregnated vaginal ring that delivers 6–9 μg estradiol daily for 3 months
- See the Menopause entry for oral and transdermal regimens (in lactating women, use topical first because oral/transdermal routes may decrease milk supply).
- The topical regimen is conjugated estrogen cream (Premarin) 2–4 g intravaginally once a day in cycles of 3 weeks on/1 week off; maintenance dose is once a week.

How Long to Treat

- Indefinitely as needed

Special Considerations

- Postmenopausal women not on HRT should also be evaluated for other complications of estrogen deficiency.

When to Consult, Refer, Hospitalize

- If signs and symptoms do not resolve with treatment, refer for biopsy.

Follow-Up

- Reevaluate 1–2 months after treatment to assess for side effects and treatment response.
- Reevaluate breastfeeding women after weaning.

Expected Course

- Resolves with ongoing or periodic treatment; typically takes 4–6 weeks for symptoms to resolve

Complications

- Superimposed infection

BARTHOLIN GLAND CYSTS AND ABSCESSES

Description

- Obstruction of a Bartholin gland (greater vestibular gland) causing a simple cyst or possible inflammation and infection; causing pain, swelling, and abscess formation

Etiology

- Obstruction of duct with retained mucus, causing a simple cyst; contributing factors include trauma, infection, epithelial hyperplasia, congenital atresia
- Infection is usually polymicrobial
- Most cysts remain minimally symptomatic smaller than 4 cm.
- Infected cysts contain mixed vaginal flora, *Neisseria gonorrhoeae, Chlamydia trachomatis, Escherichia coli*; become enlarged, acutely painful.
- Can result in chronic ductal stenosis and residual distension; frequently recurrent

Incidence and Demographics

- Most common vulvar mass
- Usually presents from ages 20–29
- Rare after age 40, presence at that age is suspicious for malignancy and requires biopsy or complete excision
- About 2% of women experience a Bartholin gland cyst or abscess

Risk Factors

- History of gonorrhea or chlamydia, at risk for STDs
- Scratching and shaving perineal area

Prevention and Screening

- Prevention of STDs

Assessment

History

- Previous episodes; prior surgical treatment (incision and drainage, marsupialization, Word catheter placement), STDs; localized edema; erythema and pain of the labia; history of vulvar abrasion, injury, or trauma
- Symptoms are pain on sides of introitus, dyspareunia, painful sitting or walking

Physical Exam

- Physical exam may show swelling on sides of the introitus; fluctuant mass at 4 o'clock or 8 o'clock, or both, but usually unilateral; if active infection, there may be redness, tenderness, edema; size can vary up to 4 cm.

Diagnostic Studies

- If drainage is present or if incision and drainage are performed, obtain wound cultures, and perform tests for gonorrhea, chlamydia.
- Consider cervical testing for gonorrhea and chlamydia.

Differential Diagnosis

- Inclusion cysts
- Lipoma
- Fibroma

- Hematoma
- Bartholin gland cancer (rare)

Management

Nonpharmacologic Treatment

- Warm soaks and sitz baths can alleviate pain, promote spontaneous ductal opening
- Cyst needs no treatment if not symptomatic
- Treatment of large, painful cyst is incision and drainage
- Word catheter can be inserted at time of incision and drainage; it can be sutured or taped into place and is allowed to drain for 2–4 weeks.

Pharmacologic Treatment

- Antibiotic treatment for both aerobic and anaerobic bacteria coverage (e.g., ceftriaxone [Rocephin] 125 mg IM one dose plus clindamycin [Cleocin] 300 mg orally four times a day for 7 days to cover skin bacterial flora, anaerobic bacteria, and possibly gonorrhea; may also need to add metronidazole (Flagyl) 500 mg orally twice a day for 7 days for treatment of trichomoniasis)

Special Considerations

- For women 40 years of age and older or postmenopausal, complex excision under general anesthesia is warranted to rule out carcinoma.

When to Consult, Refer, Hospitalize

- Refer as needed for a symptomatic or infected cyst that requires incision and drainage or other procedure.
- For a recurrent cyst, refer for excision of cyst and marsupialization to establish new ductal opening; laser incision can also be used.
- Incision and drainage and placement of the Word catheters are not beginner skills. Patients should be referred to either the collaborating physician or a gynecologist.

Follow-Up

- If incision and drainage are done, follow-up in 10 days; if a Word catheter is inserted, follow-up in 4 weeks.

Expected Course

- Abscesses often recur after incision and drainage.

Complications

- Recurrent abscess
- Labial abscesses that start initially as a papule and rapidly expand into a large abscess over 24 hours are highly suggestive of methicillin-resistant *S. aureus* (MRSA) and require immediate antibiotic coverage and incision and drainage.

BACTERIAL VAGINOSIS (BV)

Description

- A clinical syndrome caused by replacement of vaginal hydrogen peroxide–producing *Lactobacillus* species by a variety of anaerobic bacteria such as *Gardnerella vaginalis* and *Mycoplasma hominis*; not considered an STD

Etiology

- Cause not clearly known, but symptoms caused by an overgrowth of one or more anaerobic bacteria (e.g., *Prevotella* sp., *Mobiluncus* sp., *G. vaginalis, M. hominis,* replacing the normal *Lactobacillus* flora)
- *G. vaginalis* is the predominant organism.
- Primarily occurs in sexually active adolescents and adult women; not considered an STD, but is a sexually associated infection
- Women who have never been sexually active are rarely affected.

Incidence and Demographics

- In women of reproductive age, bacterial vaginosis (BV) is the most common cause of vaginal discharge.
- The most prevalent vaginitis (symptomatic) in sexually active adolescents, adults
- In the United States *G. vaginalis* accounts for about 7.4 million yearly cases of BV.
- In the obstetric setting, the incidence is about 10%–25% and in the STD clinic setting, it is about 30%–65%

Risk Factors

- Sexual activity, increasing with multiple partners and new sex partner
- Co-infection with STD
- Douching
- Black/African descent
- IUD use

Prevention and Screening

- Wearing all-cotton underwear and loose clothes.
- Avoiding douching or tampon use to decrease bacterial overgrowth.
- Advise use of condoms.

Assessment

History

- Malodorous vaginal discharge (fishy odor), primarily following coitus or before menstruation
- Itching and burning usually are not present unless there is co-infection with another pathogen.
- Patient may report vaginal irritation secondary to presence of discharge.

Physical Exam

- Introitus: presence of homogenous discharge
- Speculum exam: presence of homogenous discharges coating vaginal walls and foul (fishy) odor
- Cervix bimanual exam is normal: cervix without inflammation, discharge, or cervical motion tenderness

Diagnostic Studies

- Amsel's clinical criteria positive for diagnosis (must have three criteria):
  1. Thin, white-gray, homogeneous vaginal discharge adherent to vaginal wall
  2. Vaginal pH higher than 4.5
  3. Positive potassium hydroxide (KOH) "whiff" test: fishy odor when 10% KOH is applied to discharge
  4. Characteristic clue cells on microscopic exam

Differential Diagnosis

- *Trichomonas* vaginitis
- Cervicitis caused by *Chlamydia* or *Neisseria gonorrhoeae*
- Vulvovaginal candidiasis

Management

- Only women with symptomatic disease need treatment.
- Treatment of men is not needed because it has not been shown that treatment alters course or relapse/reinfection rate. The intravaginal route may be preferred because of a decrease in systemic side effects.

Nonpharmacologic Treatment

- Abstinence from sexual intercourse during pharmacological treatment.
- Avoiding alcohol or any alcohol-containing products while taking metronidazole, because interaction produces a profound disulfiram-like reaction such as nausea, vomiting, or hypotension

Pharmacologic Treatment

- Metronidazole 500 mg orally twice a day × 7 days, *or*
- Metronidazole gel 0.75%, 1 applicator (5 g) intravaginally q.h.s. × 5 days, *or*
- Clindamycin cream 2%, 1 applicator (5 g) intravaginally q.h.s. × 7 days
- Clindamycin 300 mg orally twice a day × 7 days

Special Considerations

- Intravaginal treatment is preferred for lactating women.
- Treatment of high-risk pregnant women (previous premature delivery) who are asymptomatic might reduce premature delivery; screening and treatment suggested early in second trimester.
- Low-risk pregnant women who have symptomatic BV should be treated; use lower doses to minimize exposure to the fetus.
- Clindamycin vaginal gel is not recommended during pregnancy; use is associated with increase in premature deliveries
- Patients allergic to metronidazole should not be given vaginal gel.
- Recent meta-analysis of metronidazole does not indicate teratogenicity in humans.
- Pregnant women at high or low risk: metronidazole 500 mg orally twice a day for 7 days, or 250 mg orally three times a day × 7 days, or clindamycin 300 mg orally twice a day for 7 days; clindamycin gel not recommended during pregnancy

When to Consult, Refer, Hospitalize

- Consult for recurrent or refractory infection

Follow-Up

- None needed except for pregnant women, 1 month following treatment

Expected Course

- Most respond promptly

Complications

- Abnormal vaginal discharge, mucopurulent cervicitis, urinary tract infections, postoperative infections, cervical dysplasia, non-puerperal endometritis, bacterial vaginosis–related PID
- Obstetric: chorioamnionitis, premature labor, premature rupture of membranes, postpartum endometritis

VAGINAL CANDIDIASIS

Description

- Vaginitis caused by *Candida* species is not considered to be a STD
- Also known as moniliasis or vaginal yeast

Etiology

- A dimorphic fungus existing as oval, budding yeast cells or chains of cells (hyphae)
- Normal flora in the vagina and skin
- Symptomatic infection typically occurring when the vaginal environment is disturbed, resulting in fungal overgrowth

Incidence and Demographics

- About 75% of all women will have at least one episode.
- Second most common cause of vaginitis (after bacterial vaginosis)

- Most cases caused by *Candida albicans* (80%–92%) with *Candida glabrata* and *Candida tropicalis* responsible for the remaining
- *C. glabrata* and *C. tropicalis* are increasing in prevalence, more often cause recurrent infections

Risk Factors

- Antibiotic, corticosteroid, or antiestrogen medications
- Sexual intercourse, oral/vaginal sex, anal/vaginal sex, contraceptives, pregnancy
- Douching, tight-fitting undergarments, obesity
- Stress and immunosuppressive disorders (e.g., HIV and diabetes mellitus)

Prevention and Screening

- Advise all women of possibility of candidiasis with antibiotic, corticosteroid, and antiestrogen use.
- Advise against douching.

Assessment

History

- Thick, white, non-odorous, cheesy vaginal discharge with or without pruritus
- Pruritus may be only symptom without discharge
- Soreness with coitus (dyspareunia); may also be the only symptom
- Obtain medication history, including recent use of over-the-counter antifungals, vaginal hygiene habits

Physical Exam

- Varying amounts of thick, white discharge without odor
- Discharge adherent to vaginal walls
- Discharge may be scant, but vulvar erythema and edema can often be present with excoriations, sometimes sufficiently severe to preclude adequate speculum exam.

Diagnostic Studies

- Litmus paper for pH: normal pH 4.0–4.5
- Wet prep: pseudohyphae may be present on normal saline slide; KOH slide demonstrates fungal hyphae, maybe spores
- STD screen as appropriate
- Fungal cultures, only necessary for recurrent episodes
- Hemoglobin A1c (HbA1c) to evaluate for diabetes mellitus

Differential Diagnosis

- Bacterial vaginosis
- Trichomonas
- Atrophic vaginitis
- chlamydia or gonorrhea

Management

- Pharmacologic treatment required only if symptomatic
- May presumptively treat (wet mount not very sensitive) if sole complaint is pruritus

Nonpharmacologic Treatment

- Proper perineal hygiene especially after bowel movements, sexual intercourse, or oral/genital sex
- Wearing looser-fitting undergarments (preferably cotton), especially in the summer
- Avoiding alcohol and large amounts of concentrated sugars
- Oatmeal baths may reduce itching.
- Sexual hygiene

Pharmacologic Treatment

- Fluconazole 150 mg orally 1 tablet, single dose
- Clotrimazole 1%, 5 g intravaginally q.h.s. × 7–14 days
- Miconazole 2% cream, 5 g intravaginally q.h.s. × 7 days
- Terconazole 0.4% cream, 5 g intravaginally q.h.s. × 7 days
- Butoconazole 2% cream, 5 g intravaginally q.h.s. × 3days
- Many of the above creams can be also given as a 1-, 3-, 10-, or 14-day treatment; also available in suppository form
- Clotrimazole, miconazole, and butoconazole are available over the counter; duration of treatment as per package instructions.

Special Considerations

- Seven-day treatment recommended for pregnant women with a history of recent candidiasis
- Pregnant women should not use fluconazole.
- For acutely symptomatic women, creams and suppositories yield quicker relief than oral fluconazole.
- Test for diabetes mellitus with persistent or recurrent infection

When to Consult, Refer, Hospitalize

- Refer to gynecologist for persistent or recurrent infection.

Follow-Up

- Only indicated if signs and symptoms fail to resolve within 2 weeks or recur

Expected Course

- Usually resolves without problem

Complications

- Refractory candidiasis

Abnormal Growths of Uterus and Ovaries

LEIOMYOMAS

Description

- Uterine fibroids, myomas, fibroid "tumors"
- Benign uterine smooth muscle connective tissue growth, responsive to estrogens
- Discrete, firm, roundish, often multiple in various anatomic locations—intramural, submucous, subserous, intraligamentous, pedunculated, and cervical
- Mostly asymptomatic and found incidentally on examination

Etiology

- Benign tumors represent localized proliferation of smooth muscle cells surrounded by a pseudocapsule of compressed muscle fibers. Etiology unknown.

Incidence and Demographics

- Only occurs in women who have a uterus; incidence increases with age
- In the United States, the incidence for Black women by 35 years old is 60% and by age 50 it increases to 80%.
- In the United States the incidence for White women by 35 years old is 40% and by age 50 it increases to 70%.

Risk Factors

- Nulliparity
- Obesity
- Black/African descent

Assessment

History

- Occasionally causes menorrhagia (with dystrophic calcification), dysmenorrhea, pelvic pain, bladder pressure, back pain (enlargement encroaches on adjacent structures, possible torsion), increasing pain in pregnancy, pregnancy losses (cavity distortion)

Physical Exam

- Enlarged, firm, irregular uterus; mobile; mostly non-tender; and negative other exam findings. Clinically useful to document size of uterus comparable to gestational size ("10–12 week's size"; "umbilicus minus 1 cm") for comparative evaluation over time.

Diagnostic Studies

- Labs: hCG, CBC (for iron-deficiency anemia), screening Pap test, and other health maintenance as indicated
- Transvaginal ultrasonography can identify characteristic fibroid changes (hypoechoic, no cysts, uniform structure), map number location, measure size, assess normalcy of adjacent structures (endometrial thickness); helpful for ruling out other concerns (such as ovarian cysts).
- Sonohysterogram to locate intramural lesions
- MRI to visualize individual myomas
- Hysterosalpingography to define extent of submucosa myomas before surgery or to evaluate uterine cavity and patency of fallopian tubes

Differential Diagnosis

- Pregnancy
- Endometriosis
- Endometrial carcinoma
- Ovarian cysts
- Uterine cancer
- Abnormal vaginal bleeding

- Adenomyosis
- Cervical cancer
- Ovarian cancer
- Leiomyosarcoma (0.5% of fibroids; very rare before age 40)

Management

Nonpharmacologic Treatment

- Heat, rest, regular complete voiding if causing pressure on bladder

Pharmacologic Treatment

- No treatment needed if asymptomatic
- Iron-replacement therapy if needed; hormonal contraception may reduce bleeding but unclear if it reduces fibroid size—may increase size in some
- NSAIDs work well for chronic pain.
- Analgesics with narcotics only for unremitting pain; needs gynecological consultation
- Reduce size medically using GnRH agonists such as leuprolide (Lupron) 3.75 mg IM monthly or 11.25 mg IM every 3 months, or DMPA; then surgical treatment may be indicated.

Special Considerations

- Patients may become pregnant in the presence of a leiomyoma.
- Pregnancy in conjunction with leiomyoma is usually unremarkable with a normal antepartum course, labor, and delivery. These patients need careful surveillance.
- The risk of spontaneous abortion or preterm labor following myomectomy is high. Use of prophylactic beta-adrenergic tocolytics is sometimes indicated.
- Vaginal birth after myomectomy is controversial.

When to Consult, Refer, Hospitalize

- Fertility concerns should be referred to gynecologist for management.
- Consult with gynecology about options to reduce bleeding (Leuprolide, surgical excision, myomectomy embolization therapy, hysterectomy) if endometrial sampling is indicated.

Follow-Up

- When symptomatic and at yearly exam
- Should monitor growth with transvaginal or pelvic ultrasound every 6 months until stable

Expected Course

- Reduction in size, symptoms after pregnancy and menopause

Complications

- Urinary incontinence, pregnancy loss, anemia

BENIGN OVARIAN GROWTHS

Description

- Functional cysts (corpus luteum cysts, theca lutein cysts) and follicular cysts produce hormones.
- Very common in adolescents; may have PMS-type prodrome; menses delayed until resolved
- Dermoid cysts (benign teratomas) are growths from germ cells; surgical excision prevents rare cancerous changes.

Etiology

- Can occur when the ovarian follicle enlarges and does not rupture or when the corpus luteum does not regress in the absence of pregnancy

- Theca lutein cysts may develop with high levels of hCG or with ovulation induction.
- May grow as large as 10–15 cm but rarely larger than 6–8 cm

Incidence and Demographics

- Most ovarian masses are not only functional but also benign.
- On ultrasound ovarian cysts are seen mostly in premenopausal women; about 18% are detected in post-menopausal women

Risk Factors

- Threefold increase in risk for smokers
- Recent obesity and obesity at age 20
- Inversely associated with ever having had a term pregnancy
- OCs tend to be protective (but benign growths still occur occasionally).

Prevention and Screening

- Screening is only necessary if patient is undergoing ovulation induction.

Assessment

History

- Discomfort with or without menstrual cycle alterations; may be incidental to visit
- Functional or follicular cysts often have hormonal effects.
- Bloating, dyspareunia, chronic lower abdominal pain and pressure, and menstrual irregularities may be evident.
- Always ask about LMP.

Physical Exam

- Exam is often unremarkable if the growth is small; unilateral or bilateral adnexal mass may be present; tenderness may be elicited

Diagnostic Studies

- hCG: rule out ectopic pregnancy; other tests as indicated by history and physical exam
- Transvaginal or pelvic ultrasound: fluid component, hypoechogenic, single cyst or simple septate area, no free fluid in cul-de-sac

Differential Diagnosis

- Ovarian cancer
- Pregnancy
- Endometrioma
- Leiomyoma
- Urinary tract disorder
- Bowel disorder
- PID
- STD
- Ectopic gestation
- PCOS

Management

Nonpharmacologic Treatment

- Between menarche and menopause, an asymptomatic, mobile, lateral simple cystic mass less than 5–6 cm confirmed by sonography can be observed; spontaneous resolution is expected. Most functional cysts or follicular cysts will regress or resorb without intervention.
- Surgical evaluation should occur for masses that persist for more than 6 weeks, enlarge, or are larger than 10 cm for dermoid cysts.

Pharmacologic Treatment

- OCs may be used to assist regression of functional and follicular cysts.
- Manage pain beginning with NSAIDs or acetaminophen; analgesics with narcotics only for unremitting pain; needs gynecological consultation

Special Considerations

- Some may rupture, causing acute pain.

When to Consult, Refer, Hospitalize

- Refer to gynecologist if markedly tender, larger than 6 cm, increases in size, or persists beyond 6 weeks.

Follow-Up

- Reevaluate size with ultrasound in 4–6 weeks.

Complications

- Usually none

POLYCYSTIC OVARY SYNDROME (PCOS)/POLYCYSTIC OVARIAN DISEASE (PCOD)/STEIN-LEVENTHAL SYNDROME

Description

- Classic presentation of hyperandrogenism (obesity, hirsutism, acne), menstrual irregularities (oligomenorrhea since menarche, amenorrhea, erratic menorrhagia, or metrorrhagia), erratic fertility patterns or infertile, insulin resistance, and hyperinsulinemia
- Polycystic ovaries are the end point of the process, not the diagnostic focal point.

Etiology

- PCOS is a result of a complex disruption of the hypothalamic-pituitary-ovarian axis and ovarian function, characterized by higher tonic levels of LH and low or low normal FSH levels.
- Familial pattern (autosomal dominant)

Incidence and Demographics

- Commonly begins in adolescence (post menarche)
- PCOS affects about 7% of women in the reproductive years

Risk Factors

- Familial/genetic component
- Weight gain with android pattern obesity

Prevention and Screening

- No prevention identified; no routine screening

Assessment

History

- History of oligomenorrhea, amenorrhea, erratic vaginal bleeding, infertility
- Cosmetically disturbing hirsutism; male pattern hair growth, hair thinning or loss, acne, and voice changes
- History of gestational diabetes mellitus or hypertension, overweight and weight gain, family history of diabetes mellitus

Physical Exam

- Central obesity common, although some patients are normal weight
- Adnexal mass may be evident
- Acanthosis nigricans, acne, hirsutism, balding, skin tags, increased BMI, clitoromegaly, thyroid enlargement

Diagnostic Studies

- Urine hCG or serum beta-hCG to rule out pregnancy
- TSH, free T4, 17-hydroxyprogesterone, serum total testosterone (elevated), DHEA-S (elevated), prolactin (to rule out pituitary tumor), fasting lipids, glucose, and 2-hour glucose tolerance test after 75 g load
- Overnight dexamethasone suppression test
- Transvaginal ultrasound revealing multiple antral follicles on a single ovary or ovarian volume larger than 10 cm^3
- MRI is *not* diagnostic; CT and ultrasound may assist in the diagnostic process but are not truly diagnostic alone.
- Consider endometrial biopsy for prolonged erratic bleeding to rule out endometrial cancer.

Differential Diagnosis

- Adrenal: tumor, Cushing's syndrome, adult-onset adrenal hyperplasia
- HAIR-AN syndrome (hyperandrogenism, insulin resistance, acanthosis nigricans)
- Ovarian: tumor, ovarian insensitivity syndrome
- Hepatic disease (alters estrogen clearance metabolism)
- Thyroid disease (may affect feedback loops)
- Prolactinoma

Management

Nonpharmacologic Treatment

- Exercise and weight loss: goal of body mass index less than 27
- Exercise and weight loss improve lipid profile, reduce hyperinsulinemia (insulin resistance uncommon with low BMI), improve fertility, improve menstrual cycles, reduce hirsutism
- Occasionally, ovarian wedge resection is needed

Pharmacologic Treatment

- Treatment with OCs or progestin can minimize menstrual irregularities and decrease risks of endometrial cancer; cycling will occur (reduces endometrial danger), may protect lipids, will not increase glucose.
- Control of lipids, blood glucose, and hypertension
- Bromocriptine (Parlodel) if prolactin level is elevated
- Metformin (Glucophage) improves insulin sensitivity, lowers LH, lowers androgen, improves fertility.

Special Considerations

- Androgen excess–related insulin resistance (reduced glucose response to insulin amount or "syndrome X/metabolic syndrome"), which spurs hyperinsulinemia (ratio of fasting glucose to fasting insulin levels lower than 3.0), increased risk of diabetes mellitus
- Also associated with hypertension, coronary artery disease, increased triglyceride level, and decreased high-density lipoprotein (HDL) levels

When to Consult, Refer, Hospitalize

- Consult with gynecologist for fertility issues and treatment with clomiphene (Clomid) to induce ovulation, antiandrogen, or other hormonal therapy.
- Consult with endocrinologist for obesity, insulin resistance, and lipid issues.

Follow-Up

- Close monitoring for excessive endometrial buildup, breast cancer
- Lipids, oral glucose tolerance testing at regular intervals

Complications

- Osteoporosis risk
- Endometrial hyperplasia/carcinoma
- Has been associated with failure of lactogenesis II and low milk supply

Other Conditions

PELVIC INFLAMMATORY DISEASE (PID)

Description

- Ascending infection and inflammation within the upper genital tract in women

Etiology

- PID has a polymicrobial etiology, with the most common pathogens being *N. gonorrhoeae, C. trachomatis* in acute PID; mixed with anaerobes, *Bacteroides* sp., staphylococci, streptococci, *Enterobacter* sp., *Haemophilus influenzae*, and others.
- Part of an ascending continuum of cervicitis, endometritis, salpingitis, and finally pelvic peritonitis

Incidence and Demographics

- Most prevalent at ages 15–29 years old
- Most common reason for gynecological hospital admission in the United States
- Lifetime prevalence for women ages 18 to 44 years old is up 4.4% in the United States.
- Women with a history of PID experience difficulties getting pregnant or become infertile because of PID; risks for tubal infertility increase with each occurrence of PID up to 40%.
- PID is uncommon in pregnancy.

Risk Factors

- Sexually active with multiple partners; change in partner within past year
- Infected partner, history of or concurrent STD, prior history of PID
- IUD, genital surgical instrumentation (dilation and curettage, induced abortion)
- Lack of condom use

Prevention and Screening

- May do STD screen for women with a new sexual partner, especially if younger than 25 years of age

Assessment

History

- Sexual partner practice history, history of STDs, prior PID, contraception, gynecologic procedures, and vaginal douching
- Presentation may be mild, nonspecific or subclinical in nature, or asymptomatic
- Speed of symptomatology is dependent on the infectious organisms involved.
- Mild to moderate: Mid-abdominal pain may be first, with dyspareunia and unusual vaginal discharge. May have some mid-cycle spotting; usually no anorexia. Pain worsens with menses.
- Severe: increasing bilateral pain, fever, and nausea with occasional vomiting as the infection worsens and progresses beyond the salpinges and into the abdominal cavity
- Fitz–Hugh–Curtis syndrome: perihepatitis including fever, chills, and pleuritic right upper quadrant pain; accounts for about 5% of PID

Physical Exam

- Classic triad of lower abdominal pain, adnexal tenderness (unilateral or bilateral), cervical motion tenderness; only one third have fever with temperature above 101°F.
- Direct abdominal tenderness (with or without rebound)
- Cervix: cervicitis (edema friability); note blood, ulcerations, nodules
- Vaginal discharge may or may not be present, may be mucopurulent
- Mild to moderate uterine tenderness
- Adnexal masses may or may not be palpable; consider tubo-ovarian abscess.
- Adnexal tenderness
- Pain response to cervical motion may be acute, startling ("chandelier sign")
- Enlarged, tender inguinal lymph nodes are often a sign of an STD or a pelvic infection. Diffuse, systemic adenopathy with flu-like symptoms: consider possibility of primary HIV infection.

Diagnostic Studies

- Diagnosis chiefly based on history and physical and less on labs, except for identification of etiologic agent
- Urine hCG, *N. gonorrhoeae*, and *Chlamydia* testing
- If lesions are noted, assess for herpes, syphilis.
- Counsel and recommend HIV screening.
- Consider cervical cytology screening after the acute infection phase is passed to minimize confounding changes affecting cytological accuracy.
- ESR is nonspecific and not reliable; WBC count is not reliable
- Vaginal wet preps should have higher than 10 WBC/HPF; look for trichomonads, which can confound the workup; confirm sexual transmission, or bacterial vaginosis, which can be an associated condition.
- Transvaginal/pelvic ultrasound can rule out pregnancy (ectopic) and identify tubal masses or ovarian abscess.

Differential Diagnosis

- Appendicitis
- Ectopic gestation
- Endometriosis
- Leiomyoma
- Acute enteritis
- Severe
- Ovarian cyst (ruptured)
- UTI/pyelonephritis
- Colitis
- Renal calculi

Management

Nonpharmacologic Treatment

- Counsel on safer sex measures

Pharmacologic Treatment

- 2021 CDC criteria for empiric treatment can be based on finding classic triad; urgent treatment is preferred even without specific lab results rather than risk a lifetime of chronic pelvic pain, scarring, infertility.
- Outpatient treatment is best with a multiple drug regimen that covers several pathogens, including *N. gonorrhoeae* and *Chlamydia*:
  - Ceftriaxone (Rocephin) 500 mg IM once, Doxycycline 100 mg orally twice a day × 14 days, and metronidazole (Flagyl) 500 mg orally twice a day × 14 days
- See 2021 CDC Guidelines for STD Treatment: Oral cephalosporins and quinolone agents are no longer a recommended treatment for gonococcal infections because of resistance.
- Concurrent treatment of all sexual partners (and the partners' sexual partners) is highly advisable.
- Patients who do not respond to oral therapy within 72 hours should be reevaluated to confirm the diagnosis and should be administered parenteral therapy on either an outpatient or inpatient basis.
- See 2021 CDC Guidelines for STD Treatment for additional alternative treatment regimens. The CDC has a free downloadable app to use at point of care: https://www.cdc.gov/std/treatment-guidelines/provider-resources.htm

How Long to Treat

- 14 days is a standard regimen

Special Considerations

- Minimal signs or symptoms do not correlate with minimal tubal scarring or other adverse sequelae.
- Avoiding alcohol or any alcohol-containing products while taking metronidazole, because interaction produces a profound disulfiram-like reaction such as nausea, vomiting, or hypotension.
- Twenty percent of patients with PID do not have positive cervical cultures for gonorrhea or chlamydia.

When to Consult, Refer, Hospitalize

- Inpatient treatment is best for a very young or unreliable patient, pregnant patient, fever with temperature above 101°F, WBC count above 11,000/mm3, evidence of peritonitis, suspected pelvic abscess, decreased bowel sounds, or anorexia; for a patient with escalating symptoms despite treatment; for non-resolving symptoms after 72 hours of treatment; or for severely immunocompromised patients.

Follow-Up

- Close follow up is needed within 72 hours to assess treatment efficacy and compliance, again after treatment is complete; if no improvement is noted, consider hospitalization.
- Treat all sex partners empirically for both chlamydia and gonorrhea.

Expected Course

- Signs and symptoms of acute infection should resolve by completion of antibiotic treatment.

Complications

- About one-third of hospitalized patients with PID have a tubo-ovarian abscess.
- Infertility that increases with each subsequent episode of PID
- Sevenfold to 10-fold increase in risk for ectopic gestation following one episode
- May produce chronic pelvic pain, dyspareunia, adhesion formation, chronic pyosalpinx, or hydrosalpinx

CARE OF THE MATERNITY PATIENT

Preconception Counseling

- Offers the opportunity to discuss with the patient planning a future pregnancy her individualized risk factors, perform preconception genetic testing for conditions such as cystic fibrosis and Tay-Sachs in specific populations, and teach the patient how to optimize her health and decrease risks in preparation for a healthy pregnancy

- To decrease the risks for neural tube defects, provide preconception supplementation with folate 400 µg daily for all women who plan to become or are at risk for becoming pregnant. The U.S. Public Health Service and CDC recommend that *all women of childbearing age consume 0.4 mg (400 µg) of folic acid daily* to prevent two common and serious birth defects: spina bifida and anencephaly.
- Encourage smoking cessation, limiting alcohol use, avoiding recreational drug use, minimizing use of over-the-counter medications, and, in conjunction with the primary care provider, if possible, lower prescribed medication doses while maintaining therapeutic level for the patient's needs.

Prenatal Care

The goal of prenatal care is to ensure the health of both mother and fetus.

- Assessment and care of the pregnant woman from conception throughout pregnancy until birth
- Prenatal care after conception should begin as soon as possible.
- Pregnancy outcome can be improved by early health intervention screening.
- The U.S. Public Health Service advises intensive intervention in early pregnancy if there are identified risk factors that can be modified (e.g., smoking, poor nutrition, psychosocial disorders, diabetes, drug or alcohol abuse).
- Use a biopsychosocial approach with a family focus.
- Care during the prenatal period includes primary and secondary prevention.
- Health promotion should be emphasized.
- Childbirth and parenting education
- Adequate nutrition, smoking cessation, drug and alcohol avoidance, exercise
- Review of current medications, including over-the-counter drugs
- Review benefits of breastfeeding and the recommendation to breastfeed exclusively for the first 6 months and continue breastfeeding with the addition of solids for a minimum of 1 year.
- Pregnant women should avoid cat-litter boxes and feces, eating uncooked meat (to avoid risk of toxoplasmosis), sushi (hepatitis A), and non-pasteurized cheeses. Limit tuna, salmon, and other high-fat fishes to once a week (because of mercury contamination).

Prenatal Screening

- To identify the patient at risk for maternal-fetal conditions and complications that require monitoring or may be treatable; identify health status of mother and baby
- Estimating the gestational age as accurately as possible
- Evaluating the health status of mother and fetus
- Empowering and encouraging the patient to care for self and baby
- Universal testing for all patients includes Pap test, urinalysis, urine culture, CBC, blood type, Rh antibody testing, STD screening, hepatitis B surface antigen (HBsAg), rubella immunity, and blood glucose.
- These tests are done as part of a prenatal blood panel at the initial visit, except for blood glucose, which is done at 24–28 weeks of gestation in low-risk patients.
- Group B beta-hemolytic streptococcus genital culture is done at 34–36 weeks of gestation.
- Hemoglobin should be checked again during the last trimester to rule out anemia.
- Patient is monitored for weight gain or loss, blood pressure, edema, uterine fundal growth, fetal growth, fetal heart tones, and fetal position.
- ConsiderTSH, anti-thyroid peroxidase (TPO) antibodies for undiagnosed hypothyroidism

FIRST PRENATAL VISIT

Assessment

History

- A complete medical, gynecological, and psychosocial history, including intimate partner violence (IPV) screening, should be obtained at the initial visit and updated throughout the pregnancy.
- Obstetrical/gynecological history: menstrual age at menarche, cycle, LMP, contraception, pregnancies, deliveries, abortions, past pregnancy or delivery complication, newborn health/complications, STD history, sexual history, medical history, social history, breastfeeding intentions/history

Physical Exam

- Height, weight, blood pressure; screen urine for protein and glucose
- Complete physical exam: check skin, hair, teeth, thyroid, lungs, heart, breasts, spine, abdomen, extremities (note varicosities, edema); perform neurological exam with special attention assessing for presence of clonus and tremors, along with sensory and motor function
- Pelvic: cervix (note color, position, status of cervical os, lesions, discharge), vagina, uterus (note size, position, tenderness, shape), ovaries (palpable, size, tenderness)
- Assess fundal height in centimeters; size equals dates.
- Fetal heart rate (when the fetal heart rate is usually heard)
- Breasts should be evaluated for growth, nipple retraction/inversion, glandular tissue, elasticity of the areola, shape and symmetry in the first and last trimester. Poor growth, nipple retraction, insufficient glandular tissue, inelasticity of the areola, and marked asymmetry are lactation risk factors.
- Pelvic/cervical examination

Diagnostic Studies

- Frequently ordered as prenatal panel
- CBC
- Blood type, Rh antibody screen
- Serology: veneral disease research laboratory (VDRL) or rapid plasm regain (RPR) titers
- Rubella titer
- Hepatitis B screen
- Urinalysis, urine culture
- Pap test (continue to follow current cervical cancer screening guidelines)
- Varicella immunity
- STD screening: chlamydia, gonorrhea, HSV if indication, HIV (opt-out approach)
- Carrier screening: cystic fibrosis and hemoglobin electrophoresis (panethnic screening because in a multiracial society)
- Uterine/fetal ultrasound as indicated: to confirm the presence of a viable intrauterine pregnancy, evaluate a suspected ectopic or molar pregnancy, provide the most accurate estimate of gestational age, assist with chorionic villus sampling, and evaluate for pelvic masses

Management

Nonpharmacologic Treatment

- Patient education as appropriate to stage of pregnancy, nutrition, exercise, psychosocial evaluation, smoking cessation

Pharmacologic Treatment

- Prenatal vitamin with folic acid 400 μg daily until 3–4 months postpartum during breastfeeding
- Elemental iron supplement (100–200 mg/day) for pregnant women with iron-deficiency anemia (hemoglobin lower than 11.0 g/dL)

When to Consult, Refer, Hospitalize

- Consult with physician for all high-risk patients for all abnormal findings during visits.
- Consult with lactation specialist for history of lactation failure or abnormal breast exam.

Follow-Up

- Usual schedule of prenatal visits: every 4 weeks until 28th week of gestation, then every 2 weeks until 36th week, then weekly until delivery
- Patients with identified risk factors can be seen as frequently as needed for careful monitoring.
- Weight checks, blood pressure, urine screen for protein and glucose, fundal height measurement and Leopold maneuvers, fetal heart tones, edema

RETURN PRENATAL VISITS

First Trimester: less than 13 Weeks

- Review of family and social conditions
- Genetic testing, chorionic villus sampling, α-fetoprotein serum levels, amniocentesis
- Weeks 11–20: Multiple markers screen should be offered; some prenatal sites offer screening for Down syndrome risk during the first trimester, measuring serum free hCG and pregnancy-associated plasma protein A (PAPP-A).

Second Trimester: 13–end of 27 Weeks

- Fetal heart tones
- Fundus at umbilicus at 20 weeks
- Quickening: fetal movement felt by mother at 18–20 weeks
- May order ultrasound if dates are in doubt or fetal growth in question
- Weeks 16–20: discuss and offer second-trimester screening for Down syndrome and birth defects with a triple (alpha-fetoprotein, hCG, and unconjugated estriol) or quad screening (alpha-fetoprotein, human chorionic gonadotropin, unconjugated estriol, and inhibin A)
- Refer for childbirth education classes.
- Discuss infant feeding: breastfeeding, bottle feeding
- Discuss symptoms to report: bleeding, cramping, fever, decreased fetal movement, dysuria.
- Weeks 24–28: Diabetes screening with glucose challenge test (50-g oral glucose load with blood glucose test 1 hour later), if abnormal, may be followed by a 3-hour glucose tolerance test (100-g oral glucose load with blood drawn fasting 1, 2, and 3 hours after ingestion of glucose); hemoglobin and hematocrit; repeat antibody screen in Rh-negative mothers before giving prophylactic Rh immunoglobulin
- Optimal timing for a single ultrasound evaluation in the absence of specific indications is at 18–20 weeks, when dating can be confirmed and anatomy assessed.

Third Trimester: 28 Weeks to Birth

- Weeks 35–36: labs: repeat hemoglobin, blood glucose; high-risk patients should be screened again for gonorrhea, chlamydia, HIV, and syphilis; vaginal and rectal cultures for group B streptococcus (linked to preterm delivery and neonatal sepsis); women testing positive for group B streptococcus will need treatment during labor before delivery.
- Evaluate blood pressure, weight gain/loss, edema, fundal height, and fetal heart tones.
- Teach signs of labor.
- Repeat breast exam.
- Discuss plans for birth control postpartum.

POSTPARTUM VISIT

The postpartum visit is usually performed no later than 6 weeks postpartum; however, patients may be assessed sooner in the event of problems or complicated associated with delivery, the postpartum period, or with breastfeeding.

Assessment

History

- Review labor and delivery record.
- Assess breastfeeding: milk supply adequacy, nipple or breast pain; encourage exclusive breastfeeding for 6 months; ask about infant's weight and growth, as well as number of wet diapers per day, to assess adequacy of mother's milk production.
- Bowels: constipation, change in elimination pattern, hemorrhoids
- Episiotomy repair: healed, problems, dehiscence, swelling
- Sexual relations: resumed, problems, dryness
- Contraception: evaluate and prescribe as needed.
- Bladder: voiding problems, incontinence, Kegel exercises
- Lochia (vaginal bleeding): resolved, clots, still bleeding
- Menses: resumed or lactational amenorrhea
- Sleeping pattern
- Nutrition
- Psychological adaptation to newborn: mother, other family members
- Screen for symptoms of postpartum depression

Physical Exam

- Vital signs, blood pressure
- Weight
- Urine: Screen for protein and glucose.
- Breast exam: Look for mastitis, redness, tenderness, masses.
- Thyroid exam: postpartum thyroiditis not uncommon

- Pelvic exam: episiotomy, uterus (involution should be nearly completed)
- Rectal exam: tone, rectoceles, hemorrhoids

Diagnostic Studies

- Pap test
- Hemoglobin if history of anemia

Management

- Estrogen-containing contraceptive methods can initiated safely by 6 weeks to 6 months postpartum for women who are breastfeeding their infants and 3 weeks postpartum for women who are not breastfeeding.
- Because of a concern about hypercoagulability during the postpartum phase, many clinicians withhold hormonal contraceptives from women after childbirth, whether or not the women are breastfeeding. The World Health Organization (WHO) reviewed available evidence on this issue and suggests that the risks of estrogen-containing contraceptives may outweigh the benefits during the first 3 weeks postpartum. After 3 weeks, however, when thrombosis risk returns to normal, postpartum women who are not breastfeeding can use estrogen-containing oral contraceptives without additional restrictions.
- Because low-dose progestins are not associated with thrombosis, the WHO recommends initiating progestin-only contraceptives at any point postpartum.
- Breastfeeding mothers may use progestin-only contraception beginning at 6 weeks postpartum.
- Mothers should continue prenatal vitamins for 3–4 months or while breastfeeding.

Follow-Up

- Routine well-woman care: Pap test in 6–12 months
- Contraception as indicated

CASE STUDIES

CASE 1

A 39-year-old, sexually active woman presents with a 3-week history of white vaginal discharge, no itching, but notices a fishy odor.

History of Present Illness (HPI): Denies abdominal pain, nausea and vomiting, fever, genital lesions, lymphadenopathy, dysuria. Patient has been in a monogamous relationship with same partner for 6 years.

1. What additional history would you obtain?

   Exam: Thin, white-gray vaginal discharge coating vaginal walls, cervix without inflammation or discharge; no cervical motion tenderness on bimanual examination.

2. What might you find on examination of vaginal fluid if this woman has bacterial vaginosis?
3. Should her partner be evaluated and treated?
4. What is the standard treatment for nonpregnant women?
5. What does the patient need to know regarding use of this medication?

CASE 2

A 30-year-old woman presents for her first prenatal visit. She has had a positive home pregnancy test. This is her third pregnancy. She reports that she has made frequent attempts to stop smoking without success.

1. What further history do you need from this patient?
2. What would you include in her physical assessment?
3. What screening tests would you order?
4. What prenatal education would she need?

CASE 3

A 52-year-old woman presents with complaints of hot flashes and no menstrual period for 4–5 months. She asks if there is a blood test to determine if she has gone through menopause and would like your advice on HRT.

HPI: LMP 4–5 months; two periods before that were late and scantier than usual. Hot flashes occur daily with profuse sweating, but she denies mood change or vaginal dryness. She has tried an herbal over-the-counter product without relief.

1. What additional history would you like before advising her on treatment?
2. What laboratory tests would you do to confirm menopause?
3. What information would you review about hormonal treatment in the management of menopause?
4. What other recommendations should you provide?

CASE STUDIES DISCUSSION

CASE 1

1. What additional history would you obtain?

   LMP, current method of contraception, use of tampons or douching, symptoms noted in partner, any recent antibiotic use

2. What might you find on examination of vaginal fluid if this woman has bacterial vaginosis?

   Thin, homogenous, white-gray discharge; pH above 4.5; clue cells visible on microscopic exam; positive KOH whiff test

3. Should her partner be evaluated and treated?

   No, treatment of men has not shown to alter relapse/reinfection rate in female partners.

4. What is the standard treatment for nonpregnant women?

   Metronidazole 500 mg orally twice a day for 7 days or metronidazole gel 0.75% intravaginal q.h.s for 5 days

5. What does the patient need to know regarding use of this medication?

   Patient is to avoid alcohol for 48 hours prior to initiating medication treatment, while taking the medication, and for 48 hours after taking the last dose because of the disulfiram like effect of this drug.

CASE 2

1. What further history do you need from this patient?

   Age at menarche, LMP, menstrual history, gynecologic history, obstetric history, past medical history, medications, social history

2. What will you include in her physical assessment?

   Height, weight, blood pressure, complete physical exam, breast exam, pelvic exam including bimanual exam for fundal height, fetal heart rate depending upon weeks of pregnancy

3. What screening tests will you order?

   Urine screen for protein and glucose followed by urinalysis and urine culture; CBC, blood type, Rh and antibody screen; RPR; rubella titer; hepatitis screen; Pap test; STD screening; varicella immunity; carrier screening

4. What prenatal education will she need?

   Include plan for smoking cessation. Provide education on the following: nutrition, exercise, changes during pregnancy, prenatal vitamin and folic acid supplementation, smoking cessation through behavior modification techniques, and usual schedule of prenatal visits.

CASE 3

1. What additional history would you like before advising her on treatment?

   Obstetric and gynecologic history; complete medical history for history of breast cancer or breast mass; migraines; osteoporosis risk factors; method of contraception; chance of pregnancy; smoking status.

2. What laboratory tests will you do to confirm menopause?

   No tests are essential; according to her history she is perimenopausal. TSH not necessary unless she is having additional symptoms of hyperthyroidism; LH, FSH, and estradiol will fluctuate. Significant elevations in FSH and LH levels may not be seen until 1 year after cessation of menses.

3. What information will you review about hormonal treatment in menopause?

   Hormone replacement is now reserved for short-term use in patients with severe symptoms. Long-term use is not cardioprotective and may increase risk for stroke, myocardial infarction, breast cancer, and perhaps dementia. Advise herbal preparations or symptomatic treatment rather than HRT at this time.

4. What other recommendations should the FNP provide?

   Calcium intake of 1,200–1,500 mg per day; vitamin D 400–800 IU per day; exercise and weight management; vaginal lubrication for intercourse if dryness occurs, Kegel exercises to prevent urinary incontinence; check active ingredient and dosage of herbal product to determine its value (black cohosh, soy in large amounts, flaxseeds may be helpful).

REFERENCES

Ajmal, M., Khan, M., & Van Fossen, K. Breast fibroadenoma. (2022). StatPearls. https://www.ncbi.nlm.nih.gov/books/NBK535345/

American Academy of Pediatrics & American College of Obstetricians & Gynecologists. (2017). *Guidelines for perinatal care* (8th ed.). Elk Grove Village, IL: American Academy of Pediatrics.

American Cancer Society. (2022). *Key statistics for cervical cancer.* https://www.cancer.org/cancer/cervicalcancer/about/keystatistics.html#:~:text=Cervical%20cancer%20is%20most%20frequently,still%20present%20as%20they%20age

American Cancer Society. (2021). *The American Cancer Society Guidelines for the Prevention and Early Detection of Cervical Cancer.* https://www.cancer.org/cancer/cervical-cancer/detection-diagnosis-staging/cervical-cancer-screening-guidelines.html.

American Cancer Society. (2020). *Cervical cancer screening recommendations.* https://www.cancer.org/health-care-professionals/american-cancer-society-prevention-early-detection-guidelines/cervical-cancer-screening-guidelines.html.

American College of Obstetricians and Gynecologists. (2021). *Updated Cervical Cancer Screening Guidelines.* https://www.acog.org/clinical/clinical-guidance/practice-advisory/articles/2021/04/updated-cervical-cancer-screening-guidelines.

American Psychiatric Association. (2022). *Diagnostic and statistical manual of mental disorders* (5th ed., text rev.). https://doi.org/10.1176/appi.books.9780890425787.

American Society for Colposcopy and Cervical Pathology. (2019). *ASCCP risk-based management consensus guidelines. https://www.asccp.org/management-guidelines.*

Berek, J. (2019). *Berek & Novak's gynecology* (16th ed.). Philadelphia, PA: Lippincott Williams & Wilkins.

Campbell-Larkin, A. (2022). Breast cancer. 5 Minute Clinical Consult. https://5minuteconsult.com/

Centers for Disease Control and Prevention. (2022). *Folic acid recommendations.* https://www.cdc.gov/ncbddd/folicacid/recommendations.html

Centers for Disease Control and Prevention. (2020a). *Birth control: Information for parents of adolescents.*https://www.cdc.gov/healthyyouth/healthservices/infobriefs/birth_control_information.htm#:~:text=There%20are%20health%20services%20available,active%20by%2012th%20grade

Centers for Disease Control and Prevention. (2023). *HIV and cervical cancer.* https://npin.cdc.gov/publication/hiv-and-cervical-cancer#:~:text=HIV%20and%20cervical%20cancer%20are,women%20living%20with%20HIV%20globally.

Centers for Disease Control and Prevention. (2020b). Update to U.S. Medical Eligibility Criteria for Contraceptive Use, 2016: Updated Recommendations for the Use of Contraception Among

Women at High Risk for HIV Infection. *MMWR: Morbidity and Mortality Weekly Reports, 69*(14);405–410. https://www.cdc.gov/mmwr/volumes/69/wr/mm6914a3.htm?s_cid=mm6914a3_w

Centers for Disease Control and Prevention. (2016). U.S. Medical Eligibility Criteria for Contraceptive Use, 2016 Recommendations and Reports. *MMWR: Morbidity and Mortality Weekly Reports, 65*(3); 1–104. https://www.cdc.gov/mmwr/volumes/65/rr/pdfs/rr6503.pdf

Centers for Disease Control and Prevention. (2015). Use of 9-valent human papillomavirus (HPV) vaccine: Updated HPV vaccination recommendations of the Advisory Committee on Immunization Practices. *MMWR: Morbidity and Mortality Weekly Reports, 64*(RR-11), 300–304. http://www.cdc.gov/mmwr/pdf/wk/mm6411.pdf#page=12

Chalasani, P. (2022). Breast cancer. Medscape. https://emedicine.medscape.com/article/1947145-overview

Chen, L., & Berek, J. S. (2022a). Endometrial carcinoma: Clinical features, diagnosis, prognosis, and screening. UpToDate. https://www.uptodate.com/contents/endometrial-carcinoma-clinical-features-diagnosis-prognosis-and-screening?search=endometrial%20cancer&topicRef=16917&source=see_link

Chen, L. & Berek, J. S. (2022b). Overview of epithelial carcinoma of the ovary, fallopian tube, and peritoneum. UpToDate. https://www.uptodate.com/contents/overview-of-epithelial-carcinoma-of-the-ovary-fallopian-tube-and-peritoneum

Committee on Adolescence. (2012). Emergency contraception. *Pediatrics.* http:// pediatrics.aappublications.org/content/early/2012/11/21/peds.2012-2962

DeCherney, A. H., Nathan, L., Laufer, N., & Roman, A. S. (2019). *Current diagnosis & treatment obstetrics and gynecology* (12th ed.). New York, NY: McGraw-Hill Lange.

Dennis, M., & Jani, A. (2022). Polycystic ovarian syndrome (PCOS). 5 Minute Clinical Consult. https://5minuteconsult.com/.

Domino, F. J., & Baldor R. A. (2014). *The 5-minute clinical consult standard* (23rd ed.). Philadelphia, PA: Lippincott Williams & Wilkins.

Dong, A. (2021). Dysmenorrhea. Medscape. https://emedicine.medscape.com/article/253812-overview#a6

Edmunds, M. W., Mayhew, M. S., & Selter, S. M. (2014). *Pharmacology for the primary care provider* (4th ed.). St. Louis, MO: Elsevier Mosby.

Erlich, D. R. (2019). Anemia, iron deficiency. 5 Minute Clinical Consult. https://5minuteconsult.com/.

Fischbach, F., & Dunning, M. B. (2015). *A manual of laboratory and diagnostic tests* (9th ed.). Philadelphia, PA: Lippincott Williams & Wilkins.

Fredrickson, E., Cawse-Lucas, J. M., & Stewart, J. (2022). Pelvic inflammatory disease. 5 Minute Clinical Consult. https://5minuteconsult.com/

Gabbe, S. G. (2020). *Obstetrics: Normal and problem pregnancies* (8th ed.). Philadelphia, PA: Elsevier.

Gilbert, D. N., Chambers, H. F., Saag, M. S., Pavia, A. T., Boucher, H. W., Black, D., Freedman, D. O., Kim, K., & Schwartz, B. S. (2021). *The Sanford guide to antimicrobial therapy* 2021 (51st ed.). Sperryville, VA: Antimicrobial Therapy, Inc.

Girerd, P. H. (2022). Bacterial vaginosis. Medscape. https://emedicine.medscape.com/article/254342-overview#a6.

Goroll, A., & Mulley, A. (2020). *Primary care medicine: Office evaluation and management of the adult patient* (7th ed.). Philadelphia, PA: Lippincott Williams & Wilkins.

Grabosch, S. (2018). Ovarian cysts. Medscape. https://emedicine.medscape.com/article/255865-overview#a6.

Harris, J. R., & Lippman, M. E., Marrow, M., & Osborne, C. K. (2014). *Diseases of the breast* (5th ed). Philadelphia, PA: Wolters Kluwer.

Hatcher, R., Trussell, J., Nelson, A., Cates, W., & Kowal, D., & Policar, M. (2017). *Contraceptive technology* (21st ed. rev.). New York, NY: Contraceptive Technology Communications.

Johnson, B., & Bouchard, K. E. (2022). Vaginitis and vaginosis. 5 Minute Clinical Consult. https://5minuteconsult.com/

King, T. L., Brucker, M. C., Osborne, K., & Jevitt, C. M. (2019). *Varney's midwifery* (6th ed.). Burlington, MA: Jones & Bartlett Learning.

Koehler, S. (2022). Fibrocystic changes of the breast. 5 Minute Clinical Consult. https://5minuteconsult.com/

Krapf, J. M. (2022). Vulvovaginitis. Medscape. https://emedicine.medscape.com/article/2188931-overview#a7

Lauters. R. A., & Olsen, K. (2022). Abnormal (Dysfunctional) uterine bleeding. 5 Minute Clinical Consult. https://5minuteconsult.com/

Lawrence, K. V. (2022). Galactorrhea. 5 Minute Clinical Consult. https://5minuteconsult.com/

Mayeaux, E. J. (N. D.). Bartholin Gland Cyst and Abscess Treatment. 5 Minute Clinical Consult. https://5minuteconsult.com/

Mazin-Mohammed, L. (2022). Cervical malignancy. 5 Minute Clinical Consult. https://5minuteconsult.com/

Meites, E., Szilagyi, P. G., Chesson, H. W., Unger, E. R., Romero, J. R., & Markowitz, L. E. (2019). Human Papillomavirus Vaccination for Adults: Updated Recommendations of the Advisory Committee on Immunization Practices. *MMWR. Morbidity and Mortality Weekly Report, 68*(32), 698–702.https://doi.org/10.15585/mmwr.mm6832a3

Monk, N., & Gibbs, L. M. (2022). Menopause. 5 Minute Clinical Consult. https://5minuteconsult.com/ National Cancer Institute. Cancer stat facts: Cervical Cancer. National Cancer Institute. https://seer.cancer.gov/statfacts/html/cervix.html

Nayar, R., & Wilbur, D. C. (2015). The Pap test and Bethesda 2014. *Acta Cytologica, 59,* 121–132.

Nayar, R., & Wilbur, D. C. (2015). *The Bethesda system for reporting cervical cytology: Definitions, criteria, and explanatory notes.* (3rd ed.). New York, NY: Springer.

Office of Disease Prevention & Health Promotion. (2022). *Healthy people 2030.* Washington, DC: US. Department of Health & Human Services. www.health.gov.

Patel, P., Lawrence, K. V. & Tahira, A. (2022). Galactorrhea. 5 Minute Clinical Consult. https://5minuteconsult.com/

Perkins, R. B., Guido, R. S., Castle, P. E., Chelmow, D., Einstein, M. H., Garcia, F., Huh, W. K., Kim, J. J., Moscicki, A. B., Nayar, R., Saraiya, M., Sawaya, G. F., Wentzensen, N., Schiffman, M., & 2019 ASCCP Risk-Based Management Consensus Guidelines Committee (2020). 2019 ASCCP Risk-Based Management Consensus Guidelines for Abnormal Cervical Cancer Screening Tests and Cancer Precursors. Journal of lower genital tract disease, 24(2), 102–131. https://doi.org/10.1097/LGT.0000000000000525

Pickering, L. K., Baker, C. J., Kimberlin, D. W., & Long, S. S. (2012). *Red Book: 2012 report of the committee on infectious diseases* (29th ed.). Elk Grove, IL: American Academy of Pediatrics.

Plaxe, S. C. & Mundt, A. J. (2022). Overview of endometrial carcinoma. *UpToDate.* https://www.uptodate.com/contents/overview-of-endometrial-carcinoma?search=endometrial%20cancer&source=search_result&selectedTitle=1~150&usage_type=default&display_rank=1#H495849057

Quinn, A. (2022). Bartholin Gland Diseases. Medscape. https://emedicine.medscape.com/article/777112-overview#a6

Rowan, S. P., Someshwar, J., & Murray, P. (2012). Contraception for primary care providers. *Adolescent Medicine, 23,* 95–110.

Saslow, D., Solomon, D., Lawson, H. W., Killackey, M., Kulasingam, S. L., Cain, J., . . . Myers, E. R. (2012). American Cancer Society, American Society for Colposcopy and Cervical Pathology, and American Society for Clinical Pathology screening guidelines for the prevention and early detection of cervical cancer. *CA: Cancer Journal for Clinicians, 62*(3), 147–172.

Steiner, M., Haskett, R. F., & Carroll, B. J. (1980). Premenstrual tension syndrome: The development of research diagnostic criteria and new rating scales. *Acta Psychiatrica Scandinavica, 62*(2), 177–190. https://doi.org/10.1111/j.1600-0447.1980.tb00605.x

U. S. Preventive Services Task Force. (2021). *USPSTF A&B Recommendations.* https://www.uspreventiveservicestaskforce.org/uspstf/recommendation-topics/uspstf-a-and-b-recommendations.

U.S. Preventive Services Task Force. (2018). *Cervical cancer: Screening.* https://www.uspreventiveservicestaskforce.org/uspstf/recommendation/cervical-cancer-screening.

U.S. Preventive Services Task Force. (2016). *Breast cancer: Screening.* https://www.uspreventiveservicestaskforce.org/uspstf/recommendation/breast-cancer-screening

U.S. Preventive Services Task Force, Curry, S. J., Krist, A. H., Owens, D. K., Barry, M. J., Caughey, A. B., Davidson, K. W., Doubeni, C. A., Epling, J. W., Jr, Kemper, A. R., Kubik, M., Landefeld, C. S., Mangione, C. M., Phipps, M. G., Silverstein, M., Simon, M. A., Tseng, C. W., & Wong, J. B. (2018a). Screening for Cervical Cancer: US Preventive Services Task Force Recommendation Statement. *Journal of the American Medical Association, 320*(7), 674–686.

U.S. Preventive Services Task Force. (2018b). *Cervical cancer: Screening.* https://www.uspreventiveservicestaskforce.org/uspstf/recommendation/cervical-cancer-screening.https://doi.org/10.1001/jama.2018.10897

Sepilian, V. P. (2022). Ectopic pregnancy. Medscape. https://emedicine.medscape.com/article/2041923-overview#a4

Singh, S. (2022). Uterine myomas. 5 Minute Clinical Consult. https://5minuteconsult.com/

Tough-DeSapri, K. A. (2019). Amenorrhea. Medscape. https://emedicine.medscape.com/article/252928-overview?icd=ssl_login_success_221012#a5

Tustison, K. S., Dupper, M. & Ballou, K. A. (2022). Endometriosis. 5 Minute Clinical Consult. https://5minuteconsult.com/

Viswanathan, M., Treiman, K. A., Kish-Doto, J., Middleton, J. C., Coker-Schwimmer, E. J., & Nicholson, W. K. (2017). Folic Acid Supplementation for the Prevention of Neural Tube Defects: An Updated Evidence Report and Systematic Review for the US Preventive Services Task Force. *Journal of the American Medical Association, 317*(2), 190–203. https://doi.org/10.1001/jama.2016.19193

Wertz. M. C. (2019). Dysmenorrhea. 5 Minute Clinical Consult. https://5minuteconsult.com/

Woo, T. M., Wynne, A. L., & Wynne, A. L. (2020). *Pharmacotherapeutics for advanced practice nurse prescribers* (5th ed). Philadelphia, PA: F. A. Davis Co.

Workowski, K. A., Bachmann, L. H., Chan, P. A., Johnston, C. M., Muzny, C. A., Park, I., Reno, H., Zenilman, J. M., & Bolan, G. A. (2021). Sexually transmitted infections treatment guidelines, 2021. *MMWR:: Morbidity and Mortality Weekly Report.* Recommendations and reports, *70*(4), 1–187.https://doi.org/10.15585/mmwr.rr7004a1

Yonkers, A. Y., & Casper, R. F. (2022) Epidemiology and pathogenesis of premenstrual syndrome and premenstrual dysphoric disorder. UpToDate. https://www.uptodate.com/contents/overview-of-endometrial-carcinoma?search=endometrial%20cancer&source=search_result&selectedTitle=1~150&usage_type=default&display_rank=1#H495849057

CHAPTER 12

MALE REPRODUCTIVE SYSTEM DISORDERS

Barbara Siebert, DNP, CRNP, FNP-BC, CNE

General Approach

DESCRIPTION

- Many complaints of the male genitourinary system are of a sensitive nature, and men are less inclined to initiate discussion or seek help for them. The family nurse practitioner should take an active role in screening for such problems with an approach that is open and nonjudgmental.
- General areas for screening: sexuality, safer sex practices, high-risk behaviors
- General history questions: past infections (sexually transmitted diseases [STDs], urinary tract infections [UTIs], prostatitis), normal voiding patterns; current symptoms in more detail
- Exam: Assessment of the male genitalia should be part of the screening/annual physical exam, even if there are no complaints, because many male genitourinary problems are asymptomatic.

RED FLAGS

- *Testicular torsion:* Rule out with any complaint of scrotal pain: acute onset of severe scrotal pain in boys or men of any age (peak ages 12 to 18), requires treatment within 4 to 12 hours surgically to preserve fertility and prevent loss of the testicle.
- *Paraphimosis:* Inability of the retracted foreskin to be reduced over the glans, can be a surgical emergency.
- *Testicular mass:* Any mass in the testicles or attached to the testicles is cancer until proven otherwise.
- *Right-sided varicoceles:* rare; associated with obstruction of the right spermatic vein and retroperitoneal neoplasms

- *Recurrent UTIs* in men: Evaluate for prostatitis.
- *Prostatic massage:* Avoid performing until acute prostatitis is excluded or treatment initiated to prevent hematogenous spread of infection.
- *Over-the-counter (OTC) medications:* Anticholinergics, parasympatholytics, and sympathomimetics precipitate or worsen urinary conditions such as benign prostatic hyperplasia; antidepressants can affect full sexual function.

Contraception

CONDOMS

- A method of pregnancy prevention used by boys and men to prevent the spillage of semen into the vaginal vault. A latex or polyurethane sheath applied before sexual intercourse/penetration that fits snugly over the entire length of the penis, with a mildly constricting ring at the base to prevent slipping off. After ejaculation, the condom holds ejaculated semen that is discarded with the condom.
- Condoms reduce the risk of exposure to STDs in man-to-woman or man-to-man contact.
- Approximately 21% of men use condoms as a contraceptive; more commonly used for prevention of STD transmission or exposure
- Effectiveness for contraception averages 88% typically, up to 97% if used properly
- Factors contributing to unsuccessful use and resultant pregnancy
    - Allergy to latex or rubber
    - Failure to use during genital foreplay when pre-ejaculate can be introduced into or near the vagina
    - Breakage or slippage of the condom during intercourse
    - Limited education about reproduction or contraception; limited access to medical care
    - Dissatisfaction with method and subsequent failure to use
- Instruction on Use
    - Apply to penis when in the erect state before contact with the partner's genitals because pre-ejaculate discharge near or in the vagina can contain semen adequate for fertilization.
    - Roll the condom to the base of the penis, leaving a small space at the tip to allow for collection of ejaculate, and decrease pressure on the condom (decreased risk of breakage).

 - ◊ Use only water-based lubricants if needed. Spermicidal cream or jelly on the penis before application of the condom and penetration or used intravaginally enhances effectiveness and reduces pregnancy risk. Do not use the same condom more than once.

- ♦ Sterilization
  - ◊ A surgical method of eliminating the transport of semen in ejaculate to prevent pregnancy, which, although possibly reversible, should be considered permanent
  - ◊ An outpatient surgical procedure performed via a scrotal incision that severs and seals the vas deferens; does not require general anesthesia
  - ◊ The most popular method of sterilization in the United States
  - ◊ Approximately 12% of men are surgically sterilized via vasectomy.
  - ◊ Failure rate is 0.1% in the first year postoperatively.
  - ◊ Sperm counts are obtained at post-procedure follow-up to confirm success of the procedure before resuming sexual intercourse.
  - ◊ Complications include potential infection and failure of sterilization.

Disorders of the Prostate Gland

BENIGN PROSTATIC HYPERPLASIA (BPH)

Description

- ♦ Nonmalignant generalized enlargement of the periurethral prostate gland related to a variety of triggers for cell growth. Believed to be under endocrine control. Enlargement mechanically obstructs urination by compressing the urethra.

Etiology

- ♦ Cause unknown; universally seen in aging
- ♦ Hyperplasia of gland due to an abnormal increase in the number of cells in prostate tissue
- ♦ Hormonal changes: Accumulation of dihydrotestosterone (DHT) and increased estrogen in aging men seem to interact in a way that causes cell proliferation.

Incidence and Demographics

- Affects approximately 8% of men aged 31 to 40; 50% of men aged 50 to 60; and nearly 90% of men more than 80 years old.
- Initially asymptomatic for men in their 40s; many develop urinary symptoms by age 60.

Risk Factors

- Increased age
- First-degree relative with BPH
- Black/African descent
- History of STDs

Prevention and Screening

- No prevention other than reducing risk factors (safer sex, change in diet)
- Early screening starting in the 40s (patient history, digital rectal exam) may allow for earlier treatment, slowing the progression of hyperplasia and possibly reduction of symptoms.

Assessment

History

- General: fever, malaise, back pain, hematuria, pain with voiding indicate infection.
- Obstructive symptoms: difficulty starting/stopping stream, hesitancy, dribbling, weakening force/size of stream, sensation of full bladder after voiding, retention.
- Irritative symptoms: urgency, frequency, nocturia, urge incontinence, dysuria
- American Urological Association (AUA) Symptom Index for Benign Prostatic Hyperplasia (Barry et al., 2017)
- 35-point scale to assess symptom severity: incomplete emptying, frequency, intermittency, urgency, weak stream, straining, nocturia
- Seven categories rated from 0 to 35 points: 0–7 = mild; 8–19 = moderate; 20–35 = severe
- The higher the points, the more severe the symptoms

- Should be completed for all patients before therapy begins
- Medications, especially cold/sinus medications: Anticholinergics impair bladder contractility, and sympathomimetics increase outflow resistance and worsen symptoms.
- Date of last digital rectal exam (DRE), prostate-specific antigen (PSA), and results
- Past Medical History (PMH): Explore for other conditions that may be associated with these symptoms: surgery, urethral instrumentation or trauma, history of type 2 diabetes, neuromuscular disease (multiple sclerosis), sexual dysfunction, psychogenic disorder, cardiovascular disease, and hypercalcemia.

Physical Exam

- Digital rectal exam (DRE): intact anal sphincter tone; prostate should be nontender, firm, smooth, and rubbery and measure 4 × 3 × 2 cm. Blunting or obliteration of the midline median sulcus indicates BPH. Finding an enlarged prostate does not always correlate with symptoms.
- Enlargement may be symmetric, nodular, or asymmetric. Any nodules should be considered possibly malignant and fully evaluated; an indurated prostate requires cancer evaluation.
- Abdomen: with urinary retention, possible distended bladder on percussion or palpation; costovertebral angle tenderness (CVAT) if renal sequelae
- Neurologic: screening exam to note nonprostate etiology for symptoms of neurogenic or myogenic etiology, detrusor muscle impairment, compression of nerves

Diagnostic Studies

- Urinalysis should be negative for hematuria, glycosuria, or infection; their presence indicates secondary UTI or another problem.
- Catheterization for a post-void residual (PVR) illustrates volume remaining in the bladder after the patient's usual void.
- Serum blood urea nitrogen (BUN) and creatinine are helpful in assessing renal function; results may be abnormal if urinary retention or obstruction has affected the upper urinary tract, as well as with underlying renal disease.
- Prostate-specific antigen (PSA) to distinguish cause (BPH or prostate cancer) of large gland; use of this test is *controversial* if the patient is asymptomatic and results are 4 to 10 ng/mL. Results higher than 10 ng/mL may be associated with cancer but are not necessarily correlated. PSA increases as the prostate gland enlarges, but do not

assume increases are due only to prostate gland enlargement. Acute urinary retention, prostatitis, urinary tract instrumentation, or prostatic infarction may elevate the PSA. *Increased levels may also be noted 1 to 24 hours post-DRE, so avoid lab work during this time period.*

- Advanced workup includes urinary flowmetry studies (flow rate), post-void residual (PVR) urine, urodynamic studies, transrectal ultrasound, intravenous pyelogram (IVP), and abdominal ultrasound.

Differential Diagnosis

Medical

- Diseases associated with increased urination (chronic heart failure [CHF])
- Type 2 diabetes mellitus

Obstructive

- Prostate cancer
- Urethral strictures or valves
- Bladder neck contracture (usually secondary to prostate surgery)
- Inability of bladder neck or external sphincter to relax appropriately during voiding

Infectious or Inflammatory

- Prostatitis
- Cystitis
- Urethritis

Neurologic

- Spinal cord injury
- Stroke
- Parkinson's disease
- Multiple sclerosis

Pharmacologic

- Diuretics
- Sympathomimetics (cold medication, decongestants, and antihistamines)
- Anticholinergics

Management

Nonpharmacologic Treatment

- The AUA recommends "watchful waiting" for:
  - monitoring of symptoms associated with mild BPH
  - without the presence of bothersome lower urinary tract symptoms or development of serious complications (AUA scores 7 and less)
- Avoid bladder irritants such as coffee, alcohol, decongestants, antihistamines, anticholinergics, and tricyclic antidepressants.
- Encourage frequent voiding to keep bladder volume low.
- Monitor voiding; watch for signs of retention.
- Limit intake of fluids in the evening; avoid large quantities over a short time.
- Eliminate prescription and OTC medications that may worsen symptoms.
- In persons with moderate to severe symptom presentation (8 points and above on AUA scale):
  - First-line medical management with alpha-adrenergic antagonists is more effective than other methods alone.
  - Use 5-alpha-reductase inhibitors to reduce prostatic volume if prostatic enlargement is present.
  - Combination therapy using alpha-adrenergic antagonists and 5-alpha-reductase inhibitors is superior to monotherapy when used for very large prostates.

Adverse Effects

- Alpha-adrenergic antagonists can cause orthostatic hypotension.

Phytotherapy

- Saw palmetto berry, bark of *Pygeum africanum*, roots of *Echinacea purpurea, Hypoxis rooperi*, pollen extract, and leaves of trembling poplar—all still being researched. Saw palmetto may provide mild improvement of peak flow rates and appears to work by blocking 5-alpha-reductase; however, use of saw palmetto remains debatable

Surgical Options

- For patients with severe symptoms, large PVR, upper UTIs, or failure of medical therapy
- Transurethral resection of the prostate (TURP) is gold standard
- Transurethral incision of the prostate (TUIP)
- Open prostatectomy

Minimally Invasive Therapy

- Nonsurgical procedures to reduce the size of the prostate include the use of heat via transurethral needle ablation (TUNA) and transurethral microwave therapy (TUMT), transurethral laser ablation using Holmium laser ablation of the tissue (TULA), transurethral laser resection/enucleation, the use of transurethral electrovaporization of the prostate (TEVP), fiber optics/laser technology, high-intensity focused ultrasound, transurethral balloon dilation of the prostate, and UroLume intraprostatic stent placement.

Pharmacologic Treatment

- For mild to moderate symptoms, see Table 12–1 for primary drugs.
- Less commonly used drugs: gonadotropin-releasing hormone (GnRH) agonists, progestational anti-androgens, flutamide (Eulexin), and testolactone (Teslac)
- Saw palmetto (160 mg twice a day) is an alternative herbal therapy; decreases testosterone uptake to decrease size of gland
- Tolterodine (Detrol) to decrease bladder contractions

TABLE 12–1. PHARMACOLOGIC MANAGEMENT OF BPH

DRUGS	DOSAGE	COMMENT
A1-ADRENERGIC BLOCKERS		
Terazosin (Hytrin)	Progressive dosing over 1 month: 1 mg × 3 days 2 mg × 11 days 5 mg × 7 days 10 mg daily	Relaxes smooth muscle around urethra Drug of choice for smaller prostate and acute irritation symptoms Decreases smooth muscle tone in bladder neck and prostate Improvement is dose dependent; takes 4–6 weeks for maximal therapeutic effect In nonhypertensive patient may cause postural hypotension, dizziness, palpitations, or syncope May be beneficial for those with concomitant BPH and hypertension; can reduce number of medications needed
Doxazosin (Cardura)	1 mg once a day h.s., may double every 1–2 weeks to max of 8 mg/day	Like terazosin
Tamsulosin	0.4 mg once a day, 30 min.	Selective; may produce fewer side effects; no
HCL (Flomax)	Before meal at same Time each day, may increase to 0.8 mg after 2–4 weeks	Cardiovascular side effects; postural hypotension not common May cause dizziness, abnormal ejaculation, rhinitis Generally, more expensive
Alfuzosin (Uroxatral)	10 mg/day orally	Selective; may produce fewer side effects Generally, more expensive
5A-REDUCTASE INHIBITOR		
Finasteride titration (Proscar)	5 mg once a day, no needed	Blocks conversion of testosterone to DHT; gland shrinks Drug of choice for large prostate and patients with contraindications or who have failed treatment with alpha-adrenergic medication Decreased hormonal (androgen) effect on prostate reduces prostate size and symptoms, resulting in increased peak urinary flow rate

Continued

TABLE 12–1. (CONTINUED)

DRUGS	DOSAGE	COMMENT
		Improvement not noted for up to 6–12 months; must be used indefinitely to sustain effect Decreased libido and ejaculate volume, erectile dysfunction Decreased PSA by up to 50%, blocking effectiveness of PSA as screening tool for CA; screen for cancer with DRE and PSA before initiating treatment
Dutasteride (Avodart)	0.5 mg/day orally	Like finasteride

How Long to Treat

- Dependent upon type and severity of symptoms and impact on daily functioning
- Medications may be prescribed until symptoms are no longer manageable and surgery considered

Special Considerations

- In the presence of concomitant diseases (diabetes mellitus; cardiovascular or neurological disease), particularly with aging of the patient, care should be coordinated with regard to medications, ability for self-care, and recommendations for procedural or surgical treatment.

When to Consult, Refer, Hospitalize

- Referral to a urologist is indicated for AUA index score of 8 or more, symptoms not responsive to medications, recurrent infections (epididymitis, repeat UTIs), elevated PSA, obstruction or acute urinary retention, bladder calculi, recurrent hematuria, renal disease, or suspicion of malignancy.

Follow-Up

- Annual evaluation, including DRE and PSA as indicated for asymptomatic or minor symptoms

- Patients who opt for the "watchful waiting" strategy should be followed every 3 to 12 months.
- Patients on medications should be seen every 2 to 4 weeks until symptoms stabilize, and then every 6 months.
- Patients receiving surgical or procedural treatments are followed by the treating urologist/surgeon.

Expected Course

- May have prolonged course of mild or stable symptoms before advancing to stage of needing nonpharmacological treatment

Complications

- Potentially serious sequelae: UTI, obstructive uropathy, urine retention, renal disease

PROSTATITIS

Description

- An inflammation and/or infection of the prostate gland traditionally categorized as acute bacterial, chronic bacterial, nonbacterial, or prostatodynia
- National Institutes of Health (NIH) prostatitis classification: (Litwin et al, 1999)
  - NIH class I: Acute bacterial prostatitis
- Febrile illness with perineal pain, dysuria, and obstructive symptoms
  - NIH class II: Chronic bacterial prostatitis
- Recurrent infection with pain and voiding disturbances
  - NIH class III: Chronic nonbacterial prostatitis/chronic pelvic pain syndrome
- NIH class IIIa: Inflammatory: significant inflammatory cells in prostatic secretions, post-prostatic massage urine, or semen
- NIH class IIIb: Noninflammatory: insignificant number of inflammatory cells
  - NIH class IV: Asymptomatic inflammatory prostatitis
- Incidental finding during prostate biopsy for infertility, cancer workup

Etiology

- Various causes: allergic, inflammatory, infectious, related to instrumentation, UTIs, STDs, prostatic abscess or calculi
- Acute infectious causes: generally gram-negative bacilli, primarily *E. coli*; may also be *Enterobacter, Klebsiella, Proteus mirabilis, Pseudomonas aeruginosa, Staphylococcus aureus, Streptococcus faecalis, Serratia, Neisseria gonorrhoeae, Ureaplasma, Trichomonas vaginalis, Chlamydia trachomatis,* and *Gardnerella vaginalis*
- Nonbacterial prostatitis causes: unknown; leading theory suggests nonrelaxation (spasm) of the internal urinary sphincter and pelvic floor striated muscles leading to increased prostatic urethral pressure and intra-prostatic urinary reflux
- Infectious causes usually occur by direct invasion from the urethra, typically a UTI.
- Men (35 years or younger) have an increased likelihood that the infectious organism is an STD (*C. trachomatis* or *N. gonorrhoeae*).

Incidence and Demographics

- 2 million cases annually in the United States
- Chronic bacterial primarily in men ages 50 and older
- All others primarily in sexually active men ages 30 to 50
- Nonbacterial: most common type, 8x greater than bacterial type, with an increased prevalence in men under 50 years old
- Acute bacterial: least common type, occurs in men across the lifespan
- Bacterial prostatitis occurs more frequently in patients with HIV.
- Prostatodynia most commonly affects ages 22 to 56.

Risk Factors

- History of or exposure to STDs (multiple sexual partners, men having sex with men, or recent new partner)
- Age 50 and over: more common cause from recurrent UTI or prostatic calculi
- Prostate biopsy, TURP, urethral dilatation, cystoscopy, urethral stricture, chronic indwelling catheter
- Instrumentation of urinary tract

- Sexual abstinence
- Trauma (e.g., bicycle, horseback riding, falls affecting the sacrum)
- Abscess elsewhere in the body
- Recurrent UTIs
- May be associated with autoimmune or neuromuscular problems, stress, allergic conditions

Prevention and Screening

- Avoidance of unsafe sexual practices decreases exposure to STDs
- Frequent voiding
- Screen with good history and DRE

Assessment

- See Table 12–2.

History

- All presentations have common symptoms of dysuria related to compression of the urethra by the inflamed prostate. All are associated with some degree of pain that is variable and may be associated with intercourse, ejaculation, and defecation.
- Acute bacterial prostatitis: characterized by its acute onset with systemic symptoms and pattern of pain and dysuria including low back pain, fever, chills, malaise, prostatodynia, perineal pain, obstructive voiding symptoms, frequency, urgency, dysuria, or nocturia
- Chronic bacterial prostatitis: characterized by remissions and exacerbations with recurrent UTIs; prostatodynia, perineal pain, dysuria, irritative voiding, lower abdominal pain, low back, scrotal and/or penile pain, pain on ejaculation, hematospermia
- Current medications (e.g., anticholinergics), other medical illness, and sexual history to assess risk of infection

TABLE 12–2.
CLINICAL PRESENTATION OF PROSTATITIS

SYMPTOMS		PHYSICAL FINDINGS
Acute	Chills, fever, malaise	Fever
Bacterial	Dysuria, urgency, burning, frequency Hematuria Pain: pelvis, perineum, lower back, scrotum, with defecation, with intercourse	Prostate very tender, boggy, warm, swollen, firm, or irregular ± urethral discharge
Chronic bacterial	± low-grade fever, dysuria, hesitancy, hematuria, hematospermia; Pain mild: perineum, scrotal, abdominal, with ejaculation	No systemic findings; prostate may be normal, indurated, mildly tender, boggy, or irregular ± prostatic stones; scrotum ± edema, erythema, and tenderness
Nonbacterial	No fever; gradual onset: dysuria, frequency, urgency; pain mild: perineum, with ejaculation; decreased libido or impotence	Urethral discharge common; prostate enlarged, boggy, and tender
Prostatodynia	No fever; dysuria, hesitancy, decreased flow, post-void dribbling; pain: perineum, back, testicle(s)	None

Physical Exam

- Evaluate for fever; abdominal exam to check for tenderness or distended bladder; exam genitalia and scrotum, and for urethral discharge, CVA tenderness to assess kidneys, and rectal exam.
- *Warning regarding prostate examinations.* Due to exquisite tenderness of the prostate gland and the risk of spreading bacterial infection into the bloodstream, examination of the prostate should be done very gently or avoided when acute prostatitis is suspected until after treatment has been initiated. Massage of the prostate is contraindicated when acute bacterial infection is suspected because this action can spread infection systemically.
- In the non-acute patient, prostatic massage *is* indicated to carry out the sequential urinalysis and culture for evaluation of prostatic secretions and as part of therapeutic treatment.

Diagnostic Studies

- Suspected acute prostatitis: urinalysis, urine and blood cultures, urine Gram stain, complete blood count (CBC) with differential
- Suspected chronic bacterial prostatitis or nonbacterial prostatitis: traditional sequential urinalysis and culture test for voided bladder (VB) specimens and expressed prostatic secretions (EPS; see Table 12–3)
- Two-sample method:
  1. Clean catch, midstream urine specimen
  2. Urine specimen after prostatic massage
- Culture any penile discharge for STDs; wet mount of EPS
- Blood cultures may be ordered for acute prostatitis.
- Chronic prostatitis is additionally evaluated with CBC, serum BUN, and creatinine, and possible IVP and/or transrectal ultrasound.
- In older adults, bladder cancer screening via urine cytology is indicated.
- PSA will be elevated with acute prostatitis; do not order PSA until at least 1 month after prostatitis is treated.
- Urodynamic testing may be helpful in evaluating suspected prostatodynia.

Differential Diagnosis

- Any of the four types of prostatitis
- Cystitis (bacterial, interstitial), epididymitis, urethritis
- Pyelonephritis

TABLE 12–3.
SEQUENTIAL LABORATORY TESTS IN PROSTATITIS (FRACTIONAL URINE EXAM)

	SPECIMEN (CULTURE EACH SAMPLE ALSO)	LOCATION
VB1	First 10 mL urine	Urine from urethra
VB2	Next 200 mL discarded; then midstream urine	Urine from bladder
EPS	Urethral secretions *after* prostatic massage	Prostatic fluid
VB3	First 10 mL urine after prostatic massage	Prostatic fluid and urine from bladder

- Malignancy
- Obstructive calculus
- Foreign body
- Acute urinary retention
- Urethral stricture
- BPH
- Renal colic

Management

Nonpharmacologic Treatment

- Avoidance of known irritants: caffeine, alcohol, OTC antihistamines or decongestants
- Avoidance of sex during first 2 or more weeks of acute illness
- Increased frequency of ejaculation in nonacute states
- Hydration maintenance (force fluids)
- Rest and sitz baths 20 minutes 2 to 3 times a day for pain as needed

Pharmacologic Treatment

- The prostate gland is difficult to penetrate with antibiotics; therefore, first-line treatment with antibiotic therapy for acute prostatitis is required for a minimum of 30 days (see Table 12–4).
- Men over age 35 are more likely to be infected with *C. trachomatis* or *N. gonorrhoeae,* requiring antibiotics according to the current recommended choices of the health department or Centers for Disease Control and Prevention (CDC, 2021; https://www.cdc.gov/std/treatment-guidelines/default.htm).
- NSAIDs are recommended for anti-inflammatory effects as well as pain relief.
- Stool softeners as needed

TABLE 12–4.
DIAGNOSIS AND MANAGEMENT OF PROSTATITIS

MICROSCOPIC	URINE CULTURES	DIAGNOSIS	TREATMENT	DURATION (VARIABLE RECOMMENDATIONS)
+WBC, bacteria in VB1, few in other specimens	# bacteria VB1 > VB2 or VB3	Urethritis	Ceftriaxone 125 mg IM × 1 or cefixime 400 mg orally × 1 or ciprofloxacin 500 mg orally × 1 PLUS azithromycin 1 g orally × 1 or doxycycline 100 mg twice a day × 1	Single-dose therapy
+WBC/RBC, bacteria in VB2, possibly VB1	# bacteria VB2 > VB1 or VB3	Cystitis	Quinolone once or twice a day or Trimethoprim-sulfamethoxazole DS (TMP/SMX) 1 tablet orally twice a day	3–7 days if uncomplicated
+WBC, bacteria in all specimens	# bacteria EPS, VB3 > VB1 or VB2	Acute prostatitis	Fluoroquinolone: ciprofloxacin 500 mg orally every 12h or levofloxacin 500 mg orally once a day	3–4 weeks
			Trimethoprim-sulfamethoxazole DS 160/800 mg (TMP/SMX) 1 tablet orally twice a day	3–4 weeks
+WBC, bacteria in EPS and VB3 only	Little/no growth in VB1 or VB2	Chronic bacterial prostatitis	First-line therapy: Fluoroquinolone: levofloxacin 750 mg orally once a day or ciprofloxacin 500 mg orally twice a day	4–12 weeks
			Second-line therapy: Organism-specific: *Chlamydia*: doxycycline 100 mg orally twice a day or azithromycin 500 mg orally daily or clarithromycin 500 mg orally daily	4–12 weeks
			Ureaplasma: tetracycline 500 mg orally twice a day	7–14 days
			Trichomonas: metronidazole (Flagyl) 2.0 g × 1 dose or 500 mg orally twice a day	7 days
+WBC in EPS, VB3 Nonbacterial organisms in EPS or VB3	No bacterial growth	Chronic nonbacterial prostatitis	No universally effective treatment; antibiotic therapy not proven to be effective	
No WBC, bacteria, or other organisms in any specimen	No bacterial growth	Prostatodynia	Nonsteroidal anti-inflammatory drugs (NSAIDs) and supportive treatments	

Special Considerations

- Patients may have concomitant urinary symptoms and infection; recurrent UTI diagnosis warrants chronic prostatitis in the differential.
- Adults age 50 years or older: Increased incidence of concomitant disease in the genitourinary (GU) system indicates greater need for advanced testing and screening for BPH, prostate or bladder cancer, and UTI.

When to Consult, Refer, Hospitalize

- Hospitalization is indicated for all patients who have systemic involvement for IV antibiotics and treatment of possible septicemia.
- Refer to a urologist if no improvement is noted within 48 hours of treatment.
- Refer patients age 50 years or older who are symptomatic or have recurrent prostatitis or acute bacterial prostatitis to a urologist, as BPH may be a compounding problem.

Follow-Up

- *Acute prostatitis*: Revaluation is done within 48 to 72 hours, then 2 to 4 weeks later (1 month after completion of treatment) for urinalysis; urine and prostatic secretion cultures 30 days after initiating treatment to monitor treatment effectiveness and assess for signs of complications.
- *Chronic bacterial prostatitis*: Check urinalysis, culture, and sensitivity every 30 days. Sequential urine tests and EPS should be repeated 4 to 6 weeks after initiation of therapy.
- Follow-up may be sooner as indicated based on the patient's responsiveness to treatment and changes in symptoms.

Expected Course

- Prostatitis requires long-term antibiotic therapy for optimal outcomes. Non-chronic prostatitis may be resolved within 6 weeks; however, chronic prostatitis requires treatment for up to 6 months. In chronic cases, treatment suppresses but does not eradicate the offending organism, hence the recurrence of symptoms.

Complications

- Potential for serious sequelae, including development of prostatic abscess, stones, ascending UTIs, epididymitis, urinary retention, renal infection, bacteremia, progressive STD complications

PROSTATE CANCER

Description

- Malignant neoplasm of the prostate gland

Etiology

- Unknown cause
- 95% develop in acinar glands of prostate (acinar adenocarcinoma)
- Two types:
  - Poorly differentiated and fast-growing
  - Androgen-dependent, well-differentiated, and slow-growing
  - Metastasizes primarily to bone

Incidence and Demographics

- Most common cancer in men; second most common cause of cancer deaths in men
- Average age at diagnosis is 71 years.
- About 80% of all clinically diagnosed cases of prostate cancer are men aged 65 years or older.
- In the United States, 200 cases/100,000 men/year
- There is a 40% greater incidence in Black men, who are diagnosed with prostate cancer at later stages and die of the disease at higher rates than White men.

Risk Factors

- Age 50 or older, exposure to chemical carcinogens, history of STDs, baseline PSA above median for age group

- Family history of carcinoma of the prostate; two times increase in risk with first-degree relative affected younger than 50 years of age
- Black men at greatest risk

Prevention and Screening

- Avoid exposure to chemical carcinogens; practice safer sex to prevent STDs.
- U.S. Preventive Services Task Force (USPSTF, 2018) current recommendations for prostate cancer screening:
- Screening for prostate cancer currently assigned a grade D recommendation (see Table 12–5).
- Evidence does not support screening for prostate cancer using the PSA test and DRE; risks of morbidity and mortality outweigh survival benefits.

Assessment

History

- Early disease is asymptomatic.
- With enlargement, frequency, nocturia, and dribbling develop (see Benign Prostatic Hyperplasia [BPH]).
- Symptoms of urethral obstruction and bone pain occur with advanced metastatic stage.
- Constitutional symptoms: anorexia, weight loss, fatigue, weakness, back pain

Physical Exam

- If symptomatic, perform a DRE to assess for prostatic masses/firmness.
- Depending on the stage of the cancer, the prostate on DRE may be normal on the palpable lateral and posterior portion of the gland, or may be asymmetrical, generally firmer with hard induration, localized nodules, and obliterated median sulcus.
- Lower-extremity edema may develop due to lymph node metastases and pathologic fractures.

TABLE 12–5.
USPSTF GRADE DEFINITIONS

GRADE	DEFINITION	SUGGESTDONS FOR PRACTICE
A	The USPSTF recommends the service. There is high certainty that the net benefit is substantial.	Offer or provide this service.
B	The USPSTF recommends the service. There is high certainty that the net benefit is moderate or there is moderate certainty that the net benefit is moderate to substantial.	Offer or provide this service.
C	The USPSTF recommends selectively offering or providing this service to individual patients, based on professional judgment and patient preferences. There is at least moderate certainty that the net benefit is small.	Offer or provide this service for select patients, depending on individual circumstances.
D	The USPSTF recommends *against* the service. There is moderate or high certainty that the service has no net benefit or that the harms outweigh the benefits.	Discourage the use of this service.
I Statement	The USPSTF concludes that current evidence is insufficient to assess the balance of benefits and harms of the service. Evidence is lacking, of poor quality, or conflicting, and the balance between benefits and harms cannot be determined.	Read the clinical considerations section of USPSTF Recommendation Statement. If the service is offered, patients should understand the uncertainty about the balance between benefits and harms.

U.S. Preventive Services Task Force. (2018). *Prostate cancer: Screening*. https://www.uspreventiveservicestaskforce.org/uspstf/recommendation/prostate-cancer-screening

Diagnostic Studies

- PSA levels above 4 ng/mL indicate possible cancer; do not always correlate with DRE. Increased levels may be noted 1 to 24 hours post-DRE, so avoid lab work during this time period if possible.
- Ejaculation may alter total and free PSA levels. Men should abstain from sex for 24 hours before serum PSA levels being drawn.
- Prostatitis and BPH can cause an increase in PSA levels.

- PSA is discredited as a screening test because PSA is normal in 40% of patients with cancer.
- CBC, urinalysis, urine culture, and sensitivity for workup of urinary symptoms
- Serum alkaline phosphatase increased with late-stage metastasis to bone
- Ultrasound with guided prostate biopsy is indicated with abnormal DRE and/or increase in PSA; bone scan.

Differential Diagnosis

- BPH
- Prostatitis
- Prostatic or bladder stones
- Bladder cancer

Management

- Treatment choice is based on the stage of the disease and age of the patient.

Nonpharmacologic Treatment

- Asymptomatic patients with life expectancy less than 10 years: watchful waiting is an option.
- Treatment options if localized include watchful waiting, radical prostatectomy, and radiation therapy.
- Disseminated disease is treated with surgical or chemical castration (hormonal therapy) or chemotherapy.

Pharmacologic Treatment

- Hormonal treatment: androgen deprivation/chemical castration—flutamide (Eulexin) 250 mg orally three times a day or leuprolide (Lupron) 1 mg SC once a day along with flutamide 7.5 mg IM monthly

How Long to Treat

- Radiation and chemotherapy treatments vary depending on staging.

Special Considerations

- Concurrent with treatment of the cancer is the need for addressing the effects of the diagnosis, sequelae of the disease, and side effects of treatments. These include coping with a chronic terminal illness, loss of self-image or self-esteem, transient or permanent incontinence (2% to 5%), loss of libido, and impotence. Impotence occurs in 40% postoperatively and 25% to 35% postradiation; hormonal treatment may additionally result in gynecomastia, cardiovascular complications, or hot flashes.

When to Consult, Refer, Hospitalize

- All patients with PSA above 10, abnormalities on DRE, and/or symptomatic are referred to a urologist for advanced workup, TRUS (trans-urethral ultrasound) with biopsy, chest X-ray, and bone scans.

Follow-Up

- Urologist, oncologist, and radiation oncologist as indicated
- For early stages, initially every 3 to 6 months for 5 years for PSA and DRE; annual bone scan if indicated; hemoglobin and liver function tests (LFTs) for monitoring status and potential progression

Expected course

- May be cured if detected and treated early; terminal if late staging

Complications

- Incontinence
- Erectile dysfunction
- Pain

- Pathologic fractures related to bone metastases
- Death

Disorders of the Scrotal Contents

CRYPTORCHIDISM

Description

- Failure of one or both testicles to descend into the scrotum

Etiology

- Partial lack of or response to gonadotropin and androgenic hormones during fetal development (testes descend by seventh fetal month)
- Mechanical factors, including elevated intra-abdominal pressure and retraction on the epididymis by the cremasteric muscles and gubernaculum
- May also have neural involvement
- Ectopic sites: superficial inguinal canal (most common site), perineal (rare), femoral (rare), penile (rare), transverse or paradox descent (rare), pelvis (rare)

Incidence and Demographics

- 3% to 4% full-term male infants, decreases to 0.8% to 1.0% by 1 year of age
- 20% to 30% of premature boys
- 6% of fathers of boys with undescended testicles had cryptorchidism; increased incidence in siblings.
- 20% are nonpalpable, with 25% of those absent at surgical exploration.
- Can be unilateral or bilateral
- Spontaneous testicular descent occurs by age 1 to 3 months in 50% to 70% of full-term male infants with cryptorchidism.

Risk Factors

- Prematurity; small for gestational age (SGA)
- Twins
- Family history

Associated Conditions

- Inguinal hernia/hydrocele; abnormalities of vas deferens and epididymis; intersex abnormalities; hypogonadotropic hypogonadism; germinal cell aplasia; prune-belly syndrome; meningomyelocele; hypospadias; Wilms tumor; Prader-Willi syndrome; Kallmann syndrome; cystic fibrosis

Prevention and Screening

- Careful examination during newborn exam and well child visits: important to document presence and position of testicles

Assessment

History

- Has the parent noted both testicles being present in the scrotal sac during the bath or while changing the infant's diaper?
- Prematurity
- Family history of cryptorchidism

Physical Exam

- Warm hands and the position of the patient (tailor position or sitting cross-legged, standing, or kneeling) may facilitate examination.
- Examine scrotum: testicles palpable and asymmetric size or nonpalpable; differentiate between retractile or gliding testis vs. true undescended testis (0.5% to 1%)
- Position of testicle if palpable outside scrotum (ectopic)
- Check for hernias and hydrocele.

Diagnostic Studies

- In boys 3 months old or younger with bilateral nonpalpable undescended testicles, hormone levels are helpful to determine whether the testes are present; check luteinizing hormone (LH), follicle stimulating hormone (FSH), and testosterone.
    - 3 months of age, use a human chorionic gonadotropin (hCG) stimulation test to determine presence/absence of testicular tissue, administer hCG 2,000 IU/day × 3 days, and check testosterone before and after stimulation.
- Lab studies: Urinary 17-ketosteroids, gonadotropins, and serum testosterone may help in tracing the cause.
- Various radiographic studies may be used on an individualized basis; however, CT scan findings in children have been found to be inconsistent. Ultrasound does not reliably localize nonpalpable testes and does not rule out an intra-abdominal testis; MRI has a sensitivity of 86%, a specificity of 79%, and an accuracy of 85%.
- Laparoscopy is useful to confirm testicular absence and locate abdominal testis and is a first and final step in surgical correction.
- Chromosome analysis if bilateral (may be ambiguous genitalia)

Differential Diagnosis

- Retractile testicle
- Atrophic testis
- Endocrine or chromosomal disorder
- Anorchia

Management

Nonpharmacologic Treatment

- Surgical correction: Orchiopexy should be performed by age 1. Orchiopexy permits accessible examinations to monitor for malignancy. Alterations in germ cell count in the cryptorchid testis have been identified by age 2. Laparoscopy is performed first if the testis is nonpalpable.

Pharmacologic Treatment

- Hormone stimulation (hCG or GnRH) is off-label use of hCG and has variable results; may even be harmful to testes.

When to Consult, Refer, Hospitalize

- Referral to a pediatric urologist if bilateral nonpalpable undescended testicles or if one or more testes has not descended by 6 months to 1 year of age.

Follow-Up

- Routine well-child visit schedule: Document presence of testicles and monitor for spontaneous resolution; post-operative initial follow-up within 1 month of surgery and periodically thereafter to assess testicular size and growth.
- Children need to be taught regular testicular self-exam once they enter puberty to assess for tumors.

Expected course

- 80% of retractile testicles descend by age 12 months.

Complications

- Risks if not corrected: testicular cancer 35 to 48 times more common, decreased fertility due to higher intra-abdominal temperature, cryptorchid testicle more prone to torsion, associated inguinal hernia in 25% of patients with mal-descent, approximately 20% of men with unilateral undescended testis remain infertile even after age-appropriate orchiopexy

HYDROCELE

Description

- A painless enlargement of the scrotum due to accumulation of clear fluid within the tunica vaginalis surrounding the testicles. May be unilateral or bilateral.

Etiology

- True etiology is unknown; possible causes include closure of the processus vaginalis, closure of the distal processus, failure of closure of processus vaginalis, infection, tumors, trauma
- Two types:
    - *Communicating* (associated with inguinal hernias): incomplete closure of tunica vaginalis; fluid descends from the peritoneal cavity
    - *Noncommunicating*: increased fluid production or decreased reabsorption within the scrotum; may be secondary to other scrotal disorders such as hernia, epididymitis, orchitis, tumors, trauma, or radiation

Incidence and Demographics

- Occur in 0.5% to 1.0% of male population; approximately half coincide with a hernia
- Predominantly in childhood (up to 6% of male infants), but may occur at any age

Risk Factors

- Previous scrotal or genitourinary disorder (epididymitis, orchitis, trauma, testicular tumor)
- 50% associated with inguinal hernia
- Peritoneal dialysis, Ehlers-Danlos syndrome, ventriculoperitoneal shunt, exstrophy of the bladder

Associated Conditions

- Testicular tumors, trauma, ventriculoperitoneal shunt, nephrotic syndrome, renal failure with peritoneal dialysis

Prevention and Screening

- Prevention only by repairing inguinal hernia
- Examination of scrotum on well child visits; periodic genital exam in adults

Assessment

History

- Acute or subacute onset of scrotal swelling or swelling in the inguinal canal
- Sensation of heaviness and bulkiness of the scrotum
- Duration of symptoms, including presence during childhood, recent trauma or infection
- Usually not painful
- Absence of other symptoms such as fever, dysuria, pain, impotency, or altered urinary patterns helps determine diagnosis

Physical Exam

- Nontender, scrotal firmness variable from soft to tense, depending upon the amount of fluid in the sac
- Swelling in the scrotum or inguinal canal; fluid collection in the scrotum that transilluminates
- Pear-shaped, fluid-filled sac with the smaller pole superiorly, usually located behind the testicles
- May be unilateral or bilateral

Diagnostic Studies

- Transillumination: transilluminates as translucent red glow with visible testicular shadow
- Doppler ultrasound indicated if any doubt of diagnosis, to rule out testicular torsion, incarcerated hernia, or cancer, particularly in a young man with sudden development and no apparent cause
- Routine aspiration of a hydrocele for the primary purpose of diagnosis is not recommended and should be discouraged.

Differential Diagnosis

- Varicocele
- Spermatocele

- Epididymitis
- Testicle trauma
- Indirect inguinal hernia
- Tumor
- Cryptorchidism
- Orchitis
- Testicular torsion

Management

Nonpharmacologic Treatment

- Many hydroceles will resolve spontaneously during the first year of life.
- Surgical correction is considered in cases of extreme size, discomfort, cosmetically bothersome, or if a hernia is present.
- Although rarely done, when indicated, aspiration of the hydrocele with installation of a sclerosing agent (talc) has been used successfully in the treatment of adults with hydrocele.
- Important to note: aspiration of the hydrocele is frequently followed by reaccumulation of fluid (recurrence rate of 34%) or infection; therefore, it is not routinely performed.

Special Considerations

- Occurs with inguinal hernias

When to Consult, Refer, Hospitalize

- Referral to a urologist or surgeon is recommended if large
- Refer to urologist if persists past 6 to 8 months of age

Follow-Up

- Initially every 3 to 6 months to assess for changes and determine if surgery is necessary
- Patients/parents monitor for symptoms (i.e., pain or changes in hydrocele size, contour, or weight; new symptoms)

Expected Course

- Pediatric: noncommunicating hydrocele present at birth usually resolves during the first year of life
- Adult: usually does not resolve on its own, but may not need treatment unless causing discomfort or in the presence of an underlying tumor

Complications

- For patients with surgical treatment, there is the potential for recurrence of hydrocele, wound infections, hematoma, or hematocele.

SPERMATOCELE

Description

- A painless cyst in the scrotal sac containing milky fluid with sperm
- Most are small, measuring less than 1 cm, but can be as large as 8 to 10 cm, which are easily mistaken for hydrocele.

Etiology

- Unknown etiology
- Diverticulum in epididymis, leading to accumulation of spermatic fluid

Incidence and Demographics

- Incidence less than 1%

Risk Factors

- None

Prevention and Screening

- No prevention
- Periodic genital exam in adults

Assessment

History

- Often asymptomatic
- Usually a random finding by the patient or examiner
- May be similar to hydrocele in that the patient notes an increased bulk or weight to the scrotum;
- Rarely can become twisted (torsion) or infected with subsequent symptoms of pain, edema, and warmth

Physical Exam

- Spermatoceles are attached to the epididymis, located above and behind the testicle.
- Palpable as round, mobile, and non-tender cysts less than 1 cm
- One or more may be present.

Diagnostic Studies

- Transillumination will reveal the mass.
- Ultrasound is indicated to clarify if any suspicion of cancer exists (ages 18 to 35 with lump newly developed or sudden onset) or if thorough scrotal examination is hindered by the lump or edema.

Differential Diagnosis

- Varicocele
- Hydrocele
- Tumor

Management, Special Considerations, Consultation, and Follow-Up

- Same as hydrocele

VARICOCELE

Description

- Abnormal venous dilatation in the scrotum (varicose veins in the scrotum)

Etiology

- Etiology is unknown, but there are several theorized causes:
  - Incompetent valves in the scrotal veins
  - Increased hydrostatic pressure in the left renal vein, inferior vena cava, and internal spermatic veins
  - Increased mechanical pressure from the superior mesenteric artery

Note: Right-sided varicoceles are rare and associated with obstruction of the right spermatic vein and retroperitoneal neoplasms.

Incidence and Demographics

- Affects 20% of the general male population
- Usually seen in older adolescents but can occur in any age group
- Almost always left-sided
- Can be associated with pathology in adult and prepubescent boys

Risk Factors

- None

Prevention and Screening

- No prevention
- Monthly testicular self-exam (TSE) and periodic clinical genitalia exam in the adult male

Assessment

History

- Asymptomatic or a sense of heaviness or dull aching in the scrotum

Physical Exam

- The characteristic presentation is a scrotum with a soft, irregular mass that feels like a "bag of worms" located above and behind the testicle and epididymis.
- It is nontender, worsens in the standing position, and often improves in the reclining position.
- Coughing or performing the Valsalva maneuver will accentuate the varicocele.
- If only palpable during a Valsalva maneuver, it is graded I; if palpable on standing, it is graded II; and, if visible on inspection alone, it is graded III.
- 97% occur on the left side of the scrotum.

Diagnostic Studies

- No testing may be needed to make the diagnosis in its classic presentation.
- Studies used to confirm the diagnosis include ultrasound, thermography, echo Doppler, and others, but these are done when a referral to a urologist is indicated.

Differential Diagnosis

- Hernia
- Epididymitis
- Hydrocele
- Spermatocele
- Tumor
- Epididymal cyst

Management

Nonpharmacologic Treatment

- Athletic supporters may provide increased comfort for patients with varicoceles.
- Surgery to correct the blood flow may be an option, depending on the grading of the varicoceles. Options include ligation, laparoscopic varicocelectomy, percutaneous varicocele occlusion, and others, and are done upon referral to a urologist or surgeon.

Special Considerations

- Right-sided varicocele is uncommon; can indicate retroperitoneal malignancy
- Sperm concentration and motility are significantly decreased in 65% to 75% of patients. Infertility is often a result and can be reversed in a high percentage of patients by correction of the varicocele as soon as identified.

When to Consult, Refer, Hospitalize

- Referral is indicated for patients who have suspected infertility, a varicocele that does not disappear in the supine position, and—most importantly—if it occurs on the right side.

Follow-Up

- No firm guidelines; return if there is an increase in pain, size, change in urinary patterns, pain with bowel movements, fever, warmth to scrotum, interference with sexual intercourse
- Early treatment and close monitoring for the younger patient (adolescents) may improve long-term fertility.
- Annual exam is adequate for asymptomatic patients.
- Post-procedure monitoring is indicated for recurrence of symptoms or development of complications.

Expected Course

- Variable and unpredictable
- Varicoceles have been found in 37% of patients with infertility, suggesting an association.
- Not associated with sexual dysfunction or increased risk of testicular cancer

Complications

- Infertility
- Post-procedure (i.e., wound infection)

EPIDIDYMITIS

Description

- An acute bacterial intra-scrotal infection associated with painful enlargement of the epididymis
- Most cases of acute epididymitis are infectious and can be divided into two categories with different age distributions and causes:
    - Sexually transmitted forms typically occur in men younger than 40 years old, are associated with urethritis, and result from *Chlamydia trachomatis* or *Neisseria gonorrhoeae*.
    - Non–sexually-transmitted forms typically occur in older men, are associated with urinary tract infections and prostatitis, and are caused by gram-negative rods.
- The route of infection is probably via the urethra to the ejaculatory duct and then down the vas deferens to the epididymis.

Etiology

- In men and boys younger than age 35, STDs are the most common cause, primarily *C. trachomatis,* then *N. gonorrhoeae.*
- Assess for serous urethral discharge (chlamydia) or purulent discharge (gonorrhea).
- In men who have sex with men, practicing anal intercourse, *Escherichia coli* or *Haemophilus Influenzae* is the common etiology; in heterosexual men over 35 years old, causative organisms are those associated with UTIs.

- Sterile epididymitis linked to vigorous physical activity (bicycle riding), trauma, andTB (rare causes)
- Gram-negative rods, *E. coli*, *Pseudomonas aeruginosa*, or coliform bacteria are common causes in men who have epididymitis that is associated with UTI (reflux of infected urine), are over 35 years old, have had instrumentation, or have anatomic abnormalities.

Incidence and Demographics

- Most common intra-scrotal inflammation in men in the United States
- More than 600,000 health care visits/year

Risk Factors

- Exposure to STDs up to 30 days before onset of symptoms
- Anatomic abnormalities
- Instrumentation/surgery

Prevention and Screening

- Safe sex practices
- Antibiotics prior to instrumentation or urethral manipulation

Assessment

History

- Presents equally on the left or right
- Testicular pain and edema that is commonly gradual in onset; symptoms may follow acute physical strain (heavy lifting), trauma, or sexual activity; associated symptoms of urethritis (pain at tip of penis and urethral discharge) or cystitis (irritating voiding symptoms) may occur; pain develops in scrotum and may radiate along the spermatic cord or to flank. On occasion, edema may double the size of the testicle in 3 to 4 hours.
- Half of all cases present with fever, urethral discharge, or voiding complaints. Associated nausea and vomiting are unusual.

- Explore the past medical history (PMH) for previous urinary symptoms or diagnoses, procedures, instrumentation of the urinary tract, or trauma to the scrotum.
- Explore the social history for information on new sexual partners, sexual practices, and use of scrotal support or protectors during sports.

Physical Exam

- Scrotal pain radiates up the spermatic cord or into the groin region; may begin acutely over several hours; there is scrotal swelling and heaviness.
- Epididymis is cord-like and palpable separately from the testicle; initially normal size, consistency, and position on exam, but later the two may appear as one enlarged, with a tender mass becoming less distinguishable with time.
- Epididymis is markedly tender to palpation.
- Pain may be relieved by elevating the scrotum (Prehn's sign—elevation of the scrotum above the pubic symphysis improves pain from epididymitis) but is not reliable.
- Cremasteric reflex present (contraction of scrotum after light stroke to thigh) on affected side (differentiates epididymitis from testicular torsion); if cremasteric reflex is absent, suspect testicular torsion.
- The prostate may be tender on a rectal examination.

Diagnostic Studies

- Gram stain of urethral exudate or intraurethral swab to diagnose gonococcal infection if present; culture of same specimen for *N. gonorrhoeae* and *C. trachomatis,* white cells without visible organisms on urethral smear represent non-gonococcal urethritis, and *C. trachomatis* is the most likely pathogen.
- Urinalysis, possible urine culture to diagnose concurrent UTI particularly in non–sexually-transmitted types
- Syphilis serology
- CBC positive leukocytosis
- HIV testing with counseling
- Ultrasound of the scrotum or radionuclide scanning may also be needed to rule out other possibilities.

Differential Diagnosis

- Tumor
- Abscess
- Cyst
- Testicular torsion
- Testicular infarction
- Testicular cancer
- Mumps orchitis
- Hydrocele
- Varicocele

Management

Nonpharmacologic Treatment

- Bed rest and restriction on activity
- Scrotal elevation (place a folded towel under genitals and across thighs)
- Ice pack/warm compress
- Athletic scrotal supporter
- Avoidance of sexual activity and physical strain until resolved

Pharmacologic Treatment

- Initiate treatment empirically, before culture results are available (see Table 12–6).
- Treat sexual partners if condition is likely due to an STD and contact was within last 60 days preceding symptoms.

How Long to Treat

- Until fever and local inflammation have subsided, bed rest and elevation of scrotum should be maintained. Antibiotic therapy should be continued for 10 days.

TABLE 12–6.
PHARMACOLOGIC TREATMENT OF EPIDIDYMITIS

INDICATION	MEDICATION
Age younger than 35 years old with high likelihood of *N. gonorrhoeae and/or C. trachomatis*	Ceftriaxone (Rocephin) 500 mg IM single dose plus doxycycline 100 mg orally four times a day × 10 days. If cephalosporin allergy: Gentamicin 240mg IM in a single dose plus azithromycin 2 g orally once Evaluate and treat all sexual partner(s) from the preceding 60 days. Men who engage in insertive anal intercourse receive ceftriaxone 500 mg* IM once and levofloxacin 500 orally daily × 10 days. *Administer 1 gm of Ceftriaxone for persons weighing more than 150 kg. If symptoms fail to improve in 3 days of antibiotic treatment, reevaluation is required.
Age over 35 years old with high likelihood of enteric organisms *or* allergies to cephalosporins or tetracycline	Gentamicin 240mg IM in a single dose plus azithromycin 2 g orally once
Fever and inflammation	Analgesics (e.g., NSAIDs, acetaminophen)

Centers for Disease Control and Prevention. (2021). Sexually transmitted diseases treatment guidelines, 2021. *MMWR: Morbidity and Mortality Weekly Report, 70*(RR-4), 1–187. https://www.cdc.gov/std/treatment-guidelines/STI-Guidelines-2021.pdf

Special Considerations

- Differentiate from other cause of acute scrotal pain, testicular torsion
- Prostatic massage is contraindicated in epididymitis due to the potential risk of spread of local infection systemically.

When to Consult, Refer, Hospitalize

- Referral to urologist is indicated for the patient who is not improving within 3 days of antimicrobial therapy or has worsening symptoms.

Follow-Up

- In 72 hours to ensure that infection is resolving

Expected Course

- Failure to improve within 3 days of antimicrobial therapy requires reevaluation of both the diagnosis and therapy.
- Swelling and tenderness that persist after completion of antimicrobial therapy should be reevaluated, noting that swelling may take weeks to months to be resolved.

Complications

- Prompt treatment usually results in a favorable outcome; delayed or inadequate treatment may result in:
  - Epididymo-orchitis,
  - Chronic pain (chronic epididymitis),
  - Abscess formation,
  - Infertility (possibly up to 50% if bilateral), or
  - Testicular atrophy.

TESTICULAR TORSION

Description

- Spermatic cord compression by twisting of the spermatic cord within the scrotum, resulting in compromised blood flow to the testicles. Constitutes a surgical emergency to prevent necrotic testicles.

Etiology

- Congenital, anatomically abnormal, free-floating testicle without fixation in the scrotum, which twists around blood supply to testicle, resulting in ischemia and potential infarction of the testicle
- May be precipitated by trauma, sudden movements that pull on the cremasteric muscle (jumping into cold water, riding bicycle), sexual activity, cold, exercise
- May occur when contents of scrotum shift in the relaxed state during sleep
- Torsion is usually spontaneous and idiopathic
- One-third of patients with testicular torsion have had prior episode of testicular pain

Incidence and Demographics

- Most commonly occurs in boys ages 12 to 18, with peak incidence at age 14, but can occur at any age; 1 in 4,000 men and boys younger than age 25
- Occurs from newborn period to seventh decade
- 40% occur during sleep

Risk Factors

- Age
- Paraplegics
- Previous contralateral testicular torsion

Prevention and Screening

- No prevention except surgical correction of defect if discovered
- High index of suspicion in young men with acute scrotal pain

Assessment

History

- Typically presents with sudden-onset, acute, profound pain that is localized to the testicles or radiating to the groin and lower abdomen; nausea and vomiting in 50% of patients
- No dysuria, fever, or urethral discharge; no irritative voiding symptoms
- A quick history should explore precipitating events (e.g., exercise, sleep, cold exposure), current medical history and medications, sexual partners, and STD exposure.
- Torsion of the testicular appendage (not entire testicle) presents with less-severe pain and more gradual onset of symptoms, and is not a surgical emergency

Physical Exam

- Typically lying still, in acute distress; first symptom is pain, usually sudden, but may have a gradual onset

- Acute tenderness of testicle with swelling and erythema
- Scrotum is enlarged, red, edematous, and painful.
- Testicle is horizontal, elevated in the scrotum, with negative (absent) cremasteric reflex.
- Prehn's sign is negative (no relief with elevating testicle above pubic symphysis).
- Epididymis very tender, out of normal position due to twisting of spermatic cord
- If only the testicular appendage is twisted, there will be a "blue dot" sign at the superior aspect of the testicle—a small, palpable lump on the superior pole of the epididymis when skin is pulled taut.
- Nausea and vomiting common due to pain
- Fever may occur, but not typical

Diagnostic Studies

- Begin immediate surgical treatment in unequivocal cases. Consider the risk of time lost for testing vs. preservation of testicle.
- Urinalysis usually not helpful unless to quickly rule out infectious component in differential diagnosis
- Doppler ultrasound with color is best; radionuclide scrotal imaging is also used

Differential Diagnosis

- Epididymitis
- Torsion of testicular appendage
- Trauma
- Orchitis
- Hernia (incarcerated or strangulated)

Management

- An acute urological emergency, may result in loss of the testicle.
- 80% salvage rate of testicle if corrected within 4 hours; only 20% if within 12 hours; necrosis of the testicle usually occurs after 6 to 8 hours.

Nonpharmacologic Treatment

- Pre-operatively, elevate the scrotum, apply ice pack
- Manual reduction followed by surgical treatment (orchidopexy)

Special Considerations

- Advise patients that both testicles will be surgically secured within the scrotum to prevent reoccurrence and that there is a risk of decreased fertility or infertility.

When to Consult, Refer, Hospitalize

- *Note*: immediate surgical consult

Follow-Up

- The surgeon follows the patient 1 to 2 weeks post-operatively
- Annual visits to evaluate atrophy of testicles, particularly before puberty

Expected Course

- Potential outcomes depend on timing of treatment. The testicle may be gangrenous and removed; saved, but atrophied; or minimally affected. Atrophy of the twisted testicle or the unaffected testicle may occur, affecting spermatogenesis and fertility, but testosterone production is unchanged.

Complications

- Impaired fertility; abnormal spermatogenesis
- Atrophy of the salvaged testicle in up to two-thirds of patients within 2 to 3 years

TESTICULAR CANCER

Description

- Carcinoma of the testicles that is categorized as either germinal or nongerminal

Etiology

- Although the cause of testicular cancer is unknown, both congenital and acquired factors have been associated with tumor development. The strongest association has been with cryptorchid testis. Approximately 7% to 10% of testicular tumors develop in patients who have a history of cryptorchidism. Seminoma is the most common form (95%) of tumor rising from this condition. Almost all cases of germ cell tumors (GCTs) show chromosome 12p abnormalities; increased expression of p53 protein is found in many GCTs.

Incidence and Demographics

- Testicular cancer is rare in children, but 66% of testicular tumors in children are malignant.
- 1% to 2% of all male cancers; most common cancer of boys and men ages 15 to 35 years
- GCTs account for 95% of all cases and are subcategorized as seminomatous (one-third to one-half) or nonseminomatous.
- Leydig cell neoplasms account for 5%.
- Most commonly occurs in men ages 20 to 40 years, but also seen in men over 60 years old and boys in childhood.

Risk Factors

- White, Scandinavian, and Swiss; higher social class, rural resident, and unmarried
- History of undescended testicles (cryptorchidism)
- Family history
- Klinefelter syndrome, XY dysgenesis, Down syndrome, testicular atrophy
- Exposure to maternal intrapartum estrogen (diethylstilbestrol [DES]), infertility, preterm birth

Prevention and Screening

- Teach adolescent boys to do regular testicular self-exams (TSE).
- Teach adolescent boys to tell parents about any abnormal findings and to seek treatment immediately.
- Encourage annual clinical screening with a testicular exam.
- Screen patients with risk factors.

Assessment

History

- Frequently incidental finding on routine exam or patient notes painless swelling, sense of heaviness, or thickening in scrotum or testicle
- Testicles may be tender, especially if associated with bleeding within the tumor or if epididymitis is present concurrently.
- Associated symptoms reflective of metastasis include gynecomastia; supraclavicular lymphadenopathy; abdominal or neck mass; or pain in the groin, flank, or back.
- Less than 10% with seminoma have symptoms of distant metastases at time of diagnosis.
- Inquire about medications and PMH, particularly relating to the associated symptoms.

Physical Exam

- Scrotal exam reveals hydrocele in up to 20% of patients with testicular cancer.
- Tumors are often found on the lower pole but can be anywhere on the testicles.
- Tumors are firm, ± tender, one or more present, on one or both testicles.
- Transillumination will not reveal the normal rosy glow; there is darkness of the tumor.
- Inguinal lymphadenopathy may or may not be present.

Diagnostic Studies

- Serum alpha-fetoprotein reflects presence of nonseminomatous germ cell tumors, lactate dehydrogenase (LDH), hCG, and chest X-ray

- Serum beta-hCG positive in 70% to 100% of seminomatous testicular carcinoma
- Scrotal ultrasound is the gold standard; it distinguishes between most of the differential diagnoses.
- Staging determined with chest X-ray, CT scan of abdomen and pelvis, pedal lymphangiography; MRI of brain/lung and bone scan for patients with metastasis or elevated alkaline phosphatase

Differential Diagnosis

- Inguinal hernias
- Epididymitis
- Orchitis, hematomas
- Hydrocele
- Spermatocele

Management

- Treatment is dictated by the type of tumor, staging, and associated symptoms.

Nonpharmacologic Treatment

- Seminomas: radiation and radical inguinal orchiectomy
- Nonseminomatous: surgery, radiation, and combination chemotherapy
- Metastasized cancer is treated with both radiation and chemotherapy.

Pharmacologic Treatment

- Chemotherapy directed by the oncologist

How Long to Treat

- Directed by the oncologist

Special Considerations

- Testicular cancer in older patients most likely metastatic, usually lymphoma

When to Consult, Refer, Hospitalize

- Pediatric: All testicular masses or tumors should be referred to a pediatric urologist and oncologist.
- Adult: All undiagnosed testicular masses should be referred to a urologist.
- Management and follow-up are directed by the oncologist.

Follow-Up

Expected Course

- Localized seminomatous cancer has a 5-year survival rate over 95%.
- Disseminated disease 5-year survival is 20%.
- Nonseminomatous GCTs treated aggressively have a 5-year survival rate of 60% to 90%.

Complications

- Metastases to lung and abdomen
- Side effects of treatment (radiation, chemotherapy)
- Post-operative wound infection, urinary tract infections related to instrumentation

Penile Disorders

PHIMOSIS

Description

- In the uncircumcised male, a tightness of the distal penile foreskin that prevents it from being retracted back from over the glans penis
- Paraphimosis occurs when foreskin is retracted and remains proximal to the glans, constricting the glans penis.

Etiology

- Occurs when the orifice of the prepuce is too small to allow retraction of the foreskin
- Most cases occur in uncircumcised men, although excessive skin left after circumcision can become stenotic and cause phimosis.
- Acquired from trauma, prior infection, or poor hygiene (retained smegma and dirt) that results in inflammation and the development of adhesions
- Can be physiologic until age 7 to 10 years
- Foreskin is physiologically adherent to the glans in the newborn. In the uncircumcised male, the foreskin naturally separates as the boy gets older; forcible retraction can cause scarring.
- Geriatric patients may develop phimosis with use of condom catheters.

Incidence and Demographics

- Age 16 or older has a 1% incidence.
- Adolescence is the predominant age of occurrence.

Risk Factors

- Uncircumcised penis
- Poor hygiene
- Trauma; diabetes
- Infection of the glans (balanitis) or prepuce (posthitis)
- Sickle-cell disease

Prevention and Screening

- Teach parents proper care of uncircumcised penis; no need to retract until foreskin does so naturally
- Examine foreskin at routine well child visits
- Hygiene of the genitalia with retraction of the foreskin during washing

Assessment

History

- Inability to retract foreskin when it was previously retractable
- Ballooning of foreskin with urination
- Urinary tract infection
- Painful urination
- Patients may be asymptomatic, with phimosis discovered on examination.
- When related to an infectious or inflammatory process, a patient complains of irritation and tenderness of the glans, discomfort with voiding, or pain on erection.
- *Note*: If severe enough, outflow of urine may be compromised, presenting as a urological emergency.

Physical Exam

- The glans is nonretractable, and the prepuce is pallid, striated, and thickened.
- If actively infected, there will be erythema, smegma and/or exudate, and tenderness.
- In paraphimosis, there will be swelling and/or edema of the glans, possible ulceration, and drainage.

Diagnostic Studies

- None

Differential Diagnosis

- Balanitis
- Penile trauma, penile lymphedema, penile tourniquet syndrome due to foreign object around penis

Management

Nonpharmacologic Treatment

- Teach parents appropriate care of uncircumcised penis—gentle retraction only as far as foreskin will easily move.
- Treat the underlying cause, such as infection or inflammation, with good hygiene, sitz baths, and warm compresses.
- Surgical release or circumcision

Pharmacologic Treatment

- If concurrent infection or inflammation, treatment with topical antifungals or steroids may be sufficient to allow for retraction. To reduce swelling: topical 0.05% betamethasone (Beta-Val) twice a day for 1 month to soften phimosis and gradual traction placed on foreskin. Within 4 to 6 weeks, the phimotic ring should open.
- Use of a triple antibiotic ointment (Neosporin or Bacitracin or the generic brand) applied to the tip of the foreskin can act as a protective barrier to fecal contamination.

How Long to Treat

- Topical treatment for underlying infection or inflammation for 1 to 2 weeks

Special Considerations

- Phimosis is normal in uncircumcised men; however, once the foreskin is retractable, it is not normal for it to spontaneously adhere again.

When to Consult, Refer, Hospitalize

- Refer to urologist for surgical release or circumcision if nonresponsive to topical treatment and hygiene, urinary flow is compromised, or asymptomatic phimosis remains.
- Paraphimosis is a true *surgical emergency*; should be referred to a urologist for immediate evaluation and circumcision. Unreduced paraphimosis can lead to gangrene of the glans.

Follow-Up

Expected Course

- Resolves completely with treatment
- No sexual activity following circumcision until healing is complete

Complications

- If there is associated infectious precipitant, complications such as meatal stenosis, UTI, or premalignant changes may occur.

ERECTILE DYSFUNCTION (ED)

Description

- Inability to achieve or maintain a satisfactory erection more than 25% to 50% of the time (although may be defined by patients as premature ejaculation or the loss of orgasm, emission, libido, or erections)

Etiology

- Psychological origin is likely with loss of orgasm when libido and erection are intact, and with premature ejaculation concurrent with anxiety, depression, relationship problems, new partner, or emotional disorders.
- Medications used to treat chronic conditions—such as anabolic steroids, furosemide (Lasix), digoxin (Lanoxin), angiotensin-converting enzyme inhibitors (ACEI) such as captopril (Capoten), beta blockers such as propranolol (Inderal), cimetidine (Tagamet), centrally acting antihypertensives (reserpine, clonidine, methyldopa [Aldomet]), spironolactone, and antidepressants (monoamine oxidase [MAO] inhibitors, tricyclics, selective serotonin uptake inhibitors [SSRIs])—have been implicated in causing loss of libido and ED.
- Lifestyle issues of alcohol, drug, and cigarette use
- A gradual loss of erections over time is indicative of organic causes.
  - Hormonal and endocrine disorders of the thyroid, hypogonadism, kidney, pituitary gland or testicular function, diabetes, Addison's disease, and Cushing syndrome

- ◊ Vascular disorders such as hypertension, arterial insufficiency, venous disease, atherosclerosis
- ◊ Neurologic disorders, structural problems, spinal cord injury, and post-treatment of prostate disorders
- ◊ When ED occurs in younger men, it is associated with a significantly increased risk of future cardiac events and should be a warning sign for the primary care provider to investigate further underlying conditions.

Incidence and Demographics

- Widely unreported, estimated that 10% of the male population affected; 10 to 20 million men in the United States
- 52% of men ages 40 to 70 years
- Age-related increase, ranging from 12.4% in men aged 40 to 49 years to 46.6% in men aged 50 to 69 years

Risk Factors

- Advancing age
- Cardiovascular disease
- Diabetes mellitus
- Metabolic syndrome
- History of urologic surgery, radiation, trauma/injury to the pelvic area or spinal cord
- Medications that induce ED
- Use or abuse of alcohol, cigarettes, and drugs
- Psychological conditions: lifestyle with high levels of stress, anxiety, depression, or relationship problems

Assessment

History

- Determine the patient's perception or definition of ED (impotence) to clarify the problem and symptoms, timing, circumstances, and frequency of occurrence.

- Detailed sexual history: Determine the nature of the patient's relationship, sexual partners, lifestyle, and stress.
- Complaints include any of the following: reduced size and strength of erection, lack of ability to achieve or maintain erections adequate for intercourse, rapid loss of erection with penetration, or lack of libido.
- Inquire if there are nocturnal or morning erections, as their presence reflects an intact blood supply, nervous system, and sexual apparatus, and reduces the likelihood of organic cause.
- Associated symptoms indicative of underlying disease: decreased body hair; gynecomastia; neuropathies; anxiety; headaches; vision changes; decreased circulation; excessive dryness or skin changes; changes in testicle size, consistency, or shape; and changes in penis such as rash, discharge, or phimosis.
- Review past medical history for other diseases; testicular infections or insults; medications (prescription, OTC, and herbal); and history of smoking, drug, alcohol use.

Physical Exam

- Complete screening physical noting general appearance, generalized anxiety or hyperactivity, vital signs for postural hypotension, dry hair, loss of secondary sex characteristics, spider angiomas, hyperpigmentation, palmar erythema, or goiter
- Chest, abdomen, and extremities for cardiac abnormalities, gynecomastia, aortic or femoral bruits, peripheral vascular deficits
- Genital examination for penile circulation, discharge, fibrosis, or lesions; testicles for size, masses, varicoceles, or atrophy; DRE for prostate abnormalities, sphincter tone, and assess for Peyronie's disease (penile plaques)
- Neurologic screening for cortical, brainstem, spinal, or peripheral neuropathies, noting especially bulbocavernosi reflex, cremasteric reflex, pinprick or light touch to genital and perianal area, focal tenderness of spine, vision abnormalities

Diagnostic Studies

- Key studies to screen for underlying etiology: fasting serum glucose, prolactin, morning total testosterone level, CBC, urinalysis, and lipid profile
- If testicular atrophy is suspected, include LH and FSH
- If hypothyroidism is suspected, measure TSH.

- Other tests are added depending on findings of history and physical and results of preliminary tests
- Nocturnal penile tumescence and rigidity testing
- Urologist may include duplex ultrasonography, penile angiography, nerve conduction studies, or a trial injection of prostaglandin E_1 phentolamine, and papaverine intracorporeally to assess vascular integrity, noting penile response.

Differential Diagnosis

Endocrine Origin

- Altered thyroxine
- Testosterone
- Prolactin
- Insulin
- Estrogen levels

Neurologic Origin

- Cortical
- Brainstem
- Spinal cord
- Peripheral neuropathies

Psychological

- Anxiety
- Depression
- Schizophrenia
- Personality/relationship problems

Vascular Origin

- Arterial insufficiency
- Venous insufficiency
- Cavernosal insufficiency

Structural

- Peyronie's disease
- Microphallus
- Hypospadias
- Scarring
- Trauma

Other

- Medication side effects
- Renal failure
- Zinc deficiency

Management

Nonpharmacologic Treatment

- Modify lifestyle: stress reduction techniques; stop alcohol, drugs, and smoking
- Use of vacuum constriction device for those with venous disorders of the penis or nonresponsiveness to vasoactive injections
- Surgical treatment

Pharmacologic Treatment

- Sildenafil (Viagra): 25–50 mg 1 hour before desired erection (works within 30 minutes to 4 hours) on an empty stomach, at least 2 hours before meals. Dose variable, dependent upon concurrent disease, age; may increase dosage up to 100 mg/day.

Contraindicated for patient taking nitrites; used cautiously with unstable angina and history of stroke, myocardial infarction. Side effects: headache, flushing, nasal congestion from vasodilation; abnormalities in vision (color changes, light sensitivity, blurred vision), priapism.

- Tadalafil (Cialis): 5–20 mg at least 2 hours before sex; may take without regard to meals; may provide longer action (up to 36 hours)
- Vardenafil (Levitra): usual daily dose 5–20 mg 1 hour before sexual activity, on an empty stomach, at least 2 hours before meals; claims to provide faster onset, have fewer adverse effects
- Other oral agents controversial, including yohimbine, trazodone (Desyrel), ginkgo biloba
- Substitute or discontinue medications known to cause ED.
  - Alternative antihypertensives include calcium channel blockers, ACEIs, selective beta blockers (atenolol).
  - Trial of antidepressants other than tricyclics: nortriptyline (Pamelor), desipramine (Norpramin); substitute ranitidine (Zantac), or other H2 blocker for cimetidine (Tagamet)
- Treat abnormal hormones as follows:
  - Insufficient testosterone treated with a 3-month testosterone trial (if indicated by androgen deficiency and patient does not have prostate cancer), using testosterone injections 200 mg IMevery 3 weeks or topical patches of 2.5 to 6 mg/day
- Hyperprolactinemia treated with bromocriptine (Parlodel) initially 2.5 mg twice a day, up to 40 mg/day
- Penile injections such as alprostadil (Caverject), first dose in the office setting 1.25 to 2.5 μg with repeat dose after 1 hour if no response. Patient to remain in office until ejaculation completed. Partial response may have a second injection in 24 hours.
- Alternatives to alprostadil (Edex) are papaverine (Papacon) or phentolamine (Rogitine).
- Urethral suppository of alprostadil (Muse) in various strength pellets

How Long to Treat

- Variable depending on treatment methods

Special Considerations

- Nitrates should be withheld for 24 hours after sildenafil or vardenafil administration and for 48 hours after use of tadalafil.

- Reasons for seeking care and etiology are age-related.
- Age adolescence to 30: concerns often psychological or gender-related, as well as with primary organic origin
- Age 50 to 60 with relationship problems; most concerned about medical problems
- Age 70+ rarely seek help, most likely have physical problems
- Use of injections or oral agents require thorough patient teaching on proper use, frequency of use, side effects, and risk of priapism, and when to seek medical help, such as erection lasting more than 4 hours.

When to Consult, Refer, Hospitalize

- Patients should notify their primary care provider for immediate attention if erection lasts more than 4 hours.
- Psychotherapist for individual or couple's therapy, sex therapy
- Urologist, endocrinologist, cardiologist, neurologist referrals as indicated by diagnosis and requirements for further evaluation or advanced treatment

Follow-Up

- Varied, depending on diagnosis, underlying etiology, response to treatment, and need for therapy. Patients should be seen initially at shorter intervals to adjust and monitor responsiveness to treatment, then every 3 months.

Expected Course

- Improvement in many patients with oral medications, vacuum devices, suppository, and penile implants; 15% improve spontaneously
- 20% failure rate with vacuum device, 10% to 30% dissatisfaction with penile implants
- Alprostadil injections have 85% to 90% response rate; urethral suppository method rates are 40 to 60%; oral agent sildenafil is effective for 70% of patients at maximal dose.

Complications

- Variable, depending on underlying etiology and treatment method side effects: priapism, penile bruising, hypotension, headache, flushing, nausea, side effects of testosterone (urinary retention, acne, vomiting), penile pain and irritation, and testicular pain

Health Care for Gay and Bisexual Men

DESCRIPTION

- Men who have sex with men (MSM)

INCIDENCE AND DEMOGRAPHICS

- 2.2% of American adult men identify as gay; 1.4% identify as bisexual; and approximately 6%–7% report same sex attraction and sexual behavior with men
- Experience health disparities that are heightened with history of traumatic events, sexual abuse or family rejection early in life.
- 37% of new HIV cases are among Black MSM and 24% of cases are among Hispanic/Latinx MSM (CDC, 2019).

RISK FACTORS

HIV and STD

- MSM account for approximately 70% of all new HIV infections in the United States.
- HIV is easily transmitted by receptive anal intercourse.
- Anal intercourse carries the highest risk of HIV infection, surpassing penile–vaginal and oral intercourse.

PREVENTION AND SCREENING

- STDs commonly seen in MSM and at higher rates than seen in men having sex with women are primary and secondary syphilis, and gonorrhea commonly found in the pharynx and rectum. Gonorrhea present in these areas may be asymptomatic, necessitating the need for careful testing for gonorrhea and chlamydia based on sexual practices.
- Higher rates of viral hepatitis A, B, and C
- HPV infection can cause anogenital warts, anal dysplasia, and anal cancer. Oncogenic strain of HPV type 16 in the anal canal of MSM with HIV is35% and MSM without HIV is 12%. The incidence of MSM with HIV acquiring anal cancer is higher than MSM without HIV.

- HPV immunization with quadrivalent and nine valent vaccines is recommended for boys and young adults up to age 26. For unvaccinated adults aged 27–45 years, shared decision-making concerning HPV is recommended by the CDC.
- Anal cytology screening is highly recommended for MSM who are positive for HIV and often performed on MSM without HIV due to the increased risk of anal cancer in this population.
- Other enteric infections need to be considered when oral–anal sexual practices are reported such as giardiasis, amebiasis, and shigellosis. Meningococcal infection transmissions are also more prevalent in areas where sexual activity occurs with MSM in saunas, bathhouses, or group sex venues. Meningococcal vaccination is strongly recommended for high-risk MSM.

MENTAL HEALTH

- Higher rates of depression, anxiety, and suicide are found in MSM. Ongoing screening and risk assessment with referral to mental health resources and therapy are recommended.

SUBSTANCE USE

- Higher rates of cigarette smoking, alcohol use, and recreational illicit drug use via oral, inhalants, and IV routes. HIV, STDs, and hepatitis rates increase significantly with IV drug use, and lack of consistent condom use.

SCREENING RECOMMENDATIONS AND PREVENTION

- The CDC recommends that MSM be screened for STDs (syphilis, gonorrhea, chlamydia, and HIV annually, and more frequently as indicated based on sexual practices and number of partners).
- Testing for HIV should be done via HIV antibody-antigen assay and the nucleic acid amplification test (NAAT) should be used for gonorrhea and chlamydia via the oropharynx, rectum, urine, and urethra.
- MSM should be tested at least once during their lifetime for hepatitis B and be vaccinated against hepatitis A and B. Hepatitis C screening is also recommended annually.
- Smoking cessation counseling and pharmacotherapy is encouraged along with screening for drug and alcohol misuse with appropriate referrals offered for treatment.

- The World Health Organization, CDC, and USPSTF recommend Pre-Exposure Prophylaxis (PrEP) for MSM with HIV and for MSM at high risk for acquiring HIV infection. PrEP should be encouraged for MSM who do not use condoms or are not in a monogamous relationship with a man without HIV, and MSM who have sex with a male partner positive for HIV who is not consistently taking antiretroviral therapy.
- Post-Exposure Prophylaxis (PEP) is antiretroviral medication started within 72 hours of an exposure to HIV or highly likely/unknown high-risk exposure to HIV and taken for 28 days to reduce the risk of HIV transmission.

Health Care for Transgender and Gender-Diverse Individuals

TERMINOLOGY

- Transgender and gender-diverse individuals may identify as gender nonbinary, gender nonconforming, genderqueer, and transsexual. Transgender individuals may have a gender identity or expression, or both, that differ from those associated with the sex assigned to them at birth. Cisgender are individuals whose sexual expression and identity align with the sex assigned to them at birth.
- Transfeminine refers to individuals who identify as female or along the feminine spectrum.
- Transmasculine refers to individuals who identify as male or along the masculine spectrum.
- Many transgender individuals do not identify using a binary definition of gender.
- Transgender individuals may use pronouns of he, she, or the gender-neutral singular pronoun—they. Always ask the person what pronoun and name they prefer to use and never assume.
- Gender and sexual orientation are distinct, and both transgender and cisgender individuals may express a wide spectrum of diversity in their sexual activity and attraction.

MULTIPLE DISPARITIES

- Many disparities exist for transgender individuals due to societal stigma, discrimination, lack of understanding, lack of legal protection in the workplace, housing, educational institutions, lack of family support, socioeconomic disadvantage and when accessing health care. Inability to access safe and supportive health care providers often leads to poor health outcomes and late diagnoses.

GENDER-AFFIRMING MEDICAL AND SURGICAL INTERVENTIONS

- Some individuals may seek gender-affirming interventions to align their physical appearance with their gender, but not all will do so. The choice is theirs to make and should be supported or accepted as such.
- Types of Gender-Affirming Cosmetic and Surgical Procedures:
  - Surgical Procedures: voice surgery, facial surgery (feminization/masculinization procedures), thyroid chondroplasty, vulvoplasty, vaginoplasty, phalloplasty, scrotoplasty, vaginectomy, metoidioplasty, chest surgery, augmentation mammoplasty, hysterectomy salpingectomy, gonadectomy, orchiectomy, oophorectomy, body contouring.
  - Cosmetic procedures: laser or electrolysis facial and body hair removal, voice therapy and modification, genital tucking and packing, chest binding.
- Counseling should be offered as indicated but is not required; referral to a health care provider or a multidisciplinary team of providers who specialize in the comprehensive management of transgender health care needs that includes the provision and monitoring of hormone therapy, fertility preservation, gender reassignment surgery, and dermatology care.
  - Long-term monitoring of general health care needs with respect for the effects of use of hormone therapy, surgical procedures performed, remaining genitalia, genetic risk factors, and the screening needs of the individual includes monitoring for cancer, cardiovascular risk and other risk factors throughout the aging process.

REFERENCES

American Urological Association (AUA) Guidelines. (2014). *Evaluation and treatment of cryptorchidism: AUA guideline 2014.* Reviewed and validity confirmed 2018. https://www.auanet.org/guidelines-and-quality/guidelines/non-oncology-guidelines

Association American Urological Association (AUA) Guidelines. (2015). *Peyronie's disease: AUA guideline 2015.* https://www.auanet.org/guidelines-and-quality/guidelines/non-oncology-guidelines

American Urological Association (AUA) Guidelines. (2018). Early detection of prostate cancer: AUA guideline 2018. Published 2013; Reviewed and validity confirmed 2018. https://www.auanet.org/guidelines-and-quality/guidelines/oncology-guidelines

American Urological Association (AUA) Guidelines. (2018). *Erectile dysfunction: AUA guideline 2018. https://doi.org/10.1016/j.juro.2018.05.004.* https://www.auanet.org/guidelines-and-quality/guidelines/non-oncology-guidelines

American Urological Association (AUA) Guidelines. (2019). *Diagnosis and treatment of early stage testicular cancer: AUA guideline 2019.* https://www.auanet.org/guidelines-and-quality/guidelines/testicular-cancer-guideline

American Urological Association (AUA) Guidelines. (2020). *Diagnosis and treatment of infertility in men: AUA/ASRM guideline* 2020. https://www.auanet.org/guidelines-and-quality/guidelines/non-oncology-guidelines

American Urological Association (AUA) Guidelines. (2021). *Management of lower urinary tract symptoms attributed to benign prostatic hyperplasia: AUA guideline 2021.* https://www.auanet.org/guidelines-and-quality/guidelines/non-oncology-guidelines

American Urological Association (AUA) Guidelines. (2022). *The diagnosis and management of priapism: An AUA/SMSNA guideline (2022).* https://www.auanet.org/guidelines-and-quality/guidelines/non-oncology-guidelines

Barry MJ, Fowler FJ Jr, O'leary MP, Bruskewitz RC, Holtgrewe HL, Mebust WK, & Cockett AT; Measurement Committee of the American Urological Association. (2017). The American Urological Association Symptom Index for Benign Prostatic Hyperplasia. J Urol. 197(2S): S189–S197. Doi: 10.1016/j.juro.2016.10.071. Epub 2016 Dec 22. PMID: 28012747.

Centers for Disease Control and Prevention. (2019). Human papillomavirus vaccination for adults: Updated recommendations of the advisory committee on immunization practices. *MMWR: Morbidity and Mortality Weekly Report, 68*(RR-32), 698–702. https://www.cdc.gov/mmwr/volumes/68/wr/mm6832a3.htm

Centers for Disease Control and Prevention (CDC). (2020a). HIV, HIV Basics, Prevention, PEP (Post-Exposure Prophylaxis). https://www.cdc.gov/hiv/basics/pep/about-pep.html

Centers for Disease Control and Prevention (CDC). (2020b). HIV, HIV Basics, Prevention, PrEP (Pre-Exposure Prophylaxis). https://www.cdc.gov/hiv/basics/prep/about-prep.html

Centers for Disease Control and Prevention. (2021). Sexually transmitted diseases treatment guidelines, 2021. *MMWR: Morbidity and Mortality Weekly Report, 70*(RR-4), 1–187. https://www.cdc.gov/std/treatment-guidelines/STI-Guidelines-2021.pdf

Centers for Disease Control and Prevention (CDC). (2022a). HIV and all gay and bisexual men. https://www.cdc.gov/hiv/group/msm/index.html

Centers for Disease Control and Prevention (CDC). (2022b). HIV and transgendered people. https://www.cdc.gov/hiv/group/gender/transgender/index.html

Fischbach, F., Fischbach, M., & Stout, K. (2022). *A manual of laboratory and diagnostic tests* (11th ed.). Philadelphia, PA: Lippincott Williams & Wilkins.

Gilbert, D. N., Chambers, H. F., Saag, M. S., Pavia, A. T., & Boucher, H. W. (2022). *The Sanford guide to antimicrobial therapy 2022* (52nd ed.). Sperryville, VA: Antimicrobial Therapy, Inc.

Hatcher, R., Trussell, J., Nelson, A., Cates, W., Kowal, D., & Policar, M. (2018). *Contraceptive technology.* (21st ed. rev.). New York, NY: Contraceptive Technology Communications.

Kimberlin, D. W., Brady, M. T., Jackson, M. A., & Long, S. S. (2018). *Red book: 2018 report of the Committee on Infectious Diseases* (31st ed.). Itasca, IL: American Academy of Pediatrics.

Litwin MS, McNaughton-Collins M, Fowler FJ Jr, Nickel JC, Calhoun EA, Pontari MA, Alexander RB, Farrar JT, O'Leary MP. (1999). The National Institutes of Health chronic prostatitis symptom index: development and validation of a new outcome measure. Chronic Prostatitis Collaborative Research Network. J Urol. 162(2):369–75. doi: 10.1016/s0022-5347(05)68562-x. PMID: 10411041.

McAninch, J. W., & Lue, T. F. (2020). *Smith & Tanagho's general urology* (19th ed.). New York, NY: McGraw-Hill.

National Cancer Institute. (2018a). Cancer stat facts: prostate cancer. https://seer.cancer.gov/statfacts/html/prost.html

National Cancer Institute. (2018b). Cancer stat facts: testicular cancer. https://seer.cancer.gov/statfacts/html/testis.html

Papadakis, M. A., McPhee, S. J., & Rabow, M. W. (2023). *Current medical diagnosis & treatment.* New York, NY: McGraw-Hill Education.

U.S. Preventive Services Task Force. (2011). *Clinical summary: Testicular cancer: Screening.* https://www.uspreventiveservicestaskforce.org/uspstf/recommendation/testicular-cancer-screening#fullrecommendationstart

U.S. Preventive Services Task Force. (2018). *Prostate cancer: Screening.* https://www.uspreventiveservicestaskforce.org/uspstf/recommendation/prostate-cancer-screening

U.S. Healthy People 2030. *Healthy people 2030.* Washington, DC: U.S. Department of Health and Human Services. https://health.gov/healthypeople

Visovsky, C. G., Zambroski, C. H., & Lutz, R. M. (2022). *Edmunds' pharmacology for the primary care provider* (54th ed.). St. Louis, MO: Elsevier Mosby.

CHAPTER 13

SEXUALLY TRANSMITTED DISEASES

Cara Curley, DNP, CRNP, WH-BC

General Approach

DESCRIPTION

- Sexually transmitted diseases (STDs) are also known as sexually transmitted infections (STIs).
- 20 million new infections occur annually in the United States.
- In 2020, over half (53%) of reported cases of STDs were among adolescents and young adults ages 15–24 years.
- 32% of all cases of chlamydia, gonorrhea, and P&S syphilis were among non-Hispanic Black persons, even though they made up only approximately 12% of the U.S. population. Men who have sex with men (MSM) are disproportionally impacted by STDs, including P&S syphilis and gonorrhea (CDC, 2020).
- It is important to note that these disparities are unlikely to be explained by differences in sexual behavior and rather reflect differential access to quality sexual health care.
- Acknowledging health inequities affecting STD rates is a critical first step toward empowering affected groups and the public health community to collaborate in addressing systemic inequities in the burden of disease with the goal of minimizing the health impacts of STDs on individuals and populations.
- Several factors have likely contributed to the initial decline in reported STD cases during the first part of 2020, including:
    - Reduced frequency of in-person health care services as routine visits decreased, resulting in less-frequent STD screening;
    - Diversion of public health staff STD work to respond to the coronavirus disease 2019 (COVID-19) pandemic;
    - STD test and laboratory supply shortages;
    - Lapses in health insurance coverage due to unemployment; and
    - Telemedicine practices that led to some infections not being captured in national data.

PREVENTION

- Counsel the adolescent or adult patient regarding sexual abstinence, the only certain method of prevention, followed by mutual monogamy.
- Consistent use of the male latex condom is highly protective if used consistently and correctly.
- Use of female condoms and other barrier methods of contraception for women may be somewhat protective against some, but not all, STDs.
- Safer sex practices are aimed at reducing the risk of HIV transmission for patients at highest risk through partner reduction and avoidance of certain practices.

Risk Assessment

- Risk assessments and screening tests help reduce the incidence of STDs and must be done for every sexually active adult and adolescent patient.
- Adolescents are at a higher risk for STDs.
- Obtain accurate, detailed history from patients to determine the risk for STDs. Most people do not know they are infected with STDs and underestimate their own risk level. Ask specific questions regarding type of sexual exposure in "lay terms" to obtain accurate information. Maintain confidentiality by asking partners and parents to leave the room. No parental consent is needed for adolescents to seek treatment for STDs; the age of consent for adolescents varies by state.
- The Five P's approach for health care providers obtaining sexual histories: partners, practices, protection from sexually transmitted infections, past history of STDs, and pregnancy intention (CDC, 2021b) https://www.cdc.gov/std/treatment-guidelines/STI-Guidelines-2021.pdf
- High-risk factors for STD are current STD(s), including HIV and history of STD(s); multiple sexual partners (or a new partner); individuals who exchange sex for money or drugs; drug users or partners of drug users; MSM; and lack of consistent use of barrier contraceptives.

Screening

- Routine steps for all sexually active (ever) women and men:
    - Explain importance/context of screening because many STDs are asymptomatic: "We review this information and screen all patients because many people with infections do not have symptoms and, therefore, have no idea that testing might be needed. Routine review is recommended by the CDC."

  - ◊ Give prevention information and encourage wise decisions and prevention behavior.
  - ◊ Review personal history for high-risk behaviors.
  - ◊ Provide annual chlamydia test for all patients, regardless of gender, who are 25 years of age or younger.
  - ◊ Women 21 to 29 years of age with no abnormal Pap history should have a Pap test every 3 years and an annual exam that includes a pelvic exam.
  - ◊ Women 30 to 65 years of age with no abnormal history should have a Pap test every 5 years and co-test for cervical cytology and high-risk human papillomavirus (HPV) every 5 years with an annual exam that includes a pelvic exam.
  - ◊ Provide annual test for gonorrhea (gonococcal infection [GC]) test if in an area of high GC prevalence and age 25 years or younger.
  - ◊ If in an area with high syphilis prevalence and patient is age 25 years or younger, or high-risk behavior, initial syphilis serology is recommended.
- Routine steps for high-risk women and men should include offering and encouraging HIV testing, reviewing history, and providing hepatitis B vaccination.
- Patients with known STD exposure or symptoms should be cultured from areas of exposure/penetration (e.g., anal, vaginal, oral pharyngeal, penile/urethral) and then treated.
- Routine screening of pregnant person in first trimester should include syphilis serologic test, hepatitis B antigen, and GC testing; offer HIV test, noting that certain states currently offer opt-out testing.
- Pap smear should follow the same timing regardless of pregnancy status.

Management

- Follow Centers for Disease Control and Prevention (CDC) 2021 treatment guidelines for GC infections for evaluation and management of all STDs. (CDC, 2021b)
- With patients who are likely not to return for follow-up, consider empiric treatment with CDC-recommended one-dose regimen when appropriate.
- Patients treated for STD should be counseled to have their sexual partners evaluated and treated.
- Expedited Partner Therapy (EPT) should be considered and is legal in some states. CDC has up-to-date information regarding EPT for male/female relationships. Limits still for MSM and EPT by current CDC guidelines.
- Sexually active persons should be counseled regarding dual protection against unintended pregnancy and STDs. The male latex condom is effective in providing dual protection if used correctly.

RED FLAGS

- Consult, refer, or hospitalize with unusual presentation of STDs; serious complication such as pelvic inflammatory disease (PID), pregnancy, HIV infection, recurrent infection, unable to tolerate oral medication, or allergy to medication.
- Consider referral to infectious disease specialist for pregnant women with hepatitis B virus (HBV), primary cytomegalovirus (CMV), primary genital herpes, or group B streptococcus infection, and women with syphilis and allergic to penicillin.
- With STDs in pediatric or adolescent populations, screen for child abuse.
- If patient reports sexual assault, consult local law authorities regarding procedures for obtaining evidence. Test for *Trichomonas vaginalis,* bacterial vaginosis (BV), yeast, chlamydia, gonorrhea (GC), HIV, HBV, and syphilis. Empiric antimicrobial regimen for chlamydia, gonorrhea, trichomoniasis, and BV is suggested, as well as prophylactic treatment for hepatitis B, pregnancy testing, and emergency contraception, if indicated.

Infections that Cause Vaginitis and Cervicitis in Women and Urethritis in Men

TRICHOMONIASIS

Description

- An inflammatory process of the vagina, cervix, and vulva in women and lower genitourinary tract in men caused by a flagellate protozoan

Etiology

- The causative organism is *T. vaginalis*
- Usually sexually transmitted; rarely transmitted by fomites
- All genders can be asymptomatic carriers: 70% to 85% of infected

Incidence and Demographics

- Estimated 2.6 million people infected annually, with an incidence rate of over 6 million

Risk Factors

- ◇ Multiple sexual partners (or a new partner)
- ◇ Individuals who exchange sex for money or drugs
- ◇ Drug users or partners of drug users
- ◇ MSM
- ◇ Inconsistent use of barrier contraceptives

Prevention and Screening

- Prevention is listed under General Approach
- No routine screening unless complaints of discharge or high-risk behaviors
- Diagnostic screening for complaints of discharge.
- Trichomoniasis screening should be conducted annually for HIV-infected women.

Assessment

History

- Incubation period is 4 to 20 days, with an average of 1 week.

Women

- May be asymptomatic
- Severe pruritus; malodorous, profuse, gray-yellow, or green vaginal discharge
- Dysuria, dyspareunia, postcoital spotting, possible menorrhagia, and dysmenorrhea
- Onset of symptoms following menses

Men

- Usually asymptomatic
- Dysuria, clear penile discharge, slight penile itching

Physical Exam

Women

- May have inguinal adenopathy
- External genitalia may be irritated from scratching.
- Vulva is erythematous and edematous.
- Introitus, urethra, vagina, and cervix are coated with profuse malodorous, frothy, gray-yellow, or green discharge.
- Cervix or vagina has petechiae or strawberry patch appearance (characteristic).

Men

- Slight penile erythema with clear discharge

Diagnostic Studies

Women

- Saline wet mount of vaginal discharge to identify motile trichomonads
- Vaginal pH higher than 4.5; Pap smear sometimes shows trichomonads
- Potassium hydroxide (KOH) wet mount to rule out *Candida albicans*; positive whiff test (fishy odor) when KOH applied in BV
- Use of nucleic acid amplification tests for the diagnosis should be considered if wet mount is negative

Men

- Microscopic exam of urine positive for trichomonads
- Use of nucleic acid amplification tests for the diagnosis should be considered

Differential Diagnosis

- Bacterial vaginosis
- Vulvovaginal candidiasis

- Gonorrhea
- PID
- *Chlamydia trachomatis*

Management

Nonpharmacologic Treatment

- Concurrent treatment of sex partners
- Persons with trichomoniasis and their sex partners should avoid sex until treatment is completed and symptoms are resolved.
- Screen for other STDs
- Avoid alcohol with metronidazole (Flagyl) and for 72 hours after because of disulfiram-like reaction (severe nausea and vomiting)

Pharmacologic Treatment

- First treatment choice for females: metronidazole (Flagyl) 500 mg orally twice daily for 7 days
- First treatment choice for males: metronidazole (Flagyl) 2 g orally as single dose
- Alternative regimen for male or female: tinidazole (Tindamax) 2 g orally as a single dose or metronidazole (Flagyl) 2 g orally as a single dose or https://www.cdc.gov/std/treatment-guidelines/trichomoniasis.htm

How Long to Treat

- Gender consideration: Female: 7-day regimen; if regimen fails and patient remains symptomatic, retreat with metronidazole (Flagyl) 500 mg orally twice daily for 7 more days or tinidazole (Tindamax) 2 g in a single dose. If there is treatment failure, consider culture for possible resistant strain of *T. vaginalis.* Male: metronidazole (Flagyl) 2 g orally as a single dose. If repeat screen positive, consider metronidazole (Flagyl) 500 mg orally twice daily for 7 days.

Special Considerations

- Pregnancy: treatment metronidazole (Flagyl) 500 mg orally twice daily for 7 days. Studies state tinidazole should be avoided in pregnancy
- Allergy to metronidazole: There is no effective alternative. Clotrimazole (Lotrimin) may inhibit growth of *T. vaginalis* but does not eradicate it.
- *T. vaginalis* might be an incidental finding on a Pap test, neither conventional nor liquid-based Pap smears are considered diagnostic tests for trichomoniasis. This finding should prompt consideration for standard screening.

When to Consult, Refer, Hospitalize

- Refer to infectious disease specialist in refractory cases not responding to treatment in 2 weeks.
- CDC is experienced with susceptibility testing for nitroimidazole-resistant *T. vaginalis* and can provide guidance regarding treatment in cases of drug resistance.

Follow-Up

- None is indicated for males.
- Females should be retested approximately 3 months after completion of therapy.
- Evaluate the treatment for partner(s).

Expected Course

- Response prompt, although symptoms will return with reinfection

Complications

- Nausea or vomiting from oral metronidazole and tinidazole,
- Disulfiram-like reaction from ingestion of alcohol while taking metronidazole and/or tinidazole,
- Vulvovaginal candidiasis infection following 7-day treatment course
- Associated with preterm labor and premature rupture of membranes
- PID, bartholinitis, skenitis, cystitis

GONORRHEA

Description

- A sexually transmitted bacterial disease caused by *Neisseria gonorrhoeae*
- 2020 rate of infection is 677,769 cases in the United States.

Etiology

- *N. gonorrhoeae* is gram-negative diplococci present in penial exudate and vaginal secretions of infected mucous secretions occurring only in humans.
- Causes localized inflammatory conditions: urethritis, epididymitis, proctitis, cervicitis, bartholinitis, PID (salpingitis and/or endometritis), and pharyngitis in adults; vulvovaginitis in children; and conjunctivitis in newborns and adults; presence in children almost always a result of child sexual abuse
- Gonococcal bacteremia results in the disseminated systemic condition; arthritis–dermatitis syndrome sometimes associated with endocarditis or meningitis.

Incidence and Demographics

- Transmission through intimate contact such as sexual intercourse; also, parturition
- 60% to 90% of women become infected following exposure
- Greatest incidence in sexually active people 15 to 29 years of age
- Approximately 15% of infected women may develop PID with possible sterility if untreated.
- Most infections in men have symptoms that cause them to seek treatment before serious outcome. Many infected women do not have symptoms until complications are present.
- Common sites in women are the urethra, endocervix, upper genital tract, pharynx, and rectum.
- Common sites in men are the urethra, epididymis, prostate, rectum, and pharynx.

Risk Factors

- Multiple sexual partners (or a new partner)
- Individuals who exchange sex for money or drugs

- Drug users or partners of drug users
- MSM
- Inconsistent use of barrier contraceptives

Prevention and Screening

- Prevention methods are listed under General Approach.
- Yearly screening for sexually active women 25 years old and younger if in an area of high GC prevalence or high-risk behaviors regardless of age
- Yearly screening for sexually active MSM; screen more frequently for men who have multiple or anonymous partners
- Screen all pregnant women at initial prenatal visit and again in third trimester.
- Prophylactic treatment for contacts of infectious patients
- A recent travel history with sexual contacts outside the United States should be part of any gonorrhea evaluation.

Assessment

History

- Incubation is short: urethritis is 2 to 5 days; cervicitis is 5 to 10 days.
- Women: often asymptomatic; dysuria, frequency, purulent urethral discharge, vaginal discharge, pelvic pain, spotting or abnormal menses; adolescent girls often have dissemination/progression within a week of menses
- Male: could be asymptomatic; dysuria, urinary frequency, copious purulent (blood tinged) penile discharge, testicular pain; rectal symptoms: erythematous, discharge, pain with defecation
- Both may have conjunctivitis or pharyngitis as well

Physical Exam

- Women: purulent discharge from cervix, inflammation of Bartholin's glands; positive cervical motion tenderness (CMT) and signs of PID if untreated

- Men: purulent urethral discharge; signs of prostatitis or epididymitis if untreated
- Disseminated gonorrhea: Stage 1, bacteremia with chills, fever, skin lesions (petechial or pustular skin rash); endocarditis or meningitis may occur. Stage 2, septic arthritis; knees, ankles, and wrists show erythema, edema, and pain.

Diagnostic Studies

- Cervical or urethral culture for *N. gonorrhoeae*
- Nucleic acid amplification test on urine in all patients can be used
- DNA probe (can diagnose gonorrhea and chlamydia) for all patients

Differential Diagnosis

- PID
- Nongonococcal cervicitis
- Urethritis
- Proctitis
- Nongonococcal pharyngitis
- *Chlamydia* infections
- Arthritis
- Vaginitis

Management

- *Pharmacologic Treatment*
- Uncomplicated gonococcal infections (genital, rectal, and pharyngeal)
    - ◇ Ceftriaxone (Rocephin) 500 mg IM in a single dose for patients under 150 kg or for persons weighing ≥150 kg, 1 g ceftriaxone should be administered
- If chlamydial infection has not been excluded, treat for chlamydia with doxycycline 100 mg orally 2 times/day for 7 days
- If ceftriaxone is not available:
    - ◇ Cefixime 800 mg orally in a single dose

- Mild to moderate PID treated as an outpatient: ceftriaxone 1 g IV every 24 hours, plus doxycycline 100 mg orally or IV every 12 hours plus metronidazole 500 mg orally or IV every 12 hours
  - ALTERNATIVE: Cefotetan 2 g IV every 12 hours plus doxycycline 100 mg orally or IV every 12 hours
  - or Cefoxitin 2 g IV every 6 hours plus doxycycline 100 mg orally or IV every 12 hours
- Gonococcal conjunctivitis: lavage of infected eye with saline solution once; plus ceftriaxone (Rocephin) 1 g IM
- Neonates without symptoms: ceftriaxone 25–50 mg/kg body weight by IV or IM in a single dose, not to exceed 250 mg
  - Infants with gonococcal conjunctivitis: ceftriaxone (Rocephin) 25 to 50 mg/kg IV or IM, not to exceed 250 mg in a single dose
  - Gonococcal infection in children who weigh more than 45 kg: treat the same as adults
  - Gonococcal infection in children who weigh 45 kg or less: ceftriaxone 25–50 mg/kg body weight IV or IM in a single dose, not to exceed 250 mg IM

Special Considerations

- Pregnant/lactating women should not be treated with quinolones or tetracycline. If a pregnant woman cannot tolerate cephalosporins and spectinomycin is not available, consult infectious disease specialists.
- All infants born with neonatal ophthalmia should be observed for gonococcal sepsis, disseminated infection.
- All children found to have GC infection should be tested for Chlamydia trachomatis (CT), syphilis, and HIV.
- Shared decision-making for EPT should be considered routine partner management strategy in MSM with gonococcal infections.
- All persons with a GC diagnosis should be tested for other STDs including Chlamydia trachomatis (CT), syphilis, and HIV. If HIV testing is negative, consideration for HIV pre-exposure prophylaxis (PrEP) should be made (CDC 2021a).

When to Consult, Refer, Hospitalize

- Hospitalize for disseminated gonorrhea
- Hospitalize for severe PID
- Refer patients who are unresponsive to treatment

- Consider state mandatory reporting laws if child presents with infection.
- Retest in 3 months following treatment.

Expected Course

- Usually there is prompt response to therapy.

Complications

- PID, sterility, salpingitis, epididymitis, prostatitis, disseminated gonococcal infection
- Perinatal postabortion endometritis and salpingitis, acute salpingitis, increased incidence of premature rupture of membranes, preterm delivery, chorioamnionitis, neonatal sepsis, postpartum sepsis, neonatal conjunctivitis
- May help facilitate HIV transmission

CHLAMYDIAL INFECTION

Description

- A sexually transmitted infection caused by *Chlamydia trachomatis*

Etiology

- *C. trachomatis* is an obligate intracellular parasite; transmission is by sexual or perinatal contact.
- Infection in women may ascend from cervicitis and urethritis to salpingitis and spread vertically to cause proctitis; in men, it may ascend the urogenital tract to epididymis and prostate.

Incidence and Demographics

- The most common STD: prevalence is highest in persons age 24 or younger.
- In 2020 a total of 1,579,885 cases of *C. trachomatis* infection were reported to the CDC.
- Leading cause of infertility, ectopic pregnancy, and PID. Reportable to local health authority; case report required in most U.S. states.

Risk Factors

- Multiple sexual partners (or a new partner)
- Individuals who exchange sex for money or drugs
- Drug users or partners of drug users
- MSM
- Inconsistent use of barrier contraceptives
- Presence of concomitant STD, especially *N. gonorrhoeae*

Prevention and Screening

- Prevention methods are listed under General Approach.
- Annually screen sexually active women 25 years of age or younger.
- Male screening for younger males is not routinely recommended except MSM or at-risk behaviors.
- Screen pregnant women initially and repeat in the third trimester for high-risk women.

Assessment

History

- Incubation 6 to 14 days
- May be asymptomatic
- Women: increase in mucopurulent vaginal discharge, low pelvic discomfort, dysuria, urinary frequency, spotting, and possibly dyspareunia; incubation period usually 1 week
- Men: mucopurulent urethra discharge or dysuria

Physical Exam

- Cervix with contact bleeding, mucopurulent discharge; may have positive CMT, or adnexal or uterine tenderness if untreated
- Occasional inguinal lymphadenopathy

Diagnostic Studies

- *Chlamydia* culture is definitive test but expensive.
- DNA probe
- Nucleic acid amplification (polymerase chain reaction [PCR] and ligase chain reaction (LCR) in men on first-void urine; can also be used in women but less accurate. Preferred screening through vaginal swab.

Differential Diagnosis

- PID
- Gonorrhea
- Salpingitis
- Urethritis

Management

Nonpharmacologic Treatment

- Sexual partners should be evaluated and treated.
- Patients should abstain from sexual intercourse until they and their sex partners have completed treatment; 7 days following single-dose treatment or after completion of a 7-day regimen.

Pharmacologic Treatment

- First choice: doxycycline 100 mg orally twice daily for 7 days
- Alternative: azithromycin 1 g single dose or levofloxacin 500 mg daily for 7 days

How Long to Treat

- 7-day course of doxycycline preferred

Special Considerations

- Neonatal ophthalmia and pneumonia may occur in infants born to infected mothers; consult and treat with erythromycin IV.
- Doxycycline and ofloxacin are contraindicated in pregnancy.
- Ofloxacin is contraindicated in patients 17 years or younger.
  - Pregnancy: azithromycin 1 g orally in a single dose *or* amoxicillin 500 mg orally three times daily for 7 days
- For Infants and Children Who Weigh less than 45 kg: Erythromycin base or ethyl succinate 50 mg/kg body weight/day orally divided into four doses daily for 14 days. Data are limited regarding the effectiveness and optimal dose of azithromycin for treating chlamydial infection among infants and children weighing less than45 kg.
- For children weighing 45 kg or more but younger than 8 years old: azithromycin 1 g orally in a single dose
- For children aged 8 years or older: azithromycin 1 g orally in a single dose or doxycycline 100 mg orally 2 times/day for 7 days

When to Consult, Refer, Hospitalize

- Consult with physician for PID in pregnant women, recurrent infection, conjunctivitis, or neonatal infection.
- Consider state mandatory reporting laws if child presents with infection.

Follow-Up

- Recommended repeat screening for reinfection risk for all patients at 3 months
- Pregnant women need repeat cultures approximately 4 weeks after therapy completion secondary to sequelae that can occur in both mothers and neonates if infection persists
- Testing for other STD should be completed for GC, syphilis, and HIV. If HIV negative should have discussion regarding possible HIV PrEP

Expected Course

- Prompt resolution of symptoms
- May become re-infected if sexual partners are not treated

Complications

- PID, infertility, increased incidence of ectopic pregnancy; may help facilitate HIV transmission

MUCOPURULENT CERVICITIS

Description

- A sexually transmitted infection syndrome characterized by purulent discharge visualized on the cervix or in the endocervical canal, endocervical swab, and/or sustained endocervical bleeding easily induced by gentle passage of a cotton swab through the cervical os

Etiology

- May be caused by *C. trachomatis* and *N. gonorrhoeae;* in one-third of cases, agent cannot be established
- *Ureaplasma* (related to *Mycoplasma hominis)* may be the responsible organism

Incidence and Demographics

- Common in sexually active, especially young women

Risk Factors

- Same as for chlamydia and gonorrhea
- May be associated with frequent douching or exposure to chemical irritants
    - Multiple sexual partners (or a new partner)
    - Individuals who exchange sex for money or drugs
    - Drug users or partners of drug users
    - MSM
    - Inconsistent use of barrier contraceptives

Prevention and Screening

- Prevention methods are listed under General Approach.
- Screening for *Chlamydia, N. gonorrhoeae*, BV, and trichomoniasis

Assessment

History

- Often asymptomatic, abnormal vaginal discharge, vaginal bleeding postcoital

Physical Exam

- Cervix has purulent or mucopurulent exudate and has contact bleeding.

Diagnostic Studies

- DNA probe to test for *N. gonorrhoeae* and *Chlamydia*
- Testing for *Trichomonas*
- A finding of leukorrhea (higher than10 WBC/high-power field [HPF]) on wet mount has been associated with *Chlamydia* or gonococcal infection of the cervix.
- Urine for culture and sensitivity

Differential Diagnosis

- *Gonorrhoeae*
- *Trichomonas*
- PID
- Urinary tract infection (UTI)
- *Chlamydia*

Management

Pharmacologic Treatment

- Treat according to suspicion for chlamydia and/or gonorrhea. Wait for test results if prevalence of both organisms is low and chance for follow-up is good.
- See treatment for gonococcal and chlamydial infections.

How Long to Treat

- Treatment for chlamydia and potentially gonorrhea single dose to 7 days per CDC guidelines
- Doxycycline 100 mg orally 2 times/day for 7 days or azithromycin 1 g single dose

Special Considerations

- Treat pregnant women with cephalosporin, erythromycin, or amoxicillin, not with quinolones or tetracycline.

When to Consult, Refer, Hospitalize

- Consult for recurrent infection.

Follow-Up

- Recommended for gonorrhea or chlamydia as appropriate
- If symptoms persist, patient should refrain from sexual activity and return for evaluation.
- Sexual partners should be examined and treated for STDs.

Expected Course

- Prompt response to treatment is expected.

Complications

- Depending on organism, same as for gonococcal or chlamydial infections

NONGONOCOCCAL URETHRITIS (NGU)

Description

- Inflammation of the urethra caused by a nongonorrheal infection characterized by mucopurulent or purulent discharge and burning

Etiology

- Nongonococcal urethritis (NGU) if gram-negative intracellular organisms are not identified on Gram stain
- *C. trachomatis* is the major cause (approximately 50%).
- Etiology of non-*Chlamydia*l NGU is unknown; however, *Ureaplasma urealyticum* and possible *Mycoplasma genitalium* may be present in as many as one-third of cases.
- Sometimes *T. vaginalis* (1%–8%) and herpes simplex virus (HSV) cause NGU.

Incidence and Demographics

- Most common STD syndrome in males living in industrialized countries
- NGU more common than gonococcal urethritis in most areas of United States
- Proportion of NGU cases caused by *Chlamydia* has been declining gradually.

Risk Factors

- Multiple sexual partners (or a new partner)
- Individuals who exchange sex for money or drugs
- Drug users or partners of drug users
- MSM
- Inconsistent use of barrier contraceptives

Prevention and Screening

- Prevention methods are listed under General Approach.
- Screening for gonorrhea and chlamydia (see General Approach)

Assessment

History

- Patient reports urethral discharge that is purulent or mucopurulent, dysuria, urethral itching
- Recent unprotected sexual activity or new sex partner

Physical Exam

- Urethra erythematous and positive for purulent or mucopurulent discharge

Diagnostic Studies

- Gram stain of urethral secretions has 5 or more WBCs/HPF without intracellular gram-negative diplococci
- Positive leukocyte esterase test on first-void urine, or microscopic exam of first-void urine positive for 10 or higher WBCs/HPF
- DNA probe test for *N. gonorrhoeae* and *C. trachomatis*
- Nucleic acid amplification test for *N. gonorrhoeae* and *Chlamydia* on urine sample

Differential Diagnosis

- Gonorrhea
- UTI
- Trichomoniasis

Management

Nonpharmacologic Treatment

- Sexual partners should be evaluated and treated appropriately.

Pharmacologic Treatment

- Defer treatment if no confirmation of urethritis until results of DNA probe are available.
- Treat for *Chlamydia* (see Chlamydial Infection) as indicated.
- Empiric treatment of symptoms for high-risk patients is unlikely to return for follow-up.
- Empiric treatment covers infection with gonorrhea and chlamydia (refer to those entries).

How Long to Treat

- Treatment should be initiated immediately after diagnosis.
- Doxycycline 100 mg twice daily for 7 days or alternate therapy of azithromycin 1 g oral single dose or azithromycin 500 mg single dose, then 250 mg orally daily for 4 days

Special Considerations

- None

When to Consult, Refer, Hospitalize

- Refer when persistent or recurrent urethritis following adequate treatment

Follow-Up

- Not necessary if resolves
- All sexual partners within the preceding 60 days should be referred for evaluation.

Expected Course

- Symptoms should be alleviated soon after treatment initiated.

Complications

- Epididymitis, prostatitis, and Reiter syndrome may help facilitate HIV transmission.

PELVIC INFLAMMATORY DISEASE, CANDIDIASIS, BACTERIAL VAGINOSIS

See Chapter 11, Female Reproductive System Disorders.

Viral Infections

GENITAL HERPES SIMPLEX VIRUS (HSV) INFECTION

Description

- Genital infection, mainly herpes simplex virus 2 (HSV-2) and, less often, herpes simplex virus 1 (HSV-1)
- May present as a primary, latent, or recurrent disease
- No cure

Etiology

- HSV infection is transmitted through direct contact with mucous membranes and secretions.
- Primary infection causes local viral replication, seeding of regional neural ganglia, and possible viremia.
- Herpes viruses establish lifelong latency in neural ganglia and periodically reactivate.
- Up to 50% of first-episode cases of genital herpes are caused by HSV-1, but recurrences and subclinical shedding are much less frequent for genital HSV-1 infection than genital HSV-2 infection.
- Many HSV-2 infected people have not received a diagnosis of genital herpes and are unaware of transmission.

Incidence and Demographics

- 50 million people are infected with herpes in the United States.
- HSV is endemic in the United States, with 776,000 new cases per year.
- 11.9% of people aged 14 to 49 years have HSV infections.
- The highest frequency is in people aged 15 to 29.

Risk Factors

- Listed under General Approach

Prevention and Screening

- Prevention methods listed under General Approach; however, condoms may not block transmission of some lesions.
- Infected people should abstain from all sexual activity when lesions or prodromal symptoms are present.
- Sexual transmission of HSV can occur during asymptomatic periods. Asymptomatic viral shedding is more frequent in genital HSV-2 infection than genital HSV-1 infection and is most frequent during the first 12 months after acquiring HSV-2.
- Can consider a suppressive dosing to decrease risk of viral shedding although effectiveness of this strategy in pregnancy has not been studied thus consideration and discussion should occur for discordant pregnant couples to consider risk of infection in pregnancy if person carrying pregnancy is negative
- Advise use of condoms during all sexual exposures; however, may not eliminate possibility of transmission.
- Patients should be informed about the risks of neonatal infection.
- No routine screening

Assessment

History

- Genital lesions (occurring 2 to 14 days after exposure), which are painful papules followed by vesicles, ulceration, crusting, and healing

- First-episode symptoms consist of hyperesthesia, burning, itching, dysuria, pain, and tenderness in genital area; fever, myalgia, malaise, lymphadenopathy. Healing of initial lesions takes up to 21 days (average is 12 days).
- Recurrent episodes usually have *prodrome* (unusual sensation in area before eruption of lesions), recur in same region, and length of shedding is reduced (average 7 days). Healing occurs in approximately 5 days.

Physical Exam

- Examination of genital area for characteristic herpetic lesions: tender vesicles on erythematous bases or ulcers in various stages of progression
- Enlarged lymph nodes in inguinal area

Diagnostic Studies

- Viral detection or culture from early lesion or vesicle is most sensitive and permits viral typing, which is helpful for prognostic information (HSV-1 has much lower risk for symptomatic recurrent outbreaks).

Differential Diagnosis

- Syphilis
- Chancroid
- *Molluscum contagiosum*
- Folliculitis
- Trauma, burn

Management

Nonpharmacologic Treatment

- Cool perineal compresses, sitz baths, loose-fitting clothes to help alleviate pain
- Good handwashing and hygiene to reduce autoinoculation to other body regions

Pharmacologic Treatment

- Topical acyclovir is less effective than oral; use is discouraged
- First episode:
  - acyclovir (Zovirax) 400 mg orally twice a day *or*
  - famciclovir (Famvir) 250 mg orally 3 times a day *or* valacyclovir (Valtrex) 1 g orally twice a day Treat 7–10 days.
- Recurrent infection:
  - valacyclovir 500 mg twice a day for 3 days *or*
  - acyclovir 800 mg orally 2 times a day × 5 days *or*
  - acyclovir 800 mg orally three times a day × 2 days *or*
  - famciclovir 125 mg orally twice a day × 5 days *or*
  - Famciclovir 1,000 mg orally twice a day × 1 day *or*
  - famciclovir 500 mg once, followed by 250 mg 2 times daily for 2 days or
  - valacyclovir 1 g daily for 5 days
- Analgesics such as acetaminophen, NSAIDs, and topical astringents

How Long to Treat

- For first episode: 7 to 10 days or longer if lesions not completely healed
- For recurrent episode: 1 to 5 days
- Daily suppressive therapy: after 1 year of therapy, consider discontinuation to assess rate of recurrent episodes.
- For episodic recurrent infection, start treatment during prodrome or within 1 day after onset of lesions.

Special Considerations

- HIV+ or immunocompromised: acyclovir 400 to 800 mg orally 2 to 3 times a day *or* famciclovir 500 mg orally twice a day *or* valacyclovir 500 mg orally twice a day until clinically resolved; if severe, treat as for severe infection. If resistance is suspected, consult with HIV specialist.
- All acyclovir-resistant strains are also resistant to valacyclovir; most are resistant to famciclovir.

- First clinical episode during pregnancy may be treated with acyclovir. Safety of acyclovir, valacyclovir, and famciclovir in pregnancy not established; benefits must outweigh risks.
- Suppressive dosing of pregnant patients is valacyclovir 500 mg twice a day or acyclovir 400 mg three times a day from 36 weeks gestation through delivery.
- Prophylactic administration of acyclovir intrapartum for women with a history of HSV is not recommended.
- Cesarean delivery is not always necessary with history of herpes; only recommended when active lesions visible at onset of labor. Cesarean delivery may be consider if a new diagnosis of HSV is made within short duration to delivery.
- Signs of congenital infection may occur from birth to 4 to 6 weeks (vesicles around eyes, mouth, skin; respiratory distress; central nervous system [CNS] infection; sepsis).

When to Consult, Refer, Hospitalize

- Consult if pregnant, serious infection, or infections resistant to treatment
- Hospitalize if suspected encephalitis, pneumonitis, or hepatitis, or congenital infection

Follow-Up

Expected Course

- Most symptoms reduce promptly.
- Usually none indicated unless severe recurrent episodes and treatment inadequate

Complications

- Encephalitis, blindness, pneumonitis, hepatitis, perinatal transmission

HUMAN PAPILLOMAVIRUS INFECTION

Description

- Infection with certain subtypes of the human papillomavirus (HPV or genital warts) causing flat, papular, or pedunculated growths on the genital mucosa
- Visible warts are known as condyloma acuminata.

Etiology

- Virus enters body during sexual activity, via an epithelial defect, and infects stratified squamous epithelium of lower genital tract; visible genital warts are usually caused by HPV types 6 or 11
- HPV infection usually persists throughout patient's life in dormant state and becomes infectious intermittently; generally benign, may be asymptomatic or cause minor symptoms
- Highly contagious; 90% to 100% of male partners of infected women become infected, most cases are subclinical
- HPV infections with types 16, 18, and 31 strongly associated with cervical dysplasia
- HPV implicated in epithelial cancers, especially anorectal carcinoma, vulvar or penile cancer

Incidence and Demographics

- 79 million men and women are currently infected with HPV.
- 14 million men and women are infected annually.
- About 355,000 people are infected with genital warts yearly.
- More than 40 HPV types can infect the genital area.
- Most common viral STD in the United States
- Approximately 33,700 cancers annually can be attributed to HPV.

Risk Factors

- Multiple sexual partners (or a new partner)
- Individuals who exchange sex for money or drugs
- Drug users or partners of drug users
- MSM
    - lack of barrier methods for contraception
    - early coitus
    - Growth of warts may be stimulated by oral contraceptives, pregnancy, or immunosuppression.

Prevention and Screening

- Prevention methods listed under general approach; however, condoms may not eliminate risk of transmission entirely; patient with HPV still infectious even after warts removed
- Screening of women through Pap smear following previously reviewed intervals
- As of 2016 the 9-valent HPV (9vHPV) vaccine is available dosing available in the United States
- HPV vaccine is recommended for patients 9 to 26 years of age. Shared risk decision making dosing for patients through age 45 was recommended starting in 2019. Vaccine not recommended in pregnant individuals but is considered acceptable in breastfeeding patients.
- HPV vaccine administration is a two dose series if given in 9- to14-year-olds. Second dose administered is 6 to 12 months after dose 1. If administered to patient over age 14 or immunocompromised patient, then doses should be given at months 0, 1–2, and 6. If series is interrupted, then can complete and not repeat earlier doses.

Assessment

History

- Usually asymptomatic or can cause palpable lesion, itching, burning, local pain, or bleeding
- Significant lesions in some individuals
- May be unknown history of contact, incubation period from weeks to a year or longer

Physical Exam

- Small, flesh-colored, wart-like lesions; some can become confluent as one large wart
- Some warts are flat or difficult to visualize; others are vegetative growths
- Women: warts seen on labia, perianal areas, vagina, cervix, or mouth
- Men: warts seen on shaft of penis, penile meatus, scrotum, perianal areas, and mouth

Diagnostic Studies

- Most warts are diagnosed by visualization.
- Pap smear on women detects koilocytosis, indicative of HPV.

- Should test for concomitant STDs: HIV, gonorrhea, syphilis, chlamydia
- Biopsy for detection of viral DNA available but not used clinically

Differential Diagnosis

- Condyloma latum
- Neoplasm
- Granuloma inguinale
- Moles
- HSV
- Syphilis
- Folliculitis
- Skin tags
- Keratosis
- Scabetic nodules

Management

Nonpharmacologic Treatment

- Smoking is a cofactor for cervical cancer with HPV; encourage cessation for woman infected with HPV.
- Examination of sexual partners is not recommended because partner's role in reinfection is minimal.
- Encourage continued use of condoms.

Pharmacologic Treatment

- Drugs treat symptoms and may decrease size of wart; no treatment available that completely eradicates virus
- External/perianal warts
    - Patient-applied podofilox (Condylox) 0.5% solution or gel (apply twice a day × 3 days, then off 4 days); may repeat cycle total of 4 times *or*

- ◊ Imiquimod (Aldara) 5% cream: Apply q.h.s. 3 × week; wash off after 6 to 10 hours. May use up to 16 weeks, may clear in 8 to 10 weeks.
- ◊ Provider-administered cryotherapy with liquid nitrogen, may repeat every 1 to 2 weeks
- ◊ Provider-administered podophyllin (Podofin) 10% to 25% in compound tincture of benzoin (wash off thoroughly 1 to 4 hours after application). Repeat weekly if necessary, *or*
- ◊ Provider-administered trichloroacetic acid (TCA) 80% to 90%; apply only to warts. Powder with talc or baking soda to remove untreated acid. Repeat weekly if necessary.

- *How Long to Treat*
- Depending on the size of wart and response to treatment, could take one to several treatments.

Special Considerations

- Pregnancy: Podophyllin, imiquimod, and podofilox are contraindicated.
- Some specialists recommend removal of visible warts during pregnancy.
- HIV patients may not respond well to treatment.

When to Consult, Refer, Hospitalize

- Vaginal and cervical warts: Consult with gynecologist; dysplasia must be excluded before treatment instituted.
- Warts on rectal mucosa should be referred to proctologist.
- Refer women with large warts (larger than 2 cm) to gynecologist for treatment with CO_2 laser, electrodesiccation, electrocautery, cryocautery, or LEEP (loop electrosurgical excision procedure [gynecologic surgery]).

Follow-Up

- During therapy, women should continue to have regular interval Pap smears

Expected Course

- Treatment of warts may require several visits for provider-administered treatment.
- Genital warts can resolve on their own, remain unchanged, or continue to grow untreated.
- Reoccurrence of warts is common, especially within the first 3 months following treatment.

Complications

- Cervical dysplasia and cervical squamous cell carcinoma; invasive carcinoma of vulva and penis
- Anal squamous cell carcinoma of bi-/homosexual males
- Scarring from treatment procedures

Other Sexually Transmitted Infections

SYPHILIS

Description

- Sexually transmitted disease affecting many organs throughout body, caused by *Treponema pallidum*
- Clinical stages include primary, secondary, early latent (up to 1 year duration), late latent, tertiary
- Transmitted via a syphilitic chancre during vaginal, anal, or oral sexual contact.
- Syphilitic chancres appear mainly on the external genitalia, vagina, anus, or rectum but may also appear on the lips and in the mouth.
- Chancres may go unnoticed or unrecognized; therefore, syphilis may be passed on from infected individuals who are unaware of the infection.

Etiology

- *T. pallidum:* Spirochete that invades the human body by penetrating intact skin or mucous membrane during sexual contact

- Once inside body, rapidly multiplies and spreads to regional lymph nodes
- Congenital: Occurs from transplacental passage of organism occurring any time during gestation; can result in spontaneous abortion (second trimester), stillbirth

Incidence and Demographics

- Although males have higher incidence, the rates in females have been steadily climbing.
- Approximately 133,945 new cases were reported in the United States in 2020 (CDC,2023).
- The congenital syphilis rate has increased in recent years. In 2020, rates of congenital syphilis were at 57.3 cases per 100,000 live births. This increase is likely related to an increase in infection in reproductive age females.

Risk Factors

- Multiple sexual partners (or a new partner)
- Individuals who exchange sex for money or drugs
- Drug users or partners of drug users
- MSM
- Lack of use or inconsistent use barrier methods for contraception

Prevention and Screening

- Prevention methods listed under General Approach
- Early diagnosis and treatment with partner notification and treatment
- Routine screening for persons 25 years or younger in high-prevalence areas; also screen persons with other STDs or reported high-risk behaviors
- Pregnancy: screening at first prenatal visit, then repeat for high-risk population at approximately 28 weeks and delivery

Assessment

- *History and Physical Exam* (see Table 13–1)

TABLE 13–1.
STAGES OF ACQUIRED SYPHILIS

PRIMARY	SECONDARY	LATENT	TERTIARY
Painless ulcer or chancre at site of inoculation 3–4 weeks after exposure Extragenital lesions such as lips or breast may be painful Primary chancre is highly infectious, heals spontaneously after 1–5 weeks and patient may not seek treatment	Rash is macular, papular, annular, or follicular (rarely pustular) and often present on palms and soles In warm, moist areas, may develop broad flat lesions (condyloma lata) Rash lasts 2–6 weeks and then heals spontaneously Mucous patches appear as elevated plaques covered with a white or gray pseudomembrane in mouth, throat, on cervix, and labial mucosa. Generalized lymphadenopathy Arthralgias/myalgias and "flu-like" symptoms	Begins with healing of the lesions in secondary stage Early latent less than1 year (infectious) Late latent more than1 year (noninfectious) Sometimes difficult to distinguish early latent from late latent stage due to unknown duration of symptoms Meningitis Cardiovascular disease, arthritis, neurologic lesions Often asymptomatic	Gummatous formation, cardiovascular or neurosyphilis

- Primary
  - Incubation is approximately 3 weeks and ranges from 10 to 90 days after exposure.
  - Painless, indurated ulcer (chancre) at site of inoculation *is* highly infectious, heals spontaneously after 1 to 5 weeks, and patient may not seek treatment; may be regional lymphadenopathy.
  - Extragenital (lips, breast) lesions may be painful.
- Secondary
  - May occur from 6 weeks to 6 months after primary stage; most contagious
  - Rash is macular, papular, annular, or follicular and is often present on palms and soles.
  - Rash lasts 2 to 6 weeks, then heals spontaneously.
  - Moist, raised lesions of the skin (condyloma lata) and mucous patches in mouth and throat, and on cervix
  - Generalized lymphadenopathy
  - Arthralgias/myalgias and "flu-like" symptoms

- Latent
  - Asymptomatic, begins with the end of secondary symptoms
  - Early latent less than 1 year (infectious)
  - Late latent more than 1 year (noninfectious)
  - Difficult to distinguish early latent from late latent stage if unknown duration of symptoms
- Tertiary
  - Gummatous formation, cardiovascular or neurosyphilis
- Congenital: asymptomatic until age 2; failure to thrive, skin rash, jaundice, rhinitis, hepatosplenomegaly

Diagnostic Studies

- Definitive method: darkfield microscopy and direct fluorescent antibody tests of lesion exudate or tissue

  Serologic tests: rapid plasm regain (RPR), venereal disease research laboratory test (VDRL) for initial testing and titers, fluorescent treponemal antibody absorption test (FTA-ABS), microhemagglutination assay forTreponema pallidum antibodies (MHA-TP) to confirm diagnosis in people with positive RPR orVDRL
- For sequential serologic tests, use the same test (VDRL or RPR); titer will decrease with time and treatment.
- Fourfold increase in titer indicates new infection.
- Failure to achieve fourfold decrease in titer in 1 year indicates failed treatment.
- Latent syphilis of more than 1 year's duration, cardiovascular syphilis, and neurosyphilis: serologic tests and lumbar puncture with tests on cerebrospinal fluid (CSF)
- Test for other STDs: HIV, gonorrhea, chlamydia

Differential Diagnosis

- Genital ulcers
- Genital herpes
- Chancroid
- Neoplasm

- Lymphogranuloma venereum
- Superficial fungal infections

Management

Nonpharmacologic Treatment

- Abstain from sexual activity until treatment is complete.
- Early infection (primary, secondary, and early latent) and congenital syphilis reportable in all U.S. states

Pharmacologic Treatment

- Patients exposed sexually to a patient who has syphilis in any stage should be evaluated clinically and serologically and treated in the following cases:
  - ◊ People exposed within 90 days preceding a diagnosis of primary, secondary, or early latent stages in a sex partner, even if seronegative
  - ◊ People exposed more than 90 days before the diagnosis of primary, secondary, or latent stages in a sex partner and in whom serologic test results are not available immediately and the opportunity for follow-up is uncertain
  - ◊ For purposes of partner notification and presumptive treatment of exposed sex partners, patients with unknown duration of illness and high serologic test titers (1:32 or higher) may be considered as having early syphilis.
- Patients with symptoms or history of symptoms and positive diagnostic studies; see Table 13–2

Special Considerations

- The U.S. Food and Drug Administration (FDA) issued an alert that possible false reactivity, or "false-positive" Rapid Plasma Reagin (RPR; non-treponemal) test results, when using the Bio-Rad Laboratories BioPlex 2200 Syphilis Total & RPR kit, can occur in some people who received a COVID-19 vaccine (CDC, 2021c).
- HIV-infected people
  - ◊ Serologic tests and interpretation the same as for HIV-infected patients
  - ◊ When clinical finding suggests syphilis, but serologic tested nonreactive or unclear, use alternate test such as biopsy of lesion, darkfield examination, or direct fluorescent antibody staining of lesion material

TABLE 13–2. RECOMMENDED TREATMENT OF ACQUIRED SYPHILIS

STAGE OF DISEASE	TREATMENT REGIMEN
Primary, secondary, and early latent disease	Benzathine penicillin G 2.4 million units IM in single dose Penicillin-allergic patients: doxycycline 100 mg twice a day × 28 days, or tetracycline 500 mg orally four times a day × 28 days Recommended for **syphilis in infants and children**: benzathine penicillin G 50,000 units/kg body weight IM, up to the adult dose of 2.4 million units in a single dose. From https://www.cdc.gov/std/treatment-guidelines/p-and-s-syphilis.htm
Late latent syphilis or syphilis of unknown duration	Benzathine penicillin G 2.4 million units IM × 3 each at 1-week intervals Penicillin-allergic patients: doxycycline 100 mg orally twice a day for 4 weeks, or tetracycline 500 mg orally four times a day for 4 weeks
Tertiary disease, excluding neurosyphilis	As for late latent disease, with appropriate management of complications
Neurosyphilis	Aqueous cystamine penicillin G, 18 to 24 million units/day given as 3 to 4 million units IV every 4 hours for 10 to 14 days, or procaine penicillin 2.4 million units IM a day plus probenecid (Benemid) 500 mg orally four times a day, both for 10 to 14 days

- ◊ Treatment the same as for HIV-negative patient
- ◊ Neurosyphilis must be considered in differential for HIV+ patients. CSF examination should be performed on HIV-infected people who show mental status changes or have either late latent syphilis or syphilis of unknown duration.
- ◊ Penicillin must be used to treat; if penicillin-allergic, must be desensitized
- ◊ Primary and secondary syphilis should have VDRL/RPR serology at 3, 6, 9, 12, and 24 months to evaluate for treatment failure. If titer increased fourfold, fails to decrease fourfold at 3 months, or symptoms persist, re-treatment is indicated.

- ♦ Pregnancy: Treat for appropriate stage of syphilis.
  - ◊ Some experts recommend a second dose of benzathine penicillin 2.4 million units IM 1 week after initial dose for pregnant women with primary, secondary, or early latent syphilis. If penicillin-allergic, desensitize patient to penicillin.
  - ◊ Women treated in second trimester are at risk for premature labor and/or fetal distress.

- Infants born to mothers with positive nontreponemal and treponemal tests
    - If infant was born to mother who tests positive for syphilis but adequate treatment with penicillin is not documented, the infant should be observed for congenital syphilis (into early childhood).
    - Routine physical exams for rash, hepatomegaly, lymphadenopathy, persistent rhinitis
    - Quantitative nontreponemal test on infant's blood (not cord blood)
    - CSF testing, long bone X-rays, and other testing may be indicated.
- All patients may experience the Jarisch-Herxheimer reaction.
    - Upon treatment of primary or secondary syphilis, occurs due to lysis of treponemes
    - Experience fever, chills, headache, myalgias, rash
    - Treated with antihistamines and antipyretics

When to Consult, Refer, Hospitalize

- Consult with physician or refer to infectious disease specialist for pregnant women, congenital syphilis, neurosyphilis infection, or HIV+ patients.
- Hospitalize for parenteral therapy and for penicillin desensitization therapy.
- Consider state mandatory reporting laws if child presents with infection not related to perinatal transmission.

Follow-Up

- Primary and secondary syphilis: Examine clinically and serologically at 6 or 12 months, or more frequently if clinically indicated; if serologic titer (VDRL or RPR) has not declined by fourfold in 6 months after therapy, consider treatment a failure.
    - Treatment failure: Reevaluate for HIV infection, provide more frequent follow-up (3 months instead of 6). If additional follow-up cannot be ensured, re-treatment is recommended (three, weekly IM injections of penicillin G 2.4 million units once per week for three weeks).
    - Consider CSF examination.
- Latent syphilis: Serological testing at 6, 12, and 24 months. Evaluate for neurosyphilis and re-treat if titers increase fourfold, initial high titer (higher than 1:32) fails to decline at least fourfold within 12 to 24 months, or symptomatic.

Expected Course

- Primary stage lasts 1 to 5 weeks; secondary stage lasts 2 to 6 weeks.

Complications

- Tertiary syphilis: cardiovascular involvement causing aortitis, aortic insufficiency, aneurysm, and neurosyphilis. Recurrent secondary symptoms possible within 1 year for 25% cases.

CASE STUDIES

CASE 1

A 23-year-old sexually active male patient presents with a 4- to 5-day history of dysuria he feels is caused by a urinary tract infection.

History of Present Illness (HPI): Denies frequency, fever, flank pain, hematuria, history of urinary tract infections

1. What additional information will help you evaluate this patient?

   Exam: Mucopurulent urethral discharge, no inguinal adenopathy, no genital lesions

2. What is the differential diagnosis?
3. Should any diagnostic tests be done?
4. What are your treatment considerations?

CASE 2

A 22-year-old patient comes to the family planning clinic for a routine pelvic exam and contraception. The patient reports having had four sexual partners in the past year and only occasionally uses condoms. They request an HIV test because one of their recent partners admits to high-risk behaviors.

Past Medical History (PMH): History of a pregnancy without carrying a pregnancy, no major illnesses, does not smoke, drinks 2 to 3 beers on the weekend, lives with mother and grandmother

1. What additional information should you obtain?

   Exam Complete physical exam with no significant findings except flat-topped, fleshy-colored lesions on labia minora and thin yellow vaginal discharge

2. What screening tests should be done?
3. What treatment should be considered today?
4. What education and prevention topics should be discussed with this patient?

CASE STUDIES DISCUSSION

CASE 1

1. What additional information will help you evaluate this patient?

   Presence and characteristics of penile discharge, number of sexual partners, history of STDs

2. What is the differential diagnosis? Gonococcal urethritis, NGU, HIV

3. Should any diagnostic tests be done?

   Tests for gonorrhea and chlamydia using one of the following: Gram stain (gonorrhea only), culture using special media for each, DNA probe, nucleic acid amplification test on first-void urine

4. What are your treatment considerations?

   Consider empiric therapy for both gonorrhea and chlamydia, notify partner(s) of need for evaluation and treatment, abstain from intercourse until treatment complete (7 days), report to public health after confirmation of gonorrhea or chlamydia, no follow-up necessary if resolves, refer for persistent or recurrent urethritis, condom use, HIV screening. Consider offering PrEP to decrease risk of HIV.

CASE 2

1. What additional information should you obtain?

   History of STDs, current symptoms of STDs, signs and symptoms of primary HIV infection (fever, adenopathy, pharyngitis, rash, myalgias, diarrhea, headache, nausea and vomiting, thrush)

2. What screening tests should be done?

   Pap smear; gonorrhea and chlamydia tests; vaginal microscopy or gram stain for trichomoniasis, bacterial vaginosis, and candidiasis; syphilis serology; HIV testing; pregnancy test

3. What treatment should be considered today?

   Rule out pregnancy before treatment of HPV and other infections

4. What education and prevention topics should be discussed with this patient?

   HIV risk factors; perinatal transmission of HIV; how to change unsafe sexual behavior; additional birth control measures; annual screening for cervical cancer, gonorrhea, chlamydia, condom use, PrEP consideration to decrease risk of HIV

REFERENCES

Centers for Disease Control and Prevention. (2021a). Preventing New HIV Infections. https://www.cdc.gov/hiv/guidelines/preventing.html

Centers for Disease Control and Prevention. (2021b). Sexually transmitted infections treatment guidelines, 2021. *MMWR Morbidity and Mortality Weekly Reports, 70.* https://www.cdc.gov/std/treatment-guidelines/default.htm

Centers for Disease Control and Prevention. (2021c). FDA Alert: Possible False RPR Reactivity with SyphilisTest https://www.cdc.gov/std/fda-alert-12-20-2021.pdf

Center for Disease Control and Prevention (2023). Reported STDs in the United States, 2020. https://www.cdc.gov/nchhstp/newsroom/fact-sheets/std/std-us-2020.html#:~:text=Congenital%20syphilis%2C%20a%20disease%20that,were%20up%20235%25%20from%202016.

Cyr, S. S., Barbee, L., Workowski, K. A., Bachmann, L. H., Pham, C., Schlanger, K., . . . & Thorpe, P. (2020). Update to CDC's treatment guidelines for gonococcal infection, 2020. *MMWR Morbidity and Mortality Weekly Report, 69*(50), 1911.

Gilbert, D. N., Moellering, R. C., Eliopoulus, G. M., & Sande, M. A. (2013). *The Sanford guide to antimicrobial therapy.* Hyde Park, VT: Antimicrobial Therapy, Inc.

Gilbert, D. (2022). *The Sanford guide to HIV/AIDS & hepatitis therapy 2019* (26th ed.). Antimicrobial Therapy.

Gilbert, D. N., MD, Chambers, H. F., MD, Saag, M. S., MD, Pavia, A. T., MD, & Boucher, H. W., MD. (2022). *The Sanford guide to antimicrobial therapy 2021* (51st ed.). Antimicrobial Therapy, Inc.

Hazra, A., Collison, M. W., & Davis, A. M. (2022). CDC sexually transmitted infections treatment guidelines, 2021. *Journal of the American Medical Association, 327*(9), 870–871.

Hospital, J. H., Kleinman, K., McDaniel, L., & Molloy, M. (2020). *The Harriet Lane Handbook: The Johns Hopkins Hospital (Mobile Medicine)* (22nd ed.). Elsevier.

Kimberlin, D. W., Barnett, E. D., Lynfield, R., & Sawyer, M. H. (2021). *Red Book: 2021–2024 report of the Committee on Infectious Diseases.* American Academy of Pediatrics.

U.S. Preventive Services Task Force. (2012). *Guide to clinical preventive services.* http://www.ahrq.gov/clinic/pocketgd1011/pocketgd1011.pdf

Workowski, K. A., Bachmann, L. H., Chan, P. A., Johnston, C. M., Muzny, C. A., Park, I., . . . & Bolan, G. A. (2021). Sexually transmitted infections treatment guidelines, 2021. *MMWR Morbidity and Mortality Weekly Report, 70*(4), 1.

CHAPTER 14

MUSCULOSKELETAL DISORDERS

Courtney E. Reinisch, DNP, RN, APN-C, FNP-BC, DCC

General Approach

DESCRIPTION

- Exclude musculoskeletal emergencies, which include impairment of neurovascular status.
- Proceed to evaluate for other diagnostic possibilities.
- Assess musculoskeletal complaints by determining the following:
  - Acute or chronic
  - Articular or nonarticular in origin
  - Inflammatory or noninflammatory in origin
  - Localized or systemic in distribution
- A thorough review of systems may provide clues to other systemic diseases such as:
  - Fever (systemic lupus erythematosus [SLE], infection)
  - Nervous system (Lyme disease, vasculitis)
  - Eye (sarcoidosis, Reiter's syndrome)
  - Gastrointestinal (scleroderma, inflammatory bowel disease)
- Examine the uninvolved side initially and the painful area last.
- Diagnostic laboratory studies may be required in the evaluation of some musculoskeletal complaints.
- As part of a conservative treatment regimen, cold/ice is usually recommended in the first 48 hours after an injury and then heat.
- Treatment decisions should use shared decision-making
- Use evidence-based guidelines to direct care.

- Consult or refer to members of the multidisciplinary care team to achieve optimal outcomes.
- Systemic presentations in children may indicate a chronic pediatric condition such as inflammatory bowel disease, cystic fibrosis, juvenile arthritis, hemophilia, sickle cell disease, leukemia, osteosarcoma, and vitamin D–resistant rickets.
  - In infants and children, obtain history of mother's pregnancy and child's birth and development. (Musculoskeletal problems comprise about 10% of childhood problems and about 25% of primary care visits.)
  - History includes mechanism of injury, occupation, any sports or exercise, repetitive use, duration, and aggravating and alleviating factors. Age is important in evaluation of any musculoskeletal findings.
  - Observe gait, posture, guarding, and patient positioning; examine the affected side in comparison to the unaffected side.

RED FLAGS

- *Back pain with neurologic signs* and or bowel and bladder dysfunction including urinary retention or incontinence, saddle anesthesia, decreased anal sphincter tone, or fecal incontinence may indicate cauda equina syndrome. This is a surgical emergency and requires immediate referral for evaluation and management.
  - *Back pain in children:* urgent referral if constant, younger than age 11, lasts several weeks, wakes patient at night, limits motion, or includes fever, neurologic signs, weight loss, or history of malignancy
  - *Malignant bone tumors* may present as unexplained pain and swelling over a bone, decreased range of motion (ROM), night pain, pain with weight-bearing, weight loss, night sweats, pallor, malaise, and fever; or have a high index of suspicion for bone metastasis in patients with previous breast, lung, or prostate cancer.
  - *Osteomyelitis* may present as pain in bone, fever, difficulty bearing weight, and possible local warmth and swelling following recent trauma. Obtain a complete blood count (CBC), erythrocyte sedimentation rate (ESR), and C-reactive protein (CRP) level and refer to orthopedist. Radiologic evidence for infection changes may present 10 to 24 days after the onset of infection.

Arthritis

OSTEOARTHRITIS (OA)

Description

- Degenerative joint disease with progressive loss of articular cartilage in movable joints.
- Degeneration of cartilage, bone hypertrophy, formation of osteophytes and subchondral cysts, and development of subchondral sclerosis in synovial joints and vertebrae.
- Most common form of arthritis.
- Radiographic evidence does not equate with symptoms.

Etiology

- Results from both mechanical and biologic events that lead to degradation of articular cartilage and subchondral bone in joint

Incidence and Demographics

- Leading chronic condition among adults 65 years of age and older
- Incidence increases with advancing age and history of participation in contact sports
- 80% of adults in United States have radiographic evidence by age 75
- Rates of symptomatic hand, hip, and knee increase rapidly at age 50 and level off after age 70
- Women affected more than men
- Prevalence: Over 50 million U.S. adults are affected by osteoarthritis

Risk Factors

- Advancing age; symptom onset typically 55 to 65 years
- Athletic overuse or repetitive joint use in occupation
- Joint trauma from acute injury or metabolic disease
- Obesity, heredity, congenital musculoskeletal disorders

- Occupations increase risk—construction, firefighting, farming, mining, forestry
- Metabolic disorders (e.g., gout) or endocrine disorders (e.g., hyperparathyroidism)

Prevention and Screening

- Maintain physical activity.
- Maintain ideal body weight; avoid obesity.
- Maintain control of metabolic and endocrine disorders.

Assessment

History

- (see Table 14–1)
- Gradual onset of joint pain, tenderness, and stiffness; worsens with activity and relieved by rest

TABLE 14–1.
DIFFERENTIATING CHARACTERISTICS OF OSTEOARTHRITIS AND RHEUMATOID ARTHRITIS

CHARACTERISTICS	OSTEOARTHRITIS	RHEUMATOID ARTHRITIS
Radiographic appearance	Joint-space narrowing, osteophytes, subchondral bone sclerosis, subchondral cysts	Periarticular osteopenia or osteoporosis, soft tissue swelling, marginal bony erosions
Morning stiffness	Lasts more than 30 minutes	Lasts less than 1 hour before improving
Joint involvement	Usually weight-bearing (spine, hips, knees), or distal finger joints (DIP)	Multiple joints, symmetric joint involvement (especially of hands)
Laboratory findings	ESR less than 20–40 mm/hour; RF negative	Positive serum RF, may have positive ANA, elevated ESR
Clinical findings	Joint pain, bony tenderness and hypertrophy, crepitus, may have some deformity; no warmth or redness	Joint deformity, muscle atrophy, soft tissue nodules (rheumatoid nodules), soft tissue swelling, warmth, redness of joints

ANA = antinuclear antibody; ESR = erythrocyte sedimentation rate; DIP = distal interphalangeal; RF = rheumatoid factor

- Morning stiffness common; usually lasts less than 30 minutes
- Joint instability in later stages, especially with osteoarthritis of the knees
- Perform review of systems for systemic symptoms to exclude other types of arthritis.

Physical Exam

- Usually localized to affected joints
- Bony hypertrophy of joint, tenderness at joint line; limited ROM
- Common in hands:
    - proximal interphalangeal (PIP) joint swelling = Bouchard's nodes;
    - distal interphalangeal (DIP) joint swelling = Heberden's nodes
- Coarse crepitus in joint with movement; soft tissue swelling may be present
- Joint effusion, if present, usually mild
- Evaluate cardiac and pulmonary status and other body systems as indicated by history to exclude other types of arthritis

Diagnostic Studies

- Plain radiographs: unequal and narrowed joint space, subchondral bony sclerosis, sharp articular margins, cysts or osteophytes
- Bone densitometry (dual X-ray absorptiometry [DEXA] scans), peripheral ultrasonography, quantitative computed tomography (QCT)
- Laboratory findings may be normal or show markers of systemic inflammation or autoimmune disease.

Differential Diagnosis

- Rheumatoid arthritis
- Psoriatic arthritis
- Gout, pseudogout
- Septic arthritis
- Reiter's disease, lupus
- Fibromyalgia

- Tendonitis, soft tissue injury
- Osteoporosis
- Multiple myeloma is considered in a differential diagnosis of osteoarthritis. Note that multiple myeloma is now known as plasma cell myeloma.

Management

Goals are to relieve symptoms, maintain/improve function, and avoid adverse effects of medication.

Nonpharmacologic Treatment

- Physical activity/therapy with supervised walking
- Occupational therapy
- Arthritis self-management programs and water aquatics courses
- Ambulation aids (canes, braces, walkers)
- Weight-loss of 10% of body weight is associated with 50% reduction in pain scores
- Refer for orthopedic consultation for surgical management if all other modalities fail and joint symptoms prevent normal activities. (Kolansinski et al., 2020)

Pharmacological Treatment

- Use pharmacologic agents when nonpharmacologic methods do no provide adequate pain relief.
- Oral and topical nonsteroidal anti-inflammatories (NSAIDs) can be used. Selection of agent may be dependent on the number of joints involved.
- NSAID use can be limited by the presence of gastrointestinal (GI), renal, and cardiovascular symptoms.
- The risk of GI bleed is reduced with co-administration with a protein pump inhibitor (PPI)
- Cyclooxygenase 2 (COX-2) inhibitors may decrease risk of GI bleeding.
- Avoid NSAIDS and aspirin in patients taking anticoagulants and
    - Monitor creatinine for patients taking angiotensin-converting enzyme inhibitors (ACEIs) or angiotensin II receptor blockers (ARBS) for hypertension.

- Duloxetine maybe considered for patients who cannot tolerate NSAIDs.
    - Oral duloxetine: Initial: 30 mg once daily for 1 week, then increase to 60 mg once daily as tolerated; maximum dose: 60 mg/day. Doses to 120 mg/day may increase benefit but are associated with an increase in adverse effects.
- Topical analgesic creams such as capsaicin 0.025% two to three times a day as needed
- Diclofenac gel 1% four times a day for knee or hand
- Narcotic analgesics are rarely indicated.
- Intra-articular corticosteroid injections for joint effusion and inflammation limited to a few joints
- Hyaluronic acid injections are considered controversial as have demonstrated only small benefit beyond placebo (Kolansinski et al., 2020)

How Long to Treat

- While symptomatic

Special Considerations

- Presence of radiographic changes does not correlate with presence or severity of symptoms.

When to Consult, Refer, Hospitalize

- Consult with physician or orthopedic specialist for intra-articular corticosteroid or hyaluronic acid injections.
- Patients with functional impairment (i.e., inability to perform normal activities of daily living) and moderate to severe pain unrelieved by other nonpharmacologic and pharmacologic therapies should be considered for joint replacement; refer to orthopedic surgeon.

Follow-Up

- Appointments as needed based on pain and disability
- If patient is taking NSAIDS, monitor for liver or kidney dysfunction and/or GI bleeding

Expected Course

- Chronic, often progressive

Complications

- Joint destruction, chronic pain, limitation of mobility

RHEUMATOID ARTHRITIS (RA)

Description

- Chronic, systemic, autoimmune inflammatory disease that affects mainly the synovial joints in a symmetric distribution; small-joint destruction and extra-articular symptoms are prominent.
- Juvenile idiopathic arthritis (JIA) is an autoimmune disorder with a genetic predisposition; presentation is an interaction of genetic, immune, and environmental factors.

Etiology

- Probably autoimmune but no specific inciting factor yet identified
- Genetic, environmental factors affect progression and extent of disease
- Pathology consists of initial changes in the synovium microvasculature, swelling of endothelial cells, and synovial hyperplasia forming a pannus. Inflammatory cells invade and joint symptoms develop secondary to the inflammatory process.

Incidence and Demographics

- Worldwide incidence 0.24% to 1%
- Global prevalence is estimated as 0.24%
- In children symptoms are present in first 1 to 3 years; then a second, less-dominant wave in 8- to 10-year-olds with girls predominantly affected.
- JIA is a diagnosis of exclusion in children younger than 16 years of age who have chronic synovial inflammation of at least one joint for 6 weeks. JIA is categorized:
  - Systemic arthritis: arthritis in one or more joints and fever of 2 weeks' duration
  - Polyarthritis, RF positive or negative: arthritis in five or more joints

- ◇ Oligoarthritis, persistent or extended
- ◇ Enthesitis-related arthritis
- ◇ Psoriatic arthritis
- ◇ Undifferentiated arthritis

Risk Factors

- Genetics
- Family history
- Age
- Gender, female to male ratio: 2:1
- Lifestyle factors: cigarette smoking

Assessment

- Early diagnosis (within first few months of symptoms) important for improved prognosis
- Important to exclude septic arthritis; typical presentation: sudden onset of pain, swelling, warmth, and redness in one large weight-bearing joint, may have fever

History

- History of joint pain, swelling, location in peripheral joints, morning stiffness lasting more than 30 minutes
- Duration of symptoms; if fewer than 6 weeks an acute viral polyarthritis may be the cause.
- Prodromal systemic symptoms: malaise, fever, weight loss
- Articular inflammation, swelling, pain, erythema, and warmth
- Involvement usually symmetrical; 75% of joints involved are knees, followed by ankles and elbows.
- In children, joint pain, one or more joints affected, swelling or effusion, and two of the following: limitation of ROM, tenderness or pain in motion, warmth; usually involves large joints or hands; if systemic: fever, rash
- Perform review of systems to identify any associated symptoms of systemic involvement; physical/emotional stress may trigger

Physical Exam

- Edema, erythema, warmth, nodules in any joint; effervescent, pale-pink/salmon-colored macular rash
- Joints are tender, may feel warm to touch, bright erythema and significant palpable heat in joint usually indicative of infection
- Subcutaneous nodules over bony prominences or extensor surfaces
- Soft tissue swelling, vasculitis, palmar erythema
- As disease progresses, joint deformities become more pronounced and joint instability develops.
- Systemic manifestations may be seen in the pulmonary, cardiac, hepatic, renal, vascular, and hematologic systems and the eyes (dry mucous membranes, ocular problems, splenomegaly, increased lymphocytes).
- In children with systemic juvenile rheumatoid arthritis (JRA), may have macular salmon-colored rash, splenomegaly, eye symptoms

Diagnostic Studies

- No single test is adequate to make diagnosis.
- Rheumatoid factor (RF) and anti-citrullinated peptide antibodies (ACPA): positive result for either increases overall diagnostic sensitivity; specificity increases when both are positive.
- ESR and serum CRP:—both are typically elevated in RA.
- Antinuclear antibody (ANA) testing. ANA is positive in one-third of RA cases
  - In children, RF and ANA may be positive.
- Synovial fluid shows inflammatory changes: sterile leukocytosis, increased polymorphonuclear cells (PMNs), negative culture.
- CBC may show anemia and thrombocytosis consistent with inflammation.
- Obtain plain radiographs of hands, wrists, and feet for baseline monitoring.
  - May show joint erosions in patient's first presentation. (Fraekel et al., 2021)

Differential Diagnosis

- Systemic lupus erythematosus (SLE)
- Seronegative spondyloarthropathy

- Psoriatic arthritis
- Septic arthritis
- Lyme disease
- Gout
- Osteoarthritis
- Lupus

Management

- Goals are early diagnosis
- Care by an expert in rheumatic disease
- Shared decision making
- Early use of disease-modifying antirheumatic drugs (DMARDs) to limit disease activity
- Prevent irreversible joint damage, maximize mobility, limit pain.

Nonpharmacologic Treatment

- Patient education regarding RA
- Rest, exercise, physical and occupational therapy
- Assistive devices (canes, splints)
- Refer to orthopedic surgeon for evaluation as needed for joint deformity.

Pharmacologic Treatment

- Methotrexate is a conventional DMARD recommended as first-line monotherapy for patients with moderate to high disease activity who have not been treated previously with a DMARD.
    - Monitor closely for bone marrow, pulmonary, hepatic, and renal toxicity.
    - Administer folic acid to reduce adverse effects.
    - Switch to subcutaneous methotrexate for patients who are not achieving target goals with oral monotherapy.
- Hydroxychloroquine (DMARD) is recommended for patients with mild symptoms.
    - Monitor eye symptoms, neuropathy, and myopathy.

- Methotrexate + tumor necrosis factor (TNF) may be used if patient fails to response to methotrexate monotherapy.
- Methotrexate + biologic may be used if patient fails to respond to a monotherapy or methotrexate +TNF.
  - Leflunomide (Arava), etanercept (Enbrel), and infliximab (Remicade) may cause hypersensitivity reaction, severe infections or sepsis, and autoimmunity (lupus-type syndrome).
  - More costly and complicated to administer.
- Corticosteroids: recommend against long-term use; switch to DMARD (Fraekel et al., 2021).

How Long to Treat

- Medications may be tapered if disease management activity goal is achieved and maintained for 6 months.
- In children, some have periods of long remissions.

Special Considerations

- Women being treated with DMARDs require preconceptual counseling
  - Pause treatment with methotrexate, hydroxychloroquine before conception to prevent fetal injury
- Pregnancy may result in remission and may allow temporary discontinuation of medications
  - Exacerbations are common in first 6 months postpartum.
  - Breastfeeding is not advised because antirheumatic medications are secreted in breast milk.

When to Consult, Refer, Hospitalize

- Rheumatologic consultation or referral is appropriate (Fraekel et al., 2021)
- All children should be referred to a pediatric rheumatologist and ophthalmologist at diagnosis.

Follow-Up

- Clinical course is highly variable; until symptoms are controlled, frequent follow-up visits are indicated; then regular evaluations at 3- to 6-month intervals.

Complications

- May be severe, including carpal tunnel syndrome, pleuritis, pericarditis, vasculitis, iridocyclitis, disability, and adverse reactions from drugs, severe joint deformity, hip disease.

GOUT

Description

- A group of metabolic diseases producing inflammatory arthritis of peripheral joints caused by deposition of uric acid or monosodium urate crystals in extracellular fluid.

Etiology

- Inborn error of purine metabolism or uric acid excretion causing hyperuricemia and uric acid crystal deposition in the joint (acute gouty arthritis)
- May be primary (hereditary) or secondary (due to other conditions that cause underexcretion or overproduction of uric acid)
- Overproduction: high intake of purine-rich foods (organ meats, shellfish, peas, lentils, beans), polycythemia vera, leukemia, multiple myeloma, hemolytic anemia, psoriasis, sarcoidosis
- Underexcretion of uric acid: reduced renal function, lactic acidosis, ketoacidosis, dehydration
- Secondary gout also associated with obesity, starvation, lead intoxication, ingestion of drugs (salicylates, diuretics, pyrazinamide, ethambutol, nicotinic acid)
- Combined overproduction/underexcretion: alcohol abuse, glucose-6-phosphatase deficiency (G-6PD), hypoxemia

Incidence and Demographics

- Men affected nine times as often as women
- Rarely affects men before adolescence or women before menopause
- Peak incidence for men is fourth to fifth decades and women is sixth to seventh decades of life
- Prevalence: three to eight million Americans affected
    - Approximately 3% of the adult American population is affected.

Risk Factors

Primary gout: Inherited

Secondary gout: Acquired

- Certain medications increase the risk for gout including diuretics, low-dose aspirin, cyclosporine, and niacin.
- Urate-lowering therapy may incite a flare, particularly during the early phase of treatment.
- Hospitalization and surgery increase risk of gout flares.
- Illnesses such as plasma cell myeloma, chronic kidney disease, and hypothyroidism increase the risk of gout.
- Heredity
- Physiologic factors—obesity, dehydration, starvation
- Alcohol consumption and purine-rich diet

Prevention and Screening

- Correct/control underlying problem.
- Avoid foods high in purines, alcohol, and causative medications.
- Maintain normal body weight.

Assessment

History

- Sudden attack of red, hot, swollen, exquisitely tender joint is common (first metatarsal phalangeal [MTP] joint very susceptible: podagra); feeling of malaise, fever; often no apparent cause
- Foot, ankle, knee, and shoulder are the most common sites; wrist, elbow, fingers also may be affected.

Physical Exam

- During acute attack, joint is red, hot, swollen, exquisitely painful; low-grade fever
- Skin desquamation and pruritus during resolution of acute attack commonly seen
- Tophi (sodium urate crystals deposited in soft tissue) present in chronic tophaceous gout, usually after 2 to 10 years from onset of acute intermittent gout
- Joint swelling, restricted range of movement caused by chronic arthritis

Diagnostic Studies

- Joint aspiration: Fluid shows presence of needle-shaped crystals (negatively birefringent) on polarized light microscopy.
- Serum uric acid above 6.8 mg/dL supports diagnosis but is not specific; elevated ESR, elevated leukocytes
- X-ray: normal in early disease; shows punched-out lesions in subchondral bone, usually first seen in first MTP joint ("Mickey Mouse" ears); soft tissue tophi may be seen if at least 5 mm in diameter
    - Ultrasound can support diagnosis.
    - Dual-energy computed tomography (DECT) can specifically identify urate deposits.

Differential Diagnosis

- Septic arthritis
- Trauma/stress fracture
- Cellulitis

- Rheumatoid arthritis
- Acute rheumatic fever
- Pyogenic arthritis

Management

Nonpharmacologic Treatment

- Dietary modification; increased fluid intake 3 liters or more per day
- Assistive devices if needed during acute phase
- Weight loss in obese patients

Pharmacologic Treatment

Acute Attack

- First-line for gout flares: oral steroids, NSAIDs, and colchicine are equivalent first-line choices.
  - Corticosteroids, use with caution and depend on comorbidities, prednisone 20–40 mg orally once a day for 2 to 3 days, then taper over 10 to 14 days; intra-articular methylprednisolone (Depo-Medrol) one 20- to 40-mg dose; IM methyl-prednisolone, one 80- to 120-mg dose
  - NSAIDs such as naproxen at full anti-inflammatory dose; naproxen 500 mg twice a day orally for first 2 to 3 days (until symptoms subside); then taper to cessation over 3 to 5 days.
- Indomethacin 50 mg orally three times a day in persons under 60 years old with neither renal nor cardiovascular comorbidities
  - Colchicine—day 1 not to exceed 1.8 mg, 1.2 mg orally as soon as symptoms appear, then 0.06 mg 1 hour later, then continue 0.6 mg once or twice daily until flare resolves
- Contraindicated with renal or hepatic impairment
- Use colchicine therapy for patients on anticoagulation therapy
  - Intraarticular glucocorticoids: option for those unable to take oral medications
  - Parenteral glucocorticoids: option for those unable to take oral options and intraarticular glucocorticoids (FitzGerald et al., 2020)

- Tophaceous gout, those with evidence of gouty joint damage on imaging, those with frequent flares, or chronic kidney disease:
  - First-line urate-lowering therapy (ULT; allopurinol less than 100 mg/day)
  - In patients with chronic kidney disease (stage ≥3), allopurinol or febuxostat are recommended
  - Treat with ULT for 3–6 months
  - Concomitant treatment with anti-inflammatory therapy is recommended when using ULT (Fitzgerald et al., 2020).

Maintenance

- Manage lifestyle factors.
  - Limit alcohol intake.
  - Limit purine intake.
  - Limit high fructose corn syrup intake.
  - Weight loss program for those who are overweight/obese
- Manage concurrent medications.
  - Switch antihypertensive from hydrochlorothiazide when possible
  - Chose losartan for hypertension management in patients with gout when feasible (Fitzgerald et al., 2020).

How Long to Treat

- Acute symptoms treated until flare resolves
- ULT is recommended at least 3–6 months, maybe indefinitely (Fitzgerald et al., 2020).

Special Considerations

- Transplant patients treated with cyclosporine have increased incidence.
- Geriatric patients: NSAIDs less well-tolerated; dosages should be reduced.

When to Consult, Refer, Hospitalize

- Consult for any complicated presentation, underlying metabolic pathology
- Refer for joint aspiration, unclear diagnosis, new/acute gout in transplant patient

Follow-Up

Expected Course

- Decrease in frequency, severity of attacks with appropriate treatment

Complications

- Kidney stones, renal obstruction or infection; joint destruction if undertreated

Conditions of the Bones

OSTEOMYELITIS

Description

- Inflammatory process of bone due to infection; can be acute or chronic
- Diagnosis is clinical with support of imaging and laboratory studies (Bury et al., 2021)

Etiology

- Bacteremia with acute or subacute hematogenous spread to bone (most common form in pediatrics)
- Direct bacterial inoculation through trauma, contact with infected tissue (most common in adults)
- Predominant organism is *Staphylococcus aureus.*
- Most common cause is contact with infected tissue, direct inoculation through trauma, and skin breakdown in vascular insufficiency.
    - Methicillin-sensitive *Staphylococcus aureus* is most frequently found cause in all types of osteomyelitis (Bury et al., 2021).
    - Followed by *Pseudomonas aeruginosa* and Methicillin-resistant *S. aureus* (Bury et al., 2021)

Incidence and Demographics

- Occurs in all ages, more common in children younger than 5 years of age
- More cases in men and boys than women and girls; cases increase with age.
- 90 per 100,000 cases in adults and 10–15 cases per 100,000 children
- Femur and tibia are most often infected, followed by humerus, calcaneus, and pelvis

Risk Factors

- Chronic disease such as cancer, diabetes, hemodialysis; sickle-cell disease
- Smoking
- Peripheral vascular disease
- Intravenous drug use

Prevention and Screening

- Careful treatment of comorbid conditions; appropriate wound care

Assessment

History

- 75% report recent trauma; 25% report recent respiratory tract infection.
- Sudden onset of high fever and pain in affected bone or joint; sudden refusal to bear weight or move extremity; localized warmth, swelling
- May have drainage from affected area (sinus tract develops).

Physical Exam

- Swelling, erythema, possible abscess formation or purulent drainage; decreased ROM; fever; point tenderness over infected bone or site of surgical hardware

Diagnostic Studies

- *Imaging*—plain film radiograph, magnetic resonance imaging (MRI), or bone scan demonstrating soft tissue infection or bony destruction, or both
- *Laboratory studies*—elevated CRP and ESR, leukocytosis, thrombocytosis, and positive blood cultures
- Note: bone biopsy with bacterial culture for definitive diagnosis (Bury et al., 2021)

Differential Diagnosis

- Soft tissue infection, cellulitis
- Gout
- Charcot arthropathy
- Sickle cell vaso-occlusive pain crisis
- Synovitis
- Malignancy
- Fracture

Management

Nonpharmacologic Treatment

- Surgical debridement, splinting, local wound care, bed rest

Pharmacologic Treatment

- Intravenous antibiotics are the mainstay of treatment; choice depends on infectious organism
- Delaying antibiotics until cultures are available is recommended except in patients in need of urgent intervention (Bury et al., 2021)

How Long to Treat

- Antibiotic therapy for 4 to 6 weeks, targeted to specific organism
- Evidence suggests oral antibiotics having similar cure rates with fewer risks compared to intravenous antibiotics (Bury et al., 2021)

Special Considerations

- Culture of draining sinus tract or superficial wound does not correlate with actual infectious organism.
- Bone biopsy should be obtained before starting antibiotics.
- Children, patients with prosthetic joints, and persons with diabetes require specialty care (Bury et al., 2021),

When to Consult, Refer, Hospitalize

- Orthopedics referral is necessary immediately.
- Consult infectious disease specialist for choice of antibiotic.
- Hospitalization as indicated for intravenous therapy or surgical management

Follow-Up

- Diagnosis and treatment plan developed by orthopedic specialist

Expected Course

- Clinical improvement should be seen within 24 to 48 hours, then gradual resolution of drainage, pain, white blood cell (WBC) count, ESR, and fever.

Complications

- Chronic osteomyelitis, need for bone and/or skin grafting, structural weakening of bone

DEVELOPMENTAL DYSPLASIA OF THE HIP

Description

- Developmental dysplasia of the hip (DDH) is a broad category of anatomic abnormalities in which the femoral head and the acetabulum are not in alignment and grow abnormally. It develops in infancy or childhood and may be present for many years before diagnosis.

- ◊ Dislocation: a loss of contact between the femoral head and acetabulum
- ◊ Dislocatable hip: a hip with instability where the femoral head is reduced at rest, but can dislocate in other positions or with maneuvers
- ◊ Subluxation: the femoral head is partially outside the acetabulum but there still remains contact
- ◊ Subluxatable hip: a hip with mild instability or laxity where the head of femur slides in and out of the acetabulum
- ◊ Dysplasia: abnormality of the shape of the joint with a shallow acetabulum
- ◊ Reducible: the hip is dislocated at rest, but the femoral head can be manipulated into the acetabulum with flexion and abduction.

Etiology

- ♦ Multifactorial (mechanical, physiologic, environmental, genetic)
- ♦ *Mechanical:* breech presentation, positioning of fetal hip against mother's sacrum; tight maternal abdomen and uterine musculature; first-born
  - ◊ Mechanical factors such as compression in utero if fetal position or oligohydramnios restricts movement in utero
- ♦ *Physiologic:* ligamentous laxity due to estrogen exposure; collagen disorders
  - ◊ Maternal hormones during pregnancy may cause temporary laxity of the hip joints.
- ♦ *Environmental:* swaddling of infant with legs in extension/adduction
  - ◊ Prevalence higher in cultures that swaddle infants for extended periods or place them on cradleboards
- ♦ *Genetic:* 20% have positive family history.

Incidence and Demographics

- ♦ Severe dysplasia in 3 to 5 per 1,000 births in the United States
- ♦ 1 to 2 per 1,000 births have DDH with dislocation
- ♦ Women more affected than men

Risk Factors

- ♦ First-born, female, breech in third trimester
- ♦ Populations who use swaddling may limit hip mobility, which may play a role in DDH

- Positive family history
  - Torticollis, or lower limb disorders such as club foot

Prevention, Screening, Physical Examination

- Avoid swaddling with legs in extension and adduction.
- Check hips at birth, 2-week, 2-month, and 4-months well baby exams.
  - Routine screening up to 2 years old:
  - Barlow and Ortolani tests in infants up to 2 or 3 months old
  - Klisic and Galeazzi tests for older infants
  - Chart screening at every visit
  - 80% of abnormal hips resolve by 2 to 8 weeks.
  - Asymmetry of the inguinal or gluteal folds is a sign.
  - In children 6–18 months old, there is limited abduction and shortening of the thigh of the affected hip.
  - Short leg with toe walking on the affected side

Assessment

History

- Prenatal and birth history
- Positive family history

Physical Exam

- Limited abduction of hip; hip instability; asymmetry of thigh folds; femoral shortening on affected side
- Unequal leg lengths; unequal knee heights when supine (Galeazzi sign); limp or "duck-like" waddle

Diagnostic Studies

- Provocation tests: click (hip relocation) felt with Ortolani maneuver; clunk felt (hip dislocation) with Barlow maneuver

- Ultrasound, which is done after 4 weeks of age to prevent false positives, is superior to radiographs.
- Radiographs may be used after 4 months of age when proximal epiphysis ossifies. (Yang et al., 2019)

Differential Diagnosis

- Unstable hip in newborn period

Management

- Goal is to prevent long-term complications and pathologic changes through early diagnosis and treatment in infancy.
- Prompt referral to an orthopedist
- Pavlik harness, worn 24 hours per day, is the treatment of choice with success rate of 80%–97%. Weekly follow-ups needed.
- Proper skin care while wearing harness.
- Surgery recommended if harness treatment is unsuccessful.

Nonpharmacologic Treatment

- Birth up to 6 months: Pavlik harness
- 6 to 18 months: Pavlik harness, closed reduction with cast
- Older than 18 months: open reduction with casting (Yang et al., 2019)

How Long to Treat

- Until corrected

Special Considerations

- About 60% of unstable hips in newborns spontaneously become normal in the first 2 to 4 weeks of life.

When to Consult, Refer, Hospitalize

- Infants or children older than 1 year with findings suggestive of DDH should be referred to a pediatric orthopedic surgeon.

Follow-Up

- Orthopedic specialist
- Recurrent DDH may occur after treatment so children will require imaging regularly until they are skeletally mature.

Expected Course

- Most cases respond to treatment.
- Earlier treatment results in better outcomes.

Complications

- Untreated cases result in permanent dislocation.
- Osteoarthritis, pain, abnormal gait, decreased agility
- Even with treatment, avascular necrosis of the femoral head may occur.

SCOLIOSIS

Description

- Lateral curvature of the spine with rotation of spinal column
- Adolescent idiopathic scoliosis (AIS) is most common type.
- Adult scoliosis is associated with degenerative changes.

Etiology

- Unclear etiology for AIS
- Genetic component
- Familial AIS

Incidence and Demographics

- 2%–3% of the population
- Estimated 6–9 million U.S. population (American Association of Neurological Surgeons [AANS], 2022)

Risk Factors

- Female gender
- Women and girls are eight times more likely than men and boys to progress to curvature requiring treatment.
- Family history

Prevention and Screening

- Screen during routine school age and adolescent physical exams with back fully exposed and no shoes.
- Observe for asymmetry of shoulders, scapulae, and pelvis.

Assessment

History

- Asymmetry of shoulder and or hip height; shirts or hemlines may be uneven
- Positive family history
- Complaints of pain

Physical Exam

- Screening done with back fully exposed and without shoes
- Observe for asymmetry of shoulders, scapulae, and hip/pelvis.
- Check for leg-length discrepancy, which may be present.
- Have patient bend forward at waist to 90° and slowly return to upright (Adams test).

- Assess for prominence of scapula or lateralization of spine.
- 90% thoracic with right curve; left thoracic curve more likely to progress.

Diagnostic Studies

- Routine X-rays are not required for mild scoliosis.
- More-severe cases require X-ray of entire length of spine (Cobb method).
- X-ray determines location and direction of curvature, measures degree of asymmetry, and evaluates vertebral bodies; view entire spine from C7 to S1.
- Repeat X-rays to monitor progression of curve.
- Consider bone age.
- Scoliometer may be helpful to detect and follow smaller curves
  - Genetic testing—The ScoliScore screens for 50 genetic markers that predict worsening curves.

Differential Diagnoses

- Neuromuscular scoliosis
- Congenital scoliosis
- Syndromic scoliosis

Management

- Goal is to prevent further deformity.
- Use Cobb method for evaluating degree of curvature; follow every 4 to 6 months in children <Tanner V.
- Curves less than 15°: Observe, follow every 4 to 6 months in children <Tanner V.
- Curves 15° or more: Refer to orthopedist to monitor for progression.
- Curves 25°–40°: bracing may prevent further progression of curve in patients who have not reached skeletal maturity (AANS, 2022).

Special Considerations

- Back pain is uncommon in adolescents with idiopathic scoliosis, so further examination is warranted if pain is present.
- Refer to orthopedist immediately for congenital or infantile congenital scoliosis.
- Scoliosis in older adults seen with deterioration of vertebral disks; surgery may relieve pain, restore stability
- Vertebral expandable prosthetic titanium rib (VEPTR) is an option for those with pulmonary side effects of scoliosis.

Follow-Up

- Close follow-up essential; can be done in primary care if curve is less than 15°, every 4 to 6 months
- Otherwise followed by the orthopedist with periodic follow-up X-rays

Expected Course

- More concern with patients with large curvature at diagnosis and patients with curvature before adolescent growth spurt; close follow-up essential
- Repeat standing posterior-anterior (PA) X-ray every 6 to 12 months in young adolescents with mild curvature; every 3 to 6 months in adolescents with large curves

Complications

- Untreated scoliosis results in unacceptable cosmetic appearance and cardiopulmonary impairment.
- Spinal osteoarthritis may occur in later life.

OSTEOPOROSIS

Description

- Skeletal condition with low bone mass, reduced bone strength, and increase risk for fracture

- Metabolic disease with bone demineralization producing diffusely decreased bone density, diminished strength; predisposes patient to pathologic fractures, severe backache, loss of height
- Bone mineral density (BMD) at least 2.5 standard deviations (SD) below peak bone density of young adult (T score); osteopenia T score is –1.5 to –2.5 of SD

Etiology

- Bone resorption by osteoclasts occurs faster than new bone matrix formation by osteoblasts and subsequent bone mineralization.
- Trabecular bone (spine, ribs, pelvis) turnover is greater than cortical bone.
- Low bone mass may be attributed to estrogen deficiency, glucocorticoid exposure, or malabsorption

Incidence and Demographics

- Primarily affects postmenopausal women 50 years old and over
- Incidence increases age 65 and over
- Prevalence among women 50 years of age and older is 12.6%.
- Prevalence among men 50 years of age and older is 4.4% (Sarafrazi et al., 2021).

Risk Factors

- Inadequate calcium intake, vitamin D deficiency; excessive alcohol, protein, or caffeine intake
- Genetic predisposition
- Low body weight (below 127 pounds)
- Advancing age
- Hyperthyroidism/hyperparathyroidism; rheumatoid arthritis
- Malignancy (multiple myeloma, leukemia)
- Early menopause (natural or surgical) with deficiency in estrogen/androgen
- Steroid use, Cushing syndrome
- Renal insufficiency

- Smoking
- Sedentary lifestyle without exposure to sun

Prevention and Screening

- Balanced diet with adequate intake of calcium and vitamin D; regular weight-bearing exercise; smoking cessation; avoiding high alcohol, protein, or caffeine intake

Screening

- BMD (bone mineral density) recommended for all women ≥65 years of age
- BMD reserved for women with increased risk factors under 65 years of age
- Screening in men reserved for those with osteopenia, history of low trauma fracture, loss of height
- Measurements of hip and spine are best determination of fracture risk.
  - Every 1–2 years for high-risk women
  - Every 10 years for low-risk women
  - FRAX (Fracture Risk Assessment Tool) estimates 10-year probability for developing osteoporotic hip fracture.

Assessment

History

- Risk factors, fracture after age 40 (spine, hip, wrist), back pain (from vertebral fracture), osteopenia on X-ray

Physical Exam

- No finding specific to osteoporosis; kyphosis common in older adults; loss of height

Diagnostic Studies

- DEXA scan shows bone density at least 2.5 SD below peak bone density, biochemical markers
- Osteopenia on X-ray (indicates loss of approximately 30% of bone mass)

Differential Diagnosis

- Endocrine disorders
- Malabsorption syndromes
- Malnutrition
- Osteomalacia
- Metastatic bone disease
- Connective tissue disorders

Management

Nonpharmacologic Treatment

- Lifestyle measures to reduce bone loss in post-menopausal women
  - Regular weight-bearing exercise 30 minutes/day, most days of the week
  - Muscle strengthening and posture exercises 2–3 days per week
  - Calcium intake or supplementation (1,000–1,500 mg/day), adequate vitamin D intake (400–800 IU/day)
  - Avoid heavy alcohol use
  - Smoking cessation
  - Counseling on fall prevention
  - Avoidance of drugs that increase bone loss

Pharmacologic Treatment

- First-line therapy with oral bisphosphonates: alendronate or risedronate
  - alendronate (Fosamax) 10 mg/day orally or alendronate sodium (Binosto) 70 mg weekly

    - ◊ risedronate (Actonel) 5 mg/day or risedronate 35 mg orally weekly
    - ◊ ibandronate (Boniva) 150 mg orally every month
- ♦ Gastrointestinal disease—zoledronate 5 mg IV annually
- ♦ Receptor activator of nuclear factor kappa (RANK/RANKL) ligand inhibitors: denosumab (Prolia) 60 mg SC every 6 months used when other osteoporosis treatment options have failed
- ♦ Teriparatide 20 mcg SC daily × 2 years (Chavarria et al., 2022)

How Long to Treat

- ♦ Until bone density is normal

Special Considerations

- ♦ Men: treat with calcium supplementation, vitamin D, bisphosphates
- ♦ Medications cannot be used in pregnancy.

When to Consult, Refer, Hospitalize

- ♦ Refer to orthopedist for suspected fracture; hospitalize for any hip fracture.

Follow-Up

- ♦ Regular follow-up for review of diet, exercise, and medications
- ♦ Repeat DEXA scan every 24 months

Expected Course

- ♦ Improvement in bone density evident 6–12 months after initiation of therapy

Complications

- ♦ Fracture (vertebral most common; hip has greatest mortality)

MALIGNANT BONE TUMORS

Description

- Neoplastic growth in a bone or bones

Etiology

- Malignant tumors of bone may originate in bone or metastasize to bone.
- In adults, most often results from seeding of another malignancy
- Metastasis from breast, lung, prostate, kidney, thyroid cancers

Incidence and Demographics

- Ewing's sarcoma most common in children, young adults
- Chondrosarcoma most common in middle to late life
- Osteosarcoma most common primary bone tumor except multiple myeloma
- Most common in children and young adults; more common in men and boys
- In the 60s to 70s age group metastatic bone cancers more common

Risk Factors

- High doses of ionizing radiation
- Certain conditions (Paget's disease, von Recklinghausen's disease, enchondromatosis) may undergo malignant transformation.

Prevention and Screening

- Early diagnosis, treatment of primary malignancy

Assessment

History

- (see Table 14–2)
- Unexplained pain and swelling over bone, decreased ROM, night pain, pain with weight-bearing
- Constitutional symptoms: weight loss, night sweats, pallor, malaise, fever

TABLE 14–2.
MALIGNANT BONE TUMORS

MALIGNANT TUMOR	TYPICAL AGE RANGE, INCIDENCE	CLINICAL PRESENTATION	RADIOGRAPHIC FINDINGS
Multiple myeloma Plasma cell malignancy (most common in adults)	Incidence 3/100,000 older than 40 Male/female 1.6:1	Bone pain Anemia, hypercalcemia, azotemia	Typical "punched-out" lytic lesions Diffuse osteoporosis
Osteosarcoma: second most common malignant tumor in adults, most common malignant bone tumor children	Peak age 10–20 50% leg 2,000–3,000 per year Male/female 1.5/1	Local pain, tenderness, swelling Night pain, pain with weight-bearing Constitutional symptoms	X-ray findings: "sunburst" pattern of radiating extensions from bone into soft tissue
Chondrosarcoma (malignant tumor of cartilage)	Middle–late adult life 90% are primary tumors; pelvis, femur, shoulder common sites Slow-growing	Acute or progressive deep pain Muscular weakness or atrophy Soft tissue mass may be palpable	Radiolucent lesions on X-ray Increased uptake on bone scan
Ewing's sarcoma: second most common malignant bone tumor in children	Most common in children, young adults More common in White men and boys	Pain, swelling, tenderness, erythema	Lytic lesion with onion-skin appearance of periosteum 53% occur on extremities

Physical Exam

- Painful mass, swelling, limited ROM of bone/joint
- Lymphadenopathy, hepatosplenomegaly

Diagnostic Studies

- X-ray may show aggressive, poorly defined lesion, irregular border, extension into soft tissue
- CT or MRI to determine extent of lesion
- Bone scan to detect metastasis
- Cytologic and pathologic examination
- CBC, liver function tests (LFTs)

Differential Diagnosis

- Benign bone tumor
- Osteomyelitis
- Metastatic disease

Management

Nonpharmacologic Treatment

- Surgery
- Radiation

Pharmacologic Treatment

- Chemotherapy
- Immunologic therapy

How Long to Treat

- Determined by oncologist

Special Considerations

- Refer for support, hospice, and pain control if necessary.

When to Consult, Refer, Hospitalize

- Refer to orthopedist for any bone lesion seen on X-ray, any constitutional signs of malignancy.
- Refer to oncology for specialty care.

Follow-Up

Expected Course

- Highly variable depending on type of tumor, patient history, tumor stage at diagnosis

Complications

- Loss of limb, metastases, death

Hip Pain in Children

INFLAMMATORY TRANSIENT SYNOVITIS

Description

- Transient synovitis
- Self-limited, unilateral inflammation of hip joint
- Children are typically well appearing

Etiology

- Unknown cause resulting in inflammation of the synovium in the hip
- Often associated with viral infections, post-vaccination, drug-mediated

Incidence and Demographics

- Most common disorder causing limp and hip pain in children
- Ages 3–8 years
- Male-to-female ratio: 2:1
- Occurs more frequently in springtime

Risk Factors

- Preceding upper respiratory tract infection
- Day care attendance
- Recent antibiotic use
- Recent immunization (especially measles, mumps, rubella [MMR])

Assessment

History

- Afebrile or low-grade fever
- No other systemic symptoms
- Insidious onset of pain, often complaining of vague "leg" pain or knee pain
- Antalgic limp or refusal to walk

Physical Exam

- Well-appearing child
- Hip held in position of flexion, abduction, and external rotation; decreased internal rotation

Diagnostic Studies

- CBC, ESR: usually normal or slightly elevated; ESR may be slightly elevated
- Blood culture and sensitivity to rule out infection
- Hip aspiration if septic arthritis suspected
- X-ray: unnecessary if hip motion is full; may show capsular swelling
- Ultrasound: can demonstrate if effusion in hip joint

Differential Diagnosis

- Septic arthritis
- Osteomyelitis
- Legg-Calvé-Perthes disease (LCPD)
- Slipped capital femoral epiphysis
- Juvenile rheumatoid arthritis

Management

Nonpharmacologic Treatment

- Rest until pain improvements

Pharmacologic Treatment

- Over-the-counter (OTC) analgesics: Acetaminophen or NSAIDS taken with food may be used for 1 to 2 weeks.

Special Considerations

- Exclude child abuse or injury as source of limp

When to Consult, Refer, Hospitalize

- Orthopedic referral needed for hip aspiration if infection is suspected.
- Hospitalize for septic joint or suspected abuse.

Follow-Up

Expected Course

- Improvement should occur in 24 to 48 hours.
- If symptoms persist beyond 1 week, reevaluation is important to exclude other diagnoses.

Complications

- 2% to 5% develop LCPD disease within 1 year
- Rarely avascular necrosis of femoral head
- May experience reoccurrence with subsequent viral infections

LEGG-CALVÉ-PERTHES DISEASE (LCPD)

Description

- Idiopathic avascular necrosis of the femoral head
- Presents as acute onset of hip pain and limp

Etiology

- Unclear
- Association with obesity, skeletal immaturity, and lower socioeconomic status

Incidence and Demographics

- Children 3 to 12 years of age; peak incidence 5–8 years
- Male-to-female ratio 3–4:1; low frequency among relatives
- Bilateral in 10%–20% of cases

Risk Factors

- History of low birth weight, delayed bone age, short stature
- 10% breech delivery
- 17% with previous trauma
- History of steroid use, sickle-cell disease, congenital hip dislocation

Prevention and Screening

- Weight loss in children with obesity may reduce risk in contralateral hip

Assessment

History

- Either insidious or sudden onset of limp, may be intermittent in early stages
- Sudden onset of groin, thigh, or knee pain
- Pain worse in morning and after activity
- Pain is not relieved with rest

Physical Exam

- Presents with painful or painless limp
- Resists internal rotation and abduction
- Leg kept in position of flexion and external rotation
- May have atrophy of quadriceps muscles

Diagnostic Studies

- X-ray AP and frog-leg views
- Early X-ray may be negative or show widening of joint space.
- Later X-ray with increased density, decreased femoral head size, and flattening of femoral head

- Ultrasound may show joint effusion early.
- MRI can identify early LCPD

Differential Diagnosis

- Septic arthritis
- Trauma
- Slipped capital femoral epiphysis
- Neoplasia
- Hemophilia
- Juvenile rheumatoid arthritis
- Acute/chronic infection

Management

Nonpharmacologic Treatment

- Rest, non-weight bearing, followed by limited activities
- Physical therapy to maintain ROM; may need crutches initially
- Containment of the femoral epiphysis with cast, brace, or orthosis

Pharmacologic Treatment

- OTC NSAIDs taken with food for pain relief

Special Considerations

- Pain often referred to knee

When to Consult, Refer, Hospitalize

- All suspected cases require orthopedic consultation.

Follow-Up

Expected Course

- Related to degree of femoral head involvement and age at onset; symptoms slowly resolve over 12 to 18 months
- Children younger than 6 years of age with better prognosis
- Children older than 8 years of age have increased risk of degenerative arthritis in adulthood and may need hip replacement

Complications

- Hip replacement

SLIPPED CAPITAL FEMORAL EPIPHYSIS (SCFE)

Description

- The femoral epiphysis slips posteriorly
- Results in limp and impaired internal rotation
- Patients present with pain in hip, groin, thigh, or knee

Etiology

- Unclear
- Multiple factors contribute to weakening of the physis and the femoral head slipping off the femoral neck

Incidence and Demographics

- Most common adolescent hip disorder; male-to-female ratio: 2:1; 2 cases per 100,000
- Peak age 12-year-old girls, 14-year-old boys
- 30% present with bilateral involvement
- 5% of cases with positive parental history of SCFE

Risk Factors

- Children younger than 10 SCFE may be associated with hypothyroidism, panhypothyroidism, hypogonadism, renal osteodystrophy, and growth hormone abnormalities.
- No prevention measures; early identification is best prognosis.
- Overweight children between 11 and 16 years of age
- Sedentary lifestyle

Assessment

History

- Pain in hip, infrequently referred pain to medial aspect of knee
- Severe pain in acute displacement
- Insidious, dull pain in gradual displacement

Physical Exam

- Presents with limp or inability to walk; walks with foot turned outward
- Local tenderness over hip
- Decreased flexion, abduction, and internal rotation
- Muscle atrophy and leg-length shortening

Diagnostic Studies

- AP, lateral, and frog-leg X-rays are diagnostic: femoral head resembles ice cream falling off cone
- Early slippage may be missed on X-ray; if suspicious, order bone scan

Differential Diagnosis

- Toxic synovitis
- LCPD
- Osteochondritis dissecans

- Chondrolysis
- Tumor
- Osteomyelitis
- JIA

Management

- Goals to prevent increased slippage and maintain hip function
- Emergent orthopedic referral for surgical management
- Child is non-weight-bearing

Nonpharmacologic Treatment

- Early disease: surgical placement of pin through femoral head and growth plate; rapid recovery with excellent prognosis
- Late disease: reconstructive surgery; poor outcome due to degenerative arthritis and need for early hip replacement

Special Considerations

- Prognosis is good if diagnosed early; avoid delay in diagnosis.

When to Consult, Refer, Hospitalize

- Emergency referral to orthopedist for surgical repair

Follow-Up

Expected Course

- Course is dependent on diagnostic timing; earlier is better.
- Anatomic position must be maintained postoperatively.
- In children younger than 10 years of age, monitor for bilateral slip.

Complications

- Avascular necrosis of femoral head
- May have slight but persistent leg-length shortening

Conditions that Cause Knee Pain

OSGOOD-SCHLATTER'S DISEASE

Description

- Overuse syndrome causing traction apophysitis of tibial tubercle (Achar & Yamanaka, 2019)

Etiology

- Repetitive microtrauma causing partial avulsion of patellar tendon insertion site on tibia (tibial apophysis)

Incidence and Demographics

- Boys 11 to 18 years old; girls 10 to 16 years old; more common in boys
- Bilateral in 25%–50% of cases
- Occurs twice as often in athletes than in nonathletes

Risk Factors

- Physically active adolescents
- Often occurs after a growth spurt in adolescents
- Sports that require running, jumping: soccer, basketball, football, ballet, figure skating, gymnastics

Prevention and Screening

- Avoiding overuse
- Adequate stretching with exercise

Assessment

History

- Pain below knee that begins during or after activity and is relieved by rest

Physical Exam

- Local tenderness and swelling over tibial tubercle
- Resisted knee extension worsens pain
- Pain is reproduced with knee extension against resistance

Diagnostic Studies

- Radiographs not necessary in typical presentation
- Ultrasound maybe considered

Differential Diagnosis

- Ewing's sarcoma
- Osteogenic sarcoma
- Patellar tendinitis

Management

Nonpharmacologic Treatment

- Application of ice
- Physical therapy for quadricep strengthening exercises and stretching of hamstrings and quadriceps
- Wear a protective pad over the tubercle

Special Considerations

- Recurrence rate 60%

When to Consult, Refer, Hospitalize

- Refer to sports medicine for possible injection if not improving over 3 months.
- Surgical management is reserved for patients who fail to respond to conservative treatment once the growth plate is fully closed.

Follow-Up

- For routine health maintenance
- Sooner if pain is not resolved or symptoms worsen, 4-week intervals

Expected Course

- Usually self-limited
- Resolves when tubercle fuses to diaphysis

Complications

- Chronic cases may require ossicle resection or excision of tibial tuberosity

KNEE INJURY

Description

- Damage to the knee or its supporting structures caused by trauma

Etiology

- Direct or indirect force to the knee
- Common in sports that require rapid changes in direction, acceleration/deceleration, knee injuries common in outpatient setting
- Often tear of ligaments or cartilage in knee
- May be fracture of the patella; children's ligaments and tendons are relatively stronger than bones; therefore children are at increased fracture risk.

Incidence and Demographics

- Common in all ages, especially adults
- Meniscus injuries are more common in adults than children

Risk Factors

- Participation in contact, running sport
- Poor conditioning
- Osteoarthritis
- Poorly fitting footwear, especially if associated with falls

Prevention and Screening

- Proper training, protective gear

History

- Gather history of trauma, repetitive motion, mechanism of injury, and previous surgeries to the affected knee.
- Ask the patient to describe hobbies, occupation, and participation in sports.
- Exclude infection by assessing for fever, recent infections, and risk for sexually transmitted diseases such as gonorrhea.

Assessment

- See Tables 14–3 and 14–4.

Collateral Ligament Injuries

- Graded on a scale of 1–3:
- Grade 1: Pain with varus/valgus stress but no instability
- Grade 2: Pain and instability at 30° of flexion during varus/valgus stress test
- Grade 3: Marked instability but no pain at 0 and 30 degrees of flexion during varus/valgus stress test

TABLE 14–3. SUMMARY OF COMMON KNEE INJURIES

INJURY	DEMOGRAPHICS	HISTORY	PHYSICAL
Fracture	Any age	Trauma Steroid use, osteoporosis Sudden swelling, pain, worse with weight-bearing	Effusion (hemarthrosis) Bony tenderness/pain to palpation Decreased ROM Difficulty bearing weight
Medial collateral ligament (MCL) injury	Adolescents and adults Contact sports	Sudden valgus stress to knee May have heard or felt "pop" Medial knee pain Localized swelling 1–4 hours	Tenderness to palpation Varying degree of joint laxity Small effusion
Lateral collateral ligament (LCL) injury	Adolescents and adults Contact sports	Direct blow to medial aspect of knee (varus stress) Similar to MCL injury but lateral	Tenderness over LCL Varying degree of joint laxity Small, if any, effusion
Anterior cruciate ligament (ACL) injury	Adolescents and adults Athletes	Pain and almost immediate swelling after sudden turning, deceleration, jumping May have heard or felt a "pop" Weight-bearing difficult due to feelings of instability	Effusion (hemarthrosis) Pain/tenderness in posterolateral joint Positive provocation tests (anterior drawer, Lachman's)
Posterior cruciate ligament (PCL) injury	Athletes, gymnasts	Forced hyperextension of knee Direct blow to anterior proximal tibia while knee is flexed and foot is planted	Mild to moderate effusion Positive posterior drawer, Godfrey's test
Meniscus tear	Adolescents, adults Athletes Older adults with osteoarthritis of knee	Pain, especially with twisting of knee (getting in and out of vehicles) Locking, catching, or giving way Harder to descend stairs than climb them	Swelling Tenderness over tibial medial or lateral joint line Positive McMurray's test

Continued

TABLE 14–3. (CONTINUED)

INJURY	DEMOGRAPHICS	HISTORY	PHYSICAL
Quadriceps rupture	Athletes Older adults with concomitant diseases (diabetes, peripheral vascular disease)	Often, fall on extended knee that forces joint into flexion Inability to straighten knee	Swelling Sometimes, palpable defect just superior to patella Inability to extend knee against resistance

TABLE 14–4. CLINICALLY RELEVANT PROVOCATIVE TESTS OF THE KNEE

TEST NAME	HOW TO PERFORM TEST
Valgus stress (tests MCL)	With patient's knee in 20°–30° of flexion, the examiner stabilizes the leg with one hand while applying inward-directed pressure to the joint. Test is repeated with knee in full extension.
Varus stress (tests LCL)	As above, but stress at joint is directed from the medial to lateral direction.
Anterior drawer (tests ACL)	With patient supine, his or her knee is flexed to 90° while examiner stabilizes patient's tibia (usually by sitting on foot/ankle). Examiner grasps proximal posterior tibia, pulling it forward. Anterior movement (translation) of tibia greater than uninvolved side is positive test.
Posterior drawer (tests PCL)	Patient and examiner in same position as for anterior drawer, but examiner pushes tibia posteriorly.
Lachman's test (more accurate than anterior drawer)	With patient supine, his or her knee is flexed to 30°. Using one hand, examiner stabilizes patient's distal femur while using other hand to pull proximal tibia anteriorly.
McMurray's test (for meniscus injury)	Patient's knee is maximally flexed, then internally rotated; as leg is passively extended, examiner simultaneously externally rotates leg while palpating tibial joint line. Repeat with leg externally rotated, internally rotating while extending. Positive test is palpable click or tibial joint line pain.

Posterior Cruciate Ligament (PCL)

- One-third of PCL tears will have a neurovascular component to the injury, so it is important to do a thorough neurological and vascular exam on the leg.
- Pain, swelling, pallor, and numbness could mean popliteal artery is involved and this requires an urgent referral within 1–2 weeks.
- Clinical examinations that support a PCL injury include a positive sag sign or a positive posterior drawer test.

Diagnostic Studies

- Joint aspiration: diagnostic and therapeutic (presence of fat globules seen with fracture; removal of effusion can improve ROM, increase patient comfort)
- X-ray: diagnose fracture, osteoarthritis
- CT: evaluate extent of fracture depression (if any), position of fracture fragments
- MRI: differentiate ligamentous, cartilaginous injuries

Differential Diagnosis

- Worsening osteoarthritis
- Septic joint
- Gout
- Tumor

Management

Nonpharmacologic Treatment

- Fracture: immobilization, no weight-bearing, surgical repair sometimes necessary
- Grade I, II collateral ligament sprains: hinged knee brace; surgery usually not required
- Grade III sprains involve complete tearing of ligament: surgery usually required
- Cruciate ligament sprains: bracing, physical therapy, surgical reconstruction may be necessary
- Meniscus tears: arthroscopic repair (preferred treatment)

- Osteoarthritis: weight loss and exercise strongly recommended (Kolansinski et al., 2020)
- Physical therapy for improving ROM, strength

Pharmacologic Treatment

- NSAIDs taken with food for 1–2 weeks regularly for inflammation and pain
- Analgesics, maybe used for short-term pain management

Special Considerations

- Active younger patients may require functional bracing to return to sports.

When to Consult, Refer, Hospitalize

- Consult for grade II, III sprains.
- Refer immediately for suspected fracture, inability to flex or extend joint, hemarthrosis, suspected septic joint or tumor.

Follow-Up

- In 2- to 4-week intervals until resolved

Expected Course

- Except for fractures, meniscus tears, complete ligamentous disruption, most knee injuries will heal in 4 to 8 weeks.

Complications

- Deformity, accelerated degenerative changes of joint, stiffness, or instability

Conditions that Cause Ankle Pain

ANKLE SPRAIN

Description

- Stretching and/or tearing of ligaments around the ankle
- Standard grading indicates extent of damage:
  - Grade I: stretching but no tearing of ligament; no joint instability (local tenderness, minimal edema, full ROM, can bear weight, discomfort)
  - Grade II: partial (incomplete) tearing of ligament; some joint instability but definite endpoint to laxity (immediate pain, localized edema, ecchymoses, pain on weight-bearing, reduced ROM)
  - Grade III: complete ligamentous tearing; joint unstable with no definite endpoint to ligamentous stressing (acute pain with injury, significant edema of foot and ankle, profound and continuing development of ecchymoses, cannot bear weight, ankle ROM restricted)

Etiology

- Most common inversion injury that affects lateral ankle
- Eversion injury affects medial ankle—second most common type

Incidence and Demographics

- Most common musculoskeletal injury
- Occurs at rate of 1 per 10,000 persons per day; men and boys affected more often

Risk Factors

- Extrinsic factors: type of activity, indoor court sports cause highest risk.
  - Outdoor courts also pose increased risk.
  - Sports requiring sudden turns, jumping; foot in supinated, plantar-flexed position
- Intrinsic factors: limited dorsiflexion, reduced proprioception, and balance deficiencies

Prevention and Screening

- Conditioning exercises for sports, avoidance of high-heeled shoes, ankle-strengthening exercises

Assessment

History

- Sudden, forced inversion or eversion of foot, often in plantar-flexed position
- Sudden onset of pain, rapid onset of swelling; often with inability to initially bear weight on affected ankle
- Possible bruising within 2–4 days
- Sensation of pop, snap, locking of joint

Physical Exam

- Edema, ecchymosis, tenderness over injured ligaments; pain aggravated by repeating motion that caused original injury
- Talar tilt test used to assess stability of calcaneofibular ligament (heel is grasped and supinated)
- Anterior drawer sign used to assess anterior talofibular ligament. (while the lower leg is held steady, the heel is grasped and pulled forward)
- Consider use of Ottawa ankle rules.

Diagnostic Studies

- X-rays not indicated in adults unless at least one of the following (Ottawa rule):
  - Unable to bear weight right after injury or when examined
  - Tenderness over posterior edge of distal 6 cm of the medial or lateral malleolus
  - Tenderness over tarsal navicular or fifth metatarsal
  - If X-rays are indicated, obtain anterior-posterior (AP), lateral, and mortise views.

Differential Diagnosis

- Syndesmosis injury
- Fracture
- Tendon rupture

Management

Nonpharmacologic Treatment

Modified RICE is recommended as a treatment for ankle sprains:

- Modified activities (previously rest)
- Ice
- Compression
- Elevation

Early motion is essential for healing, and patients should do home exercises or physical therapy.

- Splinting, weight-bearing as tolerated, ankle ROM and strengthening exercises
- Grade III injuries may require casting, surgery.

Pharmacologic Treatment

- NSAIDs taken with food or OTC analgesics

How Long to Treat

- Most Grade I or II sprains heal in 6 to 8 weeks.

Special Considerations

- Medial ankle sprains require greater force to cause injury; may have other associated injury
- Geriatric patients: older patients may require longer healing time.

When to Consult, Refer, Hospitalize

- Dislocation or subluxation
- Syndesmosis injury
- Tendon rupture
- Chronic ankle instability unresponsive to physical therapy

Follow-Up

- In 1–2 weeks if not improving after initial diagnosis

Expected Course

- Most uncomplicated sprains show improvement in 3–4 weeks and heal within 6–8 weeks.

Complications

- Syndesmosis injury, peroneal tendinitis, recurrent injury, chronic instability, avascular necrosis

SEVER'S DISEASE

Description

- Inflammatory condition causing a calcaneal apophysitis—inflammation around the Achilles tendon insertion to the posterior growth plate in skeletally immature children and adolescents (Achar & Yamanaka, 2019)
- Typically an overuse injury from participation in sports, running or jumping
- Most common cause of heel pain in children

Etiology

- Traction-induced microtrauma at insertion of Achilles tendon on the calcaneus, causing inflammation

Incidence and Demographics

- 8- to 13-year-olds, boys more commonly affected than girls
- Bilateral presentation in two-thirds of cases
- Athletes

Risk Factors

- Accelerated growth
- Tight heel cords
- Soccer players or runners

Assessment

History

- Heel pain with activity
- Bilateral or unilateral

Physical Exam

- Tenderness at insertion of the Achilles tendon on the calcaneus

Diagnostic Studies

- Radiographs not required to make diagnosis
- X-rays may show partial fragmentation and increased density of the os calcis.

Differential Diagnosis

- Bone cyst
- Stress fracture
- Strain

Management

Nonpharmacologic Treatment

- Activity modification
- Stretching, ice
- Heel cups

Pharmacologic Treatment

- NSAIDs

How Long to Treat

- Until resolved, 4 to 6 weeks

Special Considerations

- May need to modify activity, exercise, or shoes until improved

When to Consult, Refer, Hospitalize

- Achilles tendon rupture or not improving with treatment

Follow-Up

- In 2 weeks, to make sure it is resolving

Expected course

- Improvement in 2 to 4 weeks with activity modification

Complications

- Rupture of the Achilles tendon

Conditons that Cause Shoulder Pain

CLAVICLE FRACTURE

Description

- Fracture of clavicle; most frequently fractured bone during delivery

Etiology

- Birth trauma due to delivery of shoulder in vertex position and extended arms in breech delivery
- Fall on outstretched arm or on clavicle

Incidence and Demographics

- 0.2% to 4.5% of births (Hashmi et al., 2021)
- 70% middle third of clavicle
- Occurs in all ages; more common in children; in adults, usually occurs after a fall.

Risk Factors

- Large fetus, shoulder dystocia
- Breech position
- Fall on outstretched arm

Prevention and Screening

- Methods to reduce birth trauma
- Check for fractures at birth and 2-week well-child visits.

Assessment

History

- Difficult delivery, spontaneous vaginal delivery, prolonged second stage, birthweight
- Characteristic injury
- Pain, displacement, or bump on clavicle

Physical Exam

- Newborn or patient may not move arm on affected side (Erb's palsy).
- Absent Moro reflex on affected side in newborn

Diagnostic Studies

- X-rays not usually done in newborns.
- X-rays done if history of fall or trauma.

Differential Diagnosis

- Fractured humerus
- Brachial nerve palsy

Management

- Neonatal clavicle fracture is transient with good prognosis (Hashmi et al., 2021)
- Nondisplaced fracture may be treated with sling
- Callus formation occurs in 1 to 2 weeks.

Nonpharmacological Treatment

- Consider immobilization of arm and shoulder on affected side, sling or clavicular strap

Pharmacologic Treatment

- Analgesics as needed

How Long to Treat

- Until healed (4 to 6 weeks)

Special Considerations

- Check in babies with history of breech or difficult delivery, large size, mothers with gestational diabetes

When to Consult, Refer, Hospitalize

- Refer to orthopedist for any symptoms of neurovascular injury.

Follow-Up

- If not improving in 3 to 4 weeks

Expected Course

- Heals in 3 to 4 weeks in children
- Heals in 6 weeks in adults

Complications

- 10% of infants will also have concomitant brachial plexus injuries.
- Permanent bump at site of callus formation in adults; rare in children under 10 years
- Neurovascular injury

OTHER SHOULDER INJURIES

Description

- Pain in the shoulder girdle
- The shoulder is a shallow ball and socket joint relying heavily on the muscles and ligaments for stability.
- Rotator cuff tear is a common cause of impingement syndrome.

Etiology

- Traumatic, arthritic, infectious, or degenerative conditions (seeTable 14–5)

Incidence and Demographics

- Acute injuries tend to occur in adolescents and younger adults
- Chronic shoulder pain and fracture due to falls are more often found in older adults
- Lifetime prevalence 6.7%–67% (Lee et al., 2021)

TABLE 14–5.
COMMON CAUSES OF ACUTE AND CHRONIC SHOULDER PAIN

ACUTE CONDITIONS	CHRONIC CONDITIONS
Trauma: fracture (proximal humerus, greater tuberosity, clavicle, scapula)	Inflammatory conditions:
Rotator cuff strain, tear	Bursitis (subacromial and subdeltoid)
Dislocation (anterior most common)	Bicipital, rotator cuff tendinitis
Acromioclavicular separation "separated"	Impingement syndrome
Subacromial spurring	Osteoarthritis
Sternoclavicular injury	
Chronic instability	
Adhesive capsulitis (frozen shoulder)	

Risk Factors

- Repetitive overhead activity (occupational, recreational)
- Rheumatoid or osteoarthritis
- Previous shoulder injury

Prevention and Screening

- Injury prevention

Assessment

- See Table 14–6.

History

- A detailed history including hand dominance, occupation, and recreational activities is important in the initial workup.

Diagnostic Studies

- Plain X-ray: useful for evaluating fracture, acromioclavicular separation, presence of osteophytes, calcific tendinitis
- MRI: can show tendinitis, rotator cuff tear, ligamentous or cartilage injury
- Arthrogram: still used to identify extent of rotator cuff tear

Differential Diagnosis

- Septic joint
- Gout
- Complex regional pain syndrome (CRPS)
- Acromegaly

TABLE 14–6.
ASSESSMENT OF SHOULDER INJURIES

CONDITION	HISTORY	PHYSICAL FINDINGS
Fracture	Fall directly onto shoulder or outstretched arm Localized pain, swelling Decreased ROM Often, no bruising evident for first few days after injury	Patient holds arm close to body Point tenderness Varying degree of bony deformity (usually most pronounced with clavicle fracture) Decreased ROM
Rotator cuff tear	Age 40 years and older Pain may radiate into deltoid area. May have felt "pop" or "something give" in shoulder Inability to raise arm overhead Weakness or inability to externally rotate arm Inability to sleep on affected side	Weakness or inability to externally rotate shoulder Limited abduction, forward flexion of shoulder Inability to maintain resisted abduction at 90°
Dislocation	Separated shoulder Usually, direct blow or fall onto top of shoulder Pain, especially with adduction of arm Swelling Deformity depends on severity of injury. Bruising may be present.	Direct blow to shoulder or trying to avoid fall by grabbing onto something; shoulder in abducted, externally rotated position Sensation of shoulder slipping out of joint "Popping" or clicking of joint May note swelling Tenderness over acromioclavicular (AC) joint Pain with adduction (across chest) Varying degree of AC deformity (more deformity with more severe injury) Positive apprehension test: shoulder abducted to 90° and elbow flexed to 90°; shoulder then passively externally rotated; resistance by patient is a positive test Palpable clicking with ROM Deformity may be visible.

Continued

TABLE 14–6. (CONTINUED)

CONDITION	HISTORY	PHYSICAL FINDINGS
Inflammatory conditions	May progress to constant pain Pain often worse with lifting, pushing objects away Difficulty lying on affected side	Progressive pain with certain activities (usually overhead) that groove May have weak abduction Painful arc (i.e., pain at 70°–120° of abduction)
Adhesive capsulitis	Middle-aged women more likely to be afflicted May or may not have history of trauma Progressive loss of motion Pain varies from minimal to severe	Marked restriction in active and passive ROM Pain over anterior joint, rotator cuff Patient often uses scapular muscles to "increase" abduction

Management

Nonpharmacologic Treatment

- Initially, short period of rest/immobilization (no more than 14 days), then begin passive ROM exercises; progress to active, resistive exercises as healing continues.
- Surgical intervention indicated for complete rotator cuff tear, displaced fracture.
- Manipulation under anesthesia may be necessary for severe adhesive capsulitis.
- Physical therapy to maintain, improve ROM; strengthen muscles

Pharmacologic Treatment

- NSAIDs, other analgesics
- Local corticosteroid injection

How Long to Treat

- As long as symptomatic

When to Consult, Refer, Hospitalize

- Refer any fracture, suspected rotator cuff tear, AC separation with deformity, dislocation or chronic instability, adhesive capsulitis, corticosteroid injection to orthopedic
- Refer cases with rheumatoid arthritis to rheumatologist or orthopedic as indicated

Follow-Up

- Visits are variable depending on condition and severity, may be 2–4-week intervals

Expected Course

- Varies according to pathology
- Tendinitis symptoms should improve within 3 to 4 weeks of conservative therapy but may not resolve for 6 or more weeks; follow-up in 3 to 4 weeks if no improvement.
- AC separation (mild) should be reevaluated in 2 to 3 weeks; resolution usually in about 6 weeks.
- Osteoarthritis: Reevaluate 4 to 6 weeks after starting treatment.

Complications

- Permanently decreased ROM, muscular weakness

SUBACROMIAL (SHOULDER) IMPINGEMENT SYNDROME (SIS)

Description

- Pain with overhead activity
- Pain with sleeping on shoulder
- Pain with internal rotation of the shoulder

Assessment

History

- Detailed history of hand dominance, timing, duration, activities which worsen and improve symptoms

Physical Exam

- Atrophy in the supraspinatus and infraspinatus fossa
- Rolled-forward shoulder posture
- Head-forward posture
- Tenderness to the anterolateral shoulder at edge of greater tuberosity
- Lacks full active ROM and has full passive ROM
- Positive Neer impingement and Hawkins impingement signs
- Common tests for rotator cuff tear
  - Empty Can test: to test supraspinatus strength
  - Drop Arm test: patient tries to drop arm slowly from 90 degrees abduction. If the arm drops quickly, it is positive.

Diagnostic Imaging

- X-ray to exclude arthritis and fracture
- MRI to evaluate partial and full-thickness tear

Non-Pharmacologic Treatment

- Physical therapy to improve ROM and decrease motion restriction for activities of daily living (ADLs)

Pharmacologic Treatment

- NSAIDs, other analgesics
- Local corticosteroid injection

How Long to Treat

- While symptomatic

When to Consult, Refer, Hospitalize

- Consult orthopedic if no improvement after 3 months of conservative treatment including physical therapy

Follow-Up

- Visits are variable depending on condition and severity, may be 2–4-week intervals

Conditions that Cause Elbow Pain

EPICONDYLITIS

Description

- Lateral or medial epicondylitis is tendinopathy from chronic, repetitive overuse causing microtrauma at the tendon insertion site.
- Lateral epicondylitis ("tennis elbow"): involves extensor tendons of forearm; common
- Medial epicondylitis ("golfer's elbow"): involves flexor tendons of forearm; less common

Symptoms of Lateral Epicondylitis (Tennis Elbow)

- Pain with arm and wrist extended such as shaking hands, lifting objects, using a computer mouse, or hitting a racquet backhand

Symptoms of Medial Epicondylitis (Golfer's Elbow)

- Pain when arm is pronated, and wrist is flexed

Incidence and Demographics

- Common among tennis players, golfers, and manual laborers
- Incidence 1%–3% of general population

Etiology

- Overuse syndrome caused by damage to tendons, progressing to periostitis at origin on epicondyle
- Stress on tendons; may be due to repetitive motions, poor technique when playing racquet or throwing sports; most common in middle age

Risk Factors

- Weak shoulder and wrist muscles (extensors and/or flexors)
- Repetitive motion of forearm with wrist extended or flexed against resistance
- Smoking, obesity, ages 45–54

Prevention and Screening

- Strengthening of shoulder muscles and wrist extensors and flexors
- For sports, appropriate-sized grips on racquets, proper body mechanics when throwing

Assessment

History

- Pain on affected side of elbow that progresses down forearm, occasionally into wrist
- Difficulty lifting objects, even a cup of liquid
- Numbness and tingling are *not* usually associated

Physical Exam

- Lateral or medial epicondyle is tender to palpation.
- Lateral epicondylitis: pain upon grasping a weighted cup or resisted wrist extension
- Medial epicondylitis: pain with pronation, flex wrist against resistance, or squeezing hard rubber ball

Diagnostic Studies

- None indicated unless there is a history of trauma
- If failure to improve after 3 months of conservative treatment obtain three-view radiograph elbow series
- MRI for unresolved symptoms for more than 6 months to determine need for surgery

Differential Diagnosis

- Radial tunnel syndrome
- Arthritis
- Cubital tunnel syndrome

Management

Nonpharmacologic Treatment

- Rest, ice
- Avoid activities that exacerbate pain.
- Compression with counterforce bands—tennis elbow band
- Physical therapy, including ultrasound; stretching exercises after pain subsides
- Recalcitrant cases may require surgery (Bosworth procedure).

Pharmacologic Treatment

- NSAIDs
- Triamcinolone corticosteroid injection if not improving with rest and NSAIDs

How Long to Treat

- Symptoms should resolve in 3 months with conservative treatment or maximum of three injections at 6-week intervals.

Special Considerations

- More than three corticosteroid injections unlikely to improve chance of remission but more likely to cause adverse effects (tendon weakening, subcutaneous fat necrosis, hypopigmentation of skin)

When to Consult, Refer, Hospitalize

- Refer to orthopedist if no improvement after 3 months of conservative treatment.

Follow-Up

- Provide patient education about removing underlying cause of the problem to avoid recurrence.

Expected Course

- Noticeable improvement should occur within 6 weeks of treatment.

Complications

- Not common but chronic, untreated epicondylitis can progress to epicondylar spur formation and damage to collateral ligament

SUBLUXATION OF RADIAL HEAD

Description

- Subluxation of the annular ligament into the radiohumeral joint; also known as "nurse-maid's elbow"

Etiology

- Sudden longitudinal pull on the hand with elbow extended and forearm pronated
- Ligament becomes trapped when radius recoils

Incidence and Demographics

- Most common elbow injury in 2- to 4-year-olds
- Peak incidence in children younger than 4 years of age

Prevention

- Avoid pulling on child's arm, swinging child by hands, or lifting by one hand.
- Screening: No routine screening. With presenting symptoms only.

Assessment

History

- Report of child's arm being suddenly and vigorously pulled immediately followed by crying and refusal to move arm
- May have heard or felt a "click"

Physical Exam

- Child holds arm close to body in flexed, pronated position
- Flexion and extension normal; limited supination
- No swelling, deformity, point tenderness, warmth, or erythema noted

Diagnostic Studies

- X-ray if reduction unsuccessful

Differential Diagnosis

- Fracture
- Sprain/strain

Management

Nonpharmacologic Treatment

- Reduce subluxation by gentle supination with arm in 90° flexion
- "Click" usually heard or felt with immediate pain relief

Special Considerations

- Observe child after reduction to ensure use of arm
- Have child grasp a sticker with affected hand

When to Consult, Refer, Hospitalize

- Refer to orthopedist if closed reduction unsuccessful or recurrent

Follow-Up

Expected Course

- Full use returns in 30 minutes.

Complications

- Can be recurrent in some children

Conditions that Cause Wrist Pain

LIGAMENT AND TENDON INJURIES

Description

- Acute or chronic pain in the wrist due to inflammation of soft tissue

Etiology

- Trauma (radiocarpal sprain)
- Developmental (ganglion cyst)
- Overuse (de Quervain's tenosynovitis, tendinitis)

Incidence and Demographics

- Common problem that affects all ages and genders

Risk Factors

- Repetitive use of hands, wrists
- Injury to wrist
- Osteoarthritis

Prevention and Screening

- Wear protective wrist guards for sports.
- Properly position computer, keyboard, or other equipment.
- Avoid overuse.

Assessment

- (see Table 14–7)

TABLE 14–7.
COMMON CAUSES OF WRIST PAIN

CONDITION	HISTORY	PHYSICAL FINDINGS
Radiocarpal sprain	Trauma: usually forced hyperextension or flexion Pain with movement Decreased ROM	Varying degree of swelling. Numbness/ tingling are unusual more than a day or two after injury. Pain with active and passive ROM Tenderness over radiocarpal joint, but no point bony tenderness
Ganglion cyst	Usually no history of trauma May have repetitive use of hands/ wrists Progressive localized swelling that tends to fluctuate in size depending on activity Usually nonpainful	Most common on dorsum of wrist, but also seen on volar surface Encapsulated, slightly fluctuant, mobile lesion Pain may occur with compression of mass.
de Quervain's tenosynovitis	Insidious onset of burning, aching pain over radial aspect of wrist and base of thumb Common in nursing mothers (due to holding infant with thumb extended); pain often worse with grasping movements	Pain with passive, active thumb extension May have visible thickening of tendon Positive Finkelstein's test: pain with ulnar deviation of clenched fist (with thumb tucked inside fist)

Diagnostic Studies

- Clinical examination is usually sufficient to diagnose these problems.
- X-rays should be obtained if any suggestion of fracture or history of trauma
- MRI can be used to differentiate ganglion cyst from other soft tissue masses; look for more serious wrist injury (triangular fibrocartilage tear).

Differential Diagnosis

- Nerve entrapment
- Fracture
- Gout

- Rheumatoid arthritis
- Osteoarthritis

Management

Nonpharmacologic Treatment

- Splinting, moist heat, aspiration of ganglion (high recurrence rate)
- Surgical release of tendon sheath, surgical excision of ganglion

Pharmacologic Treatment

- NSAIDs
- Corticosteroid injection into first dorsal tendon sheath for de Quervain's

Special Considerations

- Women more often affected by de Quervain's, ganglion cysts

When to Consult, Refer, Hospitalize

- Consult with orthopedist for wrist condition that does not improve within 3 to 4 weeks of conservative treatment
- Refer for corticosteroid injection, any suspicion of fracture

Follow-Up

- If not improving in 4 weeks

Expected Course

- Most wrist pain resolves in 4 to 6 weeks; ganglion cysts tend to recur.

Complications

- Few, but chronic wrist pain can occur.

Other Musculoskeletal Conditions and Injuries

FRACTURES

Description

- Complete or partial break in bone
- Unstable, comminuted, or compound fractures require emergent evaluation and possibly surgical management
- Uncomplicated fractures may be managed effectively without surgical intervention

Etiology

- Trauma or extreme force to the bone is the usual cause.
- However, tumor, osteoporosis, osteomyelitis, or osteomalacia can also cause bone to break

Incidence and Demographics

- Common in children due to activity, and in advancing age
- White women 60 years of age or older have higher incidence of fracture than men.
- Vertebral fractures are most frequent, followed by wrist fracture

Risk Factors

- Trauma, falls
- Neoplasms
- Osteoporosis, osteomyelitis
- Smoking, malnutrition (vitamin D deficiency), malabsorption, chronic steroid use
- Renal osteodystrophy
- Osteogenesis imperfecta

Prevention and Screening

- Maximize bone density during adolescence/young adulthood
- Weight-bearing physical activity
- Adequate dietary intake of calcium and vitamin D
- Avoidance of smoking, excessive alcohol intake

Assessment

History

- Mechanism of injury: fall, motor vehicle accident, violence
- Localization of pain
- Pain worse with movement
- Swelling occurs rapidly, may be associated with bruising, variable degree of deformity or asymmetry
- History of past injuries or surgeries
- Additional injuries beyond the focus as there may be concomitant injuries

Physical Exam

- Point tenderness over bone; muscle weakness/pain with movement; deformity
- Assess skin, neurological, and vascular status

Diagnostic Studies

- X-ray: most cost-effective; usually adequate for showing fracture
- Bone scan: useful for identifying occult/stress fracture
- CT: for evaluating degree of displacement, compression of fracture
- MRI: identifying lesions that may affect bone
- Laboratory studies not usually indicated

Differential Diagnosis

- Sprain
- Hematoma
- Abscess
- Tumor

Management

Nonpharmacologic Treatment

- Immobilization by splinting or casting of extremity
- Ice and elevation
- Monitor and maintain neurovascular integrity.
- Displaced fractures and open fractures require surgical management.

Pharmacologic Treatment

- Analgesics, judicious use of short-acting opioid medications with acetaminophen allow for lower doses of opioids, use short term for first 48–72 hours
- NSAIDs after first 24 hours (immediate administration may increase hematoma formation due to platelet inhibition)

How Long to Treat

- Fracture immobilization and referral to orthopedic surgeon.
- Most simple fractures heal in 4 to 6 weeks; longer immobilization should be expected in presence of displaced fractures, chronic disease (diabetes, cardiovascular disease), smoking, or malignancy.

Special Considerations

- In geriatric patients, consider X-ray even if no trauma to exclude compression fracture or tumor.
- Consider stress fracture if persistent bony tenderness and negative initial X-ray.
- Epiphyseal fractures (Salter I–V) in children may disrupt growth of the bone.

When to Consult, Refer, Hospitalize

- Refer all compound, displaced, or compression fractures immediately.
- Need to hospitalize is determined by orthopedist.

Follow-Up

- In 4 to 6 weeks if improving, sooner if pain persists

Expected Course

- Fracture healing should occur in 4 to 6 weeks.
- Resolution of swelling and increase in strength take place over next 4 to 6 weeks.

Complications

- Caution decrease circulation from splinting
- Persistent deformity, arthritis, compression neuropathy, fibrous union

STRESS FRACTURE

Description

- Overuse injuries to bones caused by repetitive stress such as athletic training or military marching
- The type of stress alone would not cause fracture; it is the repetitive nature over time.

Etiology

- Microtrauma to a normal bone that exceeds that bone's capability for repair
- Fracture of a bone without trauma

Incidence and Demographics

- Less than 1% of U.S. population affected
- More common in runners, athletes who participate in jumping activities, military recruits
- Metatarsal stress fractures most common but tibial shaft, calcaneus, patella, pubic ramus, pars interarticularis also affected

Risk Factors

- Training errors (sudden increase in intensity or duration)
- Overuse
- Metabolic disorders, disordered eating
- History of prior stress fracture
- Low body mass index (BMI)
- Female gender, amenorrhea

Prevention and Screening

- Proper training, wearing appropriate footwear, using good body mechanics

Assessment

History

- Insidious onset of pain intensified by running, jogging; pain may persist for 2 to 3 weeks before patient seeks treatment

Physical Exam

- Point tenderness over fracture site
- Possible mild erythema, diffuse swelling in area lacking significant soft tissue coverage

Diagnostic Studies

- Plain radiographs are typically normal for first 2 to 3 weeks after symptom onset
- MRI useful in diagnosis and differentiation between pathologic and stress fractures

Differential Diagnosis

- Tendinopathy
- Sprain/strain
- Infection
- Neoplasm

Management

Nonpharmacologic Treatment

- Pain control
- Limit physical activity, reduce weight bearing
- Rehabilitative exercise to address biomechanical problems

Pharmacologic Treatment

- NSAIDs
- Acetaminophen

How Long to Treat

- 4 to 6 weeks

Special Considerations

- Consider in athletes, postmenopausal women with persistent bone pain without trauma

When to Consult, Refer, Hospitalize

- Consult or refer to orthopedist if any question about diagnosis, treatment

Follow-Up

- Every 1 to 3 weeks during healing period
- Stress fractures can progress to complete fractures, hence the close monitoring.

Expected Course

- Once treated, normal activities can usually be resumed in 4 to 6 weeks.

Complications

- Left untreated, can progress to full fracture

MUSCLE STRAIN

Description

- Overstretching or partial tearing of muscle fibers; graded I–III
  - ◊ Grade I: stretching, tearing of muscle fibers but fascia remains intact, no loss of muscle function; movement strong and painful
  - ◊ Grade II: tearing of muscle fibers resulting in significant hemorrhage, mild loss of muscle strength; movement strong and painful
  - ◊ Grade III: rupture of muscle, damage to fascia; movement is weak and pain free

Etiology

- Excessive stress placed on any muscle resulting in overstretching of fibers and resultant tearing and inflammation

Incidence and Demographics

- Common problem, many instances self-treated

Risk Factors

- Contact sports, running
- Lifting or moving heavy objects

Prevention and Screening

- Appropriate stretching, warm-up exercises before participating in running, sports; proper body mechanics

Assessment

History

- Sudden onset of muscle pain associated with activity; bruising, swelling, and loss of function may occur with more severe injury.
- Gradually increasing muscle pain may occur with repetitive use of specific muscle/group.

Physical Exam

- Localized tenderness, swelling, ecchymosis; pain with resisted muscle contraction and passive stretching of muscle; weakness with more severe injury.

Diagnostic Studies

- Physical exam
- MRI may be useful to identify extent of muscle involvement, but usually not necessary.

Differential Diagnosis

- Tendinitis
- Tumor

Management

Nonpharmacologic Treatment

- Rest, ice, compression (if an extremity), elevation; physical therapy to regain strength, mobility
- Transcutaneous electrical nerve stimulation (TENS) unit, acupressure improves pain relief when compared to placebo (Qaseem et al., 2020)

Pharmacologic Treatment

- NSAIDs are mainstay of treatment.
- Acetaminophen for pain relief
- Topical NSAIDs are recommended (Qaseem et al., 2020).

How Long to Treat

- Symptoms improve in 7 to 10 days.

Special Considerations

- More-active patients should not return to contact sports until they are pain free.

When to Consult, Refer, Hospitalize

- Consult with orthopedist for grade III injuries; refer for any injury involving muscle weakness.
- Refer for physical therapy for muscle strengthening

Follow-Up

- In 2 weeks if not improving

Expected Course

- Varies with degree of injury
- Mild strains resolve in 7 to 10 days; severe injuries may require 8 weeks or more of treatment

Complications

- Permanent deformity, loss of strength

BURSITIS

Description

- Inflammation or infection of synovial membrane of the bursal sac overlying bony prominences
- Common sites are shoulder (subacromial or subdeltoid), elbow (olecranon), hip (trochanteric), knee (prepatellar, pes anserine, suprapatellar), heel (retrocalcaneal)

Etiology

- Acute: trauma or infection
- Chronic: repetitive use, inflammatory conditions such as rheumatoid arthritis or gout

Incidence

- No accurate incidence is available in research literature. Estimated to account for up to 0.4% of all primary care visits.

Demographics

- Most seen in athletes or as an overuse injury

Risk Factors

- Chronic pressure on bursa (kneeling, resting point of elbow on hard surface, overhead activity)
- Rheumatoid, gouty, or inflammatory arthritis
- Baker's cyst
- Chronic or acute overuse, particularly in middle-age or older adults

Prevention and Screening

- Avoidance of activities that apply pressure to bursae
- Use of appropriate protective/padded equipment

Assessment

History

- Swelling and inflammation in superficial sites—patella, olecranon
- Sudden or gradual onset of localized painful swelling
- Increased pain and discomfort with activity

Physical Exam

- Localized fluctuant swelling (swelling over greater trochanter difficult to evaluate)
- May be warm and/or painful to touch
- Passive motion is normal, pain with active motion
- If erythema or warmth, consider septic bursitis

Diagnostic Studies

- None needed unless redness or warmth
- If redness or warmth, fluid aspiration analysis to evaluate for infection or gout; CBC

Differential Diagnosis

- Septic joint
- Gout
- Joint effusion
- Trauma
- Rheumatoid arthritis
- Cellulitis

Management

Nonpharmacologic Treatment

- Joint protection such as knee pads
- RICE protocol
- Aspiration of bursal sac to reduce pain from pressure

Pharmacologic Treatment

- If septic bursitis, oral antibiotics, often dicloxacillin or cephalexin
- NSAIDs (ibuprofen, sodium naproxen)
- Local corticosteroid injection for deeper bursae of hip or shoulder: not performed unless infection is excluded
- Retrocalcaneal injection not recommended due to risk of Achilles tendon rupture

How Long to Treat

- NSAIDs for 1 to 3 weeks until swelling subsides

Special Considerations

- Surgical drainage/removal may be necessary if infection does not respond to antibiotics, local aspiration

When to Consult, Refer, Hospitalize

- Refer to physician or other specialized health care provider for bursa aspiration, as necessary.
- Consult with physician or other health care provider for local skin infection, marked cellulitis, or signs of systemic illness associated with bursitis for parenteral antibiotics, possible hospitalization.

Follow-Up

- Provide patient education about need for joint protection.

Expected Course

- Symptoms usually improve within 2 to 3 days of aspirating/injecting bursa (if not infected).
- If infected, localized erythema should improve within 3 to 5 days.

Complications

- Chronic bursitis

CARPAL TUNNEL SYNDROME (CTS)

Description

- Entrapment neuropathy of median nerve at the wrist which produces pain, numbness, and weakness in the hand

Etiology

- Multiple causes, includes any process that encroaches on the carpal tunnel, compressing the median nerve, or causes enlargement of the median nerve
- Mnemonic for causes is PRAGMATIC: Pregnancy, Rheumatoid Arthritis, Growth hormone abnormalities, Metabolic disorders, Alcoholism, Tumors, Idiopathic, Connective tissue disorders

- Work/hobby repetitive flexion and extension of wrist: computer typists, cashiers, sorters, musicians, hairdressers, use of vibrating tools, painters, sewing
- History of trauma to wrist: fracture, dislocations

INCIDENCE AND DEMOGRAPHICS

- Affects approximately 1% of U.S. population
- Women affected more often than men; onset ages 30 to 50 years, incidence increases with age
- More common in people using forceful, repetitive wrist and hand movements or vibratory tools
- Increased incidence in patients with diabetes

Risk Factors

- Repetitive wrist flexion/extension movement; collagen vascular disease, history of Colles fracture

Prevention and Screening

- Proper ergonomics for wrist
- Treatment of underlying problem

Assessment

History

- Initially burning or aching pain, numbness, tingling that wakes patient at night and resolves after shaking the affected hand ("wake-and-shake")
- As disorder progresses, symptoms affect thumb, index and middle finger; may radiate into arm.

Physical Exam

- Tinel's sign: positive if symptoms are reproduced by tapping the median nerve at the wrist
- Phalen's sign: positive if pain within 60 seconds of bilateral wrist flexion with hands held in opposition (clinically, may be more useful than Tinel's)
- Carpal compression test: positive if numbness and tingling develop with direct pressure over carpal tunnel
- Painless thenar muscle wasting is late finding; usually no visible abnormality; pain exacerbated by extreme volar flexion
- May have decreased grip strength, decreased sensation in first three digits

Diagnostic Studies

- Electromyography/nerve conduction studies (EMG/NCS)
- Plain X-rays if any history of trauma to exclude fracture
- If secondary cause suspected, order appropriate test (e.g., thyroid-stimulating hormone [TSH], RF, hemoglobin A1c [HbA1c])

Assessment

History

- Occasionally, the pain of carpal tunnel syndrome will radiate into the forearm, shoulder, neck, and chest.

Physical Exam

- ◊ In addition to the Tinel's and Phalen's signs and nerve compression test, which are special carpal tunnel tests, a complete wrist exam including the following should be done during the physical exam:
- ◊ Inspection (SEADS—swelling, erythema, atrophy, deformity, and surgical scars), palpation of the important landmarks (scaphoid, distal radius, scapholunate ligament, hook of hamate, ulnar joint line, distal radioulnar joint), ROM, strength, and dermatomal sensation of thumb radial nerve, third finger (median nerve) and fifth finger (ulnar nerve).
- ◊ Check capillary refill and radial pulses.

Differential Diagnosis

- Cervical radiculopathy (C6, C7)
- Brachial plexopathy
- Carpal navicular fracture

Management

Nonpharmacologic Treatment

- Conservative treatment for mild disease—nighttime splinting with cock-up wrist splint to relieve compression on nerve (Wipperman & Goerl, 2016)
- Ergonomic modification of work, hobby
- Surgical release for severe disease (American Academy of Orthopaedic Surgeons [AAOS], 2016; Wipperman & Goerl, 2016)

Pharmacologic Treatment

- NSAIDs: no significant benefit shown
- Acetaminophen for pain relief
- Local corticosteroid injection into carpal tunnel as effective option (Wipperman & Goerl, 2016)

How Long to Treat

- Depends on severity of symptoms
- Generally allow 6 weeks from onset of symptoms before obtaining EMG/NCS.

Special Considerations

- Pregnancy: increased incidence likely due to fluid retention
- Lactation: may be aggravated by wrist flexion while holding nursing infant

When to Consult, Refer, Hospitalize

- Consult with hand surgeon or neurologist if patient's symptoms not improved with splinting
- Surgical release has been shown to be more effective than splinting for more severe disease (AAOS, 2016)
- Refer for EMG evaluation and corticosteroid injection

Follow-Up

Expected Course

- Mild cases usually respond to conservative measures.
- Surgical release for more severe disease, failure of conservative measures for more than 6 months, numbness, or tingling persist or increase; loss of grip/pinch strength is persistent; or there is evidence of muscle atrophy

Complications

- Permanent sensory and motor deficiencies
- Thenar muscle atrophy

LOW BACK PAIN (LBP) AND HERNIATED NUCLEUS PULPOSUS (HNP)

Description

- Common problem: goal is to exclude serious causes
  - LBP: pain in lower lumbar, lumbosacral, or sacroiliac area that may radiate down one or both buttocks/legs
  - HNP: rupture of an intervertebral disc with herniation of nucleus pulposus into spinal canal; disk compresses spinal cord or irritates associated nerve root.
  - *Spondylolysis* is an acquired condition with a bony defect of the pars interarticularis, usually at L5–S1.
  - *Spondylolisthesis* is a slip of the vertebral body in an adjacent vertebra with a bilateral pars defect at a single vertebral level.
  - *Sciatica* refers to pain and paresthesia extending down the leg in a dermatomal pattern.

Symptoms

- Back pain may be a presenting symptom in serious medical problems such as abdominal aortic aneurysm, peptic ulcer disease, kidney stones, or pancreatitis.
- Back pain with bowel and bladder symptoms such as urinary retention or incontinence, saddle anesthesia, decreased anal sphincter tone, fecal incontinence, or progressive neurological defects could indicate cauda equina syndrome and is an emergency referral.

Etiology

- LBP: ligamentous (sprain) or muscular problems (strain), osteoarthritis, other diseases (fibromyalgia, osteoporosis, osteomyelitis), tumor
- HNP: trauma, degenerative spine disease, spinal stenosis
- Spondylolysis and spondylolisthesis develop in children doing vigorous athletic activity.
- Spondylolisthesis can occur in adults with degenerative changes of the facet joints without spondylolysis of the pars.
- The most common cause of sciatica is a herniated disk at L4–5, L5–S1.

Incidence and Demographics

- Estimated that 80% of adults in United States have an episode of back pain, 10% HNP
- Most common at 20 to 40 years old, working adults
- Back pain not common in children
- Spondylolysis occurs in 5% preadolescent children, 12% in divers/gymnasts

Risk Factors

- Smoking
- Obesity
- Physically and/or psychologically strenuous work
- Sedentary work
- Job dissatisfaction
- Depression and anxiety

Prevention and Screening

- Regular exercise program
- Maintaining ideal body weight
- Proper body mechanics

Assessment

History

- (see Table 14–8)
- Assess location, duration, and severity of pain
- Assess for constitutional symptoms: weight loss, fever, or night sweats
- Symptoms suggesting more serious problem: bilateral leg weakness, bowel/bladder incontinence, saddle paresthesia, pain unrelieved by rest, pain worse at night, pain worsens with rest
- Symptoms suggesting strain: pain, stiffness associated with identified activity; worsens with activity, improves with rest
- Ask if bowel or bladder dysfunction or saddle numbness or paresthesia; indicates cauda equina syndrome, a neurologic emergency
- Assess for psychosocial distress, substance use disorder, and disability compensation
- Children: ask if trauma, recent infection, athletics, inflammatory disease, or malignancy
- Adult and geriatric patients: ask about occupation, sports, leisure activities, underlying medical problems
- Exclude urgent medical conditions with mnemonic MICE (Metastatic, Infection, Compression fracture, cauda Equina syndrome) or referred pain from pelvic, abdominal pathology
- HNP is associated with pain radiating to buttock, leg, or foot.

Physical Exam

- Note gait; check for ability to walk on heels and toes
- Palpate spinal column, note abnormal curvature
- Perform ROM extension, flexion, hyperextension, lateral bend, rotation
- Palpate paraspinal muscle tenderness, spasm

TABLE 14–8.
DIFFERENTIATING LOW BACK PAIN

CLINICAL PROBLEM	HISTORY	PHYSICAL EXAMINATION
Low back pain	Pain in back, buttocks, and/or thigh Onset after exertion and with movement No history of trauma, infection, malignancy Pain relieved by lying supine	Paravertebral tenderness, muscle spasm Loss of normal lumbar lordosis common No neurologic deficit
Herniated nucleus pulposus	Initially, back pain severe Chronic herniation usually results in leg pain greater than back pain Often, positive history of trauma, forced flexion Central herniation results in bilateral leg weakness, bowel/bladder dysfunction	L5–S1 (most common): pain in posterior thigh, posterior/lateral calf, heel; weak plantar flexion of foot; diminished ankle reflex L4–5: pain in lateral thigh, anterior calf and dorsum of foot; weak dorsiflexion of foot L3–4: pain in anterior and lateral thigh, medial calf, and foot; weak quadriceps; diminished patellar reflex
Spinal stenosis	Gradual onset of bilateral pain, claudication: leg pain, paresthesia, weakness with May have bowel and bladder Usually relieved when flexes spine or rests	X-ray: osteophytes neurogenic Weakness: foot, ankle Diminished reflexes: ankle, knee walking, standing May have atrophy in leg muscles dysfunction
Spondylosis and spondylolisthesis	Vigorous athletic activity as child Positive family history Low back pain, may radiate into buttocks Wakes patient at night	Lumbosacral tenderness Accentuation of pain with hyperextension of spine, one leg raised off ground, flexed 90° at knee and hip Reduced side bending
Low back pain in children	More common in adolescence Red flag if: constant, under age 11, last several weeks, wakes child at night, limitation of motion, fever, neurologic signs	If spinal tenderness, fever, neurologic or systemic symptoms, X-ray and labs indicated

- Check deep tendon reflexes bilaterally: knee, Achilles, Babinski
- Check strength, vibratory, and proprioceptive sensation bilaterally
- Check weakness in dorsiflexion (ankle and great toe)
- Check light touch sensation of medial, dorsal, and lateral foot, peroneal area
- With the patient on his or her back, raise one leg with knee straight until pain is experienced in the thigh, buttock, and calf. Record angle at which pain occurs. A normal (pain-free) value would be 70° to 90°, higher in people with lax ligaments.
- Then perform sciatic stretch test: dorsiflex foot at point of discomfort. Test is positive if more pain results.
- Flexing the knee will relieve the buttock pain, but this is restored by pressing on the lateral popliteal nerve.
- Severe root irritation is indicated when straight raising of the leg on the unaffected side produces pain on the affected side.

Diagnostic Studies

- X-ray studies are usually not necessary unless history of trauma, suspicion of systemic or structural changes.
- Order diagnostic imaging and testing when severe or progressive neurologic deficits present, or serious underlying conditions suspected.
- MRI: most useful for identifying HNP, diskitis, tumors
- CT: may help identify cord impingement (especially laterally), good for examination of osseous areas
- Bone scan: helpful for identifying metabolically active processes such as tumor, occult fracture, infection, abscess
- Serum studies usually not helpful but ESR elevated in infection; human leukocyte antigen B27 (HLA-B27) elevated in ankylosing spondylitis

Differential Diagnosis

Spinal Disorders

- Herniated disk
- Spondylolisthesis
- Spinal stenosis

Metabolic Disorders

- Osteoporosis
- Osteomalacia
- Paget's disease

Rheumatologic Disorders

- Rheumatoid arthritis
- Reiter syndrome
- Psoriatic arthritis
- Ankylosing spondylitis

Tumor

- Benign
- Malignant
- Metastatic

Infection

- Bacterial
- Tuberculous

Miscellaneous

- Peptic ulcer disease
- Sickle-cell disease
- Pancreatic disease
- Renal stones
- Infection
- Abdominal aortic aneurysm
- Ovarian cysts, tumors

Management

- Most LBP responds to conservative treatment within 4 to 6 weeks, in the absence of acute neurological deficit.
- 80% or more of patients with HNP also respond to conservative treatment.

Nonpharmacologic Treatment

- Activity as tolerated; encourage patient to remain active.
- Chiropractic manipulation may be helpful if no radiculopathy.
- Acupuncture and massage may offer limited improvement.
- Physical therapy to learn muscle-conditioning exercises, proper body mechanics
- Behavioral management: cognitive behavioral therapy (CBT) or mindfulness-based stress reduction (MBSR)
- Self-care advice
  - Proper lifting techniques
  - Abdominal wall and core strengthening
  - Weight loss
  - Smoking cessation

Pharmacologic Treatment

- NSAIDs or acetaminophen are first-line treatment
  - Ibuprofen 400 mg to 800 mg every 8 hours
  - Naproxen 250 mg to 500 mg every 12 hours
  - Recommend standing dose for 1 to 2 weeks and then decrease and use as needed
- Acetaminophen 650 mg every 6 hours is reasonable alternative
- Muscle relaxants may be used if LBP is not adequately managed with NSAIDs or acetaminophen
  - Cyclobenzaprine 5 to 10 mg orally three times a day
  - Tizanidine 4 to 8 mg orally three times a day as needed
  - Use lowest dose possible for shortest period
  - Caution sedation

- Opioids should not be used routinely for management of chronic back pain due to risk of harm and mild to moderate effect
- Second line therapies to consider
  - Duloxetine 30 mg orally every day × 1 week, then increase to 60 mg orally every day
  - Tramadol 50 mg orally three times a day, then decrease dose to as needed

How Long to Treat

- Most episodes resolve within 4 to 6 weeks of conservative treatment.

Special Considerations

- In jobs requiring heavy lifting and exertion, incidence is somewhat greater for women
- Pregnancy: LBP common, as is sciatica; symptoms resolve frequently after delivery

When to Consult, Refer, Hospitalize

- Refer to neurosurgeon or orthopedist for patients who do not respond to 4 weeks of conservative treatment, or with spinal instability, expanding pain that worsens at night, or signs of infection, neurologic deficit, cauda equina syndrome
- Hospitalize for abscess, tumor, signs suggestive of abdominal aneurysm

Follow-Up

- If patient in severe pain, reevaluate in 24 to 48 hours.

Expected Course

- Remitting and recurring symptoms are common; most LBP resolves in 4 to 6 weeks with conservative care; 90% resolves within 2 months

Complications

- Without neurologic deficit, few complications if diagnosed and treated, although recurrence is common

FIBROMYALGIA

Description

- Chronic pain disorder
- Disorder of pain regulation

Etiology

- Unknown

History

- Neck, shoulder, low back, and hip pain
- Pain in the trapezius, medial fat pad of the knee, lateral epicondyle of the elbow
- Fatigue, sleep disorders, numbness, chronic headache, irritable bowel syndrome (IBS)

Incidence and Demographics

- Prevalence is estimated to be 6.4% in the United States
- Most common cause of generalized muscle pain in women between the ages of 20 and 55
- Incidence increases with age

Risk Factors

- Unknown; possible genetic predisposition
- May be associated with rheumatic disease

Assessment

History

- Widespread musculoskeletal pain, bilateral involving upper and lower parts of the body
- Fatigue upon waking from sleep, morning stiffness, frequent awakenings or sleeping lightly

- Cognitive disturbances including brain fog, also known as "fibro fog"
- Other symptoms: depression, anxiety, IBS, gastrointestinal reflux disease

Physical Exam

- ACR (2016) Diagnostic criteria for fibromyalgia (see Box 14–1) met with the three following conditions:
  - ◊ Widespread pain index (WPI) is 7 symptom severity (SS) is 5 or
  - ◊ WPI is 3–6 and SS is 9
  - ◊ Symptoms have been present for 3 months
  - ◊ No other identifiable disorder explains the pain

BOX 14–1. AMERICAN COLLEGE OF RHEUMATOLOGY (ACR) PRELIMINARY DIAGNOSTIC CRITERIA (2016)

Widespread Pain Index (WPI) score will be 0 to 19	Shoulder girdle, left hip (buttock, trochanter), left jaw, left upper back shoulder girdle, right hip (buttock, trochanter), right jaw, right lower back upper arm, left upper leg, left chest neck upper arm, right upper leg, right abdomen, left lower leg, left lower arm, right lower leg, right lower arm
Symptom severity (SS) score is between 0 and 12	Fatigue, waking unrefreshed, and cognitive symptoms. For each symptom indicate the severity level over the past week: 0 no problem: 1. slight or mild problems, generally mild or intermittent 2. moderate, considerable problems, often present and/or at a moderate level 3. severe: pervasive, continuous, life-disturbing problems Considering somatic symptoms, indicate whether the patient has: 0 for no symptoms 1. a few symptoms 2. moderate number of symptoms 3. for many symptoms.

Information adapted from (Bhargava & Hurley, 2022)

Diagnostic Studies

- No specific serum; radiographic, biopsy, radionucleotide abnormalities present

Differential Diagnosis

- Polymyalgia rheumatica
- Spondylarthritis
- Inflammatory arthropathies
- Hypothyroidism

Management

Nonpharmacologic Treatment

- Interprofessional pain management team is recommended.
- Education to limit triggers
- Cognitive behavior therapy and mindfulness
- Exercise program
- Support groups
- Health diet
- Improve sleep

Pharmacologic Treatment

- Antidepressants: selective serotonin reuptake inhibitors (SSRIs) and serotonin and norepinephrine reuptake inhibitors (SNRIs)
- Cyclobenzaprine (Flexeril) 5–40 mg every night orally
- Amitriptyline (Elavil) 10–150 mg every night p.o
- Approved by the U.S. Food and Drug Administration (FDA) for fibromyalgia:
  - ◊ Pregabalin (Lyrica): Initially 75 mg twice a day, max 45 mg daily. Requires tapering if discontinued.

- ◊ Duloxetine (Cymbalta): Initially 30 mg orally for 1 week. Maximum dose 60 mg daily. Requires tapering if discontinued.
- ◊ Milnacipran (Savella): Initially 12.5 mg daily with increasing doses as needed. Maximum 200 mg daily. Requires tapering if discontinued.

How Long to Treat

- ♦ Chronic, may require years of medication

Special Considerations

- ♦ Psychosocial factors need consideration.

When to Consult, Refer, Hospitalize

- ♦ Hospitalization generally not indicated

Follow-Up

- ◊ Chronic condition will require routine follow-up

Complications

- ♦ Chronic pain, lack of "cure" may initiate depression
- ♦ Mental fog

CASE STUDIES

CASE 1

A 12-year-old child presents with pain in his right hip that has worsened over the past 2 weeks.

History of Present Illness: Prefers to play video games, does not play sports, denies trauma

Past Medical History: Tonsillectomy and adenoidectomy at age 3, above 100% for weight on growth chart, BMI higher than 32

1. What other history would you like to obtain?
2. What type of examination should be done?

   Exam: Patient has local tenderness over hip with decreased flexion, abduction, and internal rotation.

3. What diagnostic tests should be ordered?
4. What is the diagnosis and plan for management?

CASE 2

A 34-year-old with complaint of left elbow pain for the last 2 weeks.

History of Present Illness: Played in two golf tournaments 2 weeks ago. Denies trauma. Complains of dull ache in elbow joint that radiates down forearm. Denies numbness or tingling.

Past Medical History: overweight, history of "borderline hypertension"

1. What other history would you like to obtain?
2. What should be done on the physical exam?

   Exam: Medial epicondyle is tender to palpation and pain with pronation, flexing wrist against resistance, or squeezing hard rubber ball

3. What diagnostic tests should be ordered?
4. What is the diagnosis and plan for management?

CASE 3

A 15-year-old presents with complaint of bilateral knee pain during and after exercise.

History of Present Illness: Pain in anterior knee area, just below knee joints during and after exercise. Denies trauma, plays basketball on her high school team, currently practicing nightly for an upcoming tournament.

Past Medical History: Well, no history of serious illness, accidents, or medical problems

1. What other history would you like to obtain?
2. What type of examination should be done?

   Exam: No fever; no redness, edema, warmth, or effusion; ROM/ligaments all intact; bony tenderness, bilateral swelling at tibial tubercle.

3. What diagnostic tests should be ordered?
4. What is the diagnosis and plan for management?

CASE STUDIES DISCUSSION

CASE 1

12-year-old with hip pain

1. What other history would you like to obtain?

   Recent illness, description of pain, associated symptoms

2. What type of examination should be done?

   Observe gait, assess for muscle atrophy and tenderness, assess for limited range of movement. Exam reveals patient has local tenderness over hip with decreased flexion, abduction, and internal rotation.

3. What diagnostic tests should be ordered? AP and lateral of hip/frog-leg X-ray

4. What is the diagnosis and plan for management?

   Slipped capital femoral epiphysis; refer to orthopedic surgeon immediately for evaluation

CASE 2

34-year-old with elbow pain

1. What other history would you like to obtain?

   Able to lift objects, even cup or liquid; able to squeeze a hard ball; has this problem occurred before

2. What should be done on the physical exam?

   Inspect for edema, redness, palpate joint for crepitus, fluctuance. Assess for muscle atrophy and limited range of movement.

3. What diagnostic tests should be ordered? None indicated

4. What is the diagnosis and plan for management?

   Epicondylitis. Nonpharmacologic treatment will consist of RICE protocol, avoid aggravating activities, and oral NSAIDs. Symptoms should resolve in 3 months with conservative treatment.

CASE 3

15-year-old with knee pain

1. What other history would you like to obtain?

   Precipitating factors, description of pain, any redness or swelling, associated symptoms, alleviating factors

2. What type of examination should be done?

   Vital signs, inspection for redness and swelling; palpation for warmth, tenderness, effusion; assess for swelling at tibial tubercle, range of movement, ligament stability

3. What diagnostic tests should be ordered?

   None indicated unless symptoms do not improve

4. What is the diagnosis and plan for management?

   Osgood-Schlatter's disease. Avoid activities that cause pain, ice for 20 minutes after exercise, quad strengthening exercises, NSAID if necessary

REFERENCES

Achar, S., &Yamanaka, J. (2019). Apophysitis and osteochondrosis: Common causes of pain in growing bones. *American Family Physician, 99*(10): 610–618. https://www.aafp.org/pubs/afp/issues/2019/0515/p610.html

American Academy of Orthopaedic Surgeons, (2016). Management of carpal tunnel syndrome: Evidence-Based Clinical Practice Guideline. https://www.aaos.org/globalassets/quality-and-practice-resources/carpal-tunnel/cts_cpg_4-25-19.pdf

American Association of Neurological Surgeons (2022). Scoliosis. https://www.aans.org/

Bhargava, J., & Hurley, J. A. (2022). Fibromyalgia. StatPearls. https://www.ncbi.nlm.nih.gov/books/NBK540974/

Bury, D. C., Rogers, T. S., & Dickman, M. M. (2021). Osteomyelitis: Diagnosis and treatment. *American Family Physician, 104*(4). https://www.aafp.org/pubs/afp/issues/2021/1000/p395.html

Busse, J. W., Sadeghirad, B., Oparin, Y., et al. (2020) Management of acute pain from non low back, musculoskeletal injuries. A systematic review and network meta-analysis of randomized trials. *Annals of Internal Medicine,* 173. https://pubmed.ncbi.nlm.nih.gov/32805127/ doi:10.7326/M19-3601.

Chavarria, J. C., Ackert-Bicknell, C. Swanson, C., & Burger, E. (2022). Osteoporosis: An update on screening, diagnosis, evaluation, and treatment. *Orthopedics (Online).* DOI:10.3928/01477447-20220719-03

Claytor, C. M., & Bazler-Chandler, J. (2017). Chapter 38. In C. E. Burns, A. M. Dunn, M. A. Brady, et al. (Eds.), *Pediatric primary care* (6th ed.). St. Louis, MO: Elsevier Saunders.

DiFilippo, L., Vicenzi, S., Pennella, D., & Maselli, F. (2022). Treatment, diagnostic criteria & variability of terminology for lateral elbow pain: Findings from an overview of systematic reviews. *Healthcare* (Basel) *10*(6). doi:10.3390/healthcare10061095.

FitzGerald, J. D., Dalbeth, N., Mikuls, T., Bringnardello-Petersen, R., Guyatt, G., Abeles, A. M., Gelber, A. C., Harrold, L. R., Khanna, D., King, C., Levy, G., Libbey, C., Mount, D., Pillinger, M. H., Rosenthal, A., Singh, J. A., Sims, J. E., Smith, B. J., Wenger, N. S., . . . Neogi, T. (2020). 2020 American College of Rheumatology Guideline for the management of gout. *Arthritis Care & Research 72*(6). DOI:10.1002.24180.

Fraekel, L., Bathon, J. M., England, B. R., St. Clair, E. W., Arayssi, T., Caranandang, K., Deane, K. D., Genovese, M., Huston, K. K., Kerr, G. Kremer, J., Nakamura, M. C., Russell, L. A., Singh, J. A., Smith, B. J., Sparks, J. A., Venkatachalam, S., Weinblatt, M. E., Al-Gibbawi, M., . . . Akl, E. A. (2021). 2021 American College of Rheumatology Guideline for the treatment of rheumatoid arthritis. *Arthritis Care & Research, 73*(7). doi:10.1002/acr.24596.

Hashmi, H. M., Shamim, N., Kumar, V., Anjum, N., & Ahmad, K. (2021). Clavicular fractures in newborns: What happens to one of the commonly injured bones at birth? *Cureus*. https://pubmed.ncbi.nlm.nih.gov/34729262/ doi:10.7759/cureus.18372

Hellemann, D. B., & Imboden Jr., J. B. (2018). Chapter 20: Rheumatologic, immunologic & allergic disorders. In M. A. Papadakis, S. J. McPhee, & M. W. Rabow (Eds.). *Current medical diagnosis and treatment 2018* (57th ed.). NewYork: Lange/McGraw-Hill.

Kolansinski, S. L., Neogi, T., Hochberg, M. C., Oatis, C., Guyatt, G., Block, J., Leigh, C., Copenhaver, C., Dodge, C., Felson, D., Gellar, K., Harvey, W. F., Hawker, G., Herzig, E., Kwoh, C. K., Nelson, A. E., Samuels, J., Scanzello, C., White, D., . . . Reston, J. (2020). 2019 American College of Rheumatology/Arthritis Foundation Guideline for the management of osteoarthritis of the hand, hip, and knee. *Arthritis & Rheumatology, 72*(2). DOI:10.1002/art.41142.

Lee, D. Y. L., Hass, R., Wallis, J. A., O'Connor, D. A., & Buchbinder, R. (2021). Clinical practice guidelines for management of atraumatic shoulder conditions: Protocol for a systematic review. *British Medical Journal*, Open 11. doi:10.1136/bmjopen-2020-048297.

Luke, A., & Ma, C. B. (2018). Chapter 41: Sports medicine & outpatient orthopedics. In M. A. Papadakis, S. J. McPhee, & M. W. Rabow (Eds.). *Current medical diagnosis and treatment 2018* (57th ed.). New York: Lange/McGraw-Hill.

Qaseem, A., McLean, R. M., O'Gurek, D., Batur, P., Lin, K., & Kansagara, L. (2020). Nonpharmacologic and pharmacologic management of acute pain from non-low back, musculoskeletal injuries in adults: A clinical guideline from the American College of Physicians & American Academy of Family Physicians. *Annals of Internal Medicine,* (173). doi:10/7326/M19-3602.

Sarafrazi, N., Wambogo, E. A., & Shepherd, J. A., (2021). Osteoporosis or low bone mass in older adults: United States, 2017–2018. *National Center for Health Statistics* (NCHS), 405. https://www.cdc.gov/nchs/data/databriefs/db405-H.pdf.

Smith, J. M., & Varacallo, M. (2022). Osgood Schlatter disease. StatPearls. https://www.ncbi.nlm.nih.gov/books/NBK441995/

Wipperman, J., & Goerl, K. (2016) Carpal tunnel syndrome: Diagnosis and management. *American Family Physician, 94*(12). https://www.aafp.org/pubs/afp/issues/2016/1215/p993.html#:~:text=Conservative%20treatment%20may%20be%20offered,6%20are%20not%20effective%20therapies.

Yang, S., Zusman, N., Lieberman, E., & Goldstein, R. Y. (2019). Developmental dysplasia of the hip. *Pediatrics,* 143(1). https://doi.org/10.1542/peds.2018-1147

CHAPTER 15

NEUROLOGICAL DISORDERS

Joshua M. Kies, DNP, APRN, FNP-BC

General Approach

FOR ALL

- Neurological problems range from chronic to acute to lethal.
- A screening neurological exam should be done on all patients with symptoms suspicious for a neurological disorder or injury and would include: mental status (level of consciousness, orientation, memory, cognitive function, language, Glasgow Coma Scale [GCS]); motor function (body position, involuntary movement, muscle tone, strength); sensory function (light touch, pain, position sense); reflexes (deep tendon reflexes [DTRs], abdominal, Babinski); cerebellar function (gait, rapid alternating movements, point-to-point movements, Romberg); cranial nerves (I–XII, motor and sensory components).
- Abnormalities should be evaluated further with additional assessment techniques (Mini-Mental State Examination [MMSE], discriminating sensory testing [stereognosis, two-point discrimination], and meningeal irritability testing) and/or referred to a neurologic specialist for diagnostic testing.

CHILDREN

- The nervous system is more difficult to examine in infants and younger children because it is less mature. Special attention is paid to head circumference and fontanels, general appearance and positioning, primitive reflexes, and developmental milestones.
- Knowledge of normal childhood developmental milestones and the patient's previous behavioral history is important to the diagnosis.
- Early recognition of problems is of utmost importance to future development and prevention of disability.

- Birth history of the patient is important, including prenatal drug exposures, gestational age, type of birth, complications, Apgar scores, incidence of trauma, congenital anomalies, birth weight, perinatal illness or injury.
- Consider a cardiac or metabolic etiology or an adverse medication reaction in the differential diagnosis whenever a neurological problem is suspected.
- Neurological "soft signs" (clumsiness, hyperkinesis, language disturbances, developmental delays, mirroring movements, echolalia, short attention spans) are more difficult to assess and diagnose but must be considered in the neurological evaluation based on patient age.
- In infants and toddlers, fontanels can provide information regarding increasing intracranial pressure (IICP) as well as hydration status and clues to development; sagittal and coronal suture separation may indicate IICP.
- The presence of two or more unusual morphologic features is uncommon and associated with an increased likelihood of possessing a clinically important underlying neurologic anomaly.

OLDER ADULTS

- 20% decrease in blood flow to the brain with changes in autoregulation; contributes to risk of orthostatic hypotension
- No changes in thinking, behavior, or intellectual function, although response time and processing of information is slower
- Greater incidence of sensory deficits with aging and chronic illness. Decreased hearing, decreased visual acuity, decreased position sense, decreased point discrimination may contribute to or mimic neurological problems.
- Consider cardiac or metabolic etiology, or adverse medication reactions, particularly for global complaints such as syncope, weakness, or change in cognition without focal (unilateral) neurological symptoms; also consider dementia, delirium, or depression.

RED FLAGS

For All

- Refer to a neurologist if unusual presentation or no response to adequate trial of standard therapy.

Children

- Obtain timely consultation and referral for the following:
  - Any acute loss of function or developmental milestone
  - Retention of normal newborn reflexes past the sixth month of life
  - A bulging fontanel, widening of suture lines, sunset eyes, frontal bossing, or head circumference growth inconsistent with percentiles in the newborn
  - Headache associated with early morning vomiting or awakening from sleep
  - Sudden onset of vomiting after head injury—*immediate referral*
  - Nuchal rigidity with fever—*immediate referral*

Adults/Older Adults

- If focal findings suggest a space-occupying lesion of the brain or spinal cord, or a peripheral compressive neuropathy, refer to neurologist or neurosurgeon.
- Acute or sudden onset of symptoms such as headache, isolated systolic hypertension, unilateral weakness, aphasia, visual changes, or change in level of consciousness require immediate consult, referral, or hospitalization, as do deficits resulting from head or spinal trauma.

General Neurological and Neurosurgical Disorders

SPINA BIFIDA OCCULTA

Description

- A midline fusion defect of the vertebral bodies without external protrusion of the spinal cord or meninges
- Occasionally accompanied by a dermoid sinus, which may have a hairy tuft, discoloration of the skin, or a lipoma
- Usually found at L5 and S1
- More benign than other variants of spina bifida (meningocele and myelomeningocele); with a normal physical and neurological exam, requires no treatment unless other symptoms occur

Etiology

- Neural tube defect (NTD) resulting from failure of the neural tube to close during the third and fourth weeks of fetal development
- NTDs include anencephaly, encephalocele, myelomeningocele, and occult spinal dysraphism.

Incidence and Demographics

- Incidence for all NTDs is 1 per 1,000 live births in the United States.

Risk Factors

- Poor prenatal care, gestational diabetes, maternal obesity, in utero exposure to some antiseizure medications
- Folic acid deficiency, maternal
- Previous delivery of an infant with NTD (2% to 4%)
- Maternal age greater than 35 years

Prevention and Screening

- Addition of folic acid to the diets of women of childbearing age, starting at or before menarche
- Alpha-fetoprotein screen prenatally at 15 to 20 weeks of gestation

Assessment

History

- History of pregnancy, birth, and delivery as well as prenatal care and maternal risk factors, especially nutrition and folic acid deficiency, gestational diabetes, maternal use of antiseizure medications or alcohol, maternal hyperthermia during days 17 to 28 of gestation which is the period of neural tube formation (Kerr et al. 2017).
- Patient history of back pain, bowel or bladder dysfunction, decreased motor strength or coordination
- History of meningitis or recurrent episodes of meningitis

Physical Exam

- Neurological exam for strength, coordination, and reflexes, especially in the lower extremities
- Gait evaluation
- Back examination for small sinus tract in the lower midline region along the vertebrae, and skin integrity at the site
- Scoliosis
- Head circumference
- Presence of other dysmorphic features
- Rectal exam to assess sphincter tone

Diagnostic Studies

- Spinal X-ray will show defect in the closure of posterior vertebral arches and laminae, typically involving L5 and S1.
- Ultrasound in the newborn period
- Magnetic resonance imaging (MRI) to rule out tethered cord, if having motor symptoms or back pain, or other brain abnormalities
- Urodynamic studies to assess bladder function, if affected

Differential Diagnosis

- Spina bifida occulta complicated by tethered cord
- Syringomyelia or diastematomyelia
- Dermal sinus tract
- Lipoma or another local tumor
- Cysts
- Sacral agenesis

Management

Nonpharmacologic Treatment

- Usually no treatment, unless complications develop, or associated defects become apparent
- Surgical release required for tethered cord.

Pharmacologic Treatment

- None

Special Considerations

- Spina bifida occulta may be an incidental finding on X-ray in many children who have no dermal sinus.

When to Consult, Refer, Hospitalize

- With a normal physical and neurological exam, no referrals are necessary.
- If a dermal sinus is found in the newborn or new symptoms (foot weakness, bowel or bladder dysfunction) develop in an older child, further evaluation is required; consult with a physician.
- Referral to a pediatric neurosurgeon is only necessary with associated defects (e.g., tethered cord).

Follow-Up

- Patients with this deformity should have routine health assessments and immunizations.
- Pay special attention to the back evaluation, history of infections, bowel and bladder function, and lower limb motor strength at each assessment.

TOURETTE SYNDROME/TICS

Description

- Tourette syndrome is a lifelong chronic condition that has four components, not all of which must be present in each case. They are motor tics, phonic tics, obsessive–compulsive disorder (10%–50% of patients), and attention-deficit/hyperactivity disorder (ADHD; 30%–60% of patients).
  - Motor tics are sudden, rapid, recurrent, purposeless, nonrhythmic, stereotyped movements.
  - Phonic tics can be simple, which include grunting, barking, and moaning; complex phonic tics include coprolalia (involuntary use of obscene language [less than 20% of patients]), echolalia (repeating what is said by another or what is heard), and palilalia (repetition of words and sounds made by the patient).
  - Tics increase in intensity and frequency during any form of physical or mental stress, anger, excitement, fatigue, and illness.
  - Motor tics tend to be unnoticed by the patient, but persist during sleep, predominately during rapid eye movement (REM) sleep.
  - Tics develop over time from simple to complex.
- Tourette syndrome differs from simple tic disorder in that tics are present for more than 1 year, during which time no more than three consecutive months pass without tics.

Etiology

- Tourette syndrome is thought to result from a complex interaction between social and environmental factors, and multiple genetic risk factors including a mutation in the *SLITRK1* gene on chromosome 13q31.1.
- Suspected to be an abnormality along the circuits connecting the brain's cortex and subcortex, which leads to failure of the filtering mechanism along a neural pathway involving abnormal regulation of dopamine uptake and release and subsequent abnormal impulse in the involved muscle group

Incidence and Demographics

- 25% of all children experience tics; most are minor and do not lead to a clinical diagnosis.
- Incidence for Tourette syndrome is 1 of every 333 children (0.3%) in the United States.
- Motor tics typically present around age 6, the most common being eye blinking.

- Phonic tics present around age 9, usually as repeated coughing, sniffing, or clearing the throat.
- Tourette syndrome affects men and boys more often than women and girls by a ratio of approximately 4:1.
- Tourette syndrome appears to be uncommon or rare among African Americans and sub-Saharan Black Africans.

Risk Factors

- Genetic predisposition
- Low birthweight
- Maternal stress during pregnancy
- Obstetrical complications (e.g., use of forceps, vacuum delivery)
- Maternal use of coffee, cigarettes, or alcohol during pregnancy
- Androgenic hormones
- Autoimmune mechanisms/pediatric autoimmune neuropsychiatric disorders associated with streptococcal infections.
- Exposure or overuse of amphetamines

Assessment

History

- Medical and developmental history of the child
- Family history, including tics and other developmental and behavioral disorders
- Psychosocial adaptation
- Environmental supports and stresses
- Prior diagnosis of comorbid conditions, including ADHD and use of amphetamines
- Child's impression of the tics, presence of aura, stresses, effects on social and emotional function
- Recent history of sore throat or throat infection, head trauma, or use of medications or drugs
- Sleep disorders including insomnia excessive daytime sleepiness, disorders of arousal, and bruxism

Physical Exam

- The child may need to be observed from another room, via videotaping, etc., as the tics wax and wane.
- Assess for comorbid conditions through a general physical and screening neurological exam.

Diagnostic Studies

- None unless to rule out comorbid conditions such as type 2 diabetes, cardiovascular disorders, and migraine
- Head computed tomography (CT) if onset of tics associated with head injury
- Throat culture and antistreptolysin O (ASO) titer if recent history of sore throat prior to onset of tics
- Urine or serum drug toxicology screen if history indicates
- Serum copper level if history of family hepatic and neurological diseases

Differential Diagnosis

- Sydenham's chorea
- Drug-induced movements
- Wilson's disease
- Neuroacanthocytosis
- Head injury
- Seizures
- Metal poisoning

Management

Nonpharmacologic Treatment

- Behavioral therapy and biofeedback
- Family support and counseling
- Individualized Educational Plans (IEPs), including classroom modifications

Pharmacologic Treatment

- Antidopaminergics: haloperidol (Haldol) or aripiprazole (Abilify) to treat motor and phonic tics
- Vesicular monoamine transporter 2 (VMAT2) inhibitors: tetrabenazine (Xenazine) or valbenazine to treat troublesome tics
- Stimulants: dextroamphetamine (Dexedrine) or methylphenidate (Ritalin) to treat comorbid ADHD; may exacerbate tics
- Alpha-adrenergic agonists: clonidine (Catapres) or guanfacine (Intuniv) to treat tics alone or with comorbid ADHD

How Long to Treat

- True Tourette syndrome is a lifelong condition, requiring constant treatment.

Special Considerations

- Monitor for tardive dyskinesia when using antidopaminergic medications.
- For best outcome, need multimodal management plan, including the patient, family, and school.

When to Consult, Refer, Hospitalize

- Consult with a physician for use of drug therapy when behavioral strategies are not working.
- Refer to neurologist if tics are hard to control or the diagnosis is not clear.

Follow-Up

- Biannually to evaluate control of tics, school performance, need for further intervention, and collaboration

Expected Course

- Approximately one-third of children outgrow tics by adulthood

Complications

- Psychosocial problems

DOWN SYNDROME (TRISOMY 21)

Description

- A congenital syndrome consisting of intellectual disability and multiple physical abnormalities, including hypotonia, flat facial profile/flat nasal bridge, up-slanting palpebral fissures, and low-set small ears
- The defects are caused by trisomy of chromosome 21.

Etiology

- 95% to 97% because of chromosomal nondisjunction in the maternal DNA
- 1% with trisomy 21 mosaicism occurring after conception; generally, less severely affected
- Down syndrome is associated with many conditions, the most common of which are:
  - Intellectual disability (100%)
  - Infant hypotonia
  - Hearing loss (38%–78%)
  - Visual problems: refractive error (35%–76%), strabismus (25%–57%), nystagmus (18%–22%), cataracts (5%)
  - Obesity (50%)
  - Congenital heart disease (50%)
  - Hypothyroidism (10%–20%)
  - Atlanto-occipital and atlanto-axial subluxation (10%–20%)
  - Gastrointestinal obstructions and atresias (12%–28%)
  - Pediatric seizure incidence (40%)
  - Adult seizure incidence (35 years of age or older) (40%–84%)
  - Genitourinary problems, including hypospadias (1 in 250 men and boys), cryptorchidism (14% to 27% of men and boys)
  - Blood dyscrasias, including leukemia, anemia

- ◊ Retinoblastoma and testicular germ cell tumors
- ◊ Kidney malformations (3.5%)

Incidence and Demographics

- Incidence 1 in 700 live births
- Incidence increases with advancing maternal age 1:100 by maternal age of 40 years or older
- Most recognized and frequent chromosomal syndrome in humans

Risk Factors

- Advanced maternal age
- Previous history of Down syndrome in first-degree relative

Prevention and Screening

- Prenatal genetic testing via amniocentesis (15–20 weeks of gestation) or chorionic villus sampling (10–13 weeks of gestation)

Assessment

History

- History of first-degree relative with Down syndrome
- Review of genetic testing report

Physical Exam

- General: hypotonia with an open mouth and protruding tongue
- Head: brachycephaly with flattened occiput, microcephaly, false fontanel
- Eyes: up-slanting palpebral fissures, inner epicanthal folds, Brushfield spots, strabismus, nystagmus

- Ears: small, prominent, low-set ears, with over-folding of the upper helix; small ear canals
- Nose: small, flat nasal bridge
- Tongue: furrowed, protruding tongue, which appears large for mouth
- Mouth: high-arched or abnormal palate
- Teeth: may have missing, irregular, or hypoplastic teeth
- Neck: excessive skin at the nape (infants), short appearance
- Lungs: Assess for signs of infections or congestive heart failure.
- Heart: Assess for murmur, arrhythmia as cardiac defects are common.
- Abdomen: In neonate, observe for distention, which could indicate obstruction or atresia.
- Genital: straight pubic hair, small penis, cryptorchidism (adolescents)
- Extremities: hand is broad with Simian palm crease, short metacarpals and phalanges; short fifth finger with clinodactyly; wide gap between first and second toes (sandal gap); hyperflexibility of joints
- Skin: fine, soft, sparse hair; hyperkeratotic dry skin; may be cyanotic

Diagnostic Studies

- Complete blood count (CBC) as newborn
- Electrocardiography (ECG) and echocardiogram within first month of life to detect associated cardiac defects
- Brainstem auditory evoked response (BAER) testing within the first 6 months of life
- Lateral cervical spine X-ray to rule out atlanto-axial instability by school age
- Diagnosis confirmed by karyotype testing, usually in utero or neonatal period

Differential Diagnosis

- Other genetic or chromosomal syndromes

Management

Nonpharmacologic Treatment

- Many infants require surgical repair of associated heart defects.
- Parents need ongoing emotional support.
- Genetic testing and counseling within family

Pharmacologic Treatment

- Specific to associated problems

How Long to Treat

- Down syndrome requires lifetime surveillance for management of the associated disabilities and emergence of new problems.

Special Considerations

- Parents need ongoing support, both emotional and financial; parents should apply for Supplemental Security Income (SSI) benefits for the child.

When to Consult, Refer, Hospitalize

- Almost always identified at birth and immediate referrals made for unstable newborn
- Otherwise, consult with physician or specialist for infant or child entering health care system.
- If stable, referrals as follows:
  - Cardiac consult within first month of life and then continued cardiac evaluation related to the high risk of mitral valve prolapse and aortic regurgitation
  - Ophthalmology consult by age 6 months and then annually
  - Audiologic evaluation, in first 6 months, then every 6 months until the age of 5, then annually; may need ear nose and throat (ENT) referral to visualize tympanic membranes (TMs) because of small canals
  - Orthopedic evaluation, as needed

- ◊ Endocrine consult if thyroid screening abnormal
- ◊ Early language and learning intervention may prove helpful.

Follow-Up

- Patients need routine health examinations, as well as routine immunizations, in the newborn period and at least every 2 years through childhood and adolescence.
- Encourage physical activity and review diet to prevent obesity.

Complications

- Wide variety of complications due to associated abnormalities, including recurrent otitis media, constipation, airway problems, joint problems
- Emergencies in the newborn period include intestinal obstruction and acute cardiac manifestations.

CEREBRAL PALSY

Description

- A group of nonprogressive, permanent disorders resulting from malfunction of the motor centers and pathways of the brain; a major cause of disability of children
- There are varying degrees and clinical manifestations.
- Symptoms generally include paralysis, weakness, incoordination, or ataxia.

Etiology

Prenatal Factors (Most Common)

- Infection, such as rubella, toxoplasmosis, herpes simplex, and cytomegalovirus
- Maternal anoxia, anemia, placental infarcts, abruptio placenta
- Prenatal cerebral hemorrhage, maternal bleeding, maternal toxemia, Rh or ABO incompatibility
- Prenatal anoxia, twisting or kinking of the cord

- Genetic factors
- Miscellaneous: toxins, drugs

Perinatal Factors

- Anoxia from any cause, including anesthetic and analgesic drugs administered during labor, prolonged labor, placenta previa or abruptio placenta, respiratory obstruction, cerebral trauma during delivery, complications of birth
- "Small for date" babies, including prematurity (78%) and intrauterine growth retardation (34%)
- Hyperbilirubinemia
- Hemolytic disorders
- Respiratory distress
- Infections
- Serum chemistry disturbances (hypoglycemia, hypocalcemia)

Postnatal Factors

- Head trauma
- Infections, including meningitis, encephalitis, and brain abscesses
- Vascular accidents
- Anoxia
- Neoplastic and late neurodevelopmental defects

Incidence and Demographics

- Cerebral palsy occurs in approximately 2 per 1,000 live births in United States.
- Prevalence of cerebral palsy is far higher in preterm compared with term infants and increases with decreasing gestational age and birth weight.

Risk Factors

- Young or advanced maternal age
- Low birth weight (incidence increases with birth weights less than 2500 g)
- Lack of prenatal care
- Antepartum hemorrhage (27%)
- Birth trauma or anoxia
- Maternal infection (28%)
- Heavy gestational alcohol consumption, smoking, and maternal obesity

Prevention and Screening

- Prenatal care, including the provision of prenatal vitamins (including magnesium sulfate)
- Prenatal screening for maternal illness and infection
- Management of maternal toxemia of pregnancy
- Developmental screening for well babies
- Immunization programs for well babies

Assessment

History

- A thorough history, including prenatal, perinatal, and postnatal risk factors
- Attention to birth trauma, prematurity, low birth weight, Apgar scores
- History of infant activity, feeding, crying, growth

Physical Exam

- Early signs
  - Asymmetric movements, hypertonia, scissoring of the lower extremities
  - Listlessness or irritability
  - Poor sucking with tongue thrust
  - Excessive, high-pitched, or feeble cry

- ◊ Long, thin infants who are slow to gain weight
- ◊ Poor head control

- ♦ Late signs
  - ◊ Failure to follow normal pattern of motor development—delayed gross motor development is universal manifestation
  - ◊ Persistence of infantile reflexes
  - ◊ Weakness
  - ◊ Preference for one hand before the infant is 12 to 15 months old
  - ◊ Abnormal postures
  - ◊ Delayed or defective speech
  - ◊ Evidence of intellectual disability
- ♦ General health
  - ◊ Functional assessment, including ability to perform normal daily activities
  - ◊ Developmental assessment; use Denver II developmental or other screening tool.
  - ◊ Ability to protect airway: gag reflex, swallowing
  - ◊ Nutritional status: growth, or weight loss
  - ◊ Neuromuscular function and mobility: range of motion, spasticity, coordination

Diagnostic Studies

- ♦ CT scan or MRI to rule out tumor
- ♦ Laboratory testing to include CBC, urinalysis, chemistry panel, toxicology screen to rule out other disorders
- ♦ Standardized testing for children 6 to 12 years of age such as gross motor function classification system (GMFCS) to monitor changes to physical abilities over time
- ♦ Psychological testing to determine cognitive functioning in an older child
- ♦ Gait analysis
- ♦ Electroencephalography (EEG0 if seizures suspected

Differential Diagnosis

- ♦ Tumors and neoplasms
- ♦ Meningitis, encephalitis

- Spastic diplegia or quadriplegia
- Dystonia and choreoathetosis
- Metabolic diseases
- Connective tissue disorders

Management

Nonpharmacologic Treatment

- Orthopedic management of scoliosis, contractures, dislocations
- Selective surgical dorsal rhizotomy to decrease spasticity
- Enrollment in a child-development program
- Physical, speech, and occupational therapy
- Assistive devices, such as braces, joint supports, walkers to assist with movement and prevent contractures
- Biofeedback (limited success)
- Family and individual counseling can be integral components of the management plan.

Pharmacologic Treatment

- See Table 15–1
- Administration of antispasticity medications, such as baclofen (Lioresal) (oral or intrathecal) or diazepam (Valium)
  - Intrathecal administration of Baclofen significantly improves absorption as the blood–brain barrier is bypassed (doses of less than 1% of the enteral dose); given through intrathecal pump; refills 3–4 times per year; battery life of 7 years and then unit replaced.
- Administration of antireflux medications: metoclopramide (Reglan) or bethanechol (Urecholine)
- Administration of seizure medications, as needed
- Injection of botulinum toxin (Botox) IM can reduce muscle tone and reduce spasticity for up to 3 to 6 months (off-label use of medication); also, effective to reduce hypersalivation and strabismus.
- Stool softeners as needed to help prevent constipation due to immobility.

TABLE 15–1.
MEDICATIONS TO TREAT SPASTICITY, DYSTONIA, AND DYSKINETIC MOVEMENTS

MEDICATION	RECOMMENDED DOSING
Spasticity	
Baclofen	20–80 mg/day orally divided three to four times a day; start 5 mg orally three times a day, may increase by 15 mg/day every 3 days. Taper required to discontinue.
Diazepam	2–10 mg orally three to four times a day; taper required to discontinue.
Dantrolene	100 mg orally three to four times a day; start 25 mg orally once a day × 7 days, then 50 mg orally three times a day × 7 days, then 100 mg orally three times a day; max dose 100 mg orally four times a day. Use lowest effective dose. Discontinue after 45 days if no response.
Tizanidine	Individualize dose orally every 6–8h as needed; start 2 mg orally x1, may repeat every 6–8 h as needed. Max 3 doses/24 h up to 36 mg/day. Taper required to discontinue.
Dystonia	
Trihexyphenidyl	5–15 mg/day orally divided three to four times a day; start 1 mg orally every day × 1, repeat in several hours as needed; taper required to discontinue.
Diazepam	2–10 mg orally three to four times a day; taper required to discontinue.
Carbamazepine	Immediate-release form: dose 400–800 mg/day orally divided two to four times a day. Start 200 mg orally twice a day; may increase by 200 mg/day every week. Max dose 1600 mg/day. Taper required to discontinue. Genetic testing may be required before treatment initiation based on at-risk ancestry for HLA-B*1502 allele
Dantrolene	100 mg orally three to four times a day; start 25 mg orally once a day × 7 days, then 50 mg orally three times a day × 7 days, then 100 mg orally three times a day; max dose 100 mg orally four times a day. Use lowest effective dose. Discontinue after 45 days if no response.
Dyskinetic Movements	
Levetiracetam	500–1500 mg orally/IV every 12 h. Start 500 mg orally/IV every 12 h, may increase by 1000 mg/day every 2 weeks. Max dose 3000 mg/day. Taper required to discontinue.
Tetrabenazine	25 100 mg/day orally divided two to three times a day; start 12.5 mg orally every AM × 1 week, then 12.5 mg orally twice a day × 1 week, then may increase by 12.5 mg/day every week. Max dose 25 mg/dose up to 100 mg/day. Consider cytochrome 450 2D6 (CYP2D6) genotyping if dosage requirement is greater than50 mg/day. Taper required to discontinue.

Continued

TABLE 15–1.
(CONTINUED)

MEDICATION	RECOMMENDED DOSING
Sodium Valproate	30–60 mg/kg/day IV divided two to three times a day; start 10–15 mg/kg/day IV divided once a day to three times a day, increase by 5–10 mg/kg/day every 7 days. Max dose 60 mg/kg/day
Carbamazepine	Immediate-release form: dose 400–800 mg/day orally divided two to four times a day. Start 200 mg orally twice a day; may increase by 200 mg/day every week. Max dose 1600 mg/day. Taper required to discontinue. Genetic testing may be required before treatment initiation based on at-risk ancestry for HLA-B*1502 allele
Gabapentin	300–1200 mg orally three times a day; start 300 mg orally three times a day. Max dose 3600 mg/day. Taper required to discontinue.
Diazepam	2–10 mg orally three to four times a day. Taper required to discontinue.

Special Considerations

- The best outcomes require a multimodal management plan, which includes the patient, family, neurology, orthopedics, nutrition, the school, and physical and occupational therapies.
- Parents need frequent support; counseling is highly recommended for all caregivers.
- Patients need to receive routine immunizations as scheduled.

When to Consult, Refer, Hospitalize

- Refer all cases to a pediatric neurologist; patient should be followed by a multidisciplinary team.
- Hospitalization is usually for amelioration of orthopedic problems.

Surgical Management

- The use of deep brain stimulation is considered first-line therapy for dystonia in children and adults.

Follow-Up

- Routine health assessments and immunizations, biannual IEP

Complications

- Scoliosis, seizures, ADHD, behavioral problems

FRAGILE X SYNDROME

Description

- Congenital syndrome characterized by intellectual disability or developmental delay, characteristic physical features, and abnormal behavioral patterns

Etiology

- The genetic defect is a discontinuous site on the long arm of the X chromosome.

Incidence and Demographics

- Frequency estimated at 1 in 4,000 to 1 in 7,000 in men and boys and 1 in 6,000 to 1 in 11,000 in women and girls
- Most common hereditary cause of intellectual disability

Risk Factors

- Family history of the syndrome

Prevention and Screening

- Genetic testing (*FMR1* gene alteration) and carrier detection for siblings and relatives of identified cases

Assessment

History

- Family history of intellectual disability or fragile X syndrome
- Developmental history, speech, or language delay
- Behavioral problems, such as hyperactivity, aversion of gaze, manneristic behavior, hand mannerisms or stereotypes, and perseverative speech
- School performance problems
- History of visual or hearing difficulties, motor, or joint instability, and/or seizures

Physical Exam

- Appearance: prominent forehead; a long, thin face and prominent jaw that appears late in childhood; large, protuberant, and slightly dysmorphic ears
- Strabismus, nystagmus, or ptosis; pale blue irises
- Heart sounds for murmurs or clicks with associated mitral valve prolapse
- Musculoskeletal exam for flat feet, scoliosis, or loose joints; in infants, hypotonia
- Genitourinary exam for macroorchidism (older than 18 years of age), inguinal hernias

Diagnostic Studies

- Echocardiography (ECG) to assess for mitral valve prolapse
- EEG if there is history of seizures or staring episodes

Differential Diagnosis

- Intellectual disability
- Klinefelter syndrome
- Cerebral gigantism (Sotos syndrome)
- Autism

Management

Nonpharmacologic Treatment

- Counseling—behavioral (address sleep disturbances and toileting issues) and developmental; IQ testing
- Speech/language therapy as needed
- Occupational therapy to address sensory integration problems
- Orthotics for flat feet if a gait disturbance is present
- Corrective lenses or corrective surgery for strabismus
- Inguinal hernia repair
- Early intervention programs for education and learning
- For children with history of low birth weight and gastrointestinal problems: monitor weight, height, and head circumference during each office visit.
- Placement of ear tubes may be necessary to treat otitis media
- EEG to identify presence of seizure activity
- Use of continuous positive airway pressure (CPAP) or tonsillectomy to treat obstructive sleep apnea

Pharmacologic Treatment

- Medications used only to treat symptoms of associated problems, such as seizures, aggression, hyperactivity, anxiety, or depression

Special Considerations

- Special classroom arrangements or learning situations
- Adolescents will need special counseling regarding sexuality and birth control.
- Patients may have trouble adjusting to social situations because of behavioral issues and may suffer from depression because of failure to fit in.

When to Consult, Refer, Hospitalize

- Refer all suspected cases to pediatric neurologist or developmental specialist.
- Refer to other specialties for associated problems (ophthalmology, orthopedics, neurology, psychology).
- Refer family for genetic counseling.

Follow-Up

- Routine health assessments and immunizations according to the recommended schedule

Expected Course

- Life into adulthood with interdisciplinary support of the family, usually in group home situation
- Life expectancy for individuals with fragile X syndrome is normal

Complications

- School failure
- Behavioral dysfunction can be significant component

HEADACHE: TENSION, MIGRAINE, CLUSTER

Description

- Head pain may be a symptom of underlying disease or pathology or the disease process itself (cluster headache, migraine). Head pain arises from extracranial structures (muscles, skin, scalp arteries), or from the posterior fossa, the dura, intracranial arteries, and cranial nerves at the base of the brain.
    - Brain tissue itself is not sensitive to pain.
- Tension, migraine, and cluster are primary headaches.
- It is unusual for new-onset primary headache syndromes to occur after age 50.
- Secondary headaches are a symptom of an underlying disorder.

- An acute and severe headache is significant and warrants immediate attention.
- The pattern of a headache may suggest the etiology, such as acute recurrent headaches. A chronic nonprogressive pattern might suggest post-concussion syndrome. A chronic progressive headache is more concerning and would possibly indicate a brain tumor or other serious etiology requiring immediate referral.
- Tension headaches are described as squeezing, band-like pain; onset usually gradual and lasting days to years; present when awakening; and may be associated with anxiety or depression, no aura or associated neurological symptoms; tension headaches are the most common type of headache.
- Medication overuse headache, previously referred to as analgesic rebound headache, is a chronic headache that can develop from the frequent use of headache medications, including OTC analgesic, triptans, ergotamine, caffeine, opiates, or benzodiazepines.
- Cluster headaches have unilateral, excruciating pain lasting 15 minutes to 3 hours, with several attacks a day for 4 to 8 weeks, followed by a cluster-free interval for months; or chronic form when a bout persists for 1 year without remission.
- Migraines may be preceded by a prodromal or "warning" feeling; then some have an aura of visual or somatosensory disturbance immediately before headache; the headache may be unilateral or bilateral, lasting hours to several days, and associated with photophobia, phonophobia, and nausea and vomiting; followed by a postdrome phase that may include the inability to concentrate, fatigue, and lack of comprehension.
    - Migraines are recurrent, throbbing headaches of suspected primary neuronal dysfunction origin that lead to an increased sensitivity to a broad range of stimuli with strong genetic factors; the once popular vascular theory of migraine origin is no longer considered viable.
    - Most primary pediatric headaches are migraines, medication overuse headaches, and tension.
    - Migraines may be classified as without aura (70%–75%) or with aura (focal neurologic dysfunction begins and ends before onset of headache).
    - Migraine variants include retinal; hemiplegic; brainstem aura (vertigo, dysarthria, ataxia, tinnitus, decreased level of consciousness); chronic; vestibular; menstrual

Etiology

- Tension headache
    - Essentially unknown cause
    - Studies have not supported "muscle tension" or increased muscle contractions.
    - Depression, anxiety, environment, or stress may play a role.

- Migraines
  - Believed to be caused by a genetically linked neurochemical, for example, serotonin, disruption that leads to an increased sensitivity to a broad range of stimuli
- Cluster
  - Unknown; may be related to hypothalamic activation with secondary activation of the trigeminal-autonomic reflex, probably via a trigeminal-hypothalamic pathway; may also be related to cyclic neurochemical imbalances causing an inflammatory response; tend to be seasonal, occurring in spring or fall
- Secondary headaches
  - Most common in older adults, often because of disease outside the central nervous system (CNS)
  - Causes include subarachnoid hemorrhage, chronic subdural hematoma, head trauma, brain tumors, giant cell (temporal) arteritis, meningitis, hypnic headache, primary cough headache, encephalitis, cervical arthritis, visual acuity problems, fever, sinusitis, pregnancy, intoxication (drugs, chemicals, carbon monoxide), hypothyroidism

Incidence and Demographics

- Headache is among the most common medical complaints.
- Incidence declines in the 6th to 10th decades.
- Tension
  - Up to 78% of adults experience tension-type headache at some time.
  - 5:4 ratio of women to men; 40% have family history
- Migraines
  - Prevalence 24% women, 7% men 30 to 39 years of age
  - Most common during ages 30 to 45, unusual to begin after age 50; unmask earlier incidence of undiagnosed migraine via focused history; rule out other causes
  - Migraine occurs in 5% of children before puberty
  - Female-to-male ratio is equal in childhood and rises to 2:1 after puberty.
  - There is a strong genetic component; family history supports the diagnosis in the child.
- Cluster
  - Rare, much more frequent in men between the ages of 20 and 40 years

Risk Factors

- Age, gender, stress, alcohol, caffeine (for all)
- Migraine triggers: foods such as chocolate and aged cheese (27%); caffeine and nicotine or withdrawal; alcohol (38%); bright light (38%); sleep disturbances (50%); missing meals (57%); emotional stress (80%); medications, hormones in women and girls (65%)

Prevention and Screening

- Because of the many causes of headache, there is no primary prevention.
- Avoid identified individual triggers.
- Keeping a headache diary helps in the identification of triggers and in the administration of prophylactic medications.

Assessment

History

- Evaluate every headache for chronology (most important item); location, duration, quality; associated activity (exertion, sleep tension, relaxation); timing of menstrual cycle; presence of associated symptoms (focal neurological deficits, vomiting, fever); and presence of triggers.
- Recent falls or head injuries, trauma, previous and current medical and nonpharmacologic management, diagnostic testing and referrals
- Activities using the trapezius muscles, such as wearing heavy backpacks
- Suspect tension headaches with gradual onset over months to years, with episodes lasting days without neurological symptoms; may be associated with anxiety, depression, and stress
- Suspect migraine with history of aura and neurologic symptoms that resolve, then actual headache accompanied by photophobia and/or nausea and vomiting; usually follows the same pattern and precipitating events each episode
- Suspect tension headache with constant, gradual onset, daily headaches; generalized, bilateral; and common around occiput, lasts for several hours, vague symptoms, no focal neurological deficits
- Suspect cluster headaches by cyclic nature of attacks

- Headache described as the "first" or "worst" of the patient's life should be evaluated to rule out potentially serious etiology.
- Functional history: Headache interferes with work, school, functional activities of daily living (ADLs), and instrumental ADLs; headaches that do not interfere with ADLs tend to be tension type.
- Sudden onset, change in character, associated neurologic symptoms, fever, neck pain, and rash or weight loss suggest a serious headache and potential emergency; a brain tumor usually causes additional symptoms within 6 months of headache onset.
- Family history of headache
- If patient is febrile, consider meningitis, brain abscesses or other infection, encephalitis, or sinusitis.
- Review of systems
  - Neurological: aura, paresthesia, paralysis, vertigo, mood, sleep changes
  - Visual symptoms: photophobia, diplopia, scotoma, scintillation, tearing
  - Any ear, nose, or throat symptoms: may indicate sinusitis
  - Gastrointestinal: nausea, vomiting, diarrhea, constipation
- See also Brain Tumor, Stroke, and Meningitis for pertinent history of these secondary causes.
  - Constitutional symptoms: fever, chills, weight changes, appetite changes

Physical Exam

- Screening neurological exam is usually normal with primary headaches; neurologic deficits suggest a secondary cause, such as subarachnoid hemorrhage (SAH), cerebrovascular accident (CVA), tumor, or subdural hematoma.
- Funduscopic exam to rule out papilledema (signals increased intracranial pressure)
- Muscle tone, reflexes, gait, sensation, coordination, and strength for any abnormality
- Auscultate for bruits, a sign of cerebrovascular disease
- Measure head circumference and check the fontanels and sutures in the young child.
- Cervical and suboccipital tenderness, range of motion (decreased in cervical arthritis)
- Temporal artery tenderness and visual changes, particularly in patients 50 years and older suggests giant cell arteritis.
- Focused physical exam, including vital signs, to rule out secondary causes or infectious process

- Rash over facial distribution of cranial nerve V with corresponding pain indicates herpes zoster.
- Examine the teeth for obvious cavities; include an assessment of jaw movement.
- ENT exam for signs of infection of the pharynx or sinuses

Diagnostic Studies

- History consistent with primary headache with normal physical exam usually does not require further diagnostic evaluation.
- For tension headaches with stress or psychogenic component, consider psychological testing.
- Visual acuity testing to screen for gross vision issues
- CBC if chronic anemia or infection is suspected
- Consider brain CT if:
  - Significant new type headache of few weeks' duration
  - New headache in patient age 50 and older
- Immediate CT if:
  - Acute, severe headache
  - Progressive headache
  - Headache with exertion, straining, sexual activity, or coughing
  - Headache accompanied by change in level of consciousness, persistent focal neurologic deficits, or fever
- Lumbar puncture (if there is a negative CT but SAH suspected, or to rule out meningitis)
- Erythrocyte sedimentation rate (ESR) to rule out giant cell arteritis in patients over age 50
- Sinus CT or X-rays if sinusitis without response to adequate antibiotics, recurrent sinus pain, vague symptoms without definite physical findings
- Cervical spine X-rays or MRI if cervical arthritis or radiculopathy is suspected
- Other diagnostic testing as directed by history and physical exam to rule out infectious, metabolic, or autoimmune process
- Evaluate for cardiovascular disease with ECG and consider risk factors before prescribing 5-hydroxytryptophan (5-HT) agonists ("triptans") or dihydroergotamine (D.H.E. 45 or Migranal).
- ECG is not useful in screening or diagnosing headaches.

Differential Diagnosis

- Transient ischemic attack
- Subarachnoid or intracranial hemorrhage/cerebral aneurysm
- Brain tumor
- Giant cell arteritis
- Subdural hematoma
- Seizure
- Post-traumatic headache
- Meningitis
- Encephalitis
- Brain abscess
- Hydrocephalus
- Sinusitis or other referred pain from ear, eyes, teeth, or temporomandibular joint (TMJ)
- Viral syndrome
- Drug-induced, caffeine withdrawal, or intoxication
- Depression and anxiety
- Post-concussive syndrome
- Stress
- Cervical radiculopathy
- Trigeminal neuralgia
- Pseudotumor cerebri or benign intracranial hypertension (cause unknown)

Management

Nonpharmacologic Treatment

- Tension headaches
  - Relaxation techniques, biofeedback, stress reduction
  - Acupuncture has been identified as a treatment option for episodic or chronic tension-type headaches and as a preventative treatment of migraine.

- ◇ Physical therapy: transcutaneous electrical nerve stimulation (TENS), massage, ultrasound
- ◇ Headache logs

- ♦ Migraine and cluster
  - ◇ Avoid food and drugs that trigger attacks.
  - ◇ Rest during periods of exercise
  - ◇ During attack, rest in quiet, dark room with head elevated; use of cold compresses
  - ◇ 100% oxygen inhaled for 10 to 15 minutes via face mask (cluster headache)
  - ◇ The use of noninvasive vagus nerve stimulation, single-pulse transcranial magnetic stimulation, or electric trigeminal nerve stimulation may be considered for patients who prefer nondrug treatments or those for whom drug treatment is unsuccessful or contraindicated.

Pharmacologic Treatment

Abortive Therapy

- ♦ Tension headaches
  - ◇ Analgesics: single-dose ibuprofen (200 or 400 mg); if nonsteroidal anti-inflammatory drugs (NSAIDs) not tolerated, single-dose acetaminophen (1,000 mg) may be used instead; acetaminophen is the preferred initial therapy during pregnancy.
  - ◇ Patients younger than age 10, ibuprofen 5–10 mg/kg/dose every 6–8 hours or acetaminophen 10–15 mg/kg/dose every 4 hours.
  - ◇ Children under 10 with headaches more than once per week may benefit from daily prophylactic therapy with cyproheptadine 0.2–0.4 mg/kg/day in two to three divided doses, starting with 4 mg at bedtime.
  - ◇ Older children can be managed with analgesics such as ibuprofen and acetaminophen.
  - ◇ Avoid opioids, including butalbital (Fiorinal and Fioricet), because of risk of habituation as well as rebound headache phenomenon.
  - ◇ If headache occurs more than once per week, preventive medication for adults and children include low-dose amitriptyline.
- ♦ Migraines and cluster headaches: Treatment very individualized:
  - ◇ Analgesics: acetaminophen, aspirin, or NSAIDs, taken as soon as possible at onset. Avoid opioids for reasons noted above.
  - ◇ 5-HT agonists (triptans) if nonnarcotic analgesics are ineffective (or if moderate to severe attack)

- ◊ The combined use of an NSAID with a triptan appears to be more effective than using either drug class alone.
- ◊ Sumatriptan (Imitrex)—oral: 50–100 mg taken as soon as possible at onset; the most effective dose of sumatriptan is 100 mg, while the 50 mg dose may provide the best combination of efficacy and tolerability. Initial dose may be repeated once after 2 hours, if needed; the maximum dose is 200 mg in 24 hours in adults.
- ◊ Injection: 6 mg subcutaneous adults; in children 6 years and older, 3–6 mg subcutaneeous; may be repeated once after 1 hour
- ◊ Intranasal: single dose of 5 or 20 mg administered in one nostril, may repeat once after 2 hours, not to exceed 40 mg in 24 hours in adults; initial dose of 5 mg administered in one nostril is recommended in children 5 years and older
- ◊ Other 5-HT agonists include zolmitriptan (Zomig), naratriptan (Amerge), rizatriptan (Maxalt)
- ◊ Ergotamine derivatives: ergotamine/caffeine (Cafergot): 1 or 2 one mg tablets taken as soon as possible at onset, may repeat at 30-minute intervals, do not exceed 6 mg per day, 10 mg per week; not recommended in children; not recommended for treatment of migraine with brainstem aura or hemiplegic migraine as they may aggravate symptoms caused by vasospasm.
- ◊ Injectable triptans at migraine doses more effective than oral agents for individual attacks (Note: First dose of injectable preparations should be given under medical supervision and, possibly, accompanied by monitoring with ECG.)
- ◊ Injectable or inhaled ergotamines and triptans are contraindicated in patients with history of uncontrolled hypertension, Prinzmetal angina, myocardial infarction, symptomatic ischemic heart disease; not recommended for treatment of migraine with brainstem aura or hemiplegic migraine as they may aggravate symptoms caused by vasospasm.
- ◊ Sumatriptan should not be used in conjunction with any vasoconstrictor medication, or within 2 weeks of taking a monoamine oxidase inhibitor.

- ♦ Treat nausea or vomiting in adults and children with promethazine (Phenergan) or metoclopramide (Reglan) 15 to 20 minutes before oral medication.
  - ◊ Prophylactic treatment for two or more migraine attacks per month that produce impairment lasting three or more days per month: daily NSAIDs, beta blockers, calcium channel blockers, tricyclic antidepressants (limited experience with selective serotonin reuptake inhibitors (SSRIs), especially in children; see Table 15–2)
  - ◊ Pharmacologic modulation of calcitonin gene–related peptide (CGRP) activity may decrease trigeminovascular pain transmission in migraine; CGRP antagonists rimegepant (Nurtec ODT) and ubrogepant (Ubrelvy) received U.S. Food and Drug Administration (FDA) approval for acute migraine treatment in 2019 and 2020; potential vasoactive effects have led to uncertainty for efficacy and safety for those with migraine with aura.
  - ◊ Topiramate, lithium carbonate, and valproate can also be effective. However, before initiating valproate, baseline liver enzyme levels must be drawn and then monitored thereafter approximately every 3 to 6 months.

TABLE 15–2.
PHARMACOLOGIC TREATMENT: PREVENTIVE THERAPY FOR MIGRAINE

GROUP	MEDICATION	USUAL DAILY ADULT DOSE	USUAL DAILY PEDS DOSE	SIDE EFFECTS
A	Divalproex sodium (Depakote)	Usual dose for age 16 or older: start with 250 mg twice a day; usual max 1 g/day	20–40 mg/kg	Gastrointestinal (GI) upset, liver disease, thrombocytopenia; need to monitor closely
A	Sodium valproate (Depacon)	800–1,500 mg/day	—	Alopecia, rash, abdominal pain, constipation, diarrhea, pancreatitis
A	Topiramate (Topamax)	100 mg divided into two doses	Similar to adult dose: 12 years and older	Anxiety, abdominal pain, diarrhea, dyspepsia, sleep disturbances
A	On a botlinum toxin A (Botox)	155 units IM in 31 sites every 12 weeks	—	Hypersensitivity reaction, anaphylaxis, headache, neck pain, pruritis, toxin effect spread
A	Propranolol	160–240 mg/day in divided doses	Less than 35 kg: 10–20 mg orally three times a day 35 kg or more: 20–40 mg orally three times a day	Heart block, Raynaud's syndrome, systemic lupus erythematosus (SLE), fatigue, dizziness, constipation, hypotension
A	Metoprolol (Toprol)	50–200 mg/day	—	Fatigue, dizziness, pruritus, bradycardia, rash, dyspnea, sleep disturbances, photosensitivity
B	Amitriptyline (Elavil)	10–100 mg orally q.h.s.	0.25–1 mg/kg/ dose ORALLY q.h.s. 2 years or older	Drowsiness, xerostomia, nausea, anxiety, rash, confusion, constipation
B	Venlafaxine (Effexor XR)	150 mg orally once a day	—	Suicidality, depression, insomnia, decreased libido, constipation, vivid dreams

Continued

TABLE 15–2. (CONTINUED)

GROUP	MEDICATION	USUAL DAILY ADULT DOSE	USUAL DAILY PEDS DOSE	SIDE EFFECTS
B	Atenolol	50–150 mg/day	—	Arrhythmia, diarrhea, dizziness, fatigue, insomnia
B	Verapamil	240 mg/day	—	Edema, hypotension, constipation, nausea, dizziness

Adapted from Evidence-based guidelines for migraine headache in the primary care setting, by U.S. Headache Consortium, 2012. Retrieved from https://americanheadachesociety.org/resources/information-for-clinicians/practice-parameters-guidelines-and-classification/

- ◇ Generally, prophylactic agent(s) should be tried for a minimum of 2 to 3 months before switching to another drug.
- ◇ Neurology referral for headaches unresponsive to treatment or prophylaxis

Preventive Therapy

- ♦ American Headache Society Guidelines (2021) based on clinical efficacy, significant adverse events, safety profile, and clinical experience of the participants:
  - ◇ Group A—medications with proven high efficacy and mild-to-moderate adverse events
  - ◇ Group B—medications with lower efficacy (i.e., limited number of studies or studies reporting conflicting results) or efficacy suggesting only "modest" improvement and mild-to-moderate adverse events
  - ◇ Group C—no dosing recommendations provided for treatments lacking relevant, randomized-controlled trials
- ♦ Secondary headaches
  - ◇ Manage and treat the underlying cause.
  - ◇ Avoid opioids if level of consciousness needs to be monitored.
  - ◇ Ibuprofen for pain and fever if not contraindicated

How Long to Treat

- Treat acute attacks until headache resolves or maximum daily dose is reached; narcotics can be used to treat intractable pain.
- Prophylaxis: Primary headache syndromes tend to decrease or resolve in late middle age or after menopause; attempt to wean periodically.

Special Considerations

- Consider cardiovascular, gastrointestinal, renal, and hepatic disease when prescribing therapy in geriatric patients.
- Increased risk of GI bleed, renal failure, edema, and elevated blood pressure with NSAIDs in older adults
- Headaches are common in the first trimester of pregnancy.
- Migraines usually do not become worse during pregnancy.
- Counsel women of childbearing age regarding headache management and pregnancy.
- Ergotamine derivatives are strong uterine stimulants.
- Ergotamine is secreted in breast milk and may cause vomiting and diarrhea in infants.

When to Consult, Refer, Hospitalize

- Consult with physician as needed if narcotic analgesics needed.
- Refer to neurologist if unable to manage symptoms using typical therapy or if patient develops symptoms of increased ICP, or if tumor, aneurysm, or arteriovenous malformation (AVM) suspected.
- Refer to neurologist if patient is experiencing multiple headaches per week, and/or is taking multiple doses of medication without benefit (e.g., rebound headaches due to medication effects).
- Refer to emergency department for severe unresponsive migraine or cluster headache with vomiting and need for IV hydration; or sudden, severe headache; or headache with change in level of consciousness.
- Refer to surgeon or ophthalmologist for temporal artery biopsy if temporal arteritis suspected.
- Refer to psychologist or therapist for relaxation therapy or psychotherapy, or when depression is suspected that does not respond to trial of antidepressants.

- Refer to interdisciplinary pain center for chronic, intractable pain, or interference with daily life.

Follow-Up

- Routine annual health assessments
- Weekly to monthly when adjusting or changing medications

Expected Course

- Tension headaches can be lifelong.
- Migraines get better in more than two-thirds of all children, but the prognosis of remission diminishes after age 18.
- In adults, migraines and cluster headaches usually resolve during middle age, or following completion of menopause.

Complications

- Unrecognized or mistreated serious headaches from secondary causes
- Lost wages and productivity, troubled relationships from chronic pain, depression, increased risk of suicide.

BRAIN TUMORS

Description

- Primary brain tumors are a diverse group of neoplasms (abnormal growths of cells) arising from structures within the cranium.
- Classified by cell of origin (see Table 15–3) and include gliomas, meningioma (rare in children), acoustic neuroma, ependymoma, craniopharyngioma, pediatric ganglioma (benign, may be accompanied by seizures)
- May be malignant or benign
- Secondary brain tumors most often metastasize from the lung, breast, and melanoma.

TABLE 15–3. PRIMARY BRAIN TUMORS

TUMOR	STRUCTURE	TREATMENT AND PROGNOSIS
Astrocytoma (Grade I, II glioma)	Glial tissue	Total excision usually not possible; may respond to radiation. Variable prognosis
Glioblastoma multiforme (Grade III, IV glioma)	Glial tissues	Total excision not possible, reoccur Radiation and chemotherapy may slow growth Poor prognosis
Oligodendroglioma (Grade II, III)	Cerebral hemispheres	Slow-growing Successful surgical treatment
Ependymoma	Glioma usually of the fourth ventricle	Presents with signs of increased intracranial pressure (IIP) Shunt, surgical resection if possible Radiation therapy
Craniopharyngioma	Sella tunica Depresses optic chiasm	Surgical resection usually incomplete Bitemporal visual field cuts Endocrine dysfunction
Meningioma	Dura or arachnoid mater	Surgical excision, difficult to completely remove posterior fossa tumors Cure with complete resection
Acoustic neuroma	Nerve sheath Vestibular branch of eighth cranial nerve at the cerebellopontine angle	Excision usually good outcome May have residual ipsilateral hearing loss, imbalance, facial weakness, or numbness
Primary cerebral lymphoma	Reticuloendothelial system in immunocompromised patients	Shunt Prognosis depends on CD4 count

Etiology

- The exact cause of brain tumors is unknown.
- Gliomas of the supporting glial tissues account for 33% of all brain tumors.
- Grades I, II (astrocytomas), III, IV (glioblastoma multiforme)
- Grades III and IV are more invasive, faster-growing, and have a poor prognosis.

- Meningiomas develop from the covering of the brain.
- 32% of diagnosed brain tumors are malignant.
- Cure is possible for certain tumor types with complete excision, except for meningiomas of the posterior fossa where complete excision is difficult.
- Presenting signs and symptoms depend on the location and size of the tumor.

Incidence and Demographics

- Second most common cause of cancer in children
- Occur in all age groups, but childhood peak in the interval between age 5 and 9 years
- Estimated incidence in children is 1.15 to 5.14/100,000
- Incidence of primary brain and nervous system tumor is 30/100,000 in the United States
- Benign primary tumors (meningiomas) 8/100,000
- Malignant primary tumors (astrocytomas and glioblastoma multiforme) 7/100,000
    - Greatest incidence in 60-to-70-year-olds; 20% of all malignant neoplasms; make up 50% to 60% of all childhood brain tumors
- Metastatic brain tumor incidence is 10 times more common than primary brain tumors

Risk Factors

- Previous radiation therapy
- Extended exposure to ionizing radiation
- Neurofibromatosis
- Increase with age
- Primary cerebral lymphoma associated with AIDS

Assessment

- Patient chief complaint may be "classic triad": morning headache, vomiting, papilledema

History

- Focused, complete neurological history including weakness, slurred speech, or word-finding difficulty, visual changes including diplopia or field cuts, hearing loss, cognitive changes, mood or personality change, drowsiness, seizures, headache
- Children: changes in behavior or school performance; past medical history (PMH), including birth history, recent illness or trauma; growth and development history, including delays; family history of neurological disease or neurofibromatosis
- Tumors are suspected in patients with progressive deficits.
- The deficit may suggest the location of the tumor (see Table 15–4).
- In children, presence of new-onset headache, especially for 1 week or intermittent for 1 month
- Headache associated with tumor is dull and aching and increases over weeks.
- Headaches are usually secondary to hydrocephalus (IICP) or posterior fossa tumors stretching pain-sensitive structures.
- New-onset seizures at any age suggests a tumor.
- Review of systems, including head, eyes, ears, nose, and throat (HEENT) for loss of sense of smell or visual field cuts, suggest pituitary adenoma or craniopharyngioma; with unilateral hearing loss consider acoustic neuroma
- History of vomiting without nausea with deficits or headache in the morning suggests increased intracranial pressure.
- Assess for symptoms of Cushing syndrome (see Chapter 17) if pituitary adenoma suspected.

Physical Exam

- Attention to head circumference, fontanels, and cranial sutures in young children
- Complete neurological exam may reveal focal cranial nerve or motor deficits.
- Other systems as indicated by history, including eye exam, eye movements, papill-edema and, in children, skin for signs of neurocutaneous disease
- If pituitary adenoma suspected, will need complete endocrine assessment; elevated blood pressure may be present
- Metastatic brain tumor: If primary tumor site unknown, evaluate for lung, breast, and melanoma.
- Gait abnormalities, incoordination, cranial nerve paralysis, optic atrophy, loss of visual fields, nystagmus, focal motor weakness and sensory abnormalities, hyperreflexia

TABLE 15–4.
LOCATION AND SIGNS AND SYMPTOMS OF INTRACRANIAL LESIONS

LOCATION	SIGNS AND SYMPTOMS
Frontal lobe	Intellectual and cognitive decline Personality change Contralateral grasp reflex Expressive aphasia Focal motor seizures, contralateral weakness Anosmia
Temporal lobe	Seizures (may be partial without loss of consciousness) Emotional and behavioral change Auditory hallucinations Visual field cuts Receptive aphasia Contralateral weakness
Parietal lobe	Contralateral sensory loss Loss/reduction of hand–eye coordination Loss of tactile discrimination (astereognosis) Contralateral field cuts Alexia, agraphia, apraxia, acalculia Right–left confusion
Occipital	Homonymous hemianopsia Visual agnosia Cortical blindness
Cerebellum and brain stem	Ataxia and incoordination Cranial nerve palsies Nystagmus Motor and sensory deficits (unilateral or bilateral) Increased intracranial pressure

Diagnostic Studies

- CT used as fast screening exam, but MRI gives better, more detailed imaging.
- MRI for suspected posterior fossa lesions and intrasellar lesions
- Angiography of intrasellar lesion with normal hormone levels to differentiate pituitary adenoma from an aneurysm
- Pituitary adenoma: adrenocorticotropic hormone (ACTH), thyroid function tests, serum glucose and electrolytes, prolactin
- Metastatic brain tumors: CT imagining of chest/abdomen/pelvis or a whole body positron emission tomography (PET)-CT should be ordered for patients without a prior history of cancer; chest X-ray, mammogram, colonoscopy as appropriate to locate primary tumor if unknown
- Open biopsy of the tumor
- EEG studies are not helpful unless seizures are presenting symptoms.
- Cranial X-rays may demonstrate nonspecific findings associated with increased ICP.

Differential Diagnosis

- Subdural hematoma
- AVM, aneurysm
- Cerebrovascular accident
- Hydrocephalus
- Pseudotumor cerebri
- Epilepsy
- Primary headache syndrome
- Abscess
- Hamartoma (causing a brain gliosis)
- Neurofibromatosis with neuromas (when indicated by history)
- Viral infections
- Progressive multifocal leukoencephalopathy
- Multiple sclerosis

Management

- Surgery, radiation, chemotherapy as indicated
- Side effects of radiation therapy are hair loss, skin and scalp changes, ototoxicity, nausea, vomiting, and malignant otitis externa.
- Patients must be monitored for panhypopituitarism if radiation to the pituitary gland.
- Side effects of chemotherapy are myelosuppression and infection, hair loss, and weight loss from nausea/vomiting.
- Patients and parents need continuous emotional support during therapy.

How Long to Treat

- Radiation therapy: 6 weeks; multiple rounds of treatment may be required based on progression of disease
- Chemotherapy: 1 to 2 years; additional cycles of chemotherapy may be required based on progression of disease

Special Considerations

- Patients who receive large-field radiation to the cerebrum are at high risk for cognitive deficits.
- All patients receiving radiation are at increased risk for recurrent tumors.
- Malignant brain tumors: Patients younger than 45 may live three times longer than patients 65 years and older
- Prognosis decreases with lower premorbid function based on the Karnofsky Performance Status.
- Coordinate obstetric and oncology care for pregnant or lactating patients.

When to Consult, Refer, Hospitalize

- Always consult with physician if unsure of symptoms or diagnosis.
- Refer to pediatric neurologist (for children and adolescents) or a neurologist (for adults and older adults) for further evaluation and treatment.
- Refer to social services, home health services, and counseling as needed.

Follow-Up

- Patient will be closely followed by neurology/surgery/oncology team.

Complications

- Persistent neurological deficits, seizures, increased ICP, and death; refer to Table 15–4

TRIGEMINAL NEURALGIA

Description

- A pain syndrome, also called *tic douloureux,* consisting of paroxysmal, severe lancinating pain of the face, usually unilateral; originates near mouth and shoots to nose, eye, or ear; may cause facial muscle spasms
- Can also occur in multiple sclerosis

Etiology

- Compression of the fifth cranial nerve root, usually by vascular structure (80%–90%) or malformation

Incidence and Demographics

- Low incidence; most common in middle age to older women, with a majority of cases beginning after the age of 50.

Risk Factors

- Pain triggers include touch, movement, cold air, chewing, brushing teeth, talking, smiling, and grimacing

Prevention and Screening

- None identified

Assessment

History

- Focused history if chief complaint is facial pain beginning near the side of the mouth, shooting up to ipsilateral eye, ear, or nostril; initially episodes may be separated by months of pain-free time
- Establish time frame, description of episode, any triggers and pain management
- Review of systems to identify any neurological deficits such as weakness, numbness, diplopia, or other symptoms of a space-occupying lesion
- Any ear, nose, throat, or dental symptoms indicating sinusitis, dental abscess, or otitis
- History of fifth cranial nerve herpes zoster or multiple sclerosis

Physical Exam

- Examine head, eyes, ears, nose, throat, mouth, neck, and cranial nerves.
- Neurologic exam if cranial nerve abnormalities
- No physical findings with classic trigeminal neuralgia except possibly poor dental hygiene or lack of shaving or makeup on affected side

Diagnostic Studies

- CT or MRI indicated if neurological deficits present to rule out space-occupying lesion
- ESR if temporal (giant cell) arteritis suspected

Differential Diagnosis

- Fifth cranial nerve tumor
- Postherpetic neuralgia
- Temporal arteritis
- Multiple sclerosis, particularly in the young or with bilateral pain
- Herpes zoster, pain may present before vesicular rash
- Sinusitis, otitis, dental causation, TMJ

- First bite syndrome
- Cluster tic syndrome

Management

Nonpharmacologic Treatment

- Avoid triggers.
- Surgical microvascular decompression, radiofrequency rhizotomy, gamma knife radiosurgery in severe cases, peripheral neurectomy

Pharmacologic Treatment

- Primary: carbamazepine (Tegretol) 100 mg twice a day, increase by 100–200 mg every 2 to 3 days up to 1,200 mg daily in divided doses; use lowest effective dose or oxcarbazepine 300 mg/day initially. Maintenance dose is 600 mg for an adult given in two divided doses
- Secondary options: oxcarbazepine; usual maintenance dose is 450–1,200 mg orally twice a day.
- Tertiary option: gabapentin (Neurontin) 300 mg three times a day; titrate up to 3,600 mg divided/day
- Botulinum toxin injections may be beneficial for some patients, limited data.

How Long to Treat

- Attempt to decrease or discontinue dose every 3 months; decrease one drug at a time.

Special Considerations

- CNS side effects: Start with lowest possible dose of medications for older adults and titrate up slowly.
- Adjust gabapentin dose for renal insufficiency.

When to Consult, Refer, Hospitalize

- Refer to neurosurgeon for surgical decompression if intractable pain with adequate trials of medication or unable to tolerate medications.
- Surgery is inappropriate for trigeminal neuralgia secondary to multiple sclerosis.

Follow-Up

- Follow every 3 months; may need more frequent follow up while pain is unmanaged.
- Monitor CBC and liver function if on antiseizure medication.

Complications

- Generally, none

BELL'S PALSY

Description

- An acute unilateral paralysis or paresis of the face in a pattern consistent with peripheral nerve dysfunction without a detectable cause; usually because of lower motor neuron facial weakness due to inflammation of the seventh cranial nerve
- Most patients have sudden onset of a unilateral facial droop, accompanied by drooling (especially in young children) and failure to completely close the affected eye; may also have discomfort behind ear or of jaw, change in hearing, loss of taste. Pain is usually transient.
- The paralysis may be difficult to assess when the patient is at rest, but evident with crying or talking.

Etiology

- Unknown, although reactivation of herpes simplex virus has been suspected in most cases
- Cases often preceded by an upper respiratory infection, Lyme disease

- Acute inflammatory response causing swelling of the facial nerve and entrapment in the foramen of the temporal bone
- Paresis typically progresses over 3–5 days; most patients fully recover in 3–4 months.

Incidence and Demographics

- 13 to 34 per 100,000 people a year; peak incidence is 10 to 40 years; no gender or race predilection
- Low rates of familial association

Risk Factors

- Trauma, diabetes mellitus, hypothyroidism, AIDS, Lyme disease, syphilis, sarcoidosis, viral infection
- Pregnancy due to increased intravascular volume, particularly during the third trimester; increases the risk for facial nerve edema and subsequent compression by three times.

Assessment

History

- In the newborn, history of birth trauma
- Abrupt onset facial paresis, face feels "pulled to side"
- Most important to establish time frame: Sudden onset over hours to a few days suggests Bell's palsy; progressive weakness over weeks indicates a tumor or other space-occupying lesion.
- Past medical history, including any recent upper respiratory infection; Lyme disease; otitis; facial trauma; and history of chronic illness, including diabetes, thyroid disease, multiple sclerosis, sarcoidosis, HIV
- Review of systems of neurological and HEENT, including facial movements; visual changes, pain, or tearing; altered hearing or otalgia; altered taste; skin rash or recent tick bite

Physical Exam

- Vital signs, noting any increase in blood pressure or temperature
- Complete HEENT exam for decreased tone, signs of infection, lesions, or rashes
- Screening neurological exam, including all cranial nerves, paying attention to eye movement, jaw strength, symmetry of the face, hearing
- Bell's palsy indicated by complete unilateral peripheral seventh nerve paresis or paralysis, with flattening of forehead furrows, inability to raise eyebrow, inability to completely close ipsilateral eye, flattening of nasolabial fold, inability to puff out cheek, drooping of mouth, inability to smile or frown; the rest of cranial nerves and neurological exam usually normal
- A central seventh nerve palsy, or only drooping of the mouth, indicates damage only to the lower branch of the facial nerve and an upper motor neuron lesion (stroke or tumor).
- Inspect eye for corneal abrasion and tearing.
- Inspect ear canal and tympanic membrane for otitis or vesicular lesions, which indicate cephalic herpes zoster.
- Palpate parotid glands for masses.
- Check for lymphadenopathy and thyroid enlargement.
- Inspect skin for rash, particularly target lesion or erythema migrans of Lyme disease (although rash may not still be present).

Diagnostic Studies

- No testing usually necessary unless diagnosis in question
- EMG and nerve conduction studies 5 to 10 days after onset of symptoms if complete paralysis or no improvement, to guide prognosis and treatment; if over 90% neural degeneration, surgical decompression may be indicated
- X-ray if temporal bone fracture suspected
- CT scan or MRI if tumor, space-occupying lesion, cerebral infarction, or hemorrhage suspected; also images of facial nerve and temporal bone
- CBC, chemistry panel, thyroid function tests, syphilis testing, HIV serology if indicated by history to rule out associated chronic diseases
- ESR if temporal (giant cell) arteritis suspected
- Lumbar puncture if meningitis or Guillain-Barre' syndrome suspected

- Lyme titer if exposure to ticks or rash suggestive of Lyme disease
- Venereal Disease Research Laboratory (VDRL) test and/or HIV screen if history warrants
- Audiology testing if hearing affected more than 1 week or acoustic neuroma suspected
- Electromyography testing occasionally used to predict prognosis and progression of disease (usually done if symptoms last longer than 6 to 12 months)

Differential Diagnosis

- Tumor
- Stroke or transient ischemic attack (TIA)
- Herpes zoster
- Temporal bone fracture or other trauma
- Giant cell arteritis
- Lyme disease
- HIV
- Sjögren syndrome
- Guillain-Barré syndrome (typically symmetric bilateral weakness)
- Neurofibromatosis
- Melkersson-Rosenthal syndrome
- Infections (otitis media, mastoiditis, meningitis, mumps, rubella, syphilis)
- Parotid gland obstruction or mass
- Multiple sclerosis or other demyelinating conditions
- Diabetic neuropathy
- Hypothyroidism
- Sarcoidosis

Management

Nonpharmacologic Treatment

- Protect eye, artificial tears during the day (up to hourly); lubricant ointment and patch eye at bedtime

- Surgical decompression not recommended
- Physical therapy for patients with incomplete recovery after 3–4 months

Pharmacologic Treatment

- Medical treatment of Bell's palsy remains controversial.
- Prednisone in children: 2 mg/kg/day (up to 60–80 mg) orally for 5 days, followed by a 5-day taper, discontinue by day 14; in adults: 60–80 mg/day orally divided for 7 days.
- Severe Bell's palsy may add valacyclovir to glucocorticoid therapy; children: valacyclovir 20 mg/kg/dose three times a day (maximum 1,000 mg per dose) orally for 7 days; in adults: valacyclovir 1,000 mg three times a day orally for 7 days
- Artificial tears to keep affected eye moist during daytime and ointment at night

How Long to Treat

- Eye protection until patient can close and protect eye
- Steroid and antiviral therapy for 7–10 days

Special Considerations

- Incomplete recovery is associated with increased age.
- Poor prognosis is associated with complete paralysis, pain, or hyperacusis at presentation; these characteristics, combined with increased age and comorbidity, should guide decision to treat with steroids and antiviral agents.

When to Consult, Refer, Hospitalize

- Refer to ophthalmologist if corneal abrasion or significant prolonged decreased lacrimation.
- Refer to neurologist if other deficits present, recurrent paresis, or paresis lasting more than 3–4 months.
- In patients older than 6 years, refer to plastic surgeon for persistent cosmetic disfigurement.
- Counseling for patient and caregivers may be beneficial for those with prolonged recovery

Follow-Up

- At 1-week intervals to ensure eye protection and recovery

Expected Course

- Most have spontaneous recovery in 2 to 3 weeks.
- 15% may have residual weakness for several months and some have permanent weakness.

Complications

- Incomplete recovery or recurrent paresis or paralysis
- Corneal abrasion
- Recurrent episodes

STROKE AND TRANSIENT ISCHEMIC ATTACK (TIA; "BRAIN ATTACK")

Description

- Strokes are ischemic or hemorrhagic.
- Interruption in blood flow to the brain causing neuronal death or infarction. Hemorrhage accounts for 13% of strokes; the bleed may be intracerebral or subarachnoid.
- Transient ischemic attack (TIA) is a temporary interruption in cerebral vascular blood flow; the deficit lasts less than 24 hours. There is no infarcted tissue.

Etiology

- Ischemic stroke
  - Lack of blood flow to brain due to hypoxia, decreased cardiac output, thrombus, or embolus
- Thrombotic stroke
  - Caused by progressive accumulation of atherosclerotic plaque that occludes an intracranial vessel
  - Most common artery involved in ischemic stroke is the middle cerebral artery

- Embolic stroke
  - Caused by atherosclerotic debris from the heart, aorta, or carotids that flow into the internal carotids and occlude the smaller vessels of the cerebral circulation
  - Usually affects more distal cerebral arteries
- Lacunar infarcts
  - Less than 15 mm; occur in the internal capsule, basal ganglia, or thalamus
  - Due to slow, progressive occlusion of a single penetrating branch of a large cerebral artery
- TIA: may be thrombotic, embolic, or lacunar in nature
- Hemorrhagic stroke
  - Intracerebral hemorrhage: spontaneous bleeding into parenchyma from microaneurysm of perforating vessels; most commonly occurs in the basal ganglia; because of hypertension, hematological disorders, or anticoagulation therapy
- Subarachnoid hemorrhage
  - Bleeding from a ruptured aneurysm in the circle of Willis or AVM

Incidence and Demographics

- Acute stroke afflicts 795,000 Americans per year; incidence increases with age.
- One-fifth will die, making stroke the fifth leading cause of death in the United States in 2020.
- 15%–30% of survivors will be permanently disabled; 26% will require nursing home placement.

Risk Factors

- Previous cerebrovascular disease, stroke, or TIA; 7% to 40% of ischemic strokes preceded by TIA within days to months
- Aging
- Traditional risks for vascular disease: hypertension, diabetes, hyperlipidemia, smoking
- Traditional risks for emboli: atrial fibrillation, cardiomyopathy, coronary artery disease

Prevention and Screening

- Manage hypertension; screening for hypertension is recommended at least every 3–5 years in the normotensive aged 18–39; treatment is recommended (Grade A) as per the U.S. Preventive Services Task Force (USPSTF).
- Benefits of screening for asymptomatic carotid stenosis by auscultation of carotid bruits or carotid ultrasound are not significant.
- High-risk patients over age 60 with other risk factors for vascular disease who have access to vascular surgery with morbidity and mortality rates of less than 3% may benefit from screening and subsequent endarterectomy.
- Antiplatelet therapy may decrease the risk of stroke in those with asymptomatic carotid artery stenosis.
- Anticoagulation is recommended for patients with atrial fibrillation, particularly those with additional risk factors.
- Evidence suggests improved glycemic control may decrease microvascular events in type 2 diabetes.
- Decreasing serum lipids may delay progression of carotid atherosclerosis and decrease cerebrovascular events.
- All patients will benefit from diet and exercise counseling and smoking cessation.

Assessment

History

- Onset, duration, and progression of symptoms are most important in determining etiology and management.
- Resolution of symptoms in minutes to 24 hours is suggestive of a TIA.
- Onset during sleep or early morning hours with progression suggests thrombotic stroke.
- Sudden onset with activity suggests embolic or hemorrhagic stroke.
- Detailed description of symptoms or deficits—including visual changes, aphasia, motor weakness, or paresthesia—may give clue to location of stroke or lesion.
- Review of systems: headache, seizure, loss of consciousness, syncope, vertigo, vomiting, cardiac symptoms:
  - Lack of headache excludes hemorrhagic stroke.
  - Vomiting is associated with increased ICP, usually because of hemorrhage.

  - ◇ Loss of consciousness is associated with hemorrhage or posterior circulation thrombosis.
  - ◇ Syncope is more often related to cardiac etiology than stroke.
  - ◇ Vertigo suggests vestibular disease but may occur with vertebrobasilar insufficiency.
- ♦ Past medical history: cardiac disease; peripheral vascular disease; diabetes; IV drug use; previous neurological conditions such as seizure, head trauma, dementia, or brain tumors give clues to etiology and possible differential diagnosis
- ♦ Review all medications, particularly those that can alter level of consciousness or cause bleeding.

Physical Exam

- ♦ Ensuring medical stabilization with attention to airway, breathing, and circulation is a vital first step.
- ♦ Complete neurological exam, including level of consciousness, cognitive ability (apraxia, agnosia, aphasia, agraphia), motor and sensory function (contralateral deficits), cranial nerve exam including funduscopic and visual deficits, reflexes (hyper-reflexia or Babinski on affected side)
- ♦ Cardiovascular exam: hypertension, orthostatic changes, atrial fibrillation, heart murmurs, carotid bruits, abdominal bruit from aneurysm
- ♦ Signs of carotid TIA: weakness of contralateral arm, leg, or face, individually or in combination; numbness or paresthesia may occur alone or in combination with motor deficit; dysphagia; monocular visual loss; carotid bruit; atherosclerotic changes on funduscopic exam. Signs and symptoms disappear as attack resolves.
- ♦ Signs of vertebrobasilar TIA: vertigo; ataxia; diplopia; dysarthria; dysphagia; dimness; blurriness, or loss of vision in one or both eyes; perioral numbness, weakness, or sensory complaints on one or both sides of the body; drop attacks with bilateral leg weakness
- ♦ Lacunar infarction: contralateral pure motor or sensory deficit, ipsilateral ataxia, dysarthria, with complete symptom resolution over 1 to 2 months
- ♦ Cerebral infarction: Deficit depends on vessel so any variety of focal neurological deficits may develop.
- ♦ Cerebellar infarction: vertigo, ataxia, nystagmus, nausea/vomiting
- ♦ Hemorrhagic CVA: typically associated with hypertension, sudden onset, symptoms usually present during activity, initial loss of or impaired consciousness, rapidly evolving hemiplegia or paresis

Diagnostic Studies

- All patients with suspected stroke require urgent noncontrast CT scan or brain MRI.
- Finger-stick blood glucose (hypoglycemia may mimic stroke symptoms), oxygen saturation monitoring.
- Lumbar puncture if CT negative for hemorrhage and subarachnoid hemorrhage suspected.
- Carotid duplex for evaluation of symptomatic carotid stenosis, if patient is surgical candidate for endarterectomy; carotid studies useless for evaluation of posterior circulation
- Angiography remains the "gold standard" for assessing carotid stenosis, as well as identifying aneurysms, AVM, and vasculitis.
- ECG, chest X-ray, echocardiogram, EEG (if seizures suspected)
- Transesophageal or transthoracic echocardiogram if intraventricular thrombus or patent foramen ovale is suspected
- Holter monitor to rule out paroxysmal arrhythmias
- CBC, ESR, troponin, coagulation studies, comprehensive metabolic panel (CMP), toxicology screen, blood alcohol content, pregnancy test (if appropriate), arterial blood gases if hypoxia is suspected, and lipid profile to evaluate cause

Differential Diagnosis

- TIA, thrombotic, embolic, or lacunar stroke
- Subarachnoid or intracerebral hemorrhage
- Cerebral aneurysm or AVM
- Intracranial tumor
- Seizure
- Migraine with aura
- Encephalopathy
- Intoxication
- Hypoglycemia
- Multiple sclerosis
- Syncope

- Vertigo
- Postural hypotension

Management

Nonpharmacologic Treatment

- Educate families and patients at risk of first or recurrent stroke about "brain attack," common signs and symptoms, and the need for same immediate response as heart attack.
- Endovascular mechanical thrombectomy may be performed in patients experiencing a large-vessel occlusion and who are either ineligible for or have contraindications to thrombolytic treatment; generally performed up to 6 hours after the onset of stroke symptoms
- Diet and exercise counseling for primary and secondary prevention; smoking cessation
- Carotid endarterectomy for symptomatic surgical candidates with carotid stenosis at or over 70% blockage
- Begin post care rehabilitation early for stroke patients to prevent complications of immobility: physical therapy (prevention of pressure ulcers, deep vein thrombosis (DVT) and pulmonary embolism, pneumonia, and muscle contractures), occupational therapy, speech therapy
- Pneumatic compression stockings should be used to decrease the likelihood of DVT.
- Emotional support of patient and family, counseling helpful for patient and caregivers

Pharmacologic Treatment

- Recombinant tissue plasminogen activator (tPA) must be administered in a hospital within 4.5 hours of onset of symptoms of ischemic stroke; contraindicated in hemorrhagic stroke. Patients awaking with focal deficits are not appropriate for tPA because duration of deficits is unknown.
- Medical management in the post-acute phase involves anticoagulation or antiplatelet agents and treatment of underlying heart disease, hypertension, diabetes, and hyperlipidemia.
- Early initiation of short-term dual antiplatelet therapy is proven beneficial for high-risk TIA or minor ischemic stroke:
    - Aspirin 160 mg to 325 mg loading dose, followed by 50–100 mg daily; plus clopidogrel (Plavix) (300–600 mg loading dose, followed by 75 mg daily) for 21 days;

high-quality evidence that this strategy reduces the risk of recurrent ischemic stroke with only a small increase in the risk of moderate or major bleeding.

- ◊ Warfarin (Coumadin): Used for patients with atrial fibrillation or prosthetic heart valves. Dose is individualized because of small therapeutic window and interactions with food and other medications. International normalized ratio (INR) is stabilized at 2–3 for atrial fibrillation or antiplatelet failure and 2.5–3.5 for prosthetic valve.

How Long to Treat

- As long as antiplatelet or anticoagulation is not contraindicated (increased risk of GI or intracerebral bleeding)

Special Considerations

- Men are at greater risk than women, although more women die of stroke because of age, population, and socioeconomic dynamics.
- Increased risk with age and poorer prognosis, increased incidence of infection, myocardial infarction, renal failure, and delirium. Consider patient's risk of falls, ability to manage a complex medication regimen, and INR monitoring when initiating warfarin therapy.
- Do not discount stroke in young people—may be hemorrhagic stroke secondary to AVM or embolic stroke secondary to unidentified patent foramen ovale (right-to-left shunt).
- In many stroke centers, tPA may be administered intra-arterially for large-vessel occlusions that do not reopen with IV tPA, up to 6 hours following the onset of stroke symptoms.

When to Consult, Refer, Hospitalize

- Send all patients with sudden onset of focal neurological deficit to emergency facility; if TIA, may need urgent workup and treatment to prevent stroke; if diagnosed as stroke and of less than 4.5 hours duration, may start tPA therapy if patient meets criteria.
- Send patients to emergency facility with sudden severe headache, decreasing level of consciousness, vomiting, or focal neurological deficits.
- Consult with physician or neurologist for evaluation and management of patient with history of TIA or previous stroke.

Follow-Up

- Patients with risk for cerebrovascular disease should be monitored every 3 to 6 months for symptoms of TIA and hypertension, and counseled regarding stroke prophylaxis, diet, exercise, and smoking cessation.

Expected Course

- Variable; most stroke recovery occurs early. The longer the deficits last, the less likely they are to resolve, although improvement may be seen for 6 months
- 27% of stroke patients die within 1 year, and 52% within 5 years.
- One in four stroke survivors will have another stroke within 5 years.
- Physical therapy improves functional recovery.
- Older age, coma, and early acute CT changes are associated with poor prognosis.

Complications

- Intracerebral hemorrhage from tPA therapy
- Myocardial infarction, infection, renal failure
- Falls, depression, dementia
- Intracerebral bleed or GI bleed from anticoagulation

ALZHEIMER'S DISEASE (AD)/MULTI-INFARCT DEMENTIA (MID)

Description

- Dementia: impairment of global intellectual and cognitive function characterized by memory loss, aphasia, agnosia, and apraxia with preservation of level of consciousness
- Multi-infarct dementia and Alzheimer's disease (AD) make up the majority of progressive, irreversible dementias.
- MID: dementing process caused by strokes characterized by stepwise decline
- AD: gradual onset and progressive decline without focal neurological deficits; most common cause of dementia
    - First stage of AD manifested by short-term memory impairment and anosognosia. ADLs become increasingly challenging. Social, occupational, and cognitive impairment manifest themselves.

  - ◊ Second stage of AD characterized by increasing loss of social and cognitive ability, with concomitant increasing behavioral changes. These can range from agitation and restlessness to outright combativeness. Eventually, the patient no longer recognizes friends and loved ones.
  - ◊ Third and last stage of AD brings the disease full cycle, as cognitive disability is eventually followed by physical decline.
- ♦ Average life expectancy after a diagnosis of AD is 8–10 years depending on the impairment level at time of diagnosis.

Etiology

- ♦ AD: uncertain cause
- ♦ More neuritic plaques and neurofibrillary tangles are found on autopsy compared to nondemented patients.
- ♦ Three single-gene mutations are associated with early-onset AD and have been identified in families with history of AD, although not all cases may be inherited.
- ♦ MID: multiple lacunar infarcts cause a 4- to 12-fold increase in diagnosis
- ♦ A correlation between obstructive sleep apnea and AD increased mental deterioration

Incidence and Demographics

- ♦ Affects 9% of those 65 years and older and increases with age
- ♦ AD-related dementia affects 6.5 million Americans in 2022.
- ♦ Often misdiagnosed or unrecognized, especially in the early stages
- ♦ AD: 60%–70% of all dementias; MID: 10% of all dementias

Risk Factors

- ♦ AD: increasing age, Down syndrome
- ♦ Familial or inherited
- ♦ MID: hypertension, previous stroke, TIA
- ♦ Diabetes mellitus

Prevention and Screening

- Routine screening in persons younger than 65 years of age is not recommended because there is no definitive treatment, and it is difficult to recognize early dementia.
- Patients 65 years of age or older should have cognitive and functional evaluation annually.
- Be aware of early symptoms to facilitate early assessment and recognition, and rule out age-related memory changes, unidentified conditions, or reversible forms of dementia (see Table 15–5).
- Interpretation: Positive findings in any of these areas generally indicate the need for further assessment for the presence of dementia.

Assessment

History

- Detailed history of present illness, including time frame and progression, any associated neurological symptoms such as amaurosis fugax, aphasia, unilateral weakness, apraxia, olfactory disfunction, sleep disturbances, seizures, and memory impairment

TABLE 15–5.
GUIDE FOR RECOGNITION AND INITIAL ASSESSMENT OF DEMENTIA

DOES THE PERSON HAVE INCREASED DIFFICULTY WITH ANY OF THE ACTIVITIES LISTED?	
Learning and retaining new information	Repeats information; has trouble remembering recent conversations, events, appointments; frequently misplaces objects
Handling complex tasks	Has trouble following a complex train of thought or performing tasks that require many steps such as balancing a checkbook or cooking a meal
Reasoning ability	Is unable to respond with a reasonable plan to problems at home or work, such as knowing what to do if the bathroom is flooded; shows uncharacteristic disregard for rules of social conduct
Special ability and orientation	Has trouble driving, organizing objects around the house, finding way around familiar places
Language	Has increasing difficulty with finding the words to express what he or she wants to say and with following conversations
Behavior	Appears more passive and less responsive; is more irritable than usual; is more suspicious than usual; misinterprets visual or auditory stimuli

- Past medical history: hypertension, strokes, head trauma
- Psychiatric history: depression, anxiety, schizophrenia
- Social history: present living situation, marital status, occupation, education, alcohol, tobacco, illicit drug use
- Medications, including over the counter, supplements, and home remedies
- Initial and periodic functional history and assessment
- Validate history with family member and/or caregiver, but also be aware of potential for self-serving motives; informants may exaggerate or deny symptoms.

Physical Exam

- Assess level of consciousness along a continuum from alert to drowsy, to stupor, to coma.
- Perform complete mental status evaluation using an instrument such as the Montreal Cognitive Assessment (MoCA); test results are not diagnostic but serve as a baseline for assessing trends in cognitive impairment.
    - Generally, a score of less than 26 on the MoCA (which tests orientation, registration, attention, and calculation, recall and language) may indicate cognitive impairment.
    - Most important part of the diagnostic evaluation is a detailed history including the perspective of a caregiver (e.g., spouse or adult child), interviewed separately from patient.
- Complete neurological exam with attention to focal neurological deficits, which may indicate MID or other neurological problem
    - MID: focal motor weakness or impaired sensation, reflex asymmetry, positive Babinski
- Assess for sensory impairments (hearing, vision) that mimic or worsen dementia.
- Pulmonary and cardiac exams (murmurs, arrhythmias, heart enlargement, orthostatic hypotension)
- Any evidence of infectious processes
- Signs of physical and mental abuse

Diagnostic Studies

- CBC, chemistry profile, thyroid function tests, vitamin B12 level, folate level to rule out causes of delirium and reversible dementia; HIV, and drug toxicity if indicated by history
- CT or MRI may show atrophy, infarcts, hematomas, or unexpected lesions.
- Other testing based on presentation

- Neuropsychological testing is recommended under certain circumstances: to differentiate depression, stroke, or delirium in unusual presentations; or identify areas of preserved cognitive function to develop a care plan.
- Sleep study if obstructive sleep apnea is suspected

Differential Diagnosis

- Delirium
- Other dementias: Lewy body dementia, frontotemporal dementia (Pick's disease)
- Depression and anxiety
- Normal pressure hydrocephalus
- Tumor
- Hearing loss
- Vitamin B12 and folate deficiency
- Parkinson's disease
- Trauma—consider subdural hematoma, falls (whether witnessed or not)
- Alcohol intoxication
- Infectious process: chronic infection, AIDS, tertiary syphilis
- Cardiovascular or cerebrovascular accidents
- Medications: polypharmacy, interactions

Management

- Foremost, rule out or treat any conditions that may contribute to cognitive impairment.
- Discontinue all unnecessary medications, especially sedatives and hypnotics.
- MID: nonpharmacologic and pharmacologic reduction of stroke risks; see Management under Stroke and Transient Ischemic Attack (TIA; "Brain Attack")

Nonpharmacologic Treatment

- Explain memory/cognition status assessment results to the patient, putting them within the context of overall patient status.

- Educate patient and family about the illness, treatment, and community resources.
- Assist with long-term planning, including financial, legal, and advance directives.
- Assess home and driving safety.
- Behavior therapy identifies causes of problem behaviors and changes the environment to reduce the behavior.
- Recreational, art, and pet therapy create pleasurable experiences for the patient.
- Recent studies show outdoor activities prove effective in treating physical aggression; massage and touch therapy are effective at treating verbal aggression.
- Reminiscence therapy
- Incontinence care; supportive care; counseling with neuropsychologist

Pharmacologic Treatment

- The mainstay of therapy for patients with AD is the use of centrally acting cholinesterase inhibitors to attempt to compensate for the depletion of acetylcholine (ACh) in the cerebral cortex and hippocampus. A partial *N*-methyl-D-aspartate (NMDA) antagonist is approved for treatment of moderate and severe AD. Various medications are used for treatment of secondary symptoms of AD, including antidepressants, anti-anxiety agents, and antipsychotic agents. Three currently approved cholinesterase Inhibitors(i.e., donepezil, rivastigmine, galantamine) inhibit acetylcholinesterase (AChE) at the synapse.
- Cognitive symptoms
  - Cholinesterase inhibitors such as donepezil (Aricept) 5 mg initially, may increase up to 23 mg orally mg/day q.h.s. in moderate to severe dementia, or galantamine 8–12 mg orally twice a day, or rivastigmine 1.5 mg to 6 mg orally twice a day
  - No evidence that cholinesterase inhibitors are neuroprotective or alter progression of the underlying disease
  - Avoid benzodiazepines, antihistamines, or other sedatives, particularly those with anticholinergic effects.
  - NMDA receptor agonists such as memantine are proposed to be neuroprotective; memantine may be useful in combination with cholinesterase inhibitors in patients with advanced AD to help restore some cognitive function.
  - Aducanumab is a recombinant monoclonal antibody that targets amyloid beta. Although not currently recommended for routine use, this therapy is showing promising results in research studies.
  - Common side effects of cholinesterase inhibitors: headache, nausea, diarrhea
  - Liver function test monitoring not required for cholinesterase inhibitors

- Psychosis and agitation
- Primary: olanzapine (Zyprexa) 2.5–5 mg twice a day, quetiapine (Seroquel) 25 mg orally q.h.s.
  - Secondary option: pimavanserin (Nuplazid) 34 mg orally once a day
- Depression
  - Sertraline (Zoloft) HCl 25–200 mg/day
  - Citalopram (Celexa) 10–40 mg/day
  - Escitalopram (Lexapro) 10–20 mg/day
- Sleep disturbances
  - Trazodone 25–75 mg at bedtime (if using other serotonin modifiers, be alert for serotonin syndrome)

How Long to Treat

- Use other medications as needed; if needed regularly, use lowest effective dose and attempt to wean periodically.

Special Considerations

- Consider language and education level when administering and interpreting mental status tests.
- Integrate cultural beliefs into the management of minority patients with dementia.

When to Consult, Refer, Hospitalize

- Consult with physician for diagnosis and long-term treatment planning.
- Refer to neurologist for unusual presentation.
- Refer to psychiatrist if unable to differentiate from depression or see intractable behaviors.
- Use social worker and multidisciplinary services for long-term care planning.
- Hospitalize with deteriorating conditions, such as exacerbation of chronic heart failure (CHF), chronic obstructive pulmonary disease (COPD), dehydration, pneumonia, or injury. Be aware that patients with dementia are likely to become more confused and delirious and fall when hospitalized.

Follow-Up

- Generally, every 60 days

Expected Course

- AD: slowly progressive
- MID: stepwise with gradual deterioration; associated with new focal deficits and decline with each additional stroke

Complications

- Depression and suicide
- Complications usually related to comorbidity or complications, because of immobility with severe end-stage dementia

DELIRIUM

Description

- Acute disorder of attention with onset of hours to days, characterized by confusion and disorientation, with fluctuation of symptoms over the course of a day that are not explained by another neurocognitive disorder.

Etiology

- Functional disorder of the brain caused by organic factors
- Any number of factors can cause delirium: polypharmacy, infections, metabolic and electrolyte abnormalities, dehydration, nutritional deficiencies, cardiopulmonary disease, urinary retention, fecal impaction, trauma, anesthesia, environmental change

Incidence and Demographics

- 14% to 56% of hospitalized patients 65 years and older

Risk Factors

- Age, frailty, visual impairment, presence of many other chronic diseases
- Dementia, stroke, or Parkinson's disease are factors present in nearly 50% of older patients with delirium

Prevention and Screening

- Eliminate unnecessary medications.
- Provide/ensure adequate hydration, nutrition, and oxygenation.
- Correct visual and auditory deficits.
- Continuity of care and environment
- Delirium initially missed by clinicians in more than 70% of cases

Assessment

History

- Detailed history of present illness, including cognition, time frame, and progression
- Comprehensive review of systems to identify underlying etiology
- Functional history and assessment
- Validate history with family member and/or caregiver.
- History of recent alcohol or illicit drug use
- Exhaustive medication reconciliation

Physical Exam

- Complete neurological exam with attention to change in level of consciousness, focal neurological deficits
- Hearing and visual impairments
- Pulmonary and cardiac exams (murmurs, arrhythmias, heart enlargement)
- Jaundiced or dusky-appearing skin (seen with chronic pulmonary disease)
- Any evidence of infectious processes

- Signs of trauma
- Evaluation for orthostatic hypotension, urinary retention, and fecal impaction
- Folstein Mini-Mental State Examination
- Geriatric Depression Scale

Diagnostic Studies

- CBC, chemistry profile, thyroid function tests, blood alcohol concentration, vitamin B12 level, folate level to identify a reversible cause for cognitive impairment or etiology
- CT to identify infarcts, space-occupying lesions
- Syphilis, HIV, and drug toxicity if indicated by history
- Urinalysis if urinary tract infection (UTI) suspected
- Arterial oxygen or pulse oximetry if hypoxemia considered
- ECG and chest X-ray identify cardiopulmonary cause
- EEG to rule out seizure disorder
- Lumbar puncture for suspected encephalopathy or meningitis

Differential Diagnosis

- Sundowning
- Focal syndromes
- Nonconvulsive status epilepticus
- Dementia
- Depression
- See Etiology above

Management

- Identify and treat underlying cause.

Nonpharmacologic Treatment

- Provide continuity of care.
- Minimize environmental stimuli.
- Provide eyeglasses or hearing aids.
- Coordinate clocks and calendars to maintain orientation.
- Maintain hydration, nutrition, oxygenation.
- Ensure adequate bowel and bladder regimen.

Pharmacologic Treatment

- Current studies demonstrate that atypical antipsychotics may be similarly effective with decreased incidence of extrapyramidal symptoms associated with conventional antipsychotics
- Atypical antipsychotics effective in treating antipsychotics include:
    - Olanzapine
    - Quetiapine
    - Risperidone

How Long to Treat

- Depends on etiology; often continue therapy until baseline cognitive function returns

Special Considerations

- Highest incidence in hospitalized older adults
- Coronavirus disease 2019 (COVID-19)–based delirium becoming clinically relevant; approximately 50% of those hospitalized for COVID-19 will experience at least one episode of delirium
- It is recommended that patients with Parkinson's disease with delirium be treated with an atypical antipsychotic medication

When to Consult, Refer, Hospitalize

- Consult physician for any primary care patient with suspected delirium.
- Hospitalize to ensure patient safety, adequate hydration, and prescribed treatment unless underlying etiology such as UTI without sepsis can be managed at home with supervision.

Follow-Up

- Regularly to monitor for recurrence

Expected Course

- Usually, reversible

Complications

- Injury due to falls
- Associated with increased morbidity and mortality

PARKINSON DISEASE

Description

- Complex neurodegenerative disease with motor, nonmotor, and neuropsychiatric symptomatology; characterized by bradykinesia, rigidity, flexed posture, loss of postural reflex, freezing, resting tremor

Etiology

- Unknown, although genetics, endogenous toxins, and exogenous toxins have been implicated
- In Parkinson's disease, depigmentation, neuronal loss, and gliosis of the substantia nigra pars compacta and pontine locus coeruleus occur, resulting in damage to dopaminergic neurons, leaving active unopposed acetylcholine neurons intact.

- Imbalance of dopamine and acetylcholine results in loss of refinement of voluntary movement.
- Pseudo-parkinsonism (reversible) can occur in patients receiving metoclopramide, neuroleptic agents, or reserpine.

Incidence and Demographics

- Prevalence 100–200 persons 40 years of age and over per 100,000, with more than 1 million people living with this disease in North America
- Men are 1.5 times more likely to acquire the disease than women; usual onset during ages 45 to 65
- Less prevalent in Black people and people of African descent than in White people and people of Asian and European descent; geographical location is a stronger determinant of Parkinson's disease than ethnicity.
- Affects 1% of those 60 years of age and older

Risk Factors

- Age
- Genetics (especially for symptom onset at ages less than 50)
- Exposure to pesticides, nitrogen dioxide in air pollution, previous traumatic brain injury, obesity, type 2 diabetes, and metabolic syndrome

Prevention and Screening

- Studies show aerobic exercise, low to moderate caffeine intake, and the use of ibuprofen may reduce risk.
- Older patients may benefit from annual assessment of mobility and cognitive and functional status.

Assessment

History

- Focused detailed history of chief complaint, including time frame and progression, aggravating and alleviating factors such as stress or rest, and interview family, patient, and caregiver

- Complete review of neurological symptoms, including weakness, paresthesia, tremor, diplopia, aphasia, mood, and cognitive changes
- Past medical history, including neurological disorders, exposure to environmental toxins, illicit drugs
- Family history of Parkinson's disease, other movement disorders, or dementia
- Medications, including over-the-counter anticholinergics, antihistamines, decongestants, or cough and cold preparations that may worsen condition
- Functional assessment: difficulty with functional and instrumental ADLs; mobility, including stair-climbing (patients with progressive supranuclear palsy will have problem descending stairs) and rising from chair
- Falls and injuries
- Review of systems for associated autonomic dysfunction, including perspiration, incontinence, constipation, and postural hypotension
- Assess for depression and mental status—may use Geriatric Depression Scale and MMSE or other tools

Physical Exam

- General: manner, affect, dress, and hygiene; speech may be flat or soft and monotone.
- Cranial nerve exam: normal in Parkinson's disease, fourth cranial nerve palsy with progressive supranuclear palsy
- Motor exam: no weakness but cogwheel rigidity (rigidity to passive movement)
  - Bradykinesia: slowness of voluntary movement and difficulty initiating movement, difficulty rising from chair, shuffling gait, problems with turns and stopping movement
  - Tremor: slow (four to six cycles per second) resting tremor present in one limb, limbs on one side, four limbs, or absent in 20% of patients with Parkinson's disease; tremor may be obvious at rest and exaggerated with stress; some tremor of mouth and lips; tremors are often unilateral at onset
  - Tremor may increase with emotional stress, decrease with voluntary activity
- Gait and posture: stooped posture with knees and hips flexed; hands held in front, close to body; instability
- "Masked facies": fixed facial expression, drooling, wide palpebral fissures, soft voice
- Meyerson's sign: repetitive tapping on bridge of the nose produces sustained blink response

- Incoordination of rapid alternating movements; decreased automatic movement, decreased blinking
- Deep tendon reflexes unaffected
- General examination: seborrheic dermatitis (found in more than 50% of those with Parkinson's disease)
- Vital signs: orthostatic hypotension

Diagnostic Studies

- Consider head CT if diagnosis unclear and stroke or space-occupying lesion is suspected.
- Complete diagnosis requires comprehensive history and neurological exam with markers of Parkinson's disease and at minimum bradykinesia plus either tremor or rigidity; also beneficial response to dopaminergic therapy

Differential Diagnosis

- Benign essential tremor
- Scans without evidence of dopaminergic deficit (SWEDD)
- Progressive supranuclear palsy
- Multiple system atrophy
- Lewy body dementia
- Corticobasal degeneration
- Brain tumor
- Drug-induced parkinsonism may be caused by multiple drug classifications; however, adverse effects of anticholinergic medications, particularly antipsychotics, are most often seen.
- Secondary parkinsonism caused by carbon monoxide poisoning; head trauma; infections
- Vascular parkinsonism
- Normal pressure hydrocephalus
- Huntington's disease
- Cerebrovascular disease
- Idiopathic and familial basal ganglia calcification

Management

- There is no cure for Parkinson's disease. Current therapy is aimed at managing symptoms to preserve independence and mobility.
- The modified Hoehn and Yahr Scale can be helpful for staging the disease and guiding pharmacological and supportive therapy.
  - Stage 1: unilateral involvement only
  - Stage 1.5: unilateral and axial involvement
  - Stage 2: bilateral involvement without impairment of balance
  - Stage 2.5: mild bilateral disease with recovery on pull test
  - Stage 3: mild to moderate bilateral disease; some postural instability; physically independent
  - Stage 4: severe disability; still able to walk or stand unassisted
  - Stage 5: wheelchair bound or bedridden unless aided

Nonpharmacologic Treatment

- Patient and family education regarding progressive nature of disease and complex pharmacologic treatments
- Nutritional counseling regarding low-protein diet and dietary management of constipation
- Compression stockings for postural hypotension
- Physical, occupational, speech therapy with appropriate assistive devices for ambulation and ADLs
- Fall precautions and home safety evaluation; installing rails, raised toilet seats, tub chairs
- Encouragement for walking, social activities, and interaction
- Tai chi, when performed for 1 hour twice per week, has been shown to reduce fall risk
- Emotional support: counseling has proved beneficial for patient and all caregivers.
- Deep brain stimulation
- Swallowing study to prevent aspiration
- Surgical interventions: unilateral stereotaxic thalamotomy or pallidotomy, implantable high-frequency thalamic stimulation to suppress resting tremor for difficult-to-control cases

Pharmacologic Treatment

- Initial symptomatic treatment based on level of motor debilitation: dopamine precursor
  - 25 mg carbidopa/100 mg levodopa (Sinemet) three to four times a day; start therapy with one-half tablet two or three times a day with meals for 1 week to establish tolerability; titrate up by one tablet every 5 to 7 days as needed and tolerated; most patients will enjoy significant therapeutic response to total daily doses of levodopa in the range of 300 mg to 600 mg; dosing is never to exceed 200 mg carbidopa and 2,000 mg levodopa per day.
  - Waning response in 40% to 50% of patients after 1 to 3 years—patients experience inconsistent effect from same dose
  - "Wearing-off" symptoms appear before next dose is due.
  - Use lowest doses possible; consider addition of dopamine agonists.
- Dopamine agonists
  - Pramipexole (Mirapex) 0.125 mg three times a day, titrate up to 1.5 mg three times a day over 7 weeks (max dose 4.5 mg/day divided); discontinue slowly.
  - Ropinirole (Requip) 0.25 mg three times a day to start, titrate up by 0.25 mg per dose each week for 4 weeks to a total daily dose of 3 mg. After week 4, dose may be increased weekly by 1.5 mg a day up to a maximum daily dose of 24 mg. Maintenance dose is 3–24 mg a day. Discontinue slowly over 1 week.
  - Transdermal rotigotine (Neupro) 4–6 mg patch every 24 hours. Titrate up starting with a 2 mg patch every 24 hours, increase dose by 2 mg/24 hours every week; max dose 6 mg/24 hours; discontinue slowly, taper dose by 2 mg/24 hours q.o.d. to discontinue
- Monoamine oxidase B (MAO-B) inhibitors:
  - Selegiline (Eldepryl) 5 mg twice a day (at low doses, is a selective MAO inhibitor and can be administered safely with levodopa)
  - Safinamide (Xadago) 50 mg a day, may be increased to 100 mg daily after 14 days based on tolerability and benefits (usually adjunctive therapy with levodopa to help with motor fluctuations)
  - Nonselective MAO inhibitors contraindicated in combination with levodopa; use can precipitate hyperpyrexia and hypertensive crisis; must be discontinued at least 14 days before initiating levodopa
- Adamantanes
  - Amantadine (Osmolex ER): 129–322 mg orally every.a.m. Begin 129 mg per day, may increase dose every week; to discontinue, taper dose over 2 weeks; monotherapy is used as alternative to early levodopa in younger patients who are at risk for dyskinesia, especially when prominent tremor is present; can also be used to help mitigate "wearing-off" symptoms in patients with advanced Parkinson's disease.

- Anticholinergic/antimuscarinic agents
  - Benztropine 0.5–2 mg every.h.s.; start with 0.5 mg and increase if needed 0.5 mg every 5–6 days up to 2 mg.
  - Trihexyphenidyl 0.5–1 mg twice a day; may increase gradually to 2 mg three times a day if clinically required.
- Catechol O-methyltransferase (COMT) inhibitor
  - Entacapone (Comtan) 200 mg twice a day up to four times a day, max 1,600 mg/day
  - Tolcapone (Tasmar) 100–200 mg three times a day, max 600 mg/day

How Long to Treat

- Medication combinations and dosages must be individualized and adjusted during the course of the disease; disease is lifelong and progressive.

Special Considerations

- Prescribe Parkinson's medications with caution in older adults, particularly those with comorbidities of heart, renal, or liver disease.
- Avoid anticholinergics in older adults, tend to be poorly tolerated, and have increased risk of side effects including confusion, agitation, arrhythmias, urinary retention.
- Differentiate Parkinson's disease from essential tremor, which may occur at any age from childhood but increases with age and affects the distal upper extremities and head; may be familial.
  - If mild, reassurance may be the only intervention needed
  - May be treated with propranolol (Inderal), primidone (Mysoline), or gabapentin (Neurontin)
  - May be disabling; refer for possible neurosurgery

When to Consult, Refer, Hospitalize

- Refer to neurologist for confirmation of diagnosis and guidance with medical management.
- Neurosurgical consultation for patients with severe symptoms refractory to medications, or unable to tolerate medications

TABLE 15–6.
TREATMENT ALGORITHM FOR PARKINSON'S DISEASE

STAGE OR PROBLEM	THERAPEUTIC ALTERNATIVES
Mild disease (Stages1 and 2)	MAO-B inhibitors such as selegiline Anticholinergics if tremor predominant amantadine (best for rigidity and bradykinesia) Group support, exercise, education, nutrition
Functionally impaired (Stage 3) Age younger than 60 years Age 60 years or older	Tremor predominant: anticholinergics (use with caution in older adults) Functional disability: sustained-release carbidopa/levodopa (lowest dose possible); dopamine agonist Sustained-release carbidopa/levodopa
Stage 4 or 5	Immediate-release carbidopa/levodopa Dopamine agonists
Poor symptom control	Increase carbidopa/levodopa dose. Add or increase dopamine agonist dose.
Suboptimal peak response	Begin combination dopaminergic therapy. Add levodopa to dopamine agonist. Add dopamine agonist to levodopa. Increase dose of levodopa/carbidopa or dopamine agonist. Switch dopamine agonists.
Wearing off	Begin combination of dopaminergic therapy; add levodopa to dopamine agonist or add dopamine agonist to levodopa. Increase frequency of levodopa dosing. Increase dose of levodopa/carbidopa (sustained or immediate release). Change to extended-release carbidopa/levodopa. Add liquid levodopa/carbidopa. Consider adding a COMT inhibitor. Avoid protein 60–90 minutes before and after taking medications. Consider inhaled levodopa. In rare cases, wearing-off episodes may be from excessive levodopa.

Continued

TABLE 15–6.
(CONTINUED)

STAGE OR PROBLEM	THERAPEUTIC ALTERNATIVES
On-off	Begin combination dopaminergic therapy. Add levodopa to dopamine agonist. Add dopamine agonist to levodopa. Modify distribution of dietary protein. (Protein may reduce absorption and influx of levodopa into the brain.) Add COMT inhibitor Add MAO-B inhibitor
Freezing	Increase or decrease carbidopa/levodopa dose. Decrease dopamine agonist dose. Gait modification, physical therapy, use of assistive devices Consider subthalmic nucleus deep brain stimulation. Consider continuous levodopa-carbidopa intestinal gel infusion (LCIG).
No "on" time	Manipulate time and dose of levodopa. Consider inhaled levodopa Minimize dietary protein Take medication on empty stomach Evaluate for gastroparesis and constipation Consider dopamine agonist such as apomorphine Consider acute akinesia, dystonia, akathisia, diphasic dyskinesia

Adapted from Liang, T. W., & Tarsy, D. (2022). *Medical management of motor fluctuations and dyskinesia in Parkinson disease*. Evidence-Based Clinical Decision Support System| *UpToDate* | Wolters-Kluwer. https://www.uptodate.com/contents/medical-management-of-motor-fluctuations-and-dyskinesia-in-parkinson-disease?search=parkinson%20treatment&source=search_result&selectedTitle=2~150&usage_type=default&display_rank=2#H615414407

Follow-Up

- Every 3 months, as well as any time a change is made in medication and/or therapy regimens
- Episodic office visit if symptoms worsen
- Annual health assessment and physical examination

Expected Course

- Progressive; up to 80% eventually develop coexisting dementia with poorer prognosis

Complications

- Related to immobility and falls; hip fractures common, pneumonia may occur in Stage 5
- Aspiration of food
- Depression and social isolation occur.

MULTIPLE SCLEROSIS (MS)

Description

- Progressive neurodegenerative disease characterized by demyelination and inflammation of the neuronal sheath in the brain and spinal cord that produces episodic neurologic symptoms such as sensory abnormalities, visual disturbances, sphincter disturbances, and weakness with or without spasticity

Etiology

- Autoimmune disease: possible causes may be genetic, viral, immunologic, or environmental; strong association with HLA-DR2 antigen

Prevalence and Demographics

- Prevalence is 100–150 per 100,000 in the United States
- Prevalence is higher in temperate zones, ranging from only 5–15 per 100,000 in tropical zones to 50–300 per 100,000 in cooler environments.
- Women-to-men ratio: 2–3:1, the reason for this is unknown
- Age at onset 15 to 45 years; greatest incidence in young adults younger than 55 years
- Late onset of MS in the sixth to seventh decades usually severe and rapidly progressive

Risk Factors

- Familial 3%–23% increased risk in first-degree relatives
- Climate or place of residence, established by residence in the first 15 years of life
- Urban dwelling, upper socioeconomic status; Western European descent
- Genetically low serum 25-hydroxyvitamin D
- History of Epstein-Barr virus (EBV)
- Environmental factors such as tobacco smoking, obesity in childhood or adolescence

Assessment

History

- Neurological history: paresthesia, weakness and spasticity, ataxia, fatigue, heat intolerance, visual changes, diplopia on lateral gaze, vestibular disturbances, trigeminal neuralgia, facial myokymia, optic neuritis, bowel and bladder dysfunction
- Time frame with exacerbations and remission
- Past medical history for differential diagnosis: SLE, Lyme disease, cerebral and spinal tumors, HIV, EBV, varicella, seizures, peripheral neuropathy, head, or spinal trauma
- Triggers may be infection, trauma, pregnancy.
- Use McDonald diagnostic criteria.

Physical Exam

- Complete neurological exam
  - Cranial nerve deficits
  - Optic neuritis: decreased visual acuity, abnormal pupillary response, hyperemia, and edema of optic disc
  - Internuclear ophthalmoplegia: cranial nerve VI palsy or weakness of the medial rectus muscle with lateral gaze, nystagmus
  - Decreased strength, increased tone, clonus, positive Babinski; weakness, numbness, tingling or unsteadiness in a limb; disequilibrium; urinary urgency, hesitancy, incontinence
  - Decreased proprioception and vibratory sensation, positive Romberg; pyramidal, sensory, or cerebellar deficits in some or all limbs
  - Lhermitte's sign: electrical sensation down the back into the legs is produced with neck flexion

Diagnostic Studies

- Brain MRI with and without contrast (gadolinium-diethylenetriamine penta-acetic acid [DTPA]) for all patients suspected of having MS; may show characteristic multiple lesions of demyelinated areas with reactive gliosis; in addition, a spinal cord MRI may be beneficial and improve diagnostic sensitivity
- Cerebrospinal fluid (CSF) analysis for lymphocytosis, immunoglobulins, and oligoclonal immune globulin G (IgG) bands
- Autoantibody testing is appropriate for patients presenting with acute CNS demyelination when clinical, imaging, or lab features are atypical of MS; aquaporin-4 (AQP4) IgG serum autoantibody and myelin oligodendrocyte glycoprotein IgG autoantibody (MOG-IgG) testing
- Visual, auditory, and sensory evoked potentials

Differential Diagnosis

- Optic neuritis
- Myelopathy
- Tumefactive demyelination
- Stroke
- Cerebral or spinal tumors
- SLE
- Lyme disease
- Peripheral neuropathy
- AIDS
- Amyotrophic lateral sclerosis

Management

- Aimed at delaying progress, managing chronic symptoms, treating acute exacerbations

Nonpharmacologic Treatment

- Physical and occupational therapy
- Mental health services for assistance with coping strategies

Pharmacologic Treatment

- Complex, treatment regimen *must* be coordinated with a neurologist.
- Early, continuous treatment is vital
- First attack or acute exacerbations; glucocorticoid treatment is used to reduce the severity of the exacerbation and to decrease the duration of the attack
    - IV methylprednisolone 1,000 mg daily for 5 days without taper, or for patients who prefer oral therapy, methylprednisolone 1,000 mg a day without taper; oral therapy requires many tablets to be taken daily, that is, up to 31 tablets of daily methylprednisolone 32 mg tablets to reach dosing of approximately 1000 mg; patient education needed.
- All patients with a diagnosis of clinically definite relapsing-remitting multiple sclerosis (RRMS) should begin disease-modifying therapy (DMT).
    - Monoclonal antibodies for RRMS such as natalizumab or rituximab are used for patients with more active disease and who are risk tolerant.
    - Oral therapies include fumarates (dimethyl fumarate) or sphingosine 1-phosphate (S1P) receptor modulators (fingolimod) used for patients with RRMS who value self-administered medication.
    - Platform injection therapies for MS include recombinant human interferon beta-1b, recombinant human interferon beta-1a (Avonex) (30 µg weekly IM), or glatiramer acetate (Copaxone) (40 mg three times per week subcutaneeous); for patients who value safety and are less concerned with convenience or achieving the highest treatment effectiveness
- Spasticity: baclofen 20–80 mg a day orally in divided doses; start with 5 mg three times a day, titrate up every 3 days
    - Clonazepam (Klonopin) can be used for patients with predominant phasic spasticity symptoms at bedtime
- Fatigue
    - Amantadine 100 mg twice a day
    - Consider selective SSRIs such as fluoxetine (Prozac) 20–80 mg daily (titrate up slowly) or sertraline (Zoloft) 50–200 mg daily (titrate up slowly).
    - Treat underlying spastic bladder, depression.

How Long to Treat

- Multiple sclerosis is not curable, and lifetime treatment to control the disease is required.
- Antibodies to interferon may develop.
- Stop interferon if progression of disabilities continues after 6 months of treatment.

Special Considerations

- New onset or exacerbations with menstrual cycle and post-partum
- Family planning and fertility should be discussed with women of childbearing age—menses may be irregular and fertility impaired because of demyelination; pregnancy while engaged in DMT may result in adverse effects for the fetus
- Consult with obstetrician regarding medications for pregnancy and lactation.
- All MS patients are encouraged to get COVID-19 vaccination

When to Consult, Refer, Hospitalize

- Refer all patients with suspected MS to neurologist for confirmation of diagnosis and development of management plan.
- Ophthalmology referral
- Continence specialist or urologist for bladder dysfunction
- Mental health referral for coping or depression for patient and all caregivers

Follow-Up

- Followed closely by neurology, primary care for routine health visits
- Periodic MRI studies to monitor for new MS lesions

Expected Course

- Progressive with exacerbations and remissions

Complications

- Hydronephrosis and renal failure secondary to urinary retention
- Falls
- Depression

VERTIGO

Description

- Sensation of motion of the body or environment when there is no movement (illusionary movement)
- Not a disorder, but a symptom of an underlying condition

Etiology

- Peripheral vestibular dysfunction
  - Benign positional vertigo: believed to be caused by free-floating calcium debris in the semicircular canal
  - Occurs with change in position with delay between movement and symptoms; symptoms may lessen or disappear with repeated movement
  - Labyrinthitis: infection of the inner ear, most likely viral, often follows an upper respiratory infection
  - Ménière's disease: classic pathogenic lesion is endolymphatic hydrops of the labyrinthine system of the inner ear; may be caused by syphilis or head trauma, or viral
- Traumatic vertigo is due to labyrinth concussion or basilar skull fracture.
- Central vestibular dysfunction is due to vertebrobasilar insufficiency, acoustic neuroma, or compression of the eighth cranial nerve by blood vessel loops, like trigeminal neuralgia.

Incidence and Demographics

- Benign positional vertigo most common in persons 60 years of age or older
- Labyrinthitis: affects any age, usually after upper respiratory infection
- Ménière's occurs at 40 to 60 years
- Central lesions less common

Risk Factors

- Age: increasing incidence with increasing age
- Upper respiratory infection
- Trauma

Assessment

History

- Detailed description of sensation without using terms "dizzy" or "vertigo"; include time frame, duration, association with movement, alleviating and precipitating factors
- Vertigo is associated with a sensation of movement.
- Dizziness or lightheadedness associated with presyncope because of cardiac origin
- Imbalance or gait instability associated with cerebellar disease or peripheral neuropathy
- Associated symptoms of hearing loss, tinnitus, nausea, and vomiting with Ménière's disease
- History of upper respiratory infection or trauma
- Time frame
  - Positional vertigo and vertebrobasilar insufficiency occur in seconds
  - Ménière's, vestibular migraine over hours
  - Labyrinthitis, traumatic vertigo, and vestibular neuritis over days
  - Acoustic neuroma, MS, cerebellar disease over months, progressive

Physical Exam

- Screening neurological exam with attention to cranial nerves
- Sustained nystagmus is indicative of vertigo but may be central or peripheral.
- Facial palsy may or may not be present with acoustic neuroma.
- Assess gait, posture, and balance.
- Dix-Hallpike maneuver: Lay patient flat with head to one side and hanging over edge of table, sit patient up quickly with head held to side, repeat with other ear down; reproduction of symptoms and nystagmus is positive for positional vertigo. Nystagmus that is purely vertical and not fatigable with subsequent trials may be due to central vestibular dysfunction.
- Otologic exam

Diagnostic Studies

- MRI if central lesion suspected
- Audiogram to evaluate sustained hearing loss, which may occur with Ménière's disease
- Depending on clinical findings and suspected underlying etiology, may consider CBC, CMP, lipid panel, thyroid function studies, ESR, rapid plasma regain (RPR)

Differential Diagnosis

- Benign positional vertigo
- Labyrinthitis
- Ménière's disease
- Cerumen impaction
- Otitis media or externa
- Sinusitis
- Vertebrobasilar insufficiency
- Vestibular migraine
- Acoustic neuroma
- Presyncope with probable cardiac etiology
- MS
- Cerebellar disease
- Peripheral neuropathy
- Herpes zoster oticus
- Aminoglycoside toxicity

Management

Nonpharmacologic Treatment

- Remove cerumen if present.
- Rest in quiet, darkened room.
- Safety precautions to change positions slowly; may need walker for support

- Bland diet with small portions; fluids if nausea and vomiting present
- Ménière's disease: low-sodium diet
- Benign positional vertigo: vestibular rehabilitation to reduce symptoms

Pharmacologic Treatment

- Meclizine (Antivert) 25–100 mg in divided doses may reduce vertigo.
- Hydrochlorothiazide/triamterene 25 mg/37.5 mg orally every. day for Ménière's
- Antibiotics may be helpful in labyrinthitis if bacterial infection suspected.

How Long to Treat

- Taper and stop meclizine when symptoms resolve, generally within 1 to 2 weeks; do not use prophylactically or as maintenance.

Special Considerations

- Older adults are more sensitive to antihistamines; use only if necessary for severe debilitating symptoms; may cause drowsiness, confusion, anticholinergic symptoms.

When to Consult, Refer, Hospitalize

- Hospitalize for dehydration and inability to take oral rehydration secondary to severe nausea and vomiting.
- Neurosurgical referral for acoustic neuroma or other space-occupying lesions
- Neurology referral if focal neurological deficits, severe headaches, seizures, or other suggestions of CNS problem, or symptoms do not resolve with treatment

Follow-Up

- As needed for recurrence or worsening symptoms

Expected Course

- Benign positional vertigo episodes may last several days; may reoccur.
- Labyrinthitis resolves in several days.
- Ménière's disease may have multiple episodes with remissions.

Complications

- Hearing loss with Ménière's disease
- Falls
- Dehydration with associated nausea and vomiting

MENINGITIS

Description

- Central nervous system infection of the covering of the brain and spinal cord by any infectious agent, including bacteria, virus, mycobacteria, spirochetes, fungi, protozoa, and parasites

Etiology

- Caused by virulent infectious organism in a susceptible host; local host defenses overcome
- Bacteria-causing meningitis varies by the age of the patient:
  - Newborns: group B *Streptococcus, Streptococcus pneumoniae, Escherichia coli, Listeria monocytogenes*
  - Babies and young children: *Haemophilus influenzae, S. pneumoniae,* group B *Streptococcus, Mycobacterium tuberculosis, Neisseria meningitidis*
  - Teens and young adults: *S. pneumoniae, N. meningitidis*
  - Older adults: *H. influenzae, S. pneumoniae,* group B *Streptococcus, L. monocytogenes, N. meningitidis*
  - Viral meningitis can be caused by any of more than 70 different strains of viruses; most common are the non-polio enteroviruses (85%). Less serious, uncomplicated cases resolve in 7–10 days.
- Most common fungal cause *Candida* sp., *Cryptococcus neoformans*

- Candidal meningitis occurs mostly in ill premature infants and immunocompromised patients
- Aseptic meningitis can be caused by *Borrelia burgdorferi* (Lyme disease) or *Treponema pallidum* (syphilis).
- Meningitis can also be caused by tuberculosis.
- *H. influenzae, N. meningitides,* and *S. pneumoniae* cause 80% of bacterial meningitis in adults and older adults.
- Gram-negative bacilli, *Acinetobacter baumannii, Klebsiella pneumoniae,* important cause in nosocomial meningitis

Incidence and Demographics

- In children, 70% of bacterial meningitis occurs before 5 years of age.
- Incidence approximately 1.1 per 100,000 people a year
- More prevalent in lower socioeconomic groups, crowded housing, urban areas
- More prevalent in college students residing on campus than those living off campus and the general population

Risk Factors

- Poverty and lack of childhood immunizations
- Crowded living conditions
- Immunodeficiency
- College students living in campus housing and soldiers in barracks
- Infectious disease close to meninges: pneumonia, pharyngitis, otitis media, sinusitis, endocarditis
- Penetrating head trauma
- Syphilis infection
- Lyme disease
- Unvaccinated individuals in high-risk categories

Prevention and Screening

- Routine administration of the *H. influenzae* type b (Hib) vaccine has significantly reduced the incidence of meningitis.
- Administration of the pneumococcal conjugate vaccine 13 (PCV13) (Prevnar 13) or PCV20 (Prevnar 20) vaccine; other vaccines to consider based on age and risk factors PCV15 (Vaxneuvance) or PPSV23 (Pneumovax23)
- Adolescents planning to attend college and reside in dormitories should receive meningococcal vaccine.
- Postexposure prophylaxis for bacterial meningitis with oral rifampin (Rifadin) for household and day care contacts, and those with direct exposure to oral secretions (kissing) of infected patient
  - *H. influenzae:* rifampin 20 mg/kg/dose orally once a day for 4 days (max dose 600 mg)
  - *N. meningitidis:* ceftriaxone 50 mg/kg/dose twice a day for 4 days (max dose 2 g)
- The American Academy of Pediatrics recommends prophylaxis to day care or nursery school contacts if two or more index cases occur in a unit within 60 days of each other.

Assessment

History

- Rapid onset within 24 to 36 hours
- Progressive, severe headache accompanied by neck and back pain with flexion
- Neurological symptoms: drowsiness, irritability, confusion, photophobia, hearing loss, focal neurologic deficits, seizures, nuchal rigidity, photophobia
- Associated symptoms: fever, nausea, vomiting, rash
- In infants, complaints of sleep disturbances, irritability, or vomiting
- Recent history of respiratory infection, head trauma, invasive neurosurgical procedures, or dental procedures
- Past medical history: meningitis, polio, immunodeficiency
- Social history: living in crowded environment, IV drug use, foreign travel
- Environmental exposure to bird or pigeon droppings (fungal) or tick bite (Lyme)
- Medications: immunosuppressants

Physical Exam

- General: fever, tachycardia, hypotension, rash
- Assess fontanels in infants for bulging, hydration status.
- Complete neurological exam: decreased level of consciousness (drowsiness or agitation); papilledema; cranial nerve III, IV, VI, VII, and/or VIII deficits; focal motor deficits; seizure; mental status
- Meningeal irritation: nuchal rigidity, positive Brudzinski's sign (adduction and flexion of legs with neck flexion), positive Kernig's sign (after flexing thighs, extension met with resistance and pain in hamstring muscles)
- Complete physical exam for sites of primary infections:
    - Head trauma or surgery, dental abscess or caries, otitis media, sinusitis, pneumonia, pancreatitis, genital lesions, skin rashes

Diagnostic Studies

- CSF analysis, culture (diagnosis usually made on Gram stain): gold standard
    - Viral infection: some lymphocytes, normal glucose, moderately high protein content, normal or mildly elevated opening pressure on lumbar puncture.
    - Bacterial infection: increased lymphocytes, decreased glucose, high protein content, markedly elevated opening pressure
- Brain CT before lumbar puncture if space-occupying lesion (brain abscess, subdural empyema, tumor, subdural hematoma) suspected with papilledema and/or focal neurological findings; lumbar puncture contraindicated with increased ICP
- Lumbar puncture (unless contraindicated) for CSF examination to diagnose, identify causative agent, and to perform in vitro susceptibility testing
- CBC with differential, platelet count, prothrombin time/partial thromboplastin time (PT/PTT), electrolyte panel, CMP (creatinine, blood urea nitrogen [BUN], glucose), ABGs (as indicated), two aerobic blood cultures ideally taken prior to start of antimicrobial therapy
- Chest and/or sinus X-ray if exam indicates source of infection

Differential Diagnosis

- Bacterial meningitis
- Aseptic meningitis

- Encephalitis (herpes, rabies)
- Brain abscess
- Noninfectious meningeal irritation (sarcoidosis, systemic lupus erythematosus, cancer, medications, and chemical irritants)
- Bacterial sinusitis or mastoiditis
- Vertebral osteomyelitis
- Amebic meningoencephalitis

Management

Nonpharmacologic Treatment

- Medical emergency; immediate transport to hospital for IV antibiotics and supportive care
- Ensure adequate airway, cardiac function, fluid support
- Educate family and significant others regarding illness, treatment, and prognosis.
- Inform family and contacts of postexposure prophylaxis.

Pharmacologic Treatment

- IV antimicrobials in acute-care setting for those with no known immune deficiency; usually ceftriaxone, cefotaxime, vancomycin, or ampicillin (some antimicrobials combined based on causative organism)
- Ceftriaxone 2 g IV twice a day or cefotaxime 2 g IV every. 4–6 hours, in addition to both of the following medications:
  - Vancomycin 15–20 mg/kg IV every 8–12 hours (max dose of 2 g per dose or a total dose of 60 mg/kg/day); dose must be adjusted to attain vancomycin serum trough levels of 15–20 µg /mL
  - Ampicillin 2 g IV every 4 hours for adults 50 years of age or older
- Acyclovir has been used in the neonate with viral meningitis.
- Administration of dexamethasone (Decadron) before or with antibiotics appears to reduce the incidence of sensorineural hearing loss without increasing mortality or complications.

How Long to Treat

- *N. meningitidis*: 7 days
- *H. influenzae*: 7 days
- *S. pneumoniae*: 10–14 days
- Gram-negative bacteria: 21 days

Special Considerations

- Rifampin is contraindicated for postexposure prophylaxis in pregnant patients; may cause birth defects and is secreted in breast milk.
- The incidence of meningitis in Black persons in the United States is higher than Whites; education programs should be targeted within minority communities to ensure that signs and symptoms are recognized early to promote the highest patient health outcomes.

When to Consult, Refer, Hospitalize

- Medical emergency: Immediately transfer all suspected meningitis cases to an acute care facility.
- Most patients with viral meningitis can be managed at home, if stable, after physician consultation.

Follow-Up

- Patients should be seen a few days after hospital discharge.
- Parents and patients should be instructed to follow-up if any new neurological sequelae present, including hearing and vision problems.

Expected Course

- Up to 85% survival with early diagnosis, treatment, and supportive care

Complications

- Mortality rate is over 50% in patients who are not diagnosed early and referred; 10% for those who receive prompt diagnosis, appropriate IV antibiotics, and supportive care. Mortality rate of bacterial meningitis in neonates is 10%–20%; in infants/children it is 3%–10%.
- Complications of meningitis include seizures (2%–8%), hearing defects (10%), intellectual disability (10%), visual abnormalities (3%–7%), language delay (15%), motor abnormalities (3%–7%), syndrome of inappropriate antidiuretic hormone secretion (SIADH), and sixth cranial nerve palsy. Occurrence of sequelae is estimated at 25%–50% of meningitis survivors.

SEIZURES AND EPILEPSY

General Information

- A seizure is a transient, sudden, paroxysmal electrical hypersynchronization of neuronal networks in the cerebral cortex that causes an alteration in neurological function.
- May involve abnormal motor activity, sensory symptoms, change in the level of alertness, an alteration in autonomic function, or a combination of these
- A seizure is not a diagnosis but rather a clinical symptom of an underlying neurological dysfunction.
- Seizures are classified by etiology: genetic, symptomatic (most common), and idiopathic.
- Neonatal seizures are rarely idiopathic, and immediate attention must be paid to identifying the underlying disorder.
- Febrile seizures occur in infants and children because of fever, not underlying neurological disorder.
- Epilepsy, or recurrent, spontaneous seizures unrelated to fever, may occur in children and adults:
    - Benign Rolandic epilepsy, associated with characteristic centro-temporal spike EEG pattern, is the most common type in children (15%).
    - Infantile spasms are myoclonic seizures occurring in the first year of life, usually in clusters, associated with an EEG pattern called hypsarrhythmia which is a high-voltage spike and wave pattern.

NEONATAL SEIZURES

Description

- Seizures in a newborn almost always reflect a significant CNS pathology.
- Seizures in this age group may present in several ways:
  - Focal clonic: rhythmic twitching of muscle groups, including the face, limbs, and trunk
  - Focal tonic: less frequent, sustained, but transient, asymmetrical, rigid posturing of the extremities or trunk, or tonic deviation of the eyes
  - Myoclonic: focal or generalized jerking of the extremities, generally involve the distal parts of the body; rate of repetition may be slow, irregular, or erratic
  - Autonomic signs: alterations in heart rate, respiration, and blood pressure, excessive salivation, or pupil dilatation
  - Electrographic-only seizures: Most neonatal seizures are characterized by the presence of an electrographic seizure on EEG with no physical clinical features.

Etiology

- Time of onset and characteristics of seizure may suggest most probable cause.
- Rarely idiopathic; typical causes of neonatal seizures include trauma from birth or from congenital malformations, including hypoxia, intracranial hemorrhage, infection, drug withdrawal, metabolic disorders, inborn errors of metabolism, neurocutaneous disorders, pyridoxine dependency, and cerebral dysgenesis
- Focal seizures may be caused by metabolic disturbances and do not necessarily imply a focal lesion.

Incidence and Demographics

- Seizures occur in an estimated 8%–10% of the population over the course of the lifetime.
- Seizures account for 1%–2% of emergency room visits per year in the United States.

Risk Factors

- Complicated labor or delivery, prematurity
- Infants of diabetic mothers
- Family history of metabolic disorder associated with seizures, maternal drug use

Prevention and Screening

- Neonatal seizures are not preventable, but the incidence of prematurity and birth trauma may be decreased with good prenatal care and maternal education.
- Hispanic and Black mothers have a disproportionally lower percentage of adequate prenatal care in the United States when compared with White mothers; early education and linkage to ongoing prenatal care in these minority populations is essential.

Assessment

History

- Prenatal and perinatal history including maternal risk factors and complications of pregnancy, labor, and delivery
- Family history of seizure disorders or metabolic disease, congenital syndromes
- Exact description of the event, movements, or reactions that has triggered the concern

Physical Exam

- Complete physical, focusing on dysmorphic features, atypical, or rhythmic movements
- Assess growth, vital signs
- Neurological exam, presence/absence of newborn reflexes, head size/shape
- Eye exam to look for chorioretinitis (inflammation that destroys superficial tissue areas visible on funduscopic exam and causes a well-defined but irregular area of white sclera that has smaller areas of dark pigment) or coloboma (developmental abnormality in which a moderate-to-large sized area of sclera with well-demarcated borders is seen below the disc)
- Any unusual skin pigmentation or body odors for metabolic disorder
- Presence of hepatosplenomegaly, signs of drug withdrawal

Diagnostic Studies

- Laboratory testing to include CBC, CMP (calcium, BUN), electrolytes, magnesium, pH, sodium bicarbonate, bilirubin, and ammonia
- Urinalysis and urine toxicology screen

- LP, if presence or suspicion of meningitis or encephalitis, or intracranial hemorrhage
- Neuroimaging to rule out brain injury or mass
- Chromosomal analysis if presence of dysmorphic features
- Metabolic screen, including amino acids, lactate, and urine organic acids
- Toxoplasmosis, rubella, cytomegalovirus, herpes simplex, HIV (TORCH) screen
- Drug screen
- EEG: Changes may not always be present.

Differential Diagnosis

- Jitteriness
- Gastroesophageal reflux disease (GERD)
- Apnea
- Idiopathic neonatal convulsions: "fifth-day fits" (potential causes hypoxemia, birth trauma, hypoglycemia, or hypocalcemia)
- Benign familial neonatal convulsions: tonic-clonic seizures begin around day 3 of life and resolve within 1–4 months; episodes typically begin with tonic stiffness and apnea followed by clonic jerking

Management

- Treatment is guided by correcting the underlying abnormality.

Nonpharmacologic Treatment

- Ensure adequate ventilation and perfusion.

Pharmacologic Treatment

- For metabolic disorders, consider calcium gluconate, magnesium sulfate, and/or pyridoxine (vitamin B6).
- Antibiotics if infection is present
- Seizure management includes the use of phenobarbital, fosphenytoin (Sesquient), or midazolam (Versed).

How Long to Treat

- Duration of therapy is based on the underlying etiology.

When to Consult, Refer, Hospitalize

- Any newborn with suspected seizures should receive prompt evaluation and admission for workup.
- An infant with a history of neonatal seizures should be followed in conjunction with a physician and a neurologist.

Follow-Up

- Infants should be followed by a neurologist at regular intervals until seizure-free and off medications; follow-up may be extended if neurological sequelae ensue.
- Infants need routine health assessments to monitor growth and development and should receive routine immunizations.
- Infants with cognitive or motor deficits should be referred to early intervention programs.

Expected Course

- Highly individual; child may develop normally following seizure period

Complications

- Mortality rate is approximately 23% but is higher (27%–34%) in preterm infants.
- Intellectual disability and motor deficits are more common sequelae.
- Prognosis is dependent upon the underlying etiology, with cerebral dysgenesis having the worst outcomes.
- The likelihood of recurrent neonatal seizures is 15% after the newborn period.

FEBRILE SEIZURES

Description

- A seizure event in infancy or early childhood, associated with fever, but without evidence of intracranial infection or defined cause
- Most common neurological disorder of infants and young children
- Febrile seizures classified as:
  - Simple: isolated, brief, generalized seizure lasting less than 15 minutes and does not recur in a 24-hour period
  - Complex: prolonged (longer than 15 minutes), multiple seizures within a 24-hour period, focal in nature

Etiology

- Febrile seizures are caused or brought on by a fever in infancy or childhood (6 months to 5 years of age).
- The most common causes are normal childhood illnesses, such as tonsillitis, upper respiratory infections, and otitis media.
- Genetic predisposition occurred in approximately 10% of parents; there is a 20% chance of occurrence in a sibling.

Incidence and Demographics

- Occur in approximately 2%–4% of all children; more common in men and boys than women and girls (1.6:1)
- Peak incidence between 12 and 18 months of age, but can occur at any time from 6 months to 5 years of age
- Usually occurs within the first 24 hours of fever
- Approximately 30% of children will experience one or more recurrences.
- Risk of recurrence is related to the age of the child, family history, and complexity of first seizure.

Risk Factors

- Very high fever (temperature over 38.8° C [101.8°F]); 25% of events occur between 38°C and 39°C (100.4°F and 102.2° F)
- Family history of febrile seizures
- Neonatal discharge from hospital 28 days or later
- Underlying neurological deficits such as cerebral palsy or neurodevelopmental delay
- Day care attendance (increased rate of febrile illness)
- Low serum sodium, zinc, or iron
- Maternal smoking and stress during pregnancy

Prevention and Screening

- Subsequent febrile seizures may be prevented by early and adequate fever control.

Assessment

History

- Family history of febrile seizures
- Complete description of the seizure(s), duration, recovery, motor involvement, etc.
- Any history of recent illness or exposure to illness, onset of headaches, vomiting, or unusual symptoms
- Recent trauma, medication exposure
- Prenatal/perinatal history, including developmental history
- Exposure to toxins such as lead
- Metabolic disorders

Physical Exam

- Document presence of fever.
- Attention to abnormal vital signs
- Complete physical exam: Identify underlying illness or infection requiring treatment.

- Complete neurological exam, including level of consciousness, presence or absence of meningismus, or a tense bulging fontanel; head circumference; focal differences in muscle tone; spontaneous movements
- Signs of physical abuse
- Neurocutaneous skin lesions
- Postictal drowsiness should resolve in 5–10 minutes; longer resolution times should prompt for CNS infection or severe systemic infection workup.

Diagnostic Studies

- Lumbar puncture: if suspicion of meningitis or for children younger than 18 months with first seizure
- Routine lab studies *not* indicated unless no source of fever can be elicited on physical examination.
- EEG not warranted.
- MRI limited to children with focal seizures, signs/symptoms of IICP, or infants with abnormally large heads.
- Serum lead level, if indicated

Differential Diagnosis

- Shaking chills
- Meningitis or encephalitis (CNS infections)
- Genetic epilepsies with febrile seizures
- Anoxia
- Trauma
- Stroke or hemorrhage
- Metabolic encephalopathy
- Neurodegenerative disorder
- Brain tumor
- Lead poisoning or other toxins

Management

Nonpharmacologic Treatment

- Because febrile seizures are very frightening to the parents, parental reassurance and education are vitally important.
- An active search for the underlying cause of the fever and appropriate treatment with each incidence

Pharmacologic Treatment

- Vigorous control of fevers by antipyretics and sponging with tepid water
  - Acetaminophen 10–15 mg/kg per dose either orally or per rectum (max neonate dose 60 mg/kg/day; max infant and child dose 75 mg/kg/day)
  - Ibuprofen 5–10 mg/kg per dose orally (max dose 40 mg/kg/day)
- Antiseizure medication therapy drug risk higher than benefits gained for most patients.
  - History of prolonged febrile seizure diazepam (Valium) rectal gel to prevent recurrences only during a febrile illness (0.5 mg/kg) given if episode lasts for more than 5 minutes; one dose will not lead to respiratory depression.
  - Midazolam (Versed) nasal spray can be used as an equally effective alternative to diazepam rectal gel.

How Long to Treat

- During febrile episodes

Special Considerations

- Seizure(s) occurring late in the course of a febrile illness raising serious concern about meningitis or encephalitis
- Relieving parental anxiety should be a focus of management.
- Small risk of developing epilepsy later in life if:
  - Abnormal development before the seizure
  - Family history of afebrile seizures
    - Complex first febrile seizure

When to Consult, Refer, Hospitalize

- Because of parental anxiety, the first febrile seizure may be evaluated at the emergency department.
- Consult with physician; however, no referrals or consultations are necessary in simple febrile seizures.
- Consult or refer to neurologist if seizures become more focal or complex.
- If the seizure is generalized, lasts longer than 20 minutes, or is focal, or the suspected disease process is complex, the child should be hospitalized.
- Continued seizures past age 6 are not compatible with febrile seizures and require a neurology referral.

Follow-Up

- Patients with febrile seizures should receive routine childhood immunizations and health assessments at regular intervals.

Expected Course

- Full return of function following resolution of fever; child will outgrow

Complications

- Permanent cognitive and/or motor damage can occur if febrile seizures are not treated in a timely and effective manner.
- Lacerated tongue, broken teeth, bones, etc., can occur if the child's seizure is not safely contained.

ROLANDIC EPILEPSY OF CHILDHOOD DESCRIPTION

- Benign childhood epilepsy with centrotemporal or Rolandic spikes (BCECTS) is the most common variant of focal epilepsy seen in children. It is a syndrome consisting of unilateral tonic-clonic contractions of the face, paresthesia of the tongue and cheek, and occasional clonic seizures of the ipsilateral upper extremity with no impairment of consciousness.

Etiology

- The etiology is not completely known; one-fourth of patients have familial history; chromosome 15q14 may be involved.
- Seizures are typically focal (e.g., twitching of the mouth); motor activity in the upper but not lower extremities is common; guttural vocalizations, speech arrest, and hyper-salivation are typical.

Incidence and Demographics

- The prevalence of epilepsy in the pediatric population is 6 per 1,000; the male-to-female ratio is 3:2.
- Patients in a recognized low socioeconomic demographic are at higher risk of negative outcomes (more disconnectedness to care, ability to afford medications, office visits (emergency department visits).
- Rolandic epilepsy occurs at 2 to 13 years, with the peak incidence at age 7 to 9 years; the majority resolve or "outgrow" by age 12 to 13 years.
- Most episodes occur during sleep; one-half have at least one secondary generalized seizure

Risk Factors

- History of previous seizures (febrile or afebrile)
- Recent withdrawal of antiseizure medications
- History of remote neurological insult such as head trauma
- Family history of seizures

Assessment

History

- Complete description of the seizures, including duration, aura, signs of infection, motor involvement, timing, or stimulus
- Family history of seizure disorders or previous history in this child
- History of any head trauma or insult

- Any recent use of medications or drugs
- Health history of the patient
- Any recent onset of headaches, weakness, or sensory deficits

Physical Exam

- Physical exam with attention to screening neurological exam (usually normal)
- Parents may need to video record an event for the provider to view.
- Signs of systemic infection; signs of physical abuse
- Skin evaluation for neurocutaneous disorders

Diagnostic Studies

- EEG, either routine or 24-hour recording: characteristic spike focus in the centrotemporal or Rolandic area with normal background activity
- CT/MRI to rule out intracranial abnormality, especially if antiseizure therapy is not effective

Differential Diagnosis

- Night terrors
- Complex partial seizures
- Simple partial seizures
- Tics
- Migraine
- Breath-holding spells
- Panayiotopoulos syndrome

Management

Nonpharmacologic Treatment

- Occasional seizures require no therapy, just careful monitoring.

Pharmacologic Treatment

- Diazepam (Valium) 0.5 mg/kg per rectum (max 20 mg) for prolonged seizures (Panayiotopoulos syndrome)
- Levetiracetam (Keppra) 50–60 mg/kg/day orally divided every 12 hours (dose dependent on age); start 20 mg/kg/day orally divided every 12 hours, increase by 20 mg/kg/day every 2 weeks (max dose 3,000 mg/day); taper dose gradually to discontinue

How Long to Treat

- If seizure-free for at least 2 years with a normal EEG, consider weaning from medication over a period of 4–6 months and supervise closely.
- Higher risk for seizure recurrence in children with developmental delay, age older than 12 years at onset, neonatal seizures, and multiple seizures before control attained

Special Considerations

- In children with poor seizure control despite appropriate medication, consider drug compliance, growth spurts, and possible other epileptic etiologies.
- People with seizures should not swim alone or play sports that are conducive to head injuries (e.g., football, lacrosse).
- Carbamazepine (Tegretol) has been historically prescribed to treat seizure activity; however, levetiracetam (Keppra) is now considered the first choice due to its safety profile, lack of drug interactions, and tolerability.

When to Consult, Refer, Hospitalize

- If epilepsy is suspected, the patient should be referred and managed by a pediatric neurologist.
- Patients with Rolandic epilepsy rarely need hospitalization.

Follow-Up

- At least annual with pediatric neurologist
- Routine health maintenance

Expected Course

- Most completely resolve by adolescence.

Complications

- Essentially none, as response to antiseizure agents is excellent

SEIZURES AND EPILEPSY IN ADULTS/OLDER ADULTS

Description

- A transient alteration in behavior, function, and/or consciousness that results from an abnormal electrical discharge of neurons in the brain
- Epilepsy refers to chronic recurrent seizures greater than 24 hours apart.
- Most older adults have partial seizures that may quickly generalize to tonic-clonic.
- The International League Against Epilepsy has classified seizures based on clinical presentation and EEG findings (see Table 15–7).

Etiology

- A seizure is a symptom of an underlying disorder; the most frequent cause of repetitive seizures is failure to take antiseizure medications.
- Cause is unknown for most epilepsy, including primary epilepsy, but is believed to be related to abnormalities of neurotransmission.
- Patients with primary epilepsy can continue to have seizures into old age.
- Secondary epilepsy is due to injury to the cerebral cortex.
- Most new-onset epilepsy in older adults is secondary to tumors, hematomas, or stroke.
- Space-occupying lesions, stroke, metabolic disorders, and alcohol withdrawal can also cause seizures.
- Vascular disease is the most common cause of onset in patients 60 years of age or older.

TABLE 15–7. SEIZURE CLASSIFICATION

SEIZURE TYPE	DESCRIPTION	MEDICATION
Focal, Aware/Impaired Awareness, Motor Onset	Observations include automatisms, atonic, clonic, epileptic spasms (degree of awareness usually not specified), hyperkinetic, myoclonic, tonic; focal to bilateral tonic-clonic	Phenytoin, carbamazepine, phenobarbital, lamotrigine
Focal, Aware/Impaired Awareness, Non-Motor Onset	Characterized by behavior arrest, awareness of autonomic functions, e.g., feeling of gastrointestinal sensations, piloerection, heart-racing; cognitive disturbances, e.g., changes in thinking; emotional disturbances, e.g., feelings of happiness or sadness, crying, laughing, grunting; sensory disturbances, e.g., feelings coldness or heat	Carbamazepine, phenytoin, phenobarbital, lamotrigine
Generalized Motor Onset	Tonic-clonic, clonic, tonic, myoclonic, myoclonic-tonic- clonic, myoclonic-atonic, atonic, epileptic spasms	Valproate, lamotrigine topiramate, clobazam
Generalized Non-Motor Onset	Types include, typical, atypical, myoclonic, and eyelid myoclonia	Valproate, lamotrigine topiramate, clobazam
Unknown Onset Motor	Seizure activity normally includes tonic-clonic and epileptic spasms	If first seizure, and less than 2 minutes in length, identify and treat underlying cause (usually identified in emergency department)
Unknown Onset Non-motor	Activity normally seen clinically includes behavior arrest	If first seizure, and less than 2 minutes in length, identify and treat underlying cause (usually identified in emergency department)
Unclassified	Due to inadequate clinical information or inability to place in other categories	See above

Incidence and Demographics

- 8%–10% of Americans will have a seizure at some time during their lives; 1.2% have epilepsy.
- Adult new-onset epilepsy is highest in persons 65 years of age or older.

Risk Factors

- Intracranial lesions, head trauma, hypo/hyperglycemia, hyponatremia, hypocalcemia, hypomagnesemia, chronic illness that predisposes metabolic abnormality; medications that lower seizure threshold (e.g., SSRIs [sertraline (Zoloft)], certain atypical antidepressants, ciprofloxacin, penicillin, metronidazole, theophylline)
- Certain triggers: sleep deprivation, menses, flashing lights, emotional stress, fever, hormonal imbalance, loud music
- Drug or alcohol intoxication or drug or alcohol withdrawal

Prevention and Screening

- Head trauma prevention: seat belt use, bicycle and motorcycle helmets
- Fall prevention for older adults, home safety counseling

Assessment

History

- Interview witness to seizure if possible. This information is most important in making diagnosis.
- Detailed history of event; include description of seizure activity, loss of consciousness, duration, incontinence, possible triggers
- Prodromal symptoms such as aura, confusion, or focal neurological symptoms
- Postictal state: antegrade amnesia, level of consciousness
- Prior seizure history, including type, frequency, duration
- Seizure medication adherence assessment: any changes, missed doses, levels
- Past medical history: previous intracranial lesions or trauma, diabetes, HIV, stroke, migraines, dementia, psychiatric illness

- Medications: ciprofloxacin (Cipro), metronidazole, theophylline, stimulants, antipsychotics can lower seizure threshold
- Diuretic, antihypertensives, diabetes medicines can cause metabolic disturbances that can cause seizure.
- Family history of seizure.

Physical Exam

- Assess for head trauma.
- Screening neurological exam may be normal, even with structural lesions.
- Focal deficits may be worse immediately after seizure.
- Evaluate cardiovascular and pulmonary status.
- Blood pressure and pulse will be elevated during and immediately after a seizure.

Diagnostic Studies

- First-time seizure: metabolic panel, toxicology if appropriate
- Brain MRI scan even with a metabolic etiology because the metabolic abnormality could lower the seizure threshold in the presence of a structural lesion
- EEG for first-time patient who has seizure with identified etiology; need not be repeated
- EEG for first-time seizure without etiology, may determine seizure type and guide treatment and prognosis; if seizures continue and EEG nondiagnostic, may consider closed-circuit video EEG
- Lumbar puncture if new neurological findings are not explained by imaging, or if fever or continued unexplained headache present

Differential Diagnosis

Causes of Seizure

- Head trauma
- Brain tumor
- Stroke
- Metabolic disorders

- Drug or alcohol withdrawal
- Withdrawal from certain medications can also cause seizure
- COVID-19 virus infection

Disorders That May Appear to be Seizures

- Syncope
- Transient ischemic attack
- Pseudo-seizures
- Panic attack, anxiety, or psychosis
- Drug intoxication
- Migraine
- Multiple sclerosis
- Postural hypotension
- Neurodegenerative dementia, including Alzheimer's disease
- Narcolepsy with cataplexy
- Paroxysmal movement disorders

Management

Nonpharmacologic Treatment

- Educate patient and family about seizure disorder and cause.
- Educate patient and family about safety management, including using any aura period to prepare for a seizure.
- Stress the importance of always keeping an extra supply of medication readily available.
- First episodes of seizures without known cause do not have to be treated with antiseizure medications.
- Educate family about acute seizure management such as protecting patient from injury by placing on left side to maintain airway if possible.
- Patients with known recurrent seizures do not need to go to the emergency department for every seizure—only if seizure lasts more than 2 minutes or breathing is impaired (aspiration).

- Advise regarding state driving regulations.
- Advise regarding swimming alone or operating dangerous equipment.
- Teach about side effects and toxic effects of medications, and not to discontinue seizure medicines abruptly, which may precipitate seizure.
- Discuss seizure triggers: sleep deprivation, alcohol, menses, stress, low-grade fever, and infection.
- Wear Medic Alert bracelet.
- Vagus nerve stimulation (VNS) is an effective adjunctive therapy for those with drug-resistant seizures or refractory seizures

Pharmacologic Treatment

- Antiseizure medication should be initiated in patients with recurrent seizures in which the cause is unknown or irreversible.
- Antiseizure medications first initiated by a neurologist: phenytoin (Dilantin), phenobarbital, carbamazepine (Tegretol), and valproic acid (Depakene), lamotrigine (Lamictal) are first-line choices (see Table 15–7)
- 40%–50% of patients can be maintained seizure-free on a single agent.
- Phenytoin initially 1,000 mg divided into doses in one day, maintenance dose 300–400 mg/day divided into two or three doses per day.
- Phenobarbital 1 mg to 5 mg/kg orally per day divided into two or three doses.
- Carbamazepine initially 100–200 mg daily divided two to three times per day, slowly increase dose every 5 days to 800 mg to 1,200 mg daily divided into three doses (dosing recommended for immediate-release formulation); if side effects become apparent, divide daily dose into four doses or consider extended-release formulation.
- Valproic acid initially 10–15 mg/kg/day in three divided doses, increase slowly at 1-week intervals by 5–10 mg/kg/day until seizures are controlled or side effects prevent further increase in dose, maximum dose 60 mg/kg/day. Before initiating, baseline liver enzyme levels (specifically alanine transaminase [ALT] and aspartate transaminase [AST]) must be drawn and then monitored thereafter, approximately every 3 to 6 months, to determine safe serum levels.
- Lamotrigine (Lamictal) as monotherapy, initially 25 mg orally daily, increasing to 50 mg per day after two weeks; then titrating up by 50 mg per day every 1 to 2 weeks to a maintenance dose of 225–375 mg daily, divided in two doses for immediate release lamotrigine, or 300–400 mg per day for extended-release formulation.

How Long to Treat

- Consider discontinuing seizure medications in those without seizures for more than 2 years.
- Obtain an EEG before stopping medication.
- 40% will have a reoccurrence, most within the first year.
- Must consider risk factors of seizure reoccurrence and medications for each patient; consult with neurologist

Special Considerations

- With first-time seizures in patients 50 years of age and older, must consider an underlying intracranial lesion or metabolic etiology
- Antiseizure medications are metabolized in the liver and involve the cytochrome P450 (CYP) enzyme system; care must be used when administering these medications with any other medications.
- Patients must be counseled about the signs and symptoms of liver disease, including nausea and vomiting, that seem protracted, abdominal pain, anorexia, fatigue, and dark urine/stools.
- Lower, less-frequent doses may be needed for patients with hepatic and renal dysfunction.
- All antiseizure medications have been associated with increased birth defects.
- Babies of epileptic mothers have two to three times the normal risk of birth defects.
- Must counsel all women of childbearing age regarding risks of medications during pregnancy.
- Seizures may increase, decrease, or remain the same during pregnancy.
- A neurologist should be consulted before pregnancy for medical management.
- Antiseizure medications, except valproic acid, alter the effectiveness of birth control pills.
- Some antiseizure medications are excreted in breast milk and may have serious adverse effects for the nursing infant.
- There is no evidence that prophylactic antiseizure therapy prevents epilepsy following head trauma or brain surgery; therefore, it is not necessary to maintain these patients on long-term antiseizure medications.
- Educate patients about specifics of state laws limiting driving for seizure patients.
- Antiseizure medications may interfere with certain anticoagulation therapies.

- Patients should track their seizure activity on a calendar
- Most antiseizure medications require serum levels to be checked regularly to ensure therapeutic levels.

When to Consult, Refer, Hospitalize

- Referral to neurologist for first-time seizures, when considering discontinuing therapy, seizures refractory to adequate trials of monotherapy, pregnancy
- Neurosurgeon for stereotaxic procedures for intractable seizures
- Status epilepticus is a medical emergency defined as two or more seizures without complete recovery or a seizure lasting more than 30 minutes; the primary care provider witnessing a seizure lasting more than 2 minutes must activate 911 and be prepared to initiate emergency procedures. IV access and administration of IV benzodiazepines (Lorazepam) should be initiated as protocols permit.

Follow-Up

- Most patients should be seen every 3 months by their primary care provider and at least annually by their neurologist; more-frequent visits are needed if medications or seizures change.
- Antiseizure medications have small therapeutic ranges; levels should be drawn when adjusting therapy and with change in seizure frequency.
- Liver enzymes must be monitored for most antiseizure medications.

Expected Course

- Variable, one seizure to intractable seizures

Complications

- Status epilepticus, airway obstruction, injury during seizure activity

CASE STUDIES

CASE 1

A 39-year-old woman presents with new onset headache over the last 2 months.

History of Present Illness (HPI): She states that, before these episodes, she never thought of herself as a "headachy" person. She relates that the headaches are "nearly always" occipital and are often accompanied by pain so severe that she feels like the top of her head will come off. When questioned, she is both photophobic and phonophobic and also experiences lightheadedness associated with the headache.

PMH: Healthy woman; premenopausal. Medications: Lisinopril 5 mg orally every day, acetaminophen 1,000 mg as needed 4–5 times a day for headache.

1. What other history is needed?
2. What type of physical exam would you do?
3. What screening tests would you do?
4. What is the most likely diagnosis?
5. How would you manage this patient?
6. What education would you give to the patient about their current medication regimen?

CASE 2

A 2-year-old boy is brought in for follow-up after management in the emergency department for multiple febrile seizures.

PMH: No prior history of virus-induced high fevers associated with seizing. No medications except over-the-counter acetaminophen liquid for fevers.

1. What other history do you want to obtain?
2. What physical examination would you perform?
3. What further diagnostic tests would you want to order?
4. How would you initially manage this patient?

CASE 3

A 78-year-old man presents with his wife and daughter complaining of an episode over the weekend of sudden-onset right-sided weakness that resolved completely in about 2 hours. He did not seek medical attention at the time because it resolved.

PMH: Smoker, 64 pack/year history. Mild hypertension diagnosed in 1985. Was told he had elevated lipids "a few years back" but refused to take medication or change his lifestyle at that time. Has not been back to see a provider since.

Medication: Hydrochlorothiazide 50 mg/day "for a year or so," 1985–1986. Occasional acetaminophen.

1. What other history is important?
2. What systems would you examine?
3. What is the most likely diagnosis?
4. What is your plan?

CASE STUDIES DISCUSSION

CASE 1

1. What other history is needed?

   Family history of headache, including migraine. Are patient's symptoms becoming progressive? History of head injury? Does she have headache with exertion (straining, sexual activity, or coughing)? Any change in mental state, focal neurologic deficits, or fever?

2. What type of physical exam would you do?

   Screening neurological exam including funduscopic, cranial nerves, motor exam, gait and coordination, reflexes (would be normal in primary headache syndrome). Focused general exam to include vital signs, HEENT, and other systems as the history suggests excluding secondary headache. Heart and lung exam routine for woman this age.

3. What screening tests would you do?

   CBC if chronic anemia or infection is suspected. Consider CT because of new-onset headache lasting more than a few weeks. Do immediate CT if headache with exertion, straining, sexual activity, or coughing; or on exam there is change in mental state, focal neurological deficits, or fever. Other diagnostic testing as directed by history and physical exam to rule out infectious, metabolic, or autoimmune process.

4. What is the most likely diagnosis? Migraine headache

5. How would you manage this patient?

   The patient has started with analgesics, Excedrin, which did not work. Can try NSAID but avoid opioids to prevent rebound headache. Move on to 5-HT agonists if nonnarcotic analgesics ineffective. Sumatriptan (Imitrex) oral: 25 mg taken as soon as possible at onset, 25–100 mg every 2 hours up to 300 mg in 24 hours. Injection: 6 mg subcutaneeous in adults.

   Perform first injection in office. Intranasal: single dose of 5, 10, or 20 mg administered in one nostril, may repeat once after 2 hours, not to exceed 40 mg in 24 hours. See her back at weekly to monthly intervals until headaches under control. Consider prophylactic treatment for attacks occurring more than twice a month, or impairing daily function, or medications contraindicated because of hypertension or cardiovascular disease.

6. What education would you give to the patient about their current medication regime?

   The patient has the potential to reach toxic levels of acetaminophen with her current medication schedule. The patient should be counseled to keep her acetaminophen intake to below 3–4 g per day depending on her hepatic status.

CASE 2

1. What other history do you want to obtain?

   How long has he been febrile? (Febrile seizure usually occurs within the first 24 hours of fever.) Any symptoms of upper respiratory infection, otitis, tonsillitis? Is there a family history of febrile seizures? Or other risk factors for febrile seizures such as neonatal discharge 28 days or more; delayed development; day care attendance; very high fever? Complete description of the seizure, duration, recovery, motor involvement, etc. Any history of recent illness or exposure to illness, onset of headaches, vomiting or unusual symptoms? Recent trauma; lead, toxin, or medication exposure? Prenatal/perinatal history, including developmental history.

2. What physical examination would you perform?

   Complete physical exam. Identify underlying illness requiring treatment; look for signs of physical abuse. Complete neurological exam, including level of consciousness, presence of meningismus, or a tense bulging fontanel; obtain head circumference. Look for neurocutaneous skin lesions.

3. What further diagnostic tests would you want to order?

   Probably none: lumbar puncture would have been done in the emergency department if any clinical suspicion of meningitis or for children under age 18 months with first seizure; MRI would be done for child with focal seizures. Consider serum lead and routine lab studies only if no source of fever can be elicited on physical examination.

4. How would you initially manage this patient?

   Because febrile seizures are very frightening to the parents, parental reassurance and education are vitally important, as is an active search for the underlying cause of the fever and appropriate treatment with each incidence. Vigorous control of fevers by antipyretics and sponging with tepid water. Acetaminophen 10–15 mg/kg per dose either orally or per rectum. Ibuprofen 5–10 mg/kg per dose orally.

CASE 3

1. What other history is important?

   Onset, duration, and progression of symptoms are most important in determining etiology and management. Resolution of symptoms in minutes to hours is suggestive of a TIA. Detailed description of symptoms or deficits including visual changes, aphasia, motor weakness, paresthesia may give clue to location of lesion. Review of systems: for associated seizure, loss of consciousness, syncope, vertigo, vomiting, chest pain. PMH: cardiac disease, peripheral vascular disease, diabetes, IV drug abuse, and previous neurological conditions such as seizure, head trauma, dementia, brain tumors.

   Review all medications including home remedies and supplements, particularly those that can alter level of consciousness or cause bleeding.

2. What systems would you examine?

   Complete neurological exam for any neurological deficits (no lasting deficits with TIA). Cardiovascular exam for hypertension, atrial fibrillation, heart murmurs, carotid bruits, abdominal bruits.

3. What is the most likely diagnosis?

   TIA; also has significant risk factors for cardiovascular and cerebrovascular disease

4. What is your plan?

   Consult with primary care physician or refer to neurologist immediately for workup that will include CT scan; consider obtaining CBC, ESR, baseline coagulation studies, chemistry panel, lipid profile, RPR, ECG, and chest X-ray in meantime. Provide initial education to patient and family about need for immediate response for subsequent episodes, which could be stroke. Also provide initial education about risk factors—smoking, hypertension, hyperlipidemia—that will need to be modified. Prescribe aspirin 325 mg daily to be started immediately, until more definitive management is begun.

REFERENCES

Alzheimer's Association. (2023). 2023 Alzheimer's disease facts and figures: Special report. *Alzheimers and Dementia, 19*(4). DOI 10.1002/alz.13016.https://www.alz.org/media/Documents/alzheimers-facts-and-figures.pdf

American Headache Society. (2020, April). *Practice parameters, guidelines and classification.* https://americanheadachesociety.org/resources/information-for-clinicians/practice-parameters-guidelines-and-classification/

American Stroke Association. (2020, December). *Transient Ischemic Attack (TIA)* www.stroke.org. https://www.stroke.org/en/about-stroke/types-of-stroke/tia-transient-ischemic-attack/what-is-a-tia#:~:text=Approximately%2015%25%20of%20all%20strokes,report%20experiencing%20a%20TIA%20first

Ashley-Koch, A., & Gregory, S. (2020, December). *Neural tube defects (Ntds).* Duke Molecular Physiology Institute https://dmpi.duke.edu/neural-tube-defects-ntds#:~:text=Neural%20tube%20defects%20(NTDs)%20are,very%20early%20in%20human%20development

Ben-Joseph, A., Marshall, C. R., Lees, A. J., & Noyce, A. J. (2020). Ethnic variation in the manifestation of Parkinson's disease: A narrative review. *Journal of Parkinson's disease, 10*(1), 31–45. https://doi.org/10.3233/JPD-191763

Benny, S. (2020). Role of serum sodium levels in recurrence and recurrent episodes of febrile seizure. *International Journal of Contemporary Pediatrics, 7*(7), 1606–1613. https://dx.doi.org/10.18203/2349-3291.ijcp20202625

Centers for Disease Control and Prevention. (2020). *Epilepsy fast facts.* https://www.cdc.gov/epilepsy/about/fast-facts.htm#:~:text=According%20to%20the%20latest%20estimates,17%20years%20have%20active%20epilepsy.&text=Think%20of%20a%20school%20with,of%20them%20could%20have%20epilepsy

Centers for Disease Control and Prevention. (2020, December). *Data and statistics on Down syndrome.* https://www.cdc.gov/ncbddd/birthdefects/downsyndrome/data.html#:~:text=Each%20year%2C%20about%206%2C000%20babies,in%20every%20700%20babies%20born.&text=Between%201979%20and%202003%2C%20the,syndrome%20increased%20by%20about%2030%25.&text=Older%20mothers%20are%20more%20likely,Down%20syndrome%20than%20younger%20mothers

Centers for Disease Control and Prevention. (2022a). *Stroke facts.* www.cdc.gov. https://www.cdc.gov/stroke/facts.htm#:~:text=Stroke%20statistics,-In%202020%2C%201&text=Every%20year%2C%20more%20than%20795%2C000,are%20first%20or%20new%20strokes.&text=About%20185%2C000%20strokes%E2%80%94nearly%201,have%20had%20a%20previous%20stroke

Centers for Disease Control and Prevention. (2022b). *Viral meningitis.* www.cdc.gov. https://www.cdc.gov/meningitis/viral.html

Centers for Disease Control and Prevention. (2022c). *Bacterial meningitis.* https://www.cdc.gov/meningitis/bacterial.html

Centers for Disease Control and Prevention. (2022d). *Data and statistics on Tourette syndrome.* https://www.cdc.gov/ncbddd/tourette/data.html#:~:text=A%20CDC%20study%20using%20parent,174%2C000%20children%20in%202016%E2%80%932019

Collier, S. (2020). *What's the best way to manage agitation related to dementia?* Harvard Health. https://www.health.harvard.edu/blog/whats-the-best-way-to-manage-agitation-related-to-dementia-2020021418816#:~:text=The%20bottom%20line,manage%20agitation%20related%20to%20dementia

Diaz-Roman, M., Pulopulos, M., Baquero, M., Salvador, A., Cuevas, A., Ferrer, I., Ciopat, O., & Gomez, E. (2021). Obstructive sleep apnea and Alzheimer's disease-related cerebrospinal fluid biomarkers in mild cognitive impairment. *Sleep, 44*(1). https://doi.org/10.1093/sleep/zsaa133

Eisen, D. P., Hamilton, E., Bodilsen, J., Koster-Rasmussen, R., Stockdale, A. J., Miner, J., Nielsen, H., Dzupova, O., Sethi, V., Copson, R. K., Harings, M., & Adegboye, O. A. (2022). Longer than 2 hours to antibiotics is associated with doubling of mortality in a multinational community-acquired bacterial meningitis cohort. *Nature.* https://www.nature.com/articles/s41598-021-04349-7

Gavidia, M. (2021). Deep brain stimulation still effective after 15 years in people with Parkinson disease, study shows. *The American Journal of Managed Care.* https://www.ajmc.com/view/deep-brain-stimulation-still-effective-after-15-years-in-people-with-parkinson-disease-study-shows

Gawlik, K. S., Bernadette Mazurek Melnyk, F., & Teall, A. M. (2020). *Evidence-based physical examination: Best practices for health & well-being assessment.* Springer Publishing Company.

Hersi, K., Gonzalez, F. J., & Kondamudi, N. P. (2021). *Meningitis—StatPearls—NCBI bookshelf.* National Center for Biotechnology Information. https://www.ncbi.nlm.nih.gov/books/NBK459360/

Ibrahim, F., & Murr, N. (2022). *Embolic stroke—StatPearls—NCBI bookshelf.* National Center for Biotechnology Information. https://www.ncbi.nlm.nih.gov/books/NBK564351/

International Classification of Headache Disorders. (2021). *Migraine.* The International Classification of Headache Disorders 3rd edition. https://ichd-3.org/

Kerr, S.M., Parker, S.E., Mitchell, A.A., Tinker, S.C., & Werler, M.M. (2017). Periconceptional maternal fever, folic acid intake, and risk for neural tube defects. *Annals Epidemiology, 27*(12): 777–782.e.1. doi: 10.1016/j.annepidem.2017.10.010

Lakhan, S. E. (2022). *Alzheimer disease medication: Cholinesterase inhibitors, N-methyl-D-Aspartate antagonists, combination drugs, monoclonal antibodies, anti-amyloid beta, nutritional supplement, and diagnostic imaging agents*. Diseases & Conditions—Medscape Reference. https://emedicine.medscape.com/article/1134817-medication

Liang, T. W., & Tarsy, D. (2022). *Medical management of motor fluctuations and dyskinesia in Parkinson disease*. UpToDate.com. https://www.uptodate.com/contents/medical-management-of-motor-fluctuations-and-dyskinesia-in-parkinson-disease?search=parkinson%20treatment&source=search_result&selectedTitle=2~150&usage_type=default&display_rank=2#H615414407

Mayo Clinic. (2022). *Parkinson's disease—diagnosis and treatment*. www.mayoclinic.org. https://www.mayoclinic.org/diseases-conditions/parkinsons-disease/diagnosis-treatment/drc-20376062

MedlinePlus. (2021). *Benign familial neonatal seizures: MedlinePlus genetics*. https://medlineplus.gov/genetics/condition/benign-familial-neonatal-seizures/

MedlinePlus. (2022). *Alpha-fetoprotein (AFP) test*. MedlinePlus—Health Information from the National Library of Medicine. https://medlineplus.gov/lab-tests/alpha-fetoprotein-afp-test/#:~:text=An%20AFP%20test%20is%20usually,release%20more%20or%20less%20AFP

National Fragile X Foundation. (2022). *Prevalence*. https://fragilex.org/understanding-fragile-x/fragile-x-101/prevalence/

National Institute of Neurological Disorders and Stroke. (2022). *Febrile seizures fact sheet*. https://www.ninds.nih.gov/febrile-seizures-fact-sheet

Padiyar, S., Nusairat, L., Kadri, A., Uba-Swaweesh, J., & Aly, H. (2020). Neonatal seizures in the U.S. national inpatient population: Prevalence and outcomes. *Pediatrics & Neonatology, 61*(3), 300–305. https://doi.org/10.1016/j.pedneo.2019.12.006

Sawires, R., Buttery, J., & Fahey, M. (2021). A review of febrile seizures: Recent advances in understanding of febrile seizure pathophysiology and commonly implicated viral triggers. *Frontiers in Pediatrics, 9*. https://doi.org/10.3389%2Ffped.2021.801321

Shahrokhi, M., & Asuncion, R. D. (2022). *Neurologic exam—StatPearls—NCBI bookshelf*. National Center for Biotechnology Information. https://www.ncbi.nlm.nih.gov/books/NBK557589/

U.S. Preventative Services Task Force. (2021). *Hypertension in adults*. United States Preventive Services Taskforce. https://www.uspreventiveservicestaskforce.org/uspstf/recommendation/hypertension-in-adults-screening

Wirrell, E. (2021). *International League Against Epilepsy classification of seizure types*. UpToDate.com. https://www.uptodate.com/contents/ilae-classification-of-seizures-and-epilepsy?search=seizure%20in%20adults&topicRef=2219&source=see_link

Xixis, K. L., Samanta, D., & Keenaghan, M. (2022). *Febrile seizure—StatPearls—NCBI bookshelf*.

CHAPTER 16

HEMATOLOGIC DISORDERS

Colleen Stellabotte, MSN, RN, CRNP

General Approach

DESCRIPTION

- The most common blood/hematologic blood disorder in all age groups is iron-deficiency anemia.
- In anemia in patients with chronic disease/chronic inflammatory disease, expand the differential diagnosis to include other causes; do not assume it is from chronic disease.
- Do not begin treatment for B12 deficiency without assessing for and treating folate deficiency.
- Physiologic anemia of the newborn occurs at 10 to 12 weeks due to rapid growth, increase in blood volume, and shortened red blood cell (RBC) survival time; hemoglobin level may reach a low of 10 g/dL in full-term infants; this is followed by a gradual increase in RBCs, with correspondingly slower Hemoglobin rise; healthy term infants do not require therapy.
- Hematopoiesis is slowed in older adults when the presence and number of progenitor cells decline; 60% of all anemias are seen in people 65 years of age or older.

DEFINITIONS

- Anemia: Hemoglobin level is lower than 12 g/dL for females and lower than 13.5 g/dL for males; or hematocrit is lower than 36% for females and lower than 40% for males. In children, specific values defining anemia vary depending on age.
- Mean corpuscular (cell) volume (MCV): represents the size of the RBC and is calculated from the Hemoglobin, Hematocrit, or RBC count; used in differentiation of types of anemia

- Ferritin*:* represents iron storage in the serum; may be elevated during infection or chronic inflammation and decreased in iron deficiency
- Hypochromic: erythrocytes containing decreased level of Hemoglobin, causing the cells to appear "paler" on smear
- Hyperchromic: erythrocytes containing increased level of Hemoglobin, causing cells to appear "darker" on smear
- Macrocytic anemia: decreased Hemoglobin/Hematocrit/RBC with associated MCV higher than 100
- Megaloblastic anemia: anemia characterized by a large, nucleated, embryonic type of cell that is a precursor of erythrocytes in an abnormal erythropoietic process seen almost exclusively in pernicious anemia
- Microcytic anemia: decreased Hemoglobin/Hematocrit/RBC with associated MCV lower than 80
- Normocytic anemia: decreased Hemoglobin/Hematocrit/RBC with associated MCV 80 to 100
- RDW*:* RBC distribution width, a statistical index of the variation in red cell widths
- Total iron-binding capacity (TIBC): amount of iron in serum plus amount of transferrin available in serum (transferrin is a transport protein that regulates iron absorption); decreased in anemia of chronic disease
- Normal ranges for RBC studies can be found in Table 16–1.

TABLE 16–1.
BLOOD VALUES HELPFUL IN DIFFERENTIATING ANEMIAS

MICROCYTIC ANEMIAS MCV <80 μM^3	NORMOCYTIC ANEMIAS MCV 80–100 μM^3	MACROCYTIC ANEMIA MCV >100 μM^3
Iron-deficiency anemia	Hemorrhage	Folate deficiency
Anemia of chronic disease	Aplastic anemia	Vitamin B12 deficiency
Thalassemia	Hemolytic anemia	
Sideroblastic	Sickle cell anemia	
	Drug induced	
	Glucose-6-phosphate dehydrogenase (G6PD) deficiency	
	Early stage of anemia of chronic disease	

RED FLAGS

- Blood values helpful in identifying anemias can be found in Table 16–1. The table identifies normal ranges; values outside these parameters require thorough investigation.
- Anemia in the presence of splenomegaly requires further diagnostic evaluation.
- Anemia of prematurity manifests at 4 to 8 weeks of age and is more severe than physiologic anemia.
  - Influencing factors include birth weight, perinatal complications, blood transfusion history, and presence of vitamin E deficiency. Nadir Hemoglobin values reach 6 g/dL.
  - Asymptomatic, growing preterm infants require no therapy; however, signs of hypoxia (apneic episodes, tachycardia, irritability, poor feeding) indicate need for evaluation and more aggressive intervention.
- Hemolytic anemia during the newborn period is due to physiologically immature liver incapable of rapidly conjugating bilirubin created by normally rapid turnover of relatively excessive RBCs.
  - Hemolysis in the neonate is accompanied by reticulocytosis, nucleated RBCs, and sometimes spherocytosis on peripheral blood smear.
  - Most common cause of hemolytic anemia in the newborn is ABO incompatibility with hyperbilirubinemia/jaundice, usually within 24 hours of birth.
  - All cases of suspected hemolytic anemia in the newborn should be evaluated in the hospital.
- Multiple myeloma is a malignant disease of the plasma cells with peak incidence during the seventh decade. It may present with bone pain of the back, chest, or extremities; weakness and fatigue; pathologic fractures; abnormal bleeding; palpable liver and spleen; Bence-Jones protein in the urine; elevated creatinine and calcium; and increased sedimentation rate. Refer for bone marrow biopsy.
- Hodgkin's lymphoma is a malignant disease with lymphoreticular proliferation and presence of Reed-Sternberg cells; there is a bimodal age distribution: 15 to 34 years of age (peak at 20) and 50 years and older (peak at 70) with male-to-female ratio of 8:1.
  - Presents with persistent fever, night sweats, persistent dry cough, unexplained pruritus, substernal discomfort, persistent painless lymphadenopathy, weight loss more than 10%, anorexia, immediate pain after alcohol ingestion; increased incidence in persons with AIDS.
  - Diagnostic tests may show mediastinal adenopathy on chest X-ray, elevated erythrocyte sedimentation rate (ESR), increased serum alkaline phosphatase and lactate dehydrogenase (LDH), lymphocytopenia, mild leukocytosis, thrombocytosis, Reed-Sternberg cells on smear.

- ◊ Refer suspected cases to hematologist for diagnosis and management with chemotherapy and radiation; prognosis is good depending on classification at diagnosis.

- ♦ Non-Hodgkin's lymphoma is a malignant disease of the lymphoreticular system differentiated from Hodgkin's lymphoma by the absence of giant Reed-Sternberg cells; increased incidence in persons with AIDS.
  - ◊ Presents similar to Hodgkin's lymphoma; prognosis not as good
  - ◊ Refer all suspected cases to hematologist for diagnosis and management.
- ♦ Deficiency of coagulant factor VIII (hemophilia A) or factor IX (hemophilia B) is rare and presents in males during first few years of life as excessive bruising, bleeding after circumcision, bleeding hours or days after injury, hematuria, or hemorrhage or hematoma after minor injury. Laboratory results include normal platelet count, greatly prolonged partial thromboplastin time (PTT), factor VIII low in hemophilia A, factor IX low in hemophilia B. Refer to hematologist for management.

Normocytic Anemias

ANEMIA OF CHRONIC DISEASE

Description

- ♦ A mild hypo-proliferative anemia associated with chronic disease, infections, and malignancies that has persisted for more than 1 to 2 months, probably a consequence of long-term disease with inflammatory process
- ♦ Diagnosis of exclusion from active blood loss or production abnormalities associated with iron or folate intake

Etiology

- ♦ The pathophysiology of anemia of chronic disease is not well understood but may be due to decreased RBC life span, erythropoietin reduction, and problems of iron transfer.
- ♦ Occurs because of renal disease, liver disease, endocrine disorders, rheumatoid arthritis, infections, some forms of cancer

Incidence and Demographics

- The second most common anemia in the world; the incidence parallels the rate of chronic inflammatory disease.
- The most common anemia in older adults

Risk Factors

- Chronic diseases: Renal, liver, endocrine disease; rheumatoid arthritis; infection; and some cancers

Prevention and Screening

- Attention to good nutrition
- Complete blood count (CBC) screening for patients with chronic disease

Assessment

History

- Chronic disease
- Fatigue, dyspnea on exertion, irritability, listlessness, easy fatigability

Physical Exam

- Perform a complete physical exam for signs of the underlying disease.
- Signs of anemia, depending on severity: pallor, tachycardia, tachypnea on exertion

Diagnostic Studies

See Table 16–2

- CBC, reticulocyte count, iron studies (serum iron, TIBC, ferritin); studies pertinent to underlying disorder; repeat iron studies important for diagnosis and management

TABLE 16–2.
NORMAL RANGES FOR RBC STUDIES

TEST	FEMALES	MALES
Hemoglobin	12–16 g/dL	13.5–17.7 g/dL
Hematocrit	36%–48%	40%–53%
RBC (106/μL)	4.0–5.4	4.5–6.0
MCV	80–100 fL	80–100 fL
MCH	26–34 pg	26–34 pg
MCHC	31%–37% g/dL	31%–37% g/dL
Reticulocyte count	0.5%–1.5% of RBC	0.5%–1.5% of RBC
Serum iron	50–170 μg/dL	65–175 μg/dL
TIBC	250–450 μg/dL	250–450 μg/dL
Ferritin	10–120 ng/mL (avg. 55)	20–250 ng/mL (avg. 125)

MCH = mean corpuscular hemoglobin; MCHC = mean corpuscular hemoglobin concentration; RBC = red blood cell; TIBC = total iron-binding capacity; fL = femtoliter (10^{-15} L); pg = picogram (10^{-12} g); ng = nanogram (10^{-9} g); μL = microliter (10^{-6}).

- Characteristic labs: Hemoglobin usually 8 to 12 g/dL, Hematocrit 25% to 35%, MCV 75 to 85 as Hemoglobin falls below 10, often low serum iron and TIBC, and normal or increased ferritin (TIBC is increased and ferritin decreased in iron deficiency); serum erythropoietin normal but not generally assessed.

Differential Diagnosis

- Iron-deficiency anemia
- Multifactorial anemia
- Chronic renal insufficiency
- Liver disease (usually alcohol related)
- Posthemorrhagic anemia
- Endocrine disorders: hypothyroidism
- AIDS
- Aplastic anemia

Management

Nonpharmacologic Treatment

- Treat underlying disease
- Ensure appropriate nutrition
- Transfusion only in severe, symptomatic cases

Pharmacologic Treatment

- Recombinant erythropoietin (Epogen, Procrit) in selected patients. Black Box warnings for patients with certain types of cancers and patients with chronic kidney disease.

How Long to Treat

- Required as long as underlying disease and anemia persist

Special Considerations

- A profile similar to that of iron deficiency may eventually develop, with patient becoming mildly microcytic and hypochromic as Hemoglobin falls below 10 g/dL.
- Patients with AIDS often have anemia of chronic disease. As disease progresses, pancytopenia may occur due to marrow damage. At that point, checking serum erythropoietin level may help determine if patient will benefit from recombinant erythropoietin injections.
- Anemia of renal disease relates to severity of renal failure due to decreased erythropoietin production and may benefit from erythropoietin.
- In patients with diabetes mellitus, anemia is frequently severe early in the disease process.

When to Consult, Refer, Hospitalize

- Refer if diagnosis is questionable.
- Refer to confirm underlying cause (e.g., rheumatologist for collagen/vascular problem, oncologist for cancer, nephrologist for renal disease, infectious disease specialist for infections).

Follow-Up

- Frequent monitoring of blood pressure, CBC, iron studies with recombinant erythropoietin therapy

Expected Course

- Anemia will improve or worsen as the underlying disease improves or progresses.
- A patient can often tolerate low Hematocrit and Hemoglobin, as low as 30% and 10 g/dL, respectively, as these develop gradually.

Complications

- Possible exacerbation of cardiopulmonary disease, particularly in older adults: (anemia results in less oxygen delivered to tissues, heart rate and cardiac output increase to compensate; heart may begin to fail).

APLASTIC ANEMIA

Description

- Aplastic anemia is characterized by intrinsic bone marrow dysfunction or failure; pluripotent stem cell expression is impaired so pancytopenia with hypercellularity of the bone marrow is seen.
- Intrinsic marrow dysfunction produces defective RBC synthesis and produces anemia, neutropenia, thrombocytopenia, and pancytopenia.

Etiology

- Autoimmune suppression of hematopoiesis is the most common cause, but may be precipitated by viral illness, autoimmune suppression, drug or chemical exposure, tumor, radiation, or inherited disorder
- Inherited: Fanconi's anemia, Schwachman-Diamond syndrome

Incidence and Demographics

- Not common in United States
- 50% idiopathic; 20% drug or chemical exposure (chloramphenicol [Chloromycetin]—rare); 10% viral

Risk Factors

- Family history, some medications (anticonvulsants, antibiotics, gold), radiation, exposure to some toxic chemicals such as insecticides, herbicides, organic solvents, paint removers, and others

Prevention and Screening

- Most cases cannot be prevented.
- There are no recommended general screening methods.
- Individuals should avoid contact exposure to certain chemicals, such as insecticides, herbicides, organic solvents, paint removers, and other toxic chemicals. This is especially important if patient already has had aplastic anemia caused by toxic chemicals. Recurrent exposure may increase the risk of a reoccurrence of the disease.
- Individuals who have had exposure to toxic chemicals or who have had aplastic anemia in the past should have regular physical examinations.
- Individuals should report the following signs and symptoms early: fever, fatigue, weight loss, weakness, sore throat, dyspnea, palpitations, and bleeding.

Assessment

History

- Insidious onset of fever, fatigue, weight loss, weakness, sore throat, dyspnea, palpitations
- Bleeding problems such as menorrhagia, rectal bleed, epistaxis
- History of potential sources of exposure to toxic agents: medications, chemical exposure at work, hobbies, etc.
- History of associated anomalies: kidney, hypospadias, short stature

Physical Exam

- General: pallor, petechiae, bruises
- Thorough physical for tumors, signs of infection, signs of bleeding
  - Cardiac exam: systolic ejection murmur may be present
  - Eyes: retinal flame hemorrhage
  - Rectal: occult or rectal bleeding

Diagnostic Studies

- Pancytopenia is pathognomonic
- Severe anemia, decreased reticulocytes
- CBC with differential, peripheral smear, bleeding studies, TIBC, urinalysis, bone marrow, liver function, computed tomography (CT) of thymus as indicated
- Lab results: normochromic, normocytic anemia; TIBC normal; hematuria
- Bone marrow shows hypoplasia, fatty infiltration

Differential Diagnosis

- Leukemia
- Hypersplenism
- Systemic lupus erythematosus (SLE)
- Myelodysplasia
- Sepsis

Management

Nonpharmacologic Treatment

- Perform education and supportive care.
- A well-balanced diet decreases risk of infection.
- Manage underlying cause.
- Perform human leukocyte antigen (HLA) testing on patients and immediate families for inherited conditions.

Pharmacologic Treatment

- Immunosuppression therapy, oxygen
- All cases: RBC and platelet transfusions, parenteral antibiotics for infection due to severe neutropenia
- Severe cases: bone marrow transplant is considered (may be age dependent)

How Long to Treat

- Lifelong treatment may be required unless effective bone marrow transplant is curative.

Special Considerations

- Must avoid further exposure to etiologic agents

When to Consult, Refer, Hospitalize

- Refer immediately to hematologist when diagnosis is suspected; work with hematologist throughout therapy.

Follow-Up

Expected Course

- Often favorable outcome, depending on age and treatment response
- Untreated cases are fatal; successful bone marrow transplant is curative.

Complications

- Infection, leukemia, heart failure, hemorrhage

Microcytic Anemias

IRON-DEFICIENCY ANEMIA

Description

- Microcytic, hypochromic anemia due to decreased iron stores, poor iron utilization, or poor iron reutilization

Etiology

- Hemorrhage, occult malignancy, increased need (pregnancy and growth spurts), impaired absorption, inadequate dietary intake

Incidence and Demographics

- Prevalent in all ages and populations in the United States
- Seen in 7% to 10% of adult population; 10% to 20% of infants and toddlers; 15% to 45% of pregnant women; 20% of women overall
- More common in women than men because of menstruation, pregnancy

Risk Factors

- Low iron stores occurs in premature and low-birth-weight (LBW) infants and when Hemoglobin is lower than normal at birth (e.g., hemorrhage and/or smaller of twins)
- Increased need for iron; demands for iron higher than normal such as LBW infants experiencing rapid catch-up growth or normal rapid growth of infancy and adolescence, pregnancy and lactation, athletes
- Insufficient intake of iron from low dietary intake, poor bioavailability of the dietary iron, or malabsorption. Low intake is most common etiologic factor seen in infants, toddlers, teens, older adults, and persons living in institutional settings.
- Increased loss of iron due to disease process, including Meckel's diverticulum, peptic ulcer disease, polyps, hemangiomas, parasitic infections, or cow's milk enteropathy. Losses may also occur from menorrhagia, chronic use of nonsteroidal anti-inflammatory drugs (NSAIDS), uncommonly recurrent epistaxis, and possibly strenuous exercise.

- Conditions such as achlorhydria, gastric surgery, celiac disease, pica that cause impaired absorption
- Conditions such as neoplasm, duodenal/gastric ulcers, diverticulosis, ulcerative colitis
- Repeated blood donations

Prevention and Screening

- Encourage breastfeeding of all infants for the first 12 months of life; after 1 year of age, limit cow and soymilk consumption to less than 24 ounces/day. Adequate diet: consume orange juice with meals to enhance iron absorption.
- Dietary supplements if patient has risk factors
- Selective screening for at-risk populations such as menstruating women and some older adults

Assessment

History

- Preterm and LBW infants
- Initially asymptomatic; insidious onset of gradually progressing fatigue, dyspnea on exertion, irritable, listless, easy fatigability, dysphagia, postural hypotension
- Possible palpitations, shortness of breath, impaired muscular performance
- Diet history: Low in iron, pica
- Drug and chemical exposure
- Family history of iron-deficiency anemia
- Review of systems (ROS) for blood loss, symptoms of gastrointestinal problems, neoplasms

Physical Exam

- Obtain height and weight for infants and children, plot on growth chart
- Observe for pallor or chlorosis (peculiar greenish pallor)
- Angular stomatitis, ulcerations, or fissure of the mouth

- Ozena: chronic atrophy of the nasal mucosa
- Dry skin and mucous membranes
- Koilonychia: thinning and flattening of the nails, then spooning
- Auscultate heart for systolic flow murmurs
- Splenomegaly
- Brittle hair, tachycardia, tachypnea

Diagnostic Studies

- CBC with differential and smear, TIBC, serum iron, ferritin, special tests to determine underlying bleed
- Laboratory findings (see Table 16–3): Hemoglobin lower than 12 g/dL in adults and older children, variable in younger children; serum ferritin level lower than 10 ng/mL in women and lower than 20 ng/mL in men; low Hematocrit; "pencil cells" on smear, MCV and MCH decrease, RDW higher than 15, increased TIBC above 400 μg/dL, low serum iron below 30 μg/dL; transferrin saturation below 15%; MCV less than 80 μg/dL; reticulocyte count elevated in cases of blood loss, decrease in iron deficiency; increased platelet count above 400,000; bone marrow absent for iron staining
- Bone marrow aspiration if severe, questionable diagnosis, or resistant to treatment

Differential Diagnosis

- Thalassemia
- G6PD deficiency
- Infection

TABLE 16–3.
COMPARISON OF DIFFERENTIAL LABORATORY FINDINGS IN MICROCYTIC ANEMIAS

LABORATORY FINDING	THALASSEMIA TRAIT	LEAD POISONING	IRON DEFICIENCY
Hemoglobin	Decreased	Decreased	Decreased
MCV	Decreased	Decreased	Decreased
Ferritin	Normal	Normal	Decreased
FEP (free erythrocyte porphyrins)	Normal	Very High	High

- Cancer
- Chronic diseases
- Lead poisoning
- Hypothyroidism
- Renal failure

Management

Nonpharmacologic Treatment

- Diagnose and treat underlying cause.
- Normal dietary intake meets only daily losses, not therapeutic; Recommended Daily Allowance (RDA) for iron is 10 mg/day for men and up to 15 mg/day for women and children; must increase iron intake
- No dairy product or antacid within 2 hours of oral iron
- Symptomatic care on treatment side effects (constipation, nausea, cramps, diarrhea)

Pharmacologic Treatment

- Oral iron supplements: up to 300 mg of elemental iron divided three to four times a day for adolescents and adults
    - 325 mg of ferrous sulfate contains 65 mg of elemental iron.
    - Liquid preparation 2 to 3 mg/kg/day for children
    - Oral iron therapy is safer and less costly than IM or IV iron.
    - Reduce dose to decrease gastrointestinal (GI) side effects, no real benefit to more expensive preparations
    - Vitamin C will help increase absorption; meals will decrease absorption by up to 50%.
- Parenteral iron if poor absorption or inability to tolerate oral iron
- Blood transfusion is not recommended for iron supplementation.

How Long to Treat

- Until deficiency corrected; expect to see improvement within 4 weeks; return to baseline blood levels in 8 weeks; continue therapy 3 to 6 months to replace iron stores

Special Considerations

- If unresponsive to therapy, reevaluate underlying cause and compliance.

When to Consult, Refer, Hospitalize

- Refer to hematologist if patient is not responsive to treatment or underlying cause cannot be determined.

Follow-Up

- Recommended after 1 month and every 6 months if stable until resolved

Expected Course

- Cure expected; increase in Hemoglobin of 1 g/week expected
- Prolonged course of treatment may be required because of noncompliance.

Complications

- May have unidentified underlying source of bleeding
- Growth delay, learning difficulty, heart failure (late, untreated)

Macrocytic Anemias

VITAMIN B12 DEFICIENCY

Description

- A megaloblastic anemia in which MCV is above 100 resulting from a deficiency of intrinsic factor, which leads to inadequate vitamin B12 absorption (below 200 pg/mL) and impaired RBC synthesis

Etiology

- Pernicious anemia: caused by congenital enzyme deficiency so B12 cannot be absorbed; overgrowth of intestinal organisms, autoimmune reaction involving gastric parietal cells, gastrectomy
- Malabsorption: GI parasites, GI surgery, Crohn's disease, chronic alcoholism, strict vegetarians (rare)
- Older adults stomach is less acidic; B12 needs acid to be absorbed

Incidence and Demographics

- Onset at age 50 to 60; median age at diagnosis is 60
- Women slightly more than men

Risk Factors

- Age (commonly presents around age 60), family history of pernicious anemia
- Chronic alcoholism
- GI surgery, Crohn's disease, immunologic diseases

Prevention and Screening

- Adequate dietary intake: meat and dairy products
- Routine screening for B12 level in dementia and malnutrition

Assessment

History

- Insidious onset of peripheral numbness, personality changes, memory loss, anorexia, diarrhea, glossitis, distal paresthesia, ataxia
- Assess for risk factors, underlying causes
- Should be considered in differential diagnosis of dementia

Physical Exam

- Characteristic beefy-red, shiny tongue
- Abdominal tenderness, organomegaly, tachycardia, tachypnea, pallor, hepatosplenomegaly
- Neurological signs: numbness, sensory ataxia, limb weakness, spasticity, changes in deep tendon reflexes, decreased vibratory sense, impaired proprioception, impaired fine motor movement, positive Romberg test, progressive mental status impairment

Diagnostic Studies

- CBC with differential, peripheral smear, LDH, serum folate, and serum B12 levels; consider methylmalonic acid (MMA) and homocysteine levels, both are elevated in B12 deficiency; consider bone marrow aspiration
- Laboratory results: serum B12 levels below 200 pg/mL; Hematocrit decreased; MCV markedly elevated; decreased reticulocyte count; WBC and platelet count reduced, elevated LDH
- On smear: a large, nucleated, embryonic type of cell that is a precursor of erythrocytes in an abnormal erythropoietic process

Differential Diagnosis

- Folic acid deficiency
- Myelodysplasia
- Liver dysfunction
- Side effects of medications
- Alcoholism
- Bleeding/hemorrhage
- Hypothyroidism

Management

Nonpharmacologic Treatment

- Education and supportive therapy; maintain balanced diet, good health, and hygiene

Pharmacologic Treatment

- Initial: 800 to 1,000 μg of vitamin B12 IM daily for 4 to 8 weeks
- Maintenance: 100 to 1,000 μg monthly
- Oral cobalamin (vitamin B12) 1,000 μg daily is alternative replacement. Note, this may be poorly absorbed.
- May require iron supplementation for the first month of therapy during rapid regeneration of RBCs

How Long to Treat

- Lifelong

Special Considerations

- If patient presents with abnormal neurological signs, the symptoms might be irreversible.
- Might have hypokalemia in first week of treatment
- Do not begin treatment for B12 deficiency without also assessing for and treating folate deficiency.
- Check serum B_{12} levels in patients with distal polyneuropathies (even if no anemia or macrocytosis seen).
- Oral B-complex vitamin only valuable when B12 deficiency is nutritional

When to Consult, Refer, Hospitalize

- Refer as needed for underlying cause; refer for follow-up endoscopy every 5 years to exclude malignancy.

Follow-Up

Expected Course

- Response rapid; good prognosis if treatment within 6 months of neurological signs

Complications

- Stomach cancer
- Permanent central nervous system (CNS) signs/symptoms

FOLIC ACID DEFICIENCY

Description

- Folic acid deficiency results in an anemia from inadequate folic acid intake. Folic acid is needed for DNA synthesis and RBC maturation. Lack of folic acid (folate) causes macrocytic, normochromic, and megaloblastic anemia.
- Also associated with increased incidence of embryonic neural tube defects

Etiology

- Folic acid–deficient diet, malabsorption syndromes, or increased demand for folic acid (pregnancy)

Incidence and Demographics

- All races and age groups
- Most common at ages 60 to 70 years

Risk Factors

- Pregnancy, older adults, alcoholics
- Malnourished or malabsorption syndromes, hemodialysis patients
- Medications that interfere with folic acid absorption (e.g., trimethoprim, phenytoin, oral birth control pills, phenobarbital, sulfamethoxazole/trimethoprim, sulfasalazine)

Prevention and Screening

- Adequate intake of folic acid: 400 μg for pregnant women, 200 μg for all others

Assessment

History

- Indigestion, constipation, diarrhea, anorexia, lethargy
- Fatigue, weakness, headache, dizziness, dyspnea on exertion, depression, apathy

Physical Exam

- Pallor, atrophic glossitis (red, shiny tongue), stomatitis
- Change in mental status, confusion but no focal neurological deficits
- Tachycardia, wide pulse pressure, heart murmur
- Peripheral neuropathy

Diagnostic Studies

- CBC, RBC folate more reliable for diagnosis than serum folate; serum B12, TIBC, LDH, RDW, MMA, and homocysteine levels
- Laboratory results: serum folate below 3 ng/mL, RBC folate below 150 ng/mL, Hematocrit decreased, Hemoglobin normal, RDW elevated, TIBC normal, LDH and MCV elevated above 100 μg/mL; MCHC normal, MMA normal, homocysteine is elevated, serum B12 normal

Differential Diagnosis

- Vitamin B12 deficiency
- Myelodysplastic syndromes

- Pernicious anemia
- Hypothyroidism

Management

Nonpharmacologic Treatment

- Education and supportive therapy; good oral hygiene
- Folate-rich diet: green leafy vegetables, red beans, wheat bran, fish, bananas, asparagus
- Need for frequent rest

Pharmacologic Treatment

- Folic acid replacement 400 µg for pregnant women, 200 µg for all others
    - Prescription supplements usually contain 1 mg folic acid but be aware that supplementation of greater than 400 µg may mask B12 deficiency.

How Long to Treat

- Until anemia corrected, usually about 2 months until folic acid stores replenished
- Depends on elimination of underlying cause

Special Considerations

- Folate body stores can be depleted in about 4 months.
- Women on birth control who are potentially childbearing should routinely take folic acid preparations to decrease incidence of embryonic neural tube defects.

When to Consult, Refer, Hospitalize

- Not usually needed; refer patients who do not improve with therapy.

Follow-Up

- In 2 months and periodically thereafter

Expected Course

- Good prognosis

Complications

- Failure to thrive
- Neural tube defects of infants born to deficient women

Hemolytic Anemias

DESCRIPTION

Hemolytic conditions produce anemias in which accelerated RBC destruction occurs as a result of an intrinsic genetic RBC defect as seen in hemoglobinopathies (sickle cell and thalassemia), metabolic enzyme deficiencies (G6PD), or cytoskeleton disorders (spherocytosis or elliptocytosis). The intrinsic destruction could also be acquired as seen in paroxysmal nocturnal hemoglobinuria or alcoholic cirrhosis. Extrinsic causes of hemolysis include antibody-mediated processes such as autoimmune reactions, drug-related reactions, transfusion reactions, and reactions to infections.

IMPORTANT FEATURES

- Peripheral blood smear shows spherocytosis and may be hyperchromic.
- Coombs test will be positive in immune hemolysis.
- An elevated reticulocyte count in a patient with anemia is the most useful indicator of hemolysis.
- Other laboratory findings include increased unconjugated bilirubin (indirect), decreased heptoglobin, possible increase in LDH, increased urine hemoglobin, or increased urine bilirubin. Hemosiderin is a delayed sign and may represent chronic hemolysis.
- Bone marrow shows normoblastic erythroid hyperplasia.

SICKLE CELL ANEMIA/TRAIT

Description

- Sickle cell disease (SSD) is a group of Hemoglobin disorders characterized by the production of hemoglobin S (HbS), the most common of which is sickle cell anemia (HbSS). Other common genotypes are sickle-cell C (HbSC) and sickle beta-thalassemia (HbS beta-thalassemia). Severe hemolytic anemia may be produced in which abnormal hemoglobin (due to DNA point mutation in the B-globin chain) leads to chronic hemolytic anemia, with recurrent painful crises in individuals who are homozygous for hemoglobin S.
- Sickle cell disorders are characterized by chronic hemolytic anemia.

Etiology

- Hemoglobin S readily deforms the RBC into a sickle shape; the sickle cells hemolyze, and clusters of sickle cells occlude small blood vessels.
- Autosomal recessive (hemoglobin S allele from each parent)
- Sickle cell trait (Hemoglobin AS) is seen when one normal Hemoglobin allele and one sickle hemoglobin–producing allele are inherited from the parents; this will not cause sickle cell disease.

Incidence and Demographics

- Present in about 1 in 400 to 500 Black people; 8% to 10% carry hemoglobin S allele
- No gender predominance; onset in first year of life

Risk Factors

- Precipitate sickle cell crisis
  - Deoxygenation of Hemoglobin molecule, as in high altitude
  - Infection
  - Dehydration
  - Overexertion/stress
  - Exposure to extreme temperatures, hot or cold

Prevention and Screening

- Screening for sickle cell trait and genetic counseling for couples at risk; prenatal diagnosis via chorionic villus sampling or amniocentesis
- National Collegiate Athletic Association (NCAA) requires all college athletes to be screened for sickle cell trait.
- Universal newborn screening
- Good health maintenance with anticipatory guidance for potential complications
- All regular immunizations, as well as pneumococcal and influenza (yearly) vaccinations
- Recognition and avoidance of known pain-precipitating factors

Assessment

History

- Hemolytic anemia starting in first year of life
- Family history of sickle cell anemia or trait
- Trait may be asymptomatic unless provoked by exertion at high altitudes or dehydration
- Sickle cell anemia: acute, sudden, excruciating episodes with pain in long bones, back, chest, abdomen; priapism; chronic leg ulcers; delayed puberty

Physical Exam

- May include chronically ill appearance, jaundice
- Splenomegaly (primarily in children)
- Hot, tender, swollen joints
- Retinopathy
- Cardiomegaly (laterally displaced point of maximum impulse [PMI]), systolic murmur
- Chronic lower leg ulcers, blood loss

Diagnostic Studies

- Hemoglobin electrophoresis: definitive diagnostic test
- CBC: Classic findings (by age 1 year) include Hematocrit in the 20s, reticulocyte count in the 20s, normal MCV, slightly elevated white blood cell (WBC) count, and elevated platelet count.
- Peripheral blood smear: fragmented cells, long crescent-shaped irreversible sickled cells, target cells, Howell-Jolly bodies, and occasional nucleated red blood cells
- Elevated LDH and indirect bilirubin during increased hemolysis
- Laboratory results: Hemoglobin decreased, MCV might be elevated slightly, chronic neutrophilia, increased platelet count, erythrocytes with classic sickle shape on peripheral smear, Hemoglobin S predominates

Differential Diagnosis

- Other hemoglobinopathies (e.g., Hemoglobin C, D, or E)
- Compound hemoglobinopathies (e.g., HbSC disease, HbS beta-thalassemia)

Management

Nonpharmacologic Treatment

- Hydration, nonpharmacologic pain modalities, patient and family education and supportive care, genetic counseling

Pharmacologic Treatment

- Hydroxyurea 500 to 750 mg daily may decrease number of painful crises.
- Do not give iron (increases HemoglobinS production).
- Manage pain (often narcotic analgesia will be needed).
- Folic acid 1 to 2 mg orally daily
- Oxygen for hypoxia
- Consider transfusion.
- Penicillin prophylaxis in childhood

How Long to Treat

- Lifelong

Special Considerations

- Individuals have different patterns of crisis.
- Crises might increase during pregnancy.

When to Consult, Refer, Hospitalize

- Refer all suspected cases to a hematologist; hospitalize for acute episodes of sickling.
- Consult with physician for specialized care in the primary care setting.
- Any temperature above 38.5°C (101.3°F) must be considered a medical emergency and hospitalized immediately.

Follow-Up

Expected Course

- Number of crises decrease in young adulthood, but complications increase.
- Life expectancy is 60 years.

Complications

- Anemia, bone infarct, cerebrovascular accident (CVA), cardiac enlargement, priapism, retinopathy, acute chest syndrome, infections, gallstones, hemosiderosis (secondary to multiple transfusions), increased fetal loss during pregnancy, sepsis

THALASSEMIA

Description

- A group of hereditary disorders with hypochromic microcytic anemia because of gene deletion or point mutation; causes abnormal synthesis of alpha- and beta-globin chains, resulting in abnormal Hemoglobin synthesis and displacement of Hemoglobin A1 with abnormal types. Microcytosis is out of proportion to the degree of anemia.

Etiology

- Autosomal recessive genetic disorder producing defective hemoglobinization of RBCs. Normal adult hemoglobin, Hemoglobin A, has four chains or globins, two alpha and two beta. Delta and gamma chains are similar to beta and are found in Hemoglobin A2 (two gamma, two delta chains) and Hemoglobin F (fetal Hemoglobin, two delta and two gamma chains). Hemoglobin cannot be formed without the alpha chains; unaffected individuals have four copies of gene for alpha globin.
- Alpha-thalassemia is a result of a gene deletion where not enough alpha chains can be synthesized.
- Beta-thalassemia results when point mutation causes decreased or no synthesis of beta chains.
- Thalassemia major (beta) occurs when unbalanced Hemoglobin chain synthesis results in severe anemia (usually presents in infants or young children).
- Thalassemia intermedia is a more minor form of beta-thalassemia; may or may not need transfusions.
- Thalassemia trait (alpha or beta) is a milder form of anemia, not requiring aggressive therapy.

Incidence and Demographics

- Alpha-thalassemia: people originating from Southeast Asia, China, and occasionally Africa
- Beta-thalassemia: people originating from the Mediterranean, less commonly, Asia and Africa; about 1,000 patients with severe thalassemia in the United States
- Trait present in 3% to 5% of at-risk populations

Risk Factors

- One or both parents with any combination of alpha- and beta-thalassemia syndromes, or both

Prevention and Screening

- Screening of prospective parents at risk (ideally before pregnancy), genetic counseling
- Prenatal diagnosis (fetal blood sampling or chorionic villus sampling) if desired

Assessment

History

- Alpha trait (one of four alpha genes affected) usually asymptomatic; alpha-thalassemia minor (two of four alpha genes affected) and beta-thalassemia (heterozygous form) are mild forms, usually asymptomatic; beta-thalassemia major (Cooley's anemia—both genes affected): easy fatigability, palpitations, shortness of breath with exertion, headaches
- Family or personal history of lifelong anemia
- Infants and children with thalassemia major will have symptoms of severe and chronic anemia: pallor, shortness of breath, and lethargy.
- Children and adults with thalassemia trait may present with history of unresponsive anemia or signs of iron toxicity.

Physical Exam

- Normal exam in thalassemia minor syndromes
- Pallor and enlarged spleen in alpha-thalassemia with one alpha-globin gene (also called Hemoglobin H disease)
- Multiple abnormalities in thalassemia major (homozygous beta-thalassemia) starting in infancy: bony deformities, jaundice, enlarged spleen, and enlarged liver

Diagnostic Studies

See Table 16–4

- CBC with attention to RBC morphology and hemoglobin electrophoresis, iron studies
- Laboratory results: microcytic, hypochromic, acanthocytes, target cells, serum iron and TIBC normal to increased, serum ferritin above 100

TABLE 16–4.
DIAGNOSTIC STUDIES USED IN THALASSEMIA

DIAGNOSTIC STUDIES	FINDINGS
Alpha-thalassemia trait	Hematocrit 28% to 40% Very low MCV (60 to 75 μg/mL) Reticulocyte count normal Iron parameters normal Mild anemia; significant microcytosis
Alpha-thalassemia minor and beta-thalassemia minor	Hematocrit 28% to 40% MCV 55 to 75 μg/mL Reticulocyte count normal or slightly elevated Iron parameters normal Hemoglobin electrophoresis shows elevation Hemoglobin A2 to 4% to 8% and occasional Hemoglobin F to 1% to 5%
Beta-thalassemia major	Hematocrit 10% MCV below 75 μg/mL Peripheral blood smear: severe poikilocytoses, hypochromia, basophilic stippling, and nucleated red blood cells; virtually no Hemoglobin A present; major Hemoglobin present in Hemoglobin F
Hemoglobin H disease	Hematocrit 22% to 32% MCV below 7 μg/mL Peripheral blood smear markedly abnormal: hypochromia, microcytosis, poikilocytosis Reticulocyte count elevated Hemoglobin electrophoresis shows Hemoglobin H as 10% to 40% of Hemoglobin

Differential Diagnosis

- Iron-deficiency anemia
- Combined hemoglobinopathies

Management

- No treatment needed for beta-thalassemia minor or alpha-thalassemia trait

Nonpharmacologic Treatment

- Severe thalassemia major: regular transfusions, bone marrow transplants in children, splenectomy if needed, patient and family education and supportive care

Pharmacologic Treatment

- Folic acid supplementation
- Iron chelation therapy with deferoxamine (Desferal)
- Appropriate immunizations (especially if splenectomy contemplated)
- Avoid iron supplements and iron-fortified foods; avoid oxidative drugs (e.g., sulfonamides).

How Long to Treat

- Lifelong

Special Considerations

- Support for family, as coping with guilt is a major problem for parents

When to Consult, Refer, Hospitalize

- Consult or refer when diagnosis is in question; refer all patients with thalassemia major or intermedia to hematologist, hospitalize for complications. Refer all patients with severe disease to specialty clinics experienced in iron chelation and transfusions.

Follow-Up

- Depends on severity of disease

Expected Course

- Thalassemia minor: benign
- Thalassemia intermedia: patients have chronic hemolytic anemia but will generally only need transfusions when under stress; live into adulthood

- Children with thalassemia major die in their teens or when even younger unless they receive regular transfusions and iron chelation therapy; with compliance, live well into adulthood

Complications

- Limited growth and bony deformities; iron overload (due to frequent transfusions), which can cause cirrhosis, diabetes, cardiac dysfunction (including arrhythmia); failure of sexual maturation; decreased life expectancy

GLUCOSE-6-PHOSPHATE DEHYDROGENASE (G6PD) DEFICIENCY

Description

- An anemia of RBC destruction (hemolysis), occurring suddenly and episodically when RBCs are under oxidative stress from acute illness or certain medications

Etiology

- Most common form of G6PD deficiency is an X-linked, recessive hereditary enzyme defect
- Lack of enzyme leaves RBCs vulnerable to attack, causing hemolysis
- Can result in neonatal hyperbilirubinemia

Incidence and Demographics

- Seen in Black people and those of Mediterranean descent
- 7% to 15% of Black males affected
- Mediterranean variant less common but poses more severe deficiency of G6PD

Risk Factors

- Episode of hemolysis may be provoked by infection; oxidant drugs, such as certain antibiotics (e.g., dapsone, nalidixic acid, nitrofurantoin, sulfonamides), antimalarials (e.g., primaquine, quinine), phenazopyridine, doxorubicin, quinidine, and others; ingestion of fava beans

Prevention and Screening

- Immunizations (influenza, pneumococcal pneumonia, hepatitis B) and measures to avoid infections
- Avoidance of known oxidant drugs
- Family and genetic counseling as indicated
- Avoidance of specific drugs listed in Box 16–1, stress, and fava beans

Assessment

History

- Family history, medication history for oxidative drugs
- May be no history of anemia or anemia is mild so patient may only have symptoms of the acute infection

Physical Exam

- Signs of mild anemia, signs of underlying infection
- Splenomegaly may be present.

BOX 16–1.
SUBSTANCES FOR PEOPLE WITH G6PD DEFICIENCY TO AVOID

ANALGESICS	ANTIMALARIALS	ANTIBIOTICS ANTIHELMINTHS	ILLNESS	OTHER
Aspirin	Primaquine	Sulfonamides B Naphthol	Diabetic ketoacidosis	Vitamin K (okay in the newborn)
Phenacetin	Chloroquine	Sulfonamides Stibophen	Hepatitis	Probenecid
	Quinacrine	Chloramphenicol Niridazole	Other	Dimercaprol (BAL)
	Pamaquine	Dapsone		Fava beans
		Nitrofurans (Macrodantin)		Mothballs (naphthalene)
		Nalidixic acid		Methylene blue
				Henna

Diagnostic Studies

- CBC, reticulocytes, indirect bilirubin, G6PD
- In infants, direct and indirect Coombs test should be done to exclude autoimmune hemolytic anemia.
- Usual laboratory results: CBC normal between episodes, along with Heinz bodies and low level of G6PD; during episodes of hemolysis, there are increased reticulocytes, increased indirect bilirubin, decreased RBC, decreased Hemoglobin, decreased Hematocrit.

Differential Diagnosis

- Suspect Mediterranean variant if anemia is severe
- Iron-deficiency anemia
- Combined anemias (e.g., G6PD deficiency and sickle cell anemia)
- Acute hemolytic transfusion reactions (Coombs positive)

Management

- Supportive
- Find and eliminate anemia trigger

Special Considerations

- Anemic episodes are self-limiting.

When to Consult, Refer, Hospitalize

- Refer severe variants with exacerbations; refer patients with combined anemias

Follow-Up

- For exacerbations

Expected Course

- There is usually a spontaneous resolution of the anemia as older RBCs with minimal enzyme activity are destroyed and then replaced with new RBCs that have enough (even though reduced) enzyme activity.

Complications

- Generally none
- Possible severe hemolytic anemia and death with the Mediterranean variant

IMMUNE HEMOLYSIS

Description

- RBC destruction occurs because of the binding of antibodies or complement components to the erythrocyte membrane. This may occur as a result of autoimmunization, alloimmunization, or drug reactions.
- Warm-reacting antibodies hemolyze optimally at 37°C.
- Cold-reacting antibodies hemolyze optimally at 30°C.

Etiology

- Immune globulin M (IgM) (cold) and IgG (warm) antibodies induce RBC destruction after binding with antigens on the RBC wall. This binding causes a complementary cascade resulting in defective RBCs, which are prematurely removed and destroyed by hepatic macrophages.

Incidence and Demographics

- Seen in all races and in all age groups
- Warm agglutinin disease associated with neoplastic or collagen vascular disorder in 40% of the cases
- Cold agglutinin disease seen in patients with lymphoproliferative disorders, infectious diseases (Epstein-Barr virus [EBV], cytomegalovirus [CMV]), and in older adults; usually a diagnosis of exclusion

Risk Factors

- SLE, rheumatoid arthritis
- Adenocarcinoma of the stomach, ovarian teratoma, chronic lymphocytic leukemia

Prevention and Screening

- Screening of prospective parents at risk (ideally before pregnancy), genetic counseling

Assessment

History

- Family or personal history of any of the above states
- Acute episodes may present with dizziness, exertional dyspnea, palpitations, and fatigue.

Physical Exam

- In warm agglutinin disease, chronic effects are mild and may present with jaundice and/or splenomegaly; acute episodes may present with pallor in addition to above symptoms.
- In cold agglutinin disease secondary to infections, symptoms are short-lived and mild in most cases. In disease associated with neoplastic or idiopathic disorders, exposure to cold may lead to severe acrocyanosis and Raynaud's-type reactions worsened by cold.

Diagnostic Studies

- CBC with attention to RBC morphology; spherocytosis dramatically increased
- In cold agglutinin disease, blood clots at times upon being removed from the vein, distorting the RBC count, MCV, and Hematocrit. Serum haptoglobin is decreased and LDH is increased.

Differential Diagnosis

- Thalassemia
- Sickle cell disease
- Paroxysmal nocturnal hemoglobinuria
- Hypersplenism

Management

- Warm agglutinin disease
  - Glucocorticoids
  - Splenectomy
  - Immunosuppressive drugs: cyclophosphamide, azathioprine
  - Transfusion
- Cold agglutinin disease
  - Identify and treat underlying cause
  - Chlorambucil (Leukeran) 2–4 mg, up to 10 mg daily
  - Advise move to a warmer climate
  - Avoid transfusions; when needed, infuse warmed, well-matched products

Special Considerations

- None

When to Consult, Refer, Hospitalize

- Consult with physician or refer to hematologist for acute episodes.

Follow-Up

Expected Course

- Warm agglutinin disease is usually chronic, so prognosis is affected by the underlying disease.

- If cold agglutinin disease is related to an infectious syndrome, complete cure occurs when the infection is cleared; otherwise, course is similar to warm agglutinin disease.

Complications

- Major cause of death related to a thromboembolic event

Other Problems of Iron and Red Blood Cells

HEMOCHROMATOSIS

Description

- An autosomal recessive inherited disorder, resulting in an excess of iron stores in the liver, pancreas, heart, kidneys, adrenals, testes, and pituitary gland as hemosiderin

Etiology

- Disorder resulting in inefficient erythropoiesis
- Most common iron storage and genetic liver disease in the United States

Incidence and Demographics

- 3 per 1,000 in the United States
- Seen in men more than women
- Presentation in men 40 years of age and over and in women 60 years of age and over

Risk Factors

- Alcohol ingestion, iron supplementation, chronic transfusions, ingestion of large amounts of vitamin C
- Type 2 diabetes, thalassemia

Prevention and Screening

- Genetic counseling
- Screening of family members of patient with hereditary hemochromatosis

Assessment

History

- Often asymptomatic
- Weakness, dyspnea on exertion, lassitude, weight loss
- Loss of libido, impotence, testicular atrophy, amenorrhea
- Slate or brown-colored skin, alopecia
- Abdominal pain

Physical Exam

- Hepatosplenomegaly, ascites, cardiomyopathy, peripheral edema, arthropathy
- Changes in skin pigmentation: slate-gray or brown

Diagnostic Studies

- Liver biopsy is the diagnostic gold standard.
- Laboratory results: blood glucose elevated, aspartate aminotransferase (AST) increased, serum albumin decreased, follicular-stimulating hormone (FSH) and luteinizing hormone (LH) decreased, serum ferritin above 300 U/L for men and above 200 U/L for women, transferrin saturation high, urinary iron present

Differential Diagnosis

- Cirrhosis
- Excessive iron ingestion
- Repeated transfusions

Management

Nonpharmacologic Treatment

- Regular diet, avoid iron-fortified foods and iron supplements, increase tea intake (chelates iron), restrict vitamin C to small amounts between meals
- Phlebotomy of 500 mL initially 1 to 2 times/week until mild anemia, then 4 to 6 times/year maintenance

Pharmacologic Treatment

- Use iron-chelating agent only if phlebotomy is not feasible or diagnosis is secondary hemochromatosis.

How Long to Treat

- Initially until patient is iron deficient (mild anemia), then lifelong maintenance therapy

Special Considerations

- Menstruation delays onset of symptoms in women.
- Problem uncommon in people with African or Asian heritage.

When to Consult, Refer, Hospitalize

- Refer to hematologist to confirm initial diagnosis and consult throughout therapy; hematology office or infusion center for phlebotomy.

Follow-Up

Expected Course

- Usually normal life expectancy; if more than 18 months needed to achieve mild anemia, life expectancy is decreased

Complications

- Cirrhosis, type 1 diabetes, hepatocellular carcinoma, arthritis, cardiomyopathy

POLYCYTHEMIA VERA

Description

- Chronic, acquired myeloproliferative disorder showing overproduction of RBC mass, resulting in an elevation in Hematocrit and RBC mass (males, Hematocrit above 51%; females, Hematocrit above 48%)

Etiology

- As a primary disorder, it is a hematologic malignancy with excessive erythroid, myeloid, and megakaryocytic elements in the bone marrow.
- Secondary causes are lung disease, heart disease, kidney disease, and possible other malignancies.

Incidence and Demographics

- Prevalence is 1–3 per 100,000.
- Most common in newborn or persons 60 years of age or older

Risk Factors

- More prevalent in people of Ashkenazi Jewish ancestry
- Smoking
- Age, 60 years of age or older

Prevention and Screening

- Cannot prevent onset
- No routine screening currently recommended

- Often found as a result of blood studies performed for other reasons
- Advise patients to seek medical attention for onset of headache; dizziness; blurred vision; tinnitus; vertigo; spontaneous bruising; menorrhagia; peripheral cyanosis; epistaxis; upper GI bleed; pruritus, especially after bathing; rib and sternal bone pain/tenderness; sweating; weight loss; and/or fatigue.

Assessment

History

- Might be no symptoms in early stages or only vague symptoms
- Headache, dizziness, blurred vision, tinnitus, vertigo
- Spontaneous bruising, menorrhagia, peripheral cyanosis, epistaxis, upper GI bleed
- Pruritus, especially after bathing
- Rib and sternal bone pain/tenderness
- Sweating, weight loss, fatigue

Physical Exam

- Plethora (reddish flush of skin) on face, hands, feet
- Elevated systolic blood pressure, epistaxis, distended retinal veins
- Hepatosplenomegaly
- Complete exam to look for underlying cause

Diagnostic Studies

- CBC with differential, serum B12, chemistries, indirect bilirubin, bone marrow aspiration, CT for underlying malignancy
- Laboratory results: increased Hemoglobin and Hematocrit, thrombocytosis, leukocytosis, increased leukocyte alkaline phosphatase, increased serum vitamin B12, indirect bilirubin elevated

Differential Diagnosis

- Secondary polycythemia
- Secondary erythrocytosis
- Spurious polycythemia
- Hemoglobinopathy

Management

Nonpharmacologic Treatment

- Phlebotomy to remove 500 mL weekly until hematocrit 45%; patient/family education and support

Pharmacologic Treatment

- Medications for hyperacidity, pruritus, uric acid reduction as needed
- Hydroxyurea—a myelosuppressive agent—may be used.

How Long to Treat

- Lifelong

Special Considerations

- Phlebotomy worsens iron deficiency, but iron supplement not recommended
- Benign polycythemia caused by high-altitude dwelling

When to Consult, Refer, Hospitalize

- Refer to hematologist for management.

Follow-Up

Expected Course

- Survival with treatment is up to 10 years; without is 6 to 18 months

Complications

- Vascular thrombosis, leukemia, hemorrhage, peptic ulcer, gout

White Blood Cell (WBC)–Related Problems

LEUKEMIAS

Description

- A collection of disorders that produce a variety of bone marrow and WBC abnormalities that may be quickly fatal or may remain asymptomatic for years
- Types include:
  - Malignant proliferation of immature lymphocytes (acute lymphocytic leukemia [ALL]) or myeloid cells (acute myeloid leukemia: AML; acute nonlymphocytic leukemia: ANLL)
  - Proliferation of mature-appearing neoplastic lymphocytes (chronic lymphocytic leukemia: CLL) or immature granulocytes (chronic myeloid leukemia: CML)
  - Rarely: proliferation of mature B cells with prominent projections (hairy cell leukemia)

Etiology

- Unknown malignancy that affects the bone marrow and other organs; may be due to exposure to chemicals and/or ionizing radiation, genetic factors (chromosomal abnormalities), or viral agents
- Commonly see elevated WBC count, abnormal WBCs on blood smear, bone marrow failure, and involvement of other organs

Incidence and Demographics

- ALL: most common childhood malignancy with peak incidence between 2 and 10 years of age, most common in White people and boys, higher incidence in industrialized countries; adult ALL approximately 100 cases/year in the United States
- AML or ANLL: Most common type of acute leukemia in adults 50% of cases under age 50
- CLL: most common form of chronic adult leukemia in developed countries, occurring during middle age and in older adults
- CML: middle age most common sixth and seventh decades
- Hairy cell leukemia: rare, disease of old age

Risk Factors

- Several immunodeficiency states have an associated risk for lymphoma and leukemia in children (Wiskott-Aldrich, X-linked agammaglobulinemia, severe combined immune deficiency, and ataxia telangiectasia).
- Chemical and/or radiation exposure
- Chromosomal abnormalities
- Cigarette smoking
- Some types increase with age.

Prevention and Screening

- Currently there is no standard screening process to detect early stages of leukemia.
- There is no way to prevent leukemia, but an individual can make lifestyle changes to lower risk.
- Educate patients to report new onset of symptoms early.
- Patients with family histories of leukemia should have regular physical examinations.
- Patients who have been treated with chemotherapy for other types of cancers should have regular physical examinations.
- Avoid exposure to chemicals such as benzene.
- Quit smoking or do not start.

Assessment

- See table 16-5 for key assessments for leukemias

Differential Diagnosis

- Aplastic anemia
- Viral diseases
- Mononucleosis
- Pertussis
- Paroxysmal nocturnal hemoglobinuria
- Gaucher's disease
- Myelodysplasia syndromes

Management

Nonpharmacologic Treatment

- Good diet, compliance with treatment, management of side effects, chronic effects of diagnosis
- Avoid activities that might cause injury; avoid medications that affect platelets (e.g., aspirin).
- Bone marrow transplantation

Pharmacologic Treatment

- Chemotherapy, infection prevention medications
- Hospitalization required for induction of chemotherapy
- Tyrosine kinase inhibitor (TKI) therapy for CML

How Long to Treat

- Goal is remission

TABLE 16–5.
LEUKEMIA COMPARISON

	ALL	AML	CLL	CML
History	Joint pain Limping Infection	Sternal tenderness	Maybe asymptomatic Dyspnea on exertion	Maybe asymptomatic Night sweats Blurred vision Respiratory distress Sternal tenderness
Physical Exam	Lymphadenopathy Hepatosplenomegaly Petechiae Purpura	Hepatosplenomegaly Bruising Pallor	Lympadenopathy Hepatosplenomegaly	Lympadenopathy Splenomegaly Priapism
Key Diagnostic findings	Peripheral blood lymphoblasts		Sustained absolute lymphocytosis Bone marrow + lymphocytes	Philadelphia chromosome in bone marrow

Special Considerations

- Children with ALL may benefit from referral to specialty centers involved in clinical trials.
- Patients with leukemia are prone to other infections.

When to Consult, Refer, Hospitalize

- Refer to hematologist upon suspicion of diagnosis and have followed by hematologist throughout therapy.

Follow-Up

Expected course

- ALL: Remission rate is very good.
- AML: Remission rate is 60% to 80%.
- CLL: Depends on stage at diagnosis; median survival about 9 years
- CML: Usually transforms into the acute phase within 2 years; then poor survival rate
- Patients who have undergone stem cell transplantation have a 10-year survival rate of 70%.

Complications

- Infections, bleeding, side effects of chemotherapy and/or radiation, relapses

Coagulation Disorders

IDIOPATHIC THROMBOCYTOPENIA PURPURA (ITP)

Description

- An autoimmune disorder characterized by accelerated, spleen-mediated platelet destruction, resulting in a decreased platelet count (below 100,000/mL) that predisposes the patient to a decreased ability for primary clotting. May be acute (with spontaneous resolution within 2 months after an acute infection—usually children) or chronic (persists 6 months or more without identifiable cause—usually adults). IgG autoantibody binds to platelets; splenic macrophages bind to antibody-tagged platelets and destroy them.

Etiology

- Unknown, perhaps autoimmune response after viral illness

Incidence and Demographics

- Occurs predominantly in pediatric population; uncommon in geriatric population
- Slight seasonal peaks in winter and spring
- Adult female-to-male ratio is 3:1; most common acquired platelet disorder of childhood

Risk Factors

- No genetic predispositions described
- Acute infection (usually viral; e.g., varicella, EBV, CMV), HIV, cardiopulmonary bypass, hypersplenism, preeclampsia
- Exposure to drugs with antiplatelet effects (aspirin, seizure medications, heparin)
- History of autoimmune diseases (rheumatoid or collagen vascular symptoms, thyroid disease, hemolytic anemia)

Prevention and Screening

- None

Assessment

History

- Insidious onset in otherwise well person
- Prolonged purpura, bruising tendency, gingival bleeding, menorrhagia, epistaxis, petechiae
- History of acute viral illness

Physical Exam

- Nonpalpable spleen is essential criterion
- Signs of GI bleeding, dysmorphic features

Diagnostic Studies

- Often diagnosed on routine CBC with differential and platelets; also get peripheral smear; consider HIV, liver function, CT abdomen, stool guaiac as needed
- Laboratory results: platelets decreased, normal RBC and WBC morphology

Differential Diagnosis

- Viral infection
- SLE
- Bone marrow disorders
- AIDS
- Drug-induced
- Hemolytic-uremic syndrome
- Liver disease
- Congenital thrombocytopenia (e.g., Fanconi's syndrome)
- Sepsis

Management

Nonpharmacologic Treatment

- Education and supportive care
- Avoid medications that increase bleeding risk.
- Decrease activities that might cause bruising and injury.
- Monitor patient for platelet count and associated symptoms.

Pharmacologic Treatment

- Acute: prednisone 1 to 2 mg/kg once a day for 4 weeks, then taper
- Chronic: 60 mg/day for 4 to 6 weeks, then taper
- Severe: IV gamma globulin (IVGG) 0.4 g/kg/day for 3 to 5 days or high-dose parenteral glucocorticoids
- Platelet transfusion only during life-threatening hemorrhage
- Splenectomy if platelets below 30,000 mcL after 6 weeks of pharmacologic treatment (splenectomy response not good if IVGG response poor)

How Long to Treat

- Until remission

Special Considerations

- Focus: bleeding, exclusion of other diagnoses

When to Consult, Refer, Hospitalize

- Any febrile child with thrombocytopenia and petechiae (with or without elevated prothrombin time [PT] and PTT) should be hospitalized and treated for presumed sepsis.
- Refer all suspected cases to hematologist; refer to surgeon for splenectomy.

Follow-Up

Expected Course

- Acute is 80% to 85% remission, 15% become chronic; chronic is 20% spontaneous remission

Complications

- Cerebral hemorrhage (1% mortality); other blood loss, pneumococcal infection

THROMBOTIC THROMBOCYTOPENIC PURPURA (TTP)

Description

- Considered a medical emergency due to systemic thrombosis
- Can be either congenital or acquired
- Primarily occurs acutely in adults (approximately 90%)
- Results in end-organ damage
- High mortality rate if not diagnosed in a timely manner
- If treated in a timely manner, survival rates up to 90%
- Rare; therefore clinical observation is imperative for making the diagnosis
- Women more than men
- Characterized by schistocytes on peripheral blood smear (hallmark finding)

Etiology

- Caused by deficient von Willebrand factor–cleaving protease (VWFCP) or ADAMTS13 activity (if less than 10% activity confirms diagnosis of TTP)
- Primarily considered an autoimmune etiology
- IgG antibodies are higher in proportion to ADAMTS13.
- Acquired thrombotic thrombocytopenic purpura (acquired TTP)
- Congenital TTP (Upshaw–Schulman syndrome)
- Pregnancy as trigger for acquired or congenital TTP

Other Thrombotic Microangiopathies (TMAs)

- Diarrhea-associated (Shiga toxin–induced) hemolytic uremic syndrome
- Atypical hemolytic uremic syndrome (aHUS)
- Pregnancy-associated TMAs
  - HELLP syndrome (hemolysis, elevated liver enzymes, and low platelets)
- Drug-induced TMAs
  - Thienopyridines (ticlopidine and clopidogrel)
  - Calcineurin inhibitors (cyclosporine and tacrolimus)

  - ◊ Mammalian target of rapamycin (mTOR) inhibitors (sirolimus and everolimus)
  - ◊ Antineoplastic agents (mitomycin and gemcitabine)
  - ◊ Quinine
- ♦ TMA after organ transplantation
  - ◊ Renal transplantation
  - ◊ Lung transplantation
  - ◊ Allogeneic hematopoietic stem cell transplantation

ASSESSMENT

History

- ♦ Bleeding history (nose bleeds, dark tarry stools, hematuria)
- ♦ Neurological changes (e.g., headaches, confusion, dizziness)
- ♦ Fatigue
- ♦ Abdominal pain

Physical

- ♦ Pallor
- ♦ Fever
- ♦ Petechiae
- ♦ Melena
- ♦ Hematuria
- ♦ Confusion
- ♦ Jaundice
- ♦ Diarrhea
- ♦ Thrombocytopenia
- ♦ Schistocytes on peripheral smear (hallmark)
- ♦ Normal coagulation studies
- ♦ High reticulocyte count
- ♦ Low to absent haptoglobin

- Coombs-negative hemolysis
- Elevated LDH

Diagnostics for Consideration Depending on Symptoms

- If suspicion of TTP, then emergent hematology referral is warranted.

Management

- Specialist referral and management for all TMAs
- TTP management includes:
  - ◊ Plasma exchange
  - ◊ Corticosteroids
  - ◊ Hemodialysis

When to Refer Consult

- Prompt referral to hematology—TTP (or other TMAs) is considered a medical emergency.

Follow-up

- Hematology follow-up is necessary.

Expected

- Relapse is common.
- Hematology follow-up is imperative.

Complications

- Microvascular thrombi affecting target organs (i.e., brain, kidneys, heart, and lungs)
- Death

CASE STUDIES

CASE 1

L.O. is a 9-month-old brought to the clinic by mother for a routine well-child checkup. L.O.'s mother states that all is going well. L.O. lives at home with mother, father, and maternal grandmother, who cares for L.O. while the parents are at work. Diet consists of table food and drinking cow's milk.

PAST MEDICAL HISTORY: Immunizations are up to date; no illnesses requiring antibiotics. Current medications: none.

Exam: This is a very plump infant who is interactive with mother and the examiner. Vital signs are within normal limits. Weight is in the 95th percentile for age, but height is in the 50th percentile. In your office setting, you obtain an Hemoglobin level, which is 9 g/dL.

1. What additional history would you like?
2. What type of anemia is most likely in this case?
3. What is the most likely cause of L.O.'s anemia?
4. What corrective actions might you recommend at this time?

CASE 2

B.C. is a 48-year-old woman who presents to your clinic complaining of feeling tired all the time. She works full time and cares for older adults, mother in the home. B.C. reports "getting plenty of sleep and eating well." B.C. finds little time for exercise and "doesn't have the energy to even go for a walk." Review of systems (ROS): pertinent only for heavy bleeding during menstrual cycle, which began about 8 months ago. B.C. reports having to stay close to home and using a hand towel to supplement peri-pads.

Past Medical History: Denies any hospitalizations or surgeries. Anemia during pregnancy. Last menstrual history (LMP): 1 week before clinic visit. Otherwise healthy; does not smoke or drink alcohol.

1. What type of physical exam would you do?
2. At this point, what might you include in your differential diagnosis?
3. What diagnostic studies would you order?

   Test results: Hemoglobin: 10 g/dL; RBC: 3.6; MCV: 72; TSH: 1.56 (normal)

4. What would your recommendations be for B.C. at this point?

CASE 3

B.W., an 85-year-old person, is brought to clinic by the patient's daughter for evaluation of possible dementia. B.W.'s daughter is worried that the patient is unable to perform self-care, as evidenced by the fact that B.W. forgets the car at church some Sundays and walks home, and by the apparent weight loss. B.W.'s daughter is concerned the patient cannot prepare meals anymore.

Past medical history: Hypertension—controlled; bladder irritability responsive to medication. No known drug allergies, currently taking enalapril (Vasotec) 5 mg once a day, oxybutynin (Ditropan) 5 mg once a day

Social history: B.W. lives alone home, one block from the church. A neighbor on the block assists with paying the bills, going to doctor's appointments, and getting medication refills. B.W. reports being able to fix meals and denies feeling hungry.

Review of systems: Denies shortness of breath, chest pain, anorexia; admits to weight loss. Denies bowel changes. Does have some trouble remembering things but has always been able to find the car because the only place the car is used for is to go to church.

1. What would you include in your differential diagnosis at this time?

   Exam: Alert, well-dressed 85-year-old who looks younger than stated age. Vital signs are WNL. Scores 27 on the MMSE. Cranial nerves II–XII are intact. Patient ambulates without assistance. Romberg's intact; no evidence of ataxia. No lymphadenopathy. Lungs are clear without adventitious breath sounds. Heart: regular rate and rhythm without murmur or gallop. Abdominal: no distention, bowel sounds positive. No palpable masses. No hepatosplenomegaly or costovertebral angle tenderness (CVAT). Genital exam: WNL. Rectal exam: normal size prostate, enlarged without nodules. Stool is brown and heme negative.

2. What diagnostic studies would you order at this time?

   B.W. returns 1 week later and has the following laboratory results: Hemoglobin: 9 g/dL; Hematocrit: 27.2%; MCV: 72; reported as hypochromic; all other parameters are WNL. He has lost 2 more pounds, even though B.W.'s daughter has been cooking and encouraging B.W. to eat. Fecal occult blood tests (FOBTs) are all positive.

3. What type of anemia does this person most likely have and what would be the next step in your diagnostic workup of this patient?

CASE STUDIES DISCUSSION

CASE 1

1. What additional history would you like?

   Diet recall, any pica, family history of anemia, any gastrointestinal ailments

2. What type of anemia is most likely in this case? Iron-deficiency anemia

3. What is the most likely cause of L.O.'s anemia?

   Inadequate dietary intake of iron due to intake of cow's milk before 12 months of age and onset of rapid growth

4. What corrective actions might you recommend at this time?

   Parental education about appropriate diet for age, referral to nutritional assistance program if needed, consider vitamin with iron supplement, follow-up in one month and then monitor at well child exams

CASE 2

1. What type of physical exam would you do?

   General appearance, presence of cyanosis or pallor, vital signs, thyroid exam, neurological exam, breath sounds, cardiac auscultation, abdominal exam, pelvic exam, rectal exam for occult blood

2. At this point, what might you include in your differential diagnosis?

   Anemia due to blood loss, hypothyroidism, fatigue due to depression (related to caregiver burden)

3. What diagnostic studies would you order?

   CBC, TSH, chemistry panel; consider lipid panel, ECG

4. What would your recommendations be for B.C. at this point?

   Iron supplementation to treat iron-deficiency anemia due to heavy periods. Consider additional laboratory studies such as serum iron, ferritin, TIBC. Workup or referral for menorrhagia. Offer support for caregiver burden. Follow-up monthly until corrected.

CASE 3

1. What would you include in your differential diagnosis at this time?

   Dementia due to Alzheimer's disease or multi-infarct dementia; reversible causes of dementia such as vitamin B12 deficiency; depression; occult malignancy; sensory deficits

2. What diagnostic studies would you order at this time?

   CBC, chemistry panel, TSH, B12 and folate levels, rapid plasma reagin (RPR) and prostrate specific antigen (PSA), FOBT × 3

3. What type of anemia does this man most likely have and what would be the next step in your diagnostic workup of this gentleman?

   Iron-deficiency anemia, probably due to blood loss. You urgently refer the patient to a surgeon or gastrointestinal specialist for colonoscopy and order iron-replacement therapy. You caution the patient to gradually increase the iron pills to three a day between meals and increase fluids and fiber to prevent constipation.

REFERENCES

Atkins, J. L., Pilling, L. C., Masoli, J. A., Kuo, C., Jeremy D Shearman, J. D., Paul C Adams, P. C., Melzer, D. . (2020) Association of hemochromatosis HFE C282Y homozygosity with hepatic malignancy. *Journal of the American Medical Association*, 324, 2048.

Bajwa, H., & Basit, H. (2023). *Thalassemia*. In: StatPearls [Internet]. Treasure Island, FL: StatPearls Publishing LLC. www.ncbi.nlm.nih.gov/books/NBK545151/

Benevolo, G., Vassallo, F, Urbino, I., Giai, V. (2021). Polycythemia vera (PV): Update on emerging treatment options. *Therapeutics and Clinical Risk Management*, 17: 209–221. doi: 10.2147/TCRM.S213020

Brodsky, R. A. (2019). Warm autoimmune hemolytic anemia. *New England Journal of Medicine*, 381, 647.

Cooper, N., Kruse, A., Kruse, C., Watson, S., Morgan, M., rovan, D., Ghanima, W., Arnold, D. M., Tomiyama, Y., Santoro, C., Michel, M., Laborde, S., Lovrencic, B., Hou, M., Bailey, T., Taylor-Stokes, G., Haenig, J., and Bussel, J. B.. (2021). Immune thrombocytopenia (ITP) World Impact Survey (iWISh): Patient and physician perceptions of diagnosis, signs and symptoms, and treatment. *American Journal of Hematology*, 96, 188.

Ganz, T. (2019). Anemia of inflammation. *New England Journal of Medicine*, 381, 1148.

Gupta, P. M., Hamner, H. C., Suchdev, P. S., Flores-Ayala, R., Zuguo Mei, Z. (2017). Iron status of toddlers, nonpregnant females, and pregnant females in the United States. *American Journal of Clinical Nutrition*, 106, 1640S.

Kleinman, R. E., & Greer, F. R. (Eds.). (2019.) American Academy of Pediatrics Committee on Nutrition. Iron. *Pediatric nutrition*. (p. 56), Itasca, IL.

Luzzatto, L., Ally, M., & Notaro, R. (2020). Glucose-6-phosphate dehydrogenase deficiency. *Blood*, 136, 1225.

Means, R. T. (2020). Iron deficiency and iron deficiency anemia: Implications and impact in pregnancy, fetal development, and early childhood parameters. *Nutrients*, 12, 447.

Mohamed, M., Thio, J., Thomas, R. S., & Phillips, J. (2020) Pernicious anemia. *British Medical Journal*, 369, m1319

Onimoe, G., & Rotz, S. (2020). Sickle cell disease: A primary care update. *Cleveland Clinic Journal of Medicine*, *87*(1), 19–27. DOI: https://doi.org/10.3949/ccjm.87a.18051

Siddiqui, A., Journeycake, J. M., Borogovac, A., & George, J. N. (2021). Recognizing and managing hereditary and acquired thrombotic thrombocytopenic purpura in infants and children. *Pediatric Blood Cancer*, 68, e28949.

Skorochod, R., Shteingart, S., & Nesher, G. (2021). Incidence of inpatient folate deficiency and effect on overall in-hospital mortality. *American Journal of Medicine*, 134, e235.

Sukumar, N., & Saravanan, P. (2019). Investigating vitamin B12 deficiency. *British Medical Journal*, 365, l1865.

Vakiti, A., & Mewawalla, P. (2023). *Acute myeloid leukemia*. In: StatPearls [Internet]. Treasure Island, FL: StatPearls Publishing LLC. www.ncbi.nlm.nih.gov/books/NBK507875/

Weiss, G., Ganz, T., & Goodnough, L. T. (2018). Anemia of inflammation. *Blood*, 133, 40.

Young, N. S. (2018). Aplastic anemia. *New England Journal of Medicine*, 379, 1643.

CHAPTER 17

ENDOCRINE DISORDERS

Eileen Amari-Vaught, Ph.D., RN, MSN, FNP-BC

General Approach

DESCRIPTION

- Defects in aspects of the endocrine regulatory systems that can cause systemic consequences, morbidity, and death
- Endocrine disorders generally manifest in one of four ways:
  1. Excess hormone (e.g., Cushing syndrome, excess cortisol secretion)
  2. Deficit hormone (e.g., diabetes mellitus [DM] type 1; insulin secretion is low, resistant, or absent)
  3. Abnormal response of end organ to the hormone (e.g., pseudohypoparathroidism)
  4. Gland enlargement (e.g., pituitary adenoma)
- Endocrine diseases may be associated with a deficiency or hypersecretion of hormones that affect target organs.
- There are basically three types of hormone:
  1. *Steroids*, such as cortisol (adrenal cortex), estrogen, progesterone (ovaries), and testosterone (testes)
  2. *Amino acids*, such as tyrosine, thyroxine (thyroid), and catecholamines (adrenal medulla)
  3. *Protein peptides*, such as insulin (pancreas)
- Regulation of hormone secretion is through a negative feedback system.
- Patients of all ages may need to carry or wear MedicAlert or similar identification for many endocrine disorders.
- According to the CDC, a total of 37.3 million people in the United States have diabetes, comprising 11.3% of the population. 28.7 million people (28.5 million adults) are diagnosed, and 8.5 million individuals are undiagnosed. 96 million people age 18 and

over have pre-diabetes (38.0% of the U.S. population). 26.4% of the population over age 65 years have pre-diabetes.

- The American Diabetes Association (ADA) estimated the total costs of diagnosed diabetes rose to $327 billion in 2017 from $245 billion in 2012, when the cost was last examined. This is a 26% increase during this 5-year period (ADA, 2018).
- Approximately, 4 out of 10 adults who died from COVID-19 in the United States had diabetes (CDC, 2020).
- The family nurse practitioner (FNP) must consider normal physiologic changes occurring with growth, development, and aging when managing various endocrine diagnoses across the life span.
- The FNP must consider lifestyle management and certain risk factors, such as obesity, when caring for persons with endocrine diseases such as DM type 2.

RED FLAGS

- *Type 1 diabetes* may present with acute diabetic ketoacidosis: nausea, fatigue, weight loss, abdominal pain, polyuria, polydipsia, hunger, vomiting, confusion, lethargy, hypotension, fruity breath odor; symptoms generally acute and may be misdiagnosed as a viral infection.
- *Type 2 diabetes* may present with hyperglycemic, hyperosmolar syndrome (HHS), characterized by confusion and lethargy, blood glucose greater than 600 mg/dL, minimal ketosis, serum osmolality greater than 320, and profound dehydration. Mortality rate 5% to 20% (approximately 10 times the mortality rates seen in DKA), generally due to precipitating cause.
- Prediabetes generally starts 8 to 10 years before diagnosis, and macrovascular and microvascular changes may begin to occur.
- *Hypoglycemia* may present as adrenergic symptoms: hunger, sweating, shakiness, tremor, anxiety, irritability or neuroglycopenic symptoms: headache, slurred speech, confusion, difficulty problem-solving, behavior change; without treatment, can progress to coma, seizures, or death.
- *Thyroid nodules* are common, but less than 10% of solitary nodules are malignant.
- *Acute adrenal insufficiency* or Addisonian crisis may present as severe abdominal pain, nausea and vomiting, hypotension, hypoglycemia, and shock; precipitated by surgery, infection, exacerbation of comorbid illness, and sudden withdrawal of long-term glucocorticoid replacement.
- *Pituitary adenoma* may present as headache with impaired vision/diplopia, amenorrhea, or galactorrhea; obtain prolactin level and MRI of brain or CT with attention to sella turcica.

RISK FACTORS

- For malignancy, include family history of thyroid cancer or multiple endocrine metaplastic type 2 carcinoma; male gender; extremes in age (younger than 15 and older than 70); exposure to radiation of head, neck, or chest; single nodule.

Disorders of the Pancreas

DIABETES MELLITUSTYPE 1

Description

- Type 1 Diabetes (T1D) is syndrome produced by disorders in metabolism of carbohydrate, protein, and fat due to absolute lack of insulin resulting in hyperglycemia. Without insulin therapy, ketoacidosis occurs rapidly. Formerly called *insulin-dependent diabetes mellitus* (IDDM), juvenile-onset. Genetically susceptible persons develop autoimmune beta cell destruction in response to some unknown environmental triggers.

Etiology

- Destruction of beta cells in pancreatic islets and absolute deficiency and/or failure to produce insulin, related to autoimmune response or environmental trigger (e.g., virus)
- Human leukocyte antigens HLA, HLA-DR3, or HLA-DR4 associated with type 1
- May be triggered in susceptive persons by viruses, toxic chemical agents, or cytotoxins
- Genetic susceptibility influenced by environmental factors
- Hyperglycemia from inability of glucose to enter cell for use as energy
- Ketoacidosis from use of free fatty acids for energy

Incidence and Demographics

- Type 1 accounts for 5% to 10% of all diabetes cases in United States.
- Usually occurs in children and adolescents at puberty between ages 8 and 14; 45% present before 10 years old. Peak incidence between 10 and 14 years of age.
- Highest prevalence in Scandinavia, where 20% of people with diabetes are type 1; Japan and China less than 1%. Highest rates of DiabetesType 1 in the United States occur in states with a large Scandanavian population such as Minnesota.

- Can develop in adulthood, very rare in older adults
- Idiopathic etiology most common in persons of Asian or African descent

Risk Factors

- First-degree relative with type 1 diabetes mellitus: A child whose mother has T1D has a 3% risk of developing T1D and a 6% risk of developing T1D if the father has T1D.
- Other autoimmune disorders
- Inhibitor immunotherapies for advanced malignancy can precipitate autoimmune disease, including T1D.

Prevention and Screening

- No prevention and no routine screening in childhood; however, consider screening first degree relative (i.e., sibling) in research setting
- Breastfeeding in the first 6 months of life appears protective.

Assessment

History

- Acute onset of polyuria, polydipsia, polyphagia, weight loss, blurred vision, fatigue, abdominal pain, nausea/vomiting, vaginal itching/infections, unhealed wounds, skin infections/rashes, dehydration, hypoglycemic or ketotic episodes
- Nightmares, night sweats, or headache may indicate nocturnal hypoglycemia in both children and adults.
- Parent report of frequent diaper changes, bed-wetting, listlessness or fatigue, frequent sick days from school or day care, changes in school performance or behavior
- Pediatric patients: birth weight and history of complications at birth, health status at birth
- Family history of diabetes

Physical Exam

- Exam may be normal, or patient may be ill-looking with fruity odor to breath
- Weight loss, thin (children and adults) or failure to thrive (infants), signs of dehydration, orthostatic hypotension
- Presence of skin infections, oral or vaginal candidiasis (more common in type 2)
- Diabetic ketoacidosis: dehydration, labored breathing, confusion/disorientation, lethargy
- Signs of complications
  - Delayed sexual maturation (adolescents)
  - Late disease: ophthalmic changes—microaneurysm with soft and hard exudates; deep retinal hemorrhages, neovascularization, cataracts, glaucoma; peripheral vascular insufficiency; diminished deep tendon reflex
  - Possible cardiovascular changes occurring in late disease: postural hypotension (a serious prognostic sign), resting tachycardia, "silent" myocardial infarctions
  - Possible peripheral vascular changes occurring in late disease: cool extremities due to decreased circulation, decreased pulses, edema, delayed capillary refill
  - Possible neurological changes occurring in late disease: diminished pain sensation, proprioception, vibration, light touch, absent lower extremity reflexes, dysfunction in extraocular movements, weakness, ataxic gait, paresthesias; may have change in level of consciousness

Diagnostic Studies

- Diagnosis of type 1 diabetes
  - HbA1C 6.5% or higher (the level at which retinopathy risk increases). No fasting needed to measure HbA1C
  - Fasting plasma glucose (FPG) 126 mg/dL (7.0 mmol/L) or higher
  - 2-h plasma glucose 200 mg/dL (11.1 mmol/L) or higher during a 75 g OGTT
  - A random plasma glucose 200 mg/dL (11.1 mmol/L) or higher *with* classic symptoms
  - When no symptoms of hyperglycemia (polyuria, polydipsia, polyphagia, etc.) are present, the diagnosis of diabetes must be confirmed on another day by repeat measurement, repeating the same test for confirmation. If results of two different tests (Hgb A1C and FPG) are available and are both indicative of diabetes, additional testing is not needed.
- May consider serum C peptide, antibodies or insulin level
- Glucose and ketones in urine

- Baseline diagnostic studies: BUN, serum creatinine, urinalysis, urine microalbumin, and fasting lipid profile; glycosylated hemoglobin (HbA1c)
- ECG and chest X-ray for coronary and pulmonary pathology in adults
- Elevated BUN and creatinine if dehydrated; hypertriglyceridemia: triglyceride levels 150 mg/dL or higher
- Thyroid-stimulating hormone (TSH) level

Differential Diagnosis

- Diabetes mellitus type 2
- Diabetes insipidus
- Latent Autoimmune Diabetes of Adulthood
- Pancreatitis or pancreatic disease
- Pheochromocytoma
- Cushing syndrome
- Acromegaly
- Liver disease
- Salicylate poisoning
- Glucosuria without hyperglycemia in renal tubular disease or benign renal glucosuria
- Secondary effects of oral contraceptives, corticosteroids, thiazides, phenytoin, nicotinic acid
- Severe stress from trauma, burns, or infection
- Urinary tract infection (UTI)

Management

Nonpharmacologic Treatment

- Patient education: basic pathophysiology, cause, general management and long-term complications of type 1 diabetes, administration of insulin, medications. For children and adolescents, treatment team should develop a treatment plan in conjunction with the parents and their child.

- Short- and long-term goals of treatment:
  - Maximize time in glucose range (70–180 mg/dl) with goal of more than 70% of the time;
  - HbA1c goal less than 7%, (less than 8% in older or high risk adults)
  - Minimize hypoglycemia episodes of less than 70 mg/dl to less than 4% of the time (less than 1% of the time in older and high risk adults)
  - Pre-prandial capillary glucose 80–130 mg/dl (90–140 mg/dl in older and high risk adults)
  - Postprandial glucose less than 180 mg/dl (less than 200 mg/dl in older and high risk adults)
  - Goals can be modified by age/life expectancy, comorbid conditions, hypoglycemia unawareness. Continuous glucose monitoring (CGM) aids in the assessment of these outcomes.
- Lifestyle modifications: diet, exercise, smoking cessation (if appropriate), alcohol avoidance
- Medical nutrition therapy prescribed by a registered dietician, following American Diabetes Association (ADA) guidelines; constant reinforcement by all providers. Medical nutrition therapy is associated with a 1.0–1.9% drop in A1C for type 1 diabetes.
- General guidelines for nutrition: Eating plans should be individualized considering culture, religion, tradition, goals and economics. Those with increased protein and fat intake should learn how to make mealtime insulin dose adjustments to compensate for delayed postprandial glucose excursions. Those with variable meal schedules should learn to dose from meal to meal based on insulin and carb ratios. For those on fast-acting insulin (such as NovoLog) and insulin glargine, or using fast-acting insulin in an insulin pump, when exact timing and amount of meals is not as critical, intensive insulin therapy education using carbohydrate-counting meal planning approach. For those on fixed doses of insulin, consistent carbohydrate intake with respect to time and amount is recommended. A well-balanced, healthy diet is recommended, with dosing adjusted to number of carbohydrates consumed at any meal and adjustments made for high or low blood sugar.
- Daily exercise regimen for adults (150 minutes per week) and physical activity for children (60 minutes per day with 3 days per week devoted to muscle and bone strengthening exercises); caution hypoglycemia risk
- Use a multidisciplinary approach to help work with the patient and the family, including the patient, parents (if appropriate), primary care provider, endocrinologist, nurse educator, psychologist, and dietician.
- Teach patient/parent recognition and management of episodes of hypoglycemia due to inadequate oral intake, increased exercise without adequate increase in caloric intake, or excess insulin.

- Self/parental glucose monitoring education: Glucose monitoring in children should be done 6–10 times per day including pre-meals and bedtime. Monitor glucose during periods where safety checks are needed such as during exercise, driving, illness, signs of hypoglycemia. Consider using continuous glucose monitoring for all youths with T1D. Severe hypoglycemia should prompt checks for blood or urine ketones to determine whether to proceed with treatment modification or urgent referral.
- Establish a dental care plan.
- Screen children beginning at ages 7 and 8 years for depression, anxiety, disordered eating and learning disabilities.
- Provide preconception counseling to all adolescent girls
- Recommended eye exams: dilated eye exam at age 10 or after puberty is reached (after patient has had diabetes 3–5 years) and then yearly.
- Neuropathy: neuropathy rarely occurs in children but annual foot exam is recommended yearly after age 10 or after onset of puberty (after patient has had diabetes 3–5 years).
- Retinopathy: Initial dilated eye exam and comprehensive eye exam recommended for all youth 3–5 years afterT1D diagnosis if they are 11 years old or have reached puberty, whichever arrives sooner. Eye exams should continue every 2 years or every 4 years if A1C target is reached or if A1C is below 8%.
- Diabetic Kidney Disease: Albuminuria by random spot check at age 10 or after puberty is reached (after patient has had diabetes for 5 years) and then yearly
- Dyslipidemia: Fasting Lipid Profile yearly beginning at age 10 when glucose control is reached. If normal, repeat in 3–5 years. If abnormal, initiate lifestyle changes. If abnormal and patient older than 10, consider a Statin. Provide reproductive counseling due to the teratogenic risks of using statins.
- Screen for hypertension: Provide lifestyle modifications or Ace inhibitors or Arbs for HTN. Provide reproductive counseling to adolescent female patients due to the teratogenic risks of these meds.
- Thyroid disease: Soon after diagnosis, measure antithyroid peroxidase and antithyroglobulin antibodies. When glycemic control reached, checkTSH. IfTSH normal, measure every 1–2 years, sooner, if symptomatic for thyroid disease. Autoimmune thyroid disease occurs in 17–30% of individuals with type 1 diabetes.
- Celiac disease: Screen for celiac disease soon after diagnosis ofT1D. Screen again 2 years later and then again at the 5 year mark. Screen more frequently with family history of celiac or if symptomatic.
- Screen for other less common autoimmune diseases such as Addison's autoimmune hepatitis, auto-immune gastritis, dermatomyositis, and myasthenia gravis

- Teach patient/parent how to modify therapy if ill. "Sick day guidelines" require continuing usual dose of insulin, frequent self monitoring of blood glucose (SMBG), and adjustment of insulin if necessary; checking urine for ketones if SMBG is higher than 250 mg/dL, increased intake of fluids
- Technology for Type 1 Diabetes:
  - Continuous glucose monitoring
  - Subcutaneous sensor measures glucose concentrations in interstitial fluid for 7–10 days.
  - Dexcom and Minimed transmit data to Smart Phones or screens of the insulin pump.
  - Cost $800-$1000 and covered by most insurance
- Referral to local support groups and American Diabetes Association
- Recommend wearing a MedicAlert or similar identification bracelet or necklace.
- Inform school, work, and/or friends of condition.
- Pneumococcal vaccine and annual influenza vaccines

Pharmacologic Treatment

- Referred to as anti-hyperglycemic agents rather than anti-diabetic agents.
- Evidence shows that best glucose control and lowest risk of hypoglycemia occur with either multiple daily injections of insulin or continuous subcutaneous administration through an insulin pump. Intensive control leads to fewer microvascular and macrovascular complications over time. The usual regimen is 50% basal insulin and 50% rapid analog insulin through a continuous pump but may vary to fit individual carbohydrate, fat and protein intake. Analog insulin is associated with lower A1C and fewer hypoglycemia episodes as compared with human insulin. Standard total insulin dose is 0.4–1.0 units/kg/day
  - Newer basal insulins (U-300 glargine and degludec) are associated with fewer hypoglycemic incidents than glargine U-100).
  - Inhaled human insulin is associated with fewer hypoglycemia incidents than rapid acting analogs. Contraindicated in patients with lung disease or who smoke.
  - Continuous glucose monitoring is considered standard of care for type 1 diabetes.
  - Hybrid closed loop pump system has been proven safe and effective for glycemic control and reduction of hypoglycemia.
- Person presenting with ketones must be started on insulin.

- Glycemic goals should be individualized, based on a patient's duration of diabetes, age, life expectancy, comorbid conditions, known cardiovascular disease (CVD) or advanced microvascular complications, unawareness of hypoglycemia, and other considerations.
- Adjust insulin doses according to glucose monitoring.
- A "honeymoon period" or remission phase after diagnosis may last from several months to 2 years.

Special Considerations

- Puberty: initially, increased caloric need, followed by decrease to 35 calories/kg of ideal body weight as growth is completed; pubertal growth spurt will require insulin adjustment (1.25–1.5 units/kg/day)
- Co-management with pediatrician or pediatric endocrinologist

When to Consult, Refer, Hospitalize

- Hospitalization is recommended for all newly diagnosed pediatric patients.
- Hospitalize adults and children with diabetic ketoacidosis (DKA) and severe infections.
- Co-manage pediatric type 1 DM patients with a pediatrician or pediatric endocrinologist.
- Refer unstable adult or geriatric patients; consider co-management of all type 1 DM patients.
- Refer all families to diabetic educator and registered dietician (RD).
- Dentist: routine checkups and for dental complaints for all ages
- Podiatrist: routine foot care in older adults and foot problems as indicated
- Consider psychological counseling if needed, to address issues of altered body image and individual and family stressors related to disease and management.

Follow-Up

- Continue ongoing follow-up/consultation with endocrinologist and diabetes educator.
- Routine diabetes visits: daily for initiation of insulin or change in regimen, at least quarterly for patients not meeting their goals, and semiannually for other patients
- HbA1c every 3 to 6 months

- Serum fructosamine: glycosylated protein (primarily albumin); normal value 1.5–2.4 mmol/L; provides index of glycemic control for preceding 2 to 3 weeks; low albumin levels will lower fructosamine levels; useful for any provider when hemolytic states (low hematocrit, sickle-cell trait, thalassemia trait, etc.) affect HbA1c measures
- Annual physical exam or routine well child exam with primary care provider
- Thyroid function tests initially, then every 2 to 3 years for adults; annually for children
- Endocrinologists generally screen those with type 1 diabetes for other autoimmune diseases such as vitamin B_{12} deficiency, celiac disease, and hypothyroidism because these are common diseases seen along with type 1 diabetes.

Expected Course

- Chronic, lifelong disease with no cure

Complications

- Hypoglycemia signs/symptoms: shakiness, weakness, sweating, headache, tachycardia, nervousness, dizziness, hunger, irritability, convulsions, coma; limiting factor in achieving control
- Somogyi effect: early morning rebound hyperglycemia due to nocturnal hypoglycemia; around 3:00 a.m. serum glucose falls and patient is hypoglycemic; counterregulatory hormones compensate by mobilizing glucose stores; patient rebounds and becomes hyperglycemic by early morning; treated with reducing or eliminating p.m. or h.s. doses to eliminate nocturnal hypoglycemia
- Dawn phenomenon: hyperglycemia due to hepatic gluconeogenesis in early morning. Peripheral tissue insulin receptors become desensitized to insulin nocturnally, believed to be due to insulin receptor desensitizing property of growth hormone. Around 3:00 a.m., blood sugar measures either normal or high normal and gets progressively higher throughout the night; is elevated at 7:00 a.m. Treatment is to increase p.m. long-acting insulin or add an h.s. dose.
- Lipodystrophy (destruction of subcutaneous fat at injection sites): seen less with use of synthetic human insulin, rather than beef or pork insulin
- Retinopathy
- Nephropathy and renal failure
- Cardiovascular disease with lipid abnormalities; premature atherosclerosis
- Cerebrovascular disease

- Diabetic ketoacidosis
- Insulin resistance with long-term, high-dose therapy
- Peripheral neuropathy
- Autonomic nervous system problems, incontinence, and erectile dysfunction
- Infections
- Foot and skin ulcerations
- Insulin allergy

INSULIN THERAPY

Insulin therapy has become more effective with advancements such as insulin analogs and combination therapy. Bolus insulin with advance infusion technology also has led to increase glycemic control and less risk of hypoglycemia. Insulin treatment is usually prandial, basal, combination basal/prandial, and premixed biphasic (see Tables 17–1, 17–2, and 17–3). Basal/prandial insulin management is general 50% basal and 50% prandial, with the prandial divided in three doses, one at each mealtime with consideration for the largest meal. For instance, if the total daily dose insulin (TDDI) is 60 units, then 30 units would be basal insulin and 5 units prandial could be given for breakfast, 10 units prandial for lunch, and 15 units prandial for dinner, assuming dinner is the meal with the highest caloric intake.

Insulin injections must be given subcutaneously with sites of injection rotated to avoid lipohypertropy. Although insulin with syringes to be drawn up from vials is still commonly used, the insulin pen provides an easy and efficient means for patients to deliver precise, accurate insulin doses.

PREDIABETES

Description

- Failing pancreatic islet-beta cell compensation; underlying insulin resistance
- Associated with 5 fold increase in risk for type II diabetes

Incidence and Demographics

- 96 million people age 18 and over have pre-diabetes (38.0% of the U.S. population). 26.4% of the population over age 65 years have pre-diabetes.

TABLE 17–1.
PRANDIAL INSULINS, GIVEN AT MEALTIMES

REGULAR/ HUMAN SHORT-ACTING		ANALOG LISPRO RAPID-ACTING	ANALOG ASPART RAPID-ACTING	ANALOG GLULISINE RAPID-ACTING
Onset	.5–1 hr	.3–.5 hr	.25 hr	.25 hr
Peak	2–3	.5–2.5	.5–1.0	1.–1.5
Duration	3–6	3–6.5	3.5	3.5
Administration	.5–.75 hr	.25 hr	.25 hr	.25 hr

TABLE 17–2.
BASAL INSULINS

	ALL	AML	CLL
Duration	24 hrs.+	up to 24 hrs	24 hrs.

TABLE 17–3.
PREMIXED/BIPHASIC INSULINS

HUMAN BIPHASIC	ANALOG BIPHASIC	ANALOG BIPHASIC	ANALOG BIPHASIC
Human insulin (70/30) NPH/Regular	Humalog 75–25 (75% insulin lispro protamine suspension and 25% insulin lispro injection)	Humalog mix 50–50 (insulin Lispro)	NovoLog 70–30 (70% insulin aspart protamine suspension and 30% insulin aspart)

TABLE 17–4.
PRANDIAL INHALED INSULINS, ADMINISTERED AT MEALTIME

INHALED INSULIN	AFREZZA (INSULIN HUMAN)	EXUBERA (INSULIN HUMAN RDNA)
Onset	12–15 mins.	12–15 mins.
Peak	1 hr.	1 hr.
Duration	Up to 3 hrs.	Up to 3 hrs.

TABLE 17–5.
ULTRA-LONG-ACTING INSULINS

BASAL INSULIN COVERING 30–42 HOURS	INSULIN GLARGINE TOUJEO: U300 (IGLAR 300) (MOST CONCENTRATED INSULIN).	INSULIN DEGLUDEC TRESIBA (IDEG U100 AND IDEG U 200)
Onset	6 hr.	2 hr.
Duration	30 hr.	42 hr.

Note: Delivers uniform absorption among patients who require larger dosages with little risk of hypoglycemia

Risk Factors

- Obesity

Prevention and Screening

- Screen all adults over age 35 years and if normal, screen again in 3 years,
- Screen adults with BMI greater than or equal to 25.
- Screen adults with one or more risk factors for diabetes.
- Screen all adults with diabetic first-degree relative, high risk ethnicity, history of cardiovascular disease, history of HTN (above 140/90 or equal) HDL less than 35, Triglycerides less than 250, Polycystic Ovary Syndrome (PCOS), physical inactivity, other clinical conditions such as acanthos nigricans).
- Risk-based screening after age 10 years or after onset of puberty

Assessment

Prediabetes is diagnosed as one of the following:

- IFG 100–125
- 2-hour PG using 75 g OGTT 140–199
- A1C 5.7–6.4
- Note the World Health Organization used 110 mg/dl as the cutoff for pre-diabetes

Management

- Prevention programs for delaying development of diabetes type II from pre-diabetes include 7% reduction in weight, 150 minutes per week (over at least three days with gaps of no more than 2 days) of physical activity at the level of brisk walking.
- Weight loss (weight loss recommendations same for prediabetes and type II diabetes)
  - Lifestyle changes: Implement lifestyle changes always choosing language that is "person" centered such as "person with obesity" rather than "obese person" to avoid defining a person by their condition. Respect privacy, report weight to patient nonjudgmentally and be mindful that patients may decline to be weighed due to past stigmatization. Evaluate systemic, structural and socioeconomic factors such as culture and food insecurity.
  - Calculate BMI annually, noting that in some populations, BMI cut off points for obesity are lower (ex. Asian and Asian American).
  - Lifestyle changes should be reinforced
    1. At diagnosis
    2. Annually for assessment
    3. When complications arise
    4. During transitions of care.
  - Weight loss interventions should include 16 sessions over a 6-month period with target calorie deficit of 500–750 K cal/day.
  - Weight loss medications (if lifestyle interventions are not sufficient for weight loss and if BMI greater than or equal to 27 kg/m^2)
    - Phentermine/topiramate and liraglutide have been shown to reduce progression to diabetes in 80% of cases
    - FDA approved weight loss medications: orlistat, phentermine/topiramate ER, naltrexone/bupropion ER, liraglutide 3 mg, and semaglutide 2.4 mg. These medications have all been shown to improve glycemic control in patients with diabetes and delay onset of Type II diabetes in those at risk. If patient shows a weight loss of more than 5% over three months, patient may continue medication. If not, discontinue.
  - Surgery (if lifestyle interventions are not sufficient)
    - Metabolic surgery if patient has type II diabetes and BMI is greater than or equal to 40 kg/m^2 (37.5 kg/m^2 in Asian or Asian American patients) or if BMI is greater than or equal to 35 kg/m^2 (32.5 kg/m^2 in Asian or Asian Americans) and non-surgical methods were ineffective.
  - Diabetes medications—no antiglycemic medications have been approved for the management of pre-diabetes by the FDA but the following have been shown

in studies to be effective and safe in halting the progression of pre-diabetes to diabetes:

- Metformin: studies have suggested metformin is useful in prediabetic patients less than 60 years old or with BMI greater than or equal to 35 Kg/m^2.
- Acarbose

- ♦ Manage blood pressure and dyslipidemia
    - ◊ Target BP of less than 130/80 using lifestyle changes (weight loss, sodium restriction, decreased alcohol intake, moderate physical activity)
    - ◊ BP medications: ACE's and ARB's preferred to prevent kidney disease for which DMII patients are at risk but beta blockers calcium channel blockers, diuretics are also first line. Consider albuminuria, ASCVD, heart failure, race, ethnicity, pill burden and cost when choosing meds for HTN management.

DIABETES MELLITUS TYPE 2

Description

- ♦ Metabolic disease-causing hyperglycemia, characterized by a relative insufficiency of insulin due to resistance to the action of insulin in target tissues, decrease in insulin receptors, and/or impairment of insulin secretion
- ♦ Formerly *non-insulin-dependent diabetes mellitus* (NIDDM), adult or maturity onset, type 2, nonketotic diabetes (because there is some endogenous insulin activity, diabetic ketoacidosis usually does not develop)

Etiology

- ♦ Genetically and clinically a heterogeneous disorder with familial pattern
- ♦ Influenced by environmental factors, lack of physical activity, diet high in refined carbohydrate and fat with low fiber
- ♦ Obesity
- ♦ No human leukocyte antigen or islet cell antibodies
- ♦ Syndrome of hyperinsulinemia and insulin resistance, resulting in hyperglycemia, hypertension, and hyperlipidemia to varying degrees in all patients
- ♦ Drug or chemical-induced (drugs used to treat psychosis, HIV, or transplant recipients)

Incidence and Demographics

- Occurs predominantly in obese adults older than 30 years but occasionally in adolescents with a genetic predisposition or obesity
- Accounts for nearly 90% of all diabetes mellitus cases in United States.

Risk Factors

- Overweight (BMI 25 kg/m2 or higher)
- First degree relative with diabetes
- High risk race/ethnicity (e.g., Black, Latino, Native American, Asian American, Pacific Islander)
- Gestational diabetes or delivered an infant whose weight was over 9 lbs
    - Previously impaired glucose tolerance
    - Hypertension BP 130/90 or higher
    - High-density lipoprotein (HDL) cholesterol less than 35 mg/dL for men or less than 50 mg/dL for women and/or triglycerides greater than 250 mg/dL

Prevention and Screening

- USPSTF: screen patients for diabetes with blood pressure of 135/80 or higher.
- Per the ADA adults older than 35 years screened every 3 years; more often with FPG near 126 mg/dL
- Per the ADA, screen youth after age 10 or after onset of puberty who are in the 85th or greater percentile for weight and who have one of the following risk factors:
    - Maternal history of diabetes or gestational diabetes
    - Family history of diabetes in a first or second degree relative
    - Belong to a high-risk race or ethnicity group (Latino, African American, Native American, Asian, Pacific Islander)
    - Signs of insulin resistance such as acanthos nigricans, PCOS, hypertension, dyslipidemia
- Screening of pregnant women for gestational diabetes at 24 to 28 weeks' gestation, or after 28 weeks if delay in seeking prenatal care.
- Secondary prevention of complications essential

Assessment

History

- More insidious onset; may not have classical signs of hyperglycemia
- Obesity, blurred vision, chronic skin infections, polyuria, polydipsia, polyphagia, weight loss, fatigue, slow-healing wounds, recurrent infections (especially *Candida* and urinary tract infections), spontaneous abortion
- History related to type 2 diabetes: more prominent macrovascular changes than microvascular, such as vascular insufficiency, cardiovascular/cerebrovascular disease, and atherosclerosis
- History of hyperosmolar, hyperglycemic syndrome (HHS): precipitating factors such as treatment with calcium channel blockers, propranolol, corticosteroids, thiazides, phenytoin

Physical Exam

- Usually discovered on routine exam with elevated glucose level
- Central obesity, hypertensive
- Acanthosis nigricans
- Acrochordons
- With more advanced stage
    - Orthostatic blood pressure changes
    - Weight loss
    - Skin infections present
    - Visual and funduscopic changes: microaneurysms with soft (cotton wool) and hard exudates, deep retinal hemorrhages, neovascularization, cataracts, glaucoma
- Oral *Candida* infections
    - Peripheral vascular: decreased circulation, cool extremities, decreased pulses, edema, capillary refill greater than 3 seconds
    - Neurologic: decreased sensation of pain, proprioception, vibration, light touch, absent lower extremity reflexes, dysfunction in extraocular movements, weakness, ataxic gait

Diagnostic Studies

- Diagnosis of type 2 diabetes
  - ◊ HbA1C 6.5% or higher
  - ◊ Fasting plasma glucose (FPG) 126 mg/dL (7.0 mmol/L) or higher
  - ◊ 2-h plasma glucose 200 mg/dL (11.1 mmol/L) or higher during an OGTT
  - ◊ A random plasma glucose 200 mg/dL (11.1 mmol/L) or higher with classic symptoms
  - ◊ When no symptoms of hyperglycemia (polyuria, weight loss, polydipsia, etc.) are present, the diagnosis of diabetes must be confirmed on another day by repeat measurement, repeating the same test for confirmation. If results of two different tests (Hgb A1C and FPG) are available and are both indicative of diabetes, additional testing is not needed.
  - ◊ Urinalysis for protein, glucose, and ketones; microalbuminuria screening at initial diagnosis (ketonuria may occur but ketone accumulation in serum is rare)
  - ◊ BUN, urine, and serum creatinine
  - ◊ Fasting serum cholesterol and lipid profile
- Adult recommendations:
  - ◊ Glycemic control: glycosylated hemoglobin A1c (HbA1c) less than 6.5% for most patients per the AACE, or greater than 6.5% as long as 6.5% can be achieved without adverse outcomes. There should be a balance between age, comorbidities, and risk of hypoglycemia when determining the A1C goal. Preprandial capillary plasma glucose 70–130 mg/dL, peak postprandial capillary plasma glucose less than 180 mg/dL
  - ◊ Blood pressure 140/80 mmHg
  - ◊ Lipids: low-density lipoproteins (LDL) less than 100 mg/dL, trigylcerides less than 150 mg/dL, high-density lipoproteins (HDL) greater than 40 mg/dL
  - ◊ ECG and chest X-ray if clinically indicated for coronary and pulmonary pathology
  - ◊ TSH
  - ◊ Glycated serum protein: index of glycemic control over past 1 to 2 weeks
  - ◊ C peptide levels normal or above normal with type 2

Diagnostic studies should also include:

- Glutamic acid decarboxylase antibodies (GADA) not present
- Tyrosine phosphatase antibodies (IA-2A) not present

Differential Diagnosis

- Diabetes Mellitus Type 1
- Diabetes insipidus
- Latent Autoimmune Diabetes of Adulthood
- Pancreatitis or pancreatic disease
- Pheochromocytoma
- Cushing syndrome
- Liver disease
- Glucosuria without hyperglycemia in renal tubular disease or benign renal glucosuria
- Secondary effects of oral contraceptives, corticosteroids, thiazides, phenytoin, nicotinic acid
- Severe stress from trauma, burns, or infection

Management

- Common treatment plan is a goal for non-pregnant adults of maximizing the time in glucose range (70–180 mg/dl) for 70% or more of the time, based on continuous glucose monitoring (CGM) or self-monitoring (preprandial glucose of 70–130 mg/dl, HbA1c less than 7.0 and minimizing hypoglycemia to a goal of 4% or less of the time. Glycemic goals should be individualized and based on ASCVD, CHF and renal status. Goals should also be based on cost, minimizing weight gain, and minimizing hypoglycemia (less than 70 mg/dl). Type II diabetes patients should self-monitor (SMBG) their blood glucose at least three times per day if on insulin and at least one or two times per day if on oral medications. SMBG plans should be individualized, and the goals differ for at risk or older adults. (Time in range is greater than 50%, HgA1C goal is less than 8%, time below 70 mg/dl is less than 1%, preprandial blood glucose target is 90–140 mg/dl) and postpradial blood glucose target is less than 200 mg/dl).
- Diet, exercise, and medication
  - Metformin is the usual initial oral medication (if not contraindicated; should not be started in patients with GFR less than 30 ml/min/1.73m^2). Providers may individualize initial oral therapy based upon comorbidities. Monitor patients taking Metformin for vitamin B12 deficiency.
  - If patient has high ASCVD, CHF risk then Metformin + [GLP1RA or SGLT2i or other oral medication]. May need dual or triple therapy depending on risk factors and goals. Consider adding insulin if severe hyperglycemia, especially if weight loss, hyper triglycerides, ketosis, polyuria or polydipsia is present. It is common to add

insulin when blood glucose is greater than or equal to 300 mg/dl or if A1C is greater than or equal to 10.

- ◊ GLP1RA or SGLT2i are both recommended second agents in patients with high ASCVD risk or CHF
- ◊ If patient does not have high risk of ASCVD, CHF or CKD, and is asymptomatic, begin Metformin and lifestyle changes and utilize dual or triple oral therapy if monotherapy is not sufficient. Reassess glycemic goals every 3 months. If symptomatic after oral therapy or trial of injectable GIP1RA, then begin basal insulin and prandial insulin if needed. Titrate insulin every 3 days and monitor for hypoglycemia.
- ◊ All changes in diabetes type II regiments should be made in partnership with patient's goals.

- ♦ Manage blood pressure and dyslipidemia
  - ◊ Target BP of less than 130/80 using lifestyle changes (weight loss, sodium restriction, decreased alcohol intake, moderate physical activity)
  - ◊ BP medications: ACE's and ARB's preferred to prevent kidney disease for which DMII patients are at risk but beta blockers calcium channel blockers, diuretics are also first line. Consider albuminuria, ASCVD, heart failure, race, ethnicity, pill burden and cost when choosing meds for HTN management. If BP greater than 150/100 then Ace or Arb + (calcium channel blocker, beta blocker or thiazide)
- ♦ Per ASCVD risks: Target HDL less than 40 mg/dL; Triglycerides less than 150 mg/dl; LDL goals are less than 100 mg/dL for high-risk patients, less than 70 for very high risk and less than 55 for extreme high risk DMII patients.

Nonpharmacologic Treatment

- ♦ Patient education: basic pathophysiology, cause, general management, and long-term complications of type 2 diabetes; oral glucose-lowering medications dosage, administration, and side effects
- ♦ Mainstay of treatment is correction of insulin resistance through diet, exercise, adequate sleep and weight loss; patients should be treated initially with medical nutritional therapy in addition to metformin.
  - ◊ Lifestyle modifications: diet, exercise, smoking cessation (if appropriate), alcohol avoidance, adequate sleep.
  - ◊ Medical nutrition therapy prescribed by a registered dietician
  - ◊ Nutrition counseling following American Diabetes Association (ADA) guidelines; weight reduction of 5 to 10 lbs increases insulin sensitivity. ABCD (adiposity based chronic disease) is a new diagnostic term by AACE to describe obesity.
  - ◊ Consistent carbohydrate intake throughout the day

  - ◊ Moderate weight loss (10 to 20 lbs) and hypocaloric diets based on average daily intake can improve blood glucose levels.
  - ◊ Daily exercise regimen for adults and physical activity for children reduce insulin resistance by increasing number of insulin receptors, increases glucose uptake for 48 to 72 hours, and contributes to lipid control and weight loss. At least 150 minutes per week of moderate intensity activity and strength training are recommended.
  - ◊ Average of 7 hours per sleep per night recommended as sleep deprivation aggravates insulin resistance, hypertension, dyslipidemia, hyperglycemia; increases inflammatory cytokines.
- ♦ SMBG should be encouraged as appropriate and when medications are initiated or altered: before each meal, at bedtime, and 2:00 a.m. to 4:00 a.m. for 3 days, then before breakfast and dinner for 7 days. Once glucose is controlled, monitor daily at random times; maintain SMBG log.
  - ◊ Continuous blood glucose monitoring is encouraged for some T2D patients with the advantage of reducing risk of hypoglycemia. Best for patients at high risk of hypoglycemia and who have not reached treatment goals in 3 months' time.
- ♦ Teach patient/parent how to modify therapy if ill. "Sick day guidelines" for adults require continuing usual dose medication, frequent SMBG, increase intake of fluids; for pediatric patients, consult with pediatrician or pediatric endocrinologist.
- ♦ Counsel regarding contraception and discuss importance of glucose control before and during pregnancy.
- ♦ Referral to local support groups and American Diabetes Association.
- ♦ Medic Alert or similar identification bracelet or necklace
- ♦ Foot care plan
- ♦ Annual influenza vaccinations
- ♦ Pneumococcal vaccinations as per schedule
- ♦ Avoid HHS with hydration

Pharmacologic Treatment

- ♦ Step approach
- ♦ Antidiabetic agents listed in Table 17–4: Start with metformin (unless contraindicated) and select second or third agent based on efficacy, comorbidities, risk of hypoglycemia, weight, side effects, and cost.
- ♦ After patient is on monotherapy, consider dual, triple, or combination with injectable to achieve desired glycemic goal.

TABLE 17–6.
COMMONLY USED ORAL ANTI-HYPERGLYCEMIC AGENTS

GENERIC AND CLASS	BRAND NAME	ACTION	DOSAGE RANGE	USUAL MAXIMUM DOSAGE	COMMENTS AND MAJOR SIDE EFFECTS
SULFONYLUREAS: PANCREATIC ISLET BETA CELL INSULIN-RELEASE STIMULATOR					
Glipizide second generation	Glucotrol Glucotrol XL	Intermediate acting Long acting	5–15 mg daily 15 mg/day or 40 mg divided 5–10 mg daily	5–40 mg/day, divided 20 mg/day	Hypoglycemia, weight gain Good in controlling postprandial hyperglycemia
Glimepiride second generation	Amaryl	Long acting	1–8 mg daily	8 mg/day	Hypoglycemia, weight gain Good in controlling postprandial hyperglycemia
MEGLITINIDES: PANCREATIC ISLET BETA CELL INSULIN-RELEASE STIMULATOR					
Repaglinide	Prandin	Short-acting	0.5–4 mg within 30 min. of meals 2–4x/day	16 mg/day	Take with meals, quick onset; hypoglycemia; many drug interactions
Nateglinide	Starlix	Short-acting	60–120 mg three times a day within 30 min. before meals	120 mg three times a day	Quick onset, which may be useful in adolescents with irregular eating schedules; do not take if a meal is skipped. Use with caution in severe renal disease. May be used as an adjunct with metformin.
BIGUANIDES: DECREASE HEPATIC GLUCOSE PRODUCTION; INCREASE ACTION ON MUSCLE GLUCOSE UPTAKE					
Metformin	Glucophage	Intermediate acting	500 mg–2.55 g divided into two or three doses	2.55 g/day	Contraindicated in renal dysfunction, chronic heart failure requiring treatment; use cautiously in many conditions that may predispose to lactic acidosis

Continued

TABLE 17–6.
(CONTINUED)

GENERIC AND CLASS	BRAND NAME	ACTION	DOSAGE RANGE	USUAL MAXIMUM DOSAGE	COMMENTS AND MAJOR SIDE EFFECTS
Metformin, Extended Release (Glucophage XL)	Glucophage XL	Intermediate-acting	500–2,000 mg 1 time daily with evening meal	Dosage may be increased from starting dose 500 mg weekly	Few GI side-effects
THIAZOLIDINEDIONES: INCREASE INSULIN ACTION ON MUSCLE AND FAT GLUCOSE UPTAKE					
Pioglitazone	Actos	Long-acting	15 or 30 mg daily	45 mg/day	Precautions with hepatic dysfunction, cardiac disease, anovulatory conditions
Rosiglitazone	Avandia	Long-acting	4–8 mg single or divided into two doses	8 mg/day	Precautions with hepatic dysfunction, cardiac disease, anovulatory conditions
ALPHA-GLUCOSIDASE INHIBITORS: DELAY CARBOHYDRATE DIGESTION AND DECREASE POSTPRANDIAL GLUCOSE					
Acarbose	Precose	Short-acting	50–100 mg three times a day	less than 60 kg: 150 mg/day divided greater than 60 kg: 300 mg/day divided	Take before meals Contraindicated in inflammatory bowel disease and other intestinal conditions; use glucose rather than sucrose for hypoglycemia
Miglitol	Glyset	Short-acting	50 mg three times a day	300 mg/day divided into three doses	Take before meals Contraindicated in inflammatory bowel disease and other intestinal conditions; use glucose rather than sucrose for hypoglycemia

DIPEPTIDYL PEPTIDASE IV (DPP-IV) INHIBITORS: INHIBIT THE DEGRADATION OF INCRETINS SUCH AS GLP-1 BY INHIBITING THE ENZYME DPP-IV					
Sitagliptin	Januvia	Long-acting	25 mg, 50 mg, 100 mg based on GFR	25 mg daily GFR less than 30 mL/ min 50 mg GFR 30–50 mL/min 100 mg GFR ≥ 50 mL/min	Avoid using in patients with a history of pancreatitis or increased risk of pancreatitis
Saxgliptin	Onglyza	Long-acting	2.5 mg or 5 mg based on GFR	2.5 mg daily GFR ≤ 50 mL/ min 5 mg daily GFR greater than 50 mL/ min	Avoid using in patients with a history of pancreatitis or increased risk of pancreatitis
Alogliptin	Nesina	Long-acting	6.25 mg or 12.5 mg or 25 mg based on GFR	6.25 mg daily ESRD or GFR less than 30 mL/min 12.5 mg daily GFR30–59 mL/min 25 mg GFR greater than 59 mL/min	Avoid using in patients with a history of pancreatitis or increased risk of pancreatitis
Linagliptin	Tradjenta	Long-acting	5 mg	5 mg daily	Avoid using in patients with a history of pancreatitis or increased risk of pancreatitis
GLIFLOZINS: SODIUM-GLUCOSE CO-TRANSPORTER-2(SGLT2) INHIBITORS: REDUCE BLOOD GLUCOSE LEVELS BY INHIBITING THE RE-ABSORPTION OF GLUCOSE IN THE KIDNEY, INCREASING GLUCOSE EXCRETION					
Dapagliflozin also combined with Metformin as: Xigdua Or also combined with DDP4 as: Otern	Farxiga	Long-acting	5–10 mg daily	10 mg daily	Renal dosing advised Contraindicated in bladder CA or low BP; may predispose to UTI

Continued

TABLE 17–6.
(CONTINUED)

GENERIC AND CLASS	BRAND NAME	ACTION	DOSAGE RANGE	USUAL MAXIMUM DOSAGE	COMMENTS AND MAJOR SIDE EFFECTS
Canagliflozin also combined with Metformin as: Invokamet	Invokana	Long-acting	100–300 mg daily	300 mg daily	Renal dosing advised Contraindicated bladder CA or low BP; may predispose to UTI
Empagliflozin also combined with DDP4 as: Glyxambi	Jardiance	Long-acting	10–25 mg daily	25 mg daily	Renal dosing advised Contraindicated in bladder CA or low BP; may predispose to UTI Lowers risk of CV death
Ertuglifozin also combined with Metformin as: Segluromet Or also combined with DDP4 as: Steglujan	Steglatro	Long-acting	5–10 mg orally daily	10 mg daily	Renal dosing advised Major side effect urinary infections
GLP-1 AGONISTS: ACT TO INCREASE INSULIN RELEASE IN THE PRESENCE OF ELEVATED GLUCOSE, DECREASING GLUCAGON SECRETION AND DELAYED GASTRIC EMPTYING					
Exenatide	Byetta Bydureon	Short-acting Very long-acting	10 mg bidac; 5 μg bidac (renal) 2 mg weekly	10 mg bidac; 5 μg bidac (renal) 2 mg weekly	Avoid using in patients with a history of pancreatitis or increased risk of pancreatitis; caution use with renal impairment, severe GI disease
Liraglutide	Victoza	Long-acting	1.2 mg daily or 1.8 mg daily	1.8 mg daily	Avoid using in patients with a history of pancreatitis or increased risk of pancreatitis, history or thyroid tumors or MEN

Albiglutide	Tanzeum	Very long-acting	30 mg or 50 mg weekly	50 mg weekly	Avoid using in patients with a history of pancreatitis or increased risk of pancreatitis, history or thyroid tumors or MEN
Dulaglutide	Trulicity	Very long-acting	0.75 mg or 1.5 mg weekly	1.5 mg weekly	Avoid using in patients with a history of pancreatitis or increased risk of pancreatitis, history or thyroid tumors or MEN
Semaglutide	Ozempic	Very long-acting	Initially 0.25 mg/week × 4 weeks, then 0.5 mg/week × 4 weeks, then 1.0 mg/week or 2.o mg/week if not at A1C goal		Several drug-drug interactions. Contraindicated in severe renal dysfunction, pancreatitis, or thyroid cancer
LONG-ACTING INSULIN COMBINATION WITH GLP-1 RA					
Glargine & Lixisenatide	Soliqua	Varies	If daily insulin dose greater than 30u, start with 30u Soliqua or if daily dose less than 30u, start with 15u Soliqua	100u/mL & 33µg/mL	Avoid if history of pancreatitis or Multiple Endocrine Neoplasia syndrome type 2 (MEN 2). May cause thyroid C-cell tumors.
Liraglutide & degludec	Xultophy	Varies	Start at 16u/ day; titrate +2/every 3–4 days till fasting prepandial glucose is at target; Do not exceed 50u.	100u/mL & 3.6mg/mL	Avoid if history of pancreatitis or Multiple Endocrine Neoplasia syndrome type 2 (MEN 2). May cause thyroid C-cell tumors.

- See table 17–4 for antidiabetic agents. Note that the FDA restricted use of rosiglitazone and issued a black box warning in 2007 due to concerns about increased cardiovascular risk. However, based on new information, the FDA has revised its guidelines and categorizes *rosiglitazone* similar to other drugs for type 2 DM. According to an FDA review, *pioglitazone* may be associated with an increased risk of bladder cancer.
    - Adding Insulin in management ofType 2 Diabetes: Start with basal and then add prandial coverage
    - Treat to the goal with basal insulin; start with 0.1–0.4 U/kg basal insulin in the evening before bedtime or 5–15 units before bedtime and adjust every two-three days in 10–20% increments based on mean fasting finger stick blood glucose (FSBG) on preceding 2 days. Basal insulin is often sufficient initially, but as diabetes progresses, may need to add prandial insulin
- Goal of therapy: individualized based on patient's age/life expectancy, comorbid conditions, disease duration, risk of hypoglycemia, established vascular complications
- If blood glucose is higher than 400 mg/dL or patient has signs of ketoacidosis, insulin therapy is required.
- In metabolic syndrome (syndrome X or insulin resistance syndrome), it is theorized that the insulin receptors' insensitivity leads to hyperinsulinemia; this leads to increased hepatic, very low-density lipoprotein (VLDL) production, which leads to increased sodium retention. Hyperinsulinemia also leads to endothelial proliferation, accelerating atherosclerosis with associated hypertension. These patients require treatment for hyperglycemia, hypertension, dyslipidemia, and weight loss.

Special Considerations

- Pregnancy: Gestational diabetes (GDM) often represents undiagnosed pre-diabetes, type II diabetes or developing type 1 diabetes. It is estimated that 5.8%–9.2% of pregnant women are diagnosed with gestational diabetes. Complications resulting from GDM include preeclampsia, fetal macrosomia (may cause shoulder dystocia and birth injury), neonatal hypoglycemia.
    - Routine screening after 24 weeks gestation in all pregnant women. Typically, screening is performed between 24- and 28-weeks' gestation but may be done after 28 weeks.
    - Criteria for diagnosis of gestational diabetes following one-step or two-step approach:
- One step: 2-h 75-g OGTT glucose load: fasting 92 mg/dL or higher, 1-h 180 mg/dL or higher, 2-h 153 mg/dL (8.5 mmol/L) or higher is positive (gestational diabetes) GDM

- Two step: 1-h 50-g OGTT; if 140mg/dl or higher, proceed to 100-g OGTT and diagnosis made if at least two of the following four plasma glucose levels are met or exceeded: fasting 95mg/dl, 1-h 180mg/dl, 2-h 155mg/dl, 3-h 140mg/dl
  - High-risk women (previous gestational diabetes, other risk factors) should be screened at the first prenatal visit.
- Positive screening necessitates a standard glucose tolerance test or fasting plasma glucose before 24 to 28 weeks.
  - Gestational diabetes is treated through a multidisciplinary approach, including nutrition therapy and insulin, if necessary.
- Pregnant patients with gestational diabetes requiring insulin management should be managed by an endocrinologist and perinatologist.
- Refer all gestational diabetic patients who require insulin therapy.
  - Screen women with GDM for persistent diabetes at 4 to 12 weeks postpartum, using the 75 g OGTT and non-pregnancy diagnostic criteria.
  - Women with a history of GDM should have lifelong screening for the development of diabetes or prediabetes at least every 1–3 years if the 4–12-week 75 g OGTT is normal
    - Women diagnosed with GDM are 10 times more likely to develop type 2 diabetes in their lifetime compared with women who were not diagnosed with GDM.
- Older adults
  - Frail or mentally disabled older adults are likely to have hypoglycemic events resulting from forgetting to take medication as prescribed; incidence of falls may increase.

When to Consult, Refer, Hospitalize

- Endocrinologist referral for uncontrolled hyperglycemia
- Pediatric endocrinologist for pediatric DM type 2 patients until stabilized
- Hospitalize for severe infections or HHS, characterized by blood glucose higher than 600 mg/dL, minimal ketosis, serum osmolality higher than 340, and profound dehydration.
- Diabetes educator for further teaching for all patients and for pregnancy/lactation
- Registered dietician for further nutritional teaching
- Ophthalmologist: initial screening and annual exam for diabetic retinopathy and visual problems; all patients older than 9 years who have diabetes for 3 to 5 years; and all patients older than 30 years
- Podiatrist for routine foot care in older adults and any patients with foot problems as indicated

Follow-Up

- When first diagnosed or when adjusting medications, see weekly, then biweekly, monthly; well-controlled diabetic patients, see every 6 months
- Annual urine protein, FPG, lipid profile, creatinine, ECG, full physical exam with funduscopic and neurologic exams, complete foot inspection
- If treated with medication, obtain HbA1c every 3 to 6 months; goal less than 7%
- Thyroid function tests yearly in pediatrics and 2 to 3 years in adults

Expected Course

- Chronic, lifelong disease that requires long-term control to minimize risk of complications

Complications

- Hyperglycemic hyperosmolar coma; Charcot foot is a weakening of bones in the foot and develops secondary to neuropathy; also see type 1 DM complications

HYPOGLYCEMIA

Description

- Plasma glucose concentration less than 70 mg/dL (value may vary by lab); may be asymptomatic; plasma glucose level of less than 30 mg/dL usually symptomatic
- Can be classified as reactive (within 5 hours of eating) or fasting (occurs more than 5 hours after a meal)
  - Reactive hypoglycemia rare; more likely is pseudo hypoglycemia (symptoms without the drop in blood glucose; unclear cause)
- An estimated 6–10% of type 1 diabetics die because of hypoglycemia
- Also occurs in type 2 diabetics, especially those using insulin therapy, sulfonureas or glinides.

Etiology

- Most caused by excess exogenous insulin in patients with diabetes taking insulin, but may result from use of some oral antihyperglycemic agents; precipitated by change in quantity and timing of activity and food
- At onset, parasympathetic nervous system is activated, causing hunger, which is followed by activation of the sympathetic nervous system (nervousness, sweating, tachycardia); known as "Whipple's triad," which consists of low plasma glucose, parasympathetic and sympathetic symptoms, and relief with ingestion of carbohydrates.
- Other causes: benign functional disturbance of insulin secretion, pancreatic beta-cell tumor (insulinoma); autoimmune process (very rare); ethanol ingestion; glucocorticoid and growth hormone deficiencies; malnutrition; gastrointestinal surgery; chronic disease states (hepatic, renal, chronic heart failure [CHF])
- In neonates, due to erythroblastosis fetalis, insulinomas, B-cell nesidioblastosis, functional B-cell hyperplasia, Beckwith syndrome, panhypopituitarism, infants of mothers with DM and gestational DM, very ill or immature, intrauterine malnutrition, metabolic defects

Incidence and Demographics

- Most prevalent in diabetic patients on insulin and sulfonylureas
- Occurs in 1 to 3 per 1,000 live births, including approximately 5% to 15% of infants with intrauterine growth retardation (IUGR)

Risk Factors

- Type 1 DM, type 2 DM on insulin or sulfonylureas
  - Insulin doses are excessive, ill-timed, or wrong type.
  - Influx of exogenous insulin is reduced due to overnight fast, other periods of fasting or skipped meal or snack.
  - Insulin-independent glucose utilization increased (ex. Exercise)
  - Sensitivity to insulin increases with improved glycemic control, after exercise, after weight loss or in the middle of the night.
  - Endogenous glucose is decreased (example after ingestion of alcohol).
  - Insulin clearance reduced (during renal failure)
  - Hypoglycemia unawareness—patient can no longer sense signs of hypoglycemia

- Enzyme defects
- Liver disease, insulinoma, kidney disease
- Medication use, such as disopyramide (Norpace), pentamidine, quinine
- Pregnancy, third trimester
- Pituitary or adrenal insufficiency
- Alcohol abuse
- Neonatal: prematurity, hypoxia, hypothermia, IUGR, maternal DM, maternal glucose infusion during labor, small-for-gestational age (SGA)

Assessment

History

- Symptom history, especially if occurs postprandially or when fasting; may follow excessive exercise
- Initial symptoms of headache, hunger, difficulty problem-solving; may be sweating, shakiness, tremor, anxiety, irritability, behavior change
- Progresses to coma and seizures without treatment
- Insulinoma: morning headaches, morning confusion, nocturnal or early morning seizures
- Infants/children: SGA (highest risk), IUGR, prematurity
  - Hypothermia, hypoxia, or drug withdrawal at birth
  - Maternal DM, gestational DM history, or glucose infusion at birth
  - History of apnea of prematurity

Physical Exam

- Altered mental status; tachycardia; hypotension; pale, cool, and clammy skin; coma; positive Babinski
- In neonates, onset may be a few hours to 1 week after birth with jitteriness; convulsions; episodic cyanosis, apnea, or tachycardia; lethargy and poor feeding; high pitched cry; diaphoresis; pallor; hypothermia

Diagnostic Studies

- Adults: serum glucose level less than 70 mg/dL indicates hypoglycemia (varies by laboratory)
- Consider drug testing for ethyl alcohol or sulfonylurea, liver function, BUN, creatinine, cortisol tests to identify associated factors in a diabetic patient.
- In nondiabetic patient, also get C peptide levels, insulin, insulin antibodies, oral glucose tolerance test
- If cause not identified, additional testing after 72-hour fast may be done by specialist.
- Neonates/children: serum glucose level less than 35 mg/dL at 1 to 3 hours of age; less than 40 mg/dL at 3 to 24 hours of age; less than 45 mg/dL after 24 hours of age

Differential Diagnosis

- Pseudohypoglycemia
- Anxiety and panic
- Pheochromocytoma
- Factitious hypoglycemia
- Other causes of coma
- See conditions listed under Etiology

Management

Nonpharmacologic Treatment

- Avoid fasting, alcohol use; snack before exercise.
- Caffeine restriction (mimics symptoms)
- Avoid simple carbohydrates or beverages with high sugar content.
- Diet: high protein with complex carbohydrates, frequent small meals approximately 6x/day
- Avoid causative agents.
- Insulinomas and nesidioblastosis: surgery
- In neonates: oral or gavage feeding of high-risk, normoglycemic neonates and monitor for hypoglycemia

Pharmacologic Treatment

- If able to take oral substances, consume three to four glucose tablets or 4 ounces juice or 6-ounce regular soda (equivalent to 10–15 g glucose) at onset of symptoms, followed by complex carbohydrates after the acute reaction is controlled.
- If unconscious or unable to swallow, home or office management could include
  - 1 mg glucagon IM or subcutaneous (adult and adolescent); 0.5–1 mg glucagon (5 to 10 years); 0.25–0.5 mg (younger than 5 years): roll on side in case of vomiting; transport to an acute care facility for further monitoring and treatment.
- If oral or gavage feedings are not tolerated in a normoglycemic, high-risk neonate, refer to neonatal specialist for further care.

Special Considerations

- Some drugs, such as beta-adrenergic antagonists, mask symptoms of hypoglycemia.
- Men can fast for 72 hours and maintain plasma glucose level above 50 mg/dL, while women exhibit progressive decrease in plasma glucose during prolonged fasting.
- Geriatric patients may have blunted autonomic response and present with confusion and impaired central nervous system (CNS) function.

When to Consult, Refer, Hospitalize

- Refer for suspected insulinoma and nesidioblastosis to adult or pediatric surgeon as appropriate.
- Consult with physician or refer to endocrinologist for any unknown or uncontrollable cause.
- Activate the emergency medical system for all unconscious patients.

Follow-Up

- Educate patient and family about prevention, symptoms, and treatment of hypoglycemia.
- Monitor insulin and sulfonylurea dosage carefully, based on patient's diet and activity.
- Monitor children with hypoglycemia for attainment of developmental milestones as intellect can be affected, especially in low-birth-weight infants and infants of diabetic mothers.

Expected Course

- Variable and dependent on etiology, but favorable prognosis with appropriate treatment

Complications

- Brain damage and tissue death from prolonged low glucose level

Thyroid Disorders

SCREENING

- The USPSTF 2015 recommendations state the optimal screening interval for thyroid dysfunction with TSH is unknown. If screening, multiple tests should be done over 3–6 months to confirm or rule out an abnormal TSH. If TSH is persistently abnormal, follow up with serum T4 to differentiate between overt and subclinical thyroid dysfunction. Screen according to the following known risk factors:
  - Risk factors for elevated TSH: female, advancing age, white race, Type 1 diabetes, Downs Syndrome, family history of thyroid disease, goiter, previous hyperthyroidism (treated with surgery), external-beam radiation of head and neck.
  - Risk factors for low TSH include female, advancing age, Black race, low iodine intake, personal or family history of thyroid disease, ingestion of iodine containing medications (ex. Amiodorone).

HYPERTHYROIDISM (THYROTOXICOSIS)

Description

- Clinical condition caused by increased level of thyroid hormones T4 (thyroxine) and T3 (triiodothyronine)
- Manifestations include excessive metabolic rate (tachycardia, atrial fibrillation, insomnia, weight loss, anxiety). Long-term manifestations can include osteoporosis and cardiovascular collapse.

Etiology

- Excessive and uncontrolled secretion of thyroid hormone from a variety of causes
- Graves' disease (autoimmune disorder with autoantibodies against the gland that catalyze accelerated hormone production and release).
- Toxic multinodular goiter (Plummer's disease)
- Solitary hyperfunctioning adenoma (toxic adenoma); transient subacute
- Subacute, painless or postpartum thyroiditis
- Drug-induced, such as iodide and iodide-containing drugs (amiodarone) and contrast media
- Exogenous ingestion of thyroid hormone (factitia)
- Rare causes: toxic thyroid carcinoma, HCG-secreting tumors (choriocarcinoma, hydatidiform mole), TSH-secreting pituitary tumors, testicular embryonal carcinoma

Incidence and Demographics

- Approximately 1.2% people in the United States
- Graves's disease accounts for more than 85% of cases of hyperthyroidism It is the most common cause of thyrotoxicosis.
- Affects women more than men, 8:1
- Typical age at onset in adulthood: mid-20s through 30s, but can occur in older adults
- Typical age at onset in childhood: 12 to 14 years, can occur at any age; less likely in neonates

Risk Factors

- Family history of thyroid disorders and autoimmune disorders
- Thyroid replacement hormone ingestion
- Other history of autoimmune disorder
- Mother with Graves's disease (neonates)
- Elevated ANA

Prevention and Screening

- MonitorTSH andT4 for patients taking thyroid replacement hormones.

Assessment

History

- Weight loss, increased appetite, nightmares, hypersensitivity to heat, fatigue, weakness, palpitations
- Mental: insomnia, irritability, nervousness, anxiety, psychosis; in older adults, severe depression
- GI: increased frequency of bowel movements, diarrhea, vomiting
- GU: Irregular menses
- Skin: pruritis
- Medication history (particularly amiodorone), past medical history, and family history of autoimmune diseases

Physical Exam

- Adrenergic: nervousness, sweating, tachycardia, palpitations, tremor, lid lag, excitability
- Skin: onycholysis, myxedema, hyperpigmentation, flushes, diaphoresis, thin/fine hair, spider angiomas, thyroid acropachy (extreme and unusual)
- Eyes (only Graves's disease): periorbital edema, exophthalmos, chemosis, ophthalmoplegia, papilledema, blurred vision, photophobia, diplopia
- Neck: goiter smooth or nodular, thyroid bruit or thrill
- Throat: Dysphagia
- Cardiac: arrhythmia, such as atrial fibrillation, sinus tachycardia, systolic flow murmurs, heart failure, widened pulse pressure
- Respiratory: dyspnea on exertion, tachypnea
- Muscle: proximal myopathy, periodic paralysis, progressive wasting of muscles
- Lymph nodes: lymphadenopathy, splenomegaly
- Bone: osteoporosis, hypercalcemia
- Reproductive: miscarriage, infertility, abnormal menses, testicular atrophy, gynecomastia

- Neurologic: hyperactive reflexes, tremors
- Thyroid storm (life-threatening, rare in children): hyperpyrexia, tachyarrhythmia, encephalopathy, shock, congestive heart failure. Often precipitated by infection, trauma, noncompliance with antithyroid drugs, ventricular fibrillation, agitation, high fever, vomiting, dehydration or other event

Diagnostic Studies

- TSH decreased or undetectable (usually less than 0.01 mU/L); free T4 (unbound thyroxine) and total T3 elevated; if free T4 normal, order total T3 (5% hyperthyroid patients have normal T4 with elevated T3)
- In Grave's Disease: Elevated thyrotropin receptor antibodies (TRAb), positive thyroid stimulating immunoglobulin (TSI)
- Subclinical hyperthyroidism occurs when TSH is decreased or undetectable but free T3 and free T4 are normal; patients may have mild or no symptoms.
- Other potential lab findings: hypercalcemia; elevated alkaline phosphatase; low hemoglobin/hematocrit
- Urine pregnancy test in females if abnormal menses present
- CT scan for unilateral eye findings to rule out tumor; ECG in the older adult patient
- A radioactive iodine uptake and scan (123I) should be ordered if the diagnosis is in question. High radioactive iodine uptake scan indicates Graves' disease or toxic multinodular goiter; low radioactive iodine uptake indicates thyroiditis.
- Radioactive iodine scans contraindicated in patients with recent exposure to high iodine content (such as contrast CT).
- For patients with palpable thyroid nodules, order ultrasound to identify suspicious nodules. Thyroid uptake and scan will show cold nodule(s) (high risk of being cancer).
- Biopsy: Patients with suspicious nodules on ultrasound should be referred for fine needle aspiration (FNA) prior to treating with radioactive iodine.

Differential Diagnosis

- Psychological disorders (e.g., anxiety, panic, psychosis)
- False elevation of T3 and T4 from Biotin supplements
- Suppression of TSH during pregnancy
- Pheochromocytoma

- Infection
- Thyrotoxic phase of Hashimoto's thyroiditis
- Hormone ingestion
- Plummer's disease
- Acromegaly
- Malignancy
- Chronic heart failure
- New onset or worsening angina
- Orbital tumors (cause exophthalmos)
- Myasthenia gravis (ophthalmoplegic changes)

Management

Nonpharmacologic Treatment

- Treatment may not be necessary in mild cases or in subclinical hyperthyroidism
- Due to complications of hypoparathyroidism and vocal cord paralysis, thyroidectomy is generally reserved for patients with severe hyperthyroidism with a large goiter.
- Educate parents about thyroid disease if appropriate.

Pharmacological Treatment

- Therapy to control symptoms
  - Propranolol (Inderal) 10–40 mg q6h to abate catecholamine symptoms; children 1 mg/kg/day
  - Atenolol 25–100 mg 1–2 times daily.; not recommended in children or pregnant women
  - Beta blockade should be used in all patients with hyperthyroidism who are symptomatic, especially in older adults and those with high heart rates (greater than 90 bpm) or with concomittent cardiovascular disease
- Antithyroid medication is often first-line therapy, depending on severity of signs and symptoms. Antithyroid medications stop the thyroid gland from overproducing thyroid hormone. There are two options for antithyroid medications:
  - Propylthiouracil (PTU) 50–150 mg q8h initially, then 50–100 mg twice a day maintenance dose

- 6 to 12 weeks to reach euthyroid state
- In adults, PTU is only preferred during the first trimester of pregnancy
  - Methimazole (Tapazole) 5–40 mg q day
- Preferred in children for the treatment of hyperthyroidism. Typical dose ranges are 0.2–0.5 mg/kg/day
- Children: 0.4 mg/kg/day in divided doses, then 0.2 mg/kg maintenance dose
- 4 to 6 weeks to reach euthyroid state
  - Once thyroid levels normalize, doses of antithyroid drugs can typically be reduced by up to 50%; continue monitoring every 6–8 weeks
- Up to 30% of patients with Graves will experience remission after 12–18 months on antithyroid therapy
  - Agranulocytosis and hepatic injury: rare side effects. For this reason, patients should have a baseline hepatic panel and CBC and should be counseled to report high fever, jaundice, abdominal pain, dark stools, or pharyngitis
- Other medications as needed
  - Diltiazem (Cardizem) for patients unable to take beta blockers
  - Multivitamin, calcium replacement, and vitamin D rebuild bone density.
- Ophthalmopathy: eye lubricants for mild cases
- Radioactive iodine (131I) is the definitive treatment choice for Graves' disease, symptomatic multinodular goiter, and single hyperfunctioning adenoma; low cost and low complication rate compared to surgery
- Patients should be referred to an endocrinology provider after initial Pharmacological Treatment to discuss definitive treatment options including radioactive iodine or surgery
- Contraindicated in pregnancy, breastfeeding and in children
- Patients will become hypothyroid after radioactive iodine treatment. This typically occurs within 2–6 months after treatment. Levothyroxine should be started based on thyroid labs.

Special Considerations

- Thyroid labs should not be ordered if patients are taking biotin as this can interfere with the thyroid assays and cause abnormal results that mimic hyperthyroidism. If patient is on biotin, stop it and repeat labs 2 days later.
- Older adults may develop arrhythmia (usually atrial fibrillation), CHF, and angina.

- The diagnosis of hyperthyroidism in pregnancy can be challenging due to increases in thyroid hormone binding globulin; a referral to an endocrinology expert is recommended.
- Nonthyroidal illnesses, such as active hepatitis, cirrhosis, nephrotic syndrome, infections, malnutrition, and severe acute illness, can affect thyroid functioning serum tests.
- PTU at lowest doses during pregnancy, does not cross placenta
- Spontaneous remission in 25% of children within 2 years, and in 50% of children within 4 to 5 years; relapse can occur in 30% to 40% of cases.
- Eye disease: Grave's opthalmopathy
  - Deposits of mucopolysacharides and infiltration of chronic inflammatory cells of orbital tissue into the extraocular muscles
  - 20–40% of Grave's patients have eye disease
  - 5–10% of Grave's patients have severe exopthalmos
  - In exophthalmos, eye is pushed forward due to thickened eye muscles and retro-orbital fat. Stage 1 (early inflammatory stage lasting 18–36 months); Stage 2 (Chronic stage characterized by fibrocystic tissue resistant to glucocorticoid treatment).
  - More severe in smokers
  - Eye disease is a contraindication for Iodine 131 treatment.
  - Clinical findings: Dalrymple sign (upper eyelid retraction); Von Graefe sign (lid lag, downward gaze); Koder sign (starting appearance); Proptosis, conjunctival chemosis, inflammation, weakness of upper gaze (Stedwag sign).
  - Long term severe exophthalmos can lead to diplopia, muscle entrapment, optic nerve compression resulting in a loss of color vision, visual acuity, and visual fields.
  - Treatment includes recommending that the patient wear glasses for eye protection, tape lids shut at night to prevent corneal drying.
  - Other therapies include methylcellulose drops and gels (artificial tears), selenium 100 µg BID to slow progression in patients with a Mourits score greater than 3, methylprednisone IV pulse × 12 weeks or oral prednisone. IV administration is considered superior to oral prednisone. If resistant to corticosteroids, then may treat with monoclonal antibodies. Progressive active exophthalmos may be treated with retrobulbar radiation.

When to Consult, Refer, Hospitalize

- Refer to endocrinologist for management of all patients; may co-manage after initial therapy.
- Hospitalize for thyroid storm. Symptoms include heart failure, severe sinus tachycardia (60%), ventricular fibrillation (13%), frequent MI, cardiogenic shock, agitation, or

delirium (63%), high fever, vomiting, diarrhea, dehydration, hepatic impairment (52%). The Burch-Wartofsky score is used to evaluate severity of thyrotoxic crisis.

- Pituitary tumor: immediate referral to neurosurgeon
- Surgical referral for thyroidectomy if radioactive iodine is not possible or if patient has large goiter or suspicious nodules found on ultrasound.
- Ophthalmologist for evaluation of eye pathology

Follow-Up

- Monitor free T4 and TSH every 4 to 8 weeks until patient becomes euthyroid or hypothyroid, then thyroid replacement therapy
- Maintenance visits every 3 months, then 6 months, then annually
- After radioactive iodine therapy, order TSH every 6 weeks, 12 weeks, 6 months, then annually
- Baseline CBC, LFT every 3 to 6 months, ECG in older adults as needed by history and physical exam.

Expected Course

- Usually requires long-term maintenance for replacement therapy, or follow-up for recurrence after remission

Complications

- Thyroid storm, immediate threat to life (admit)
- Hypothyroidism following surgery or radiation
- Severe depression post-treatment
- Visual disturbance from ophthalmopathy
- Hypoparathyroidism and vocal cord paralysis post-surgery
- Osteoporosis
- Hypercalcemia
- Increased Alkaline Phosphatase
- Decreased libido

- Erectile dysfunction
- Decreased sperm motility
- Anemia
- Cardiac arrythmia
- Neutropenia

HYPOTHYROIDISM

Description

- Decreased secretion of thyroid hormone due to dysfunction in thyroid gland or pituitary gland, occurring after the neonatal period
- Congenital hypothyroidism is present at birth.
- Affects 1% of population and 5% of individuals over age 60

Etiology

- Primary: inability of thyroid gland to produce TSH
  - Autoimmune thyroiditis (Hashimoto's) is the most common.
  - Transient hypothyroidism in acute or subacute thyroiditis (viral etiology): transient postpartum thyroiditis
  - Ablation of gland due to surgery, radiation, thioamide drugs, radioactive iodine
  - Congenital: ectopic thyroid gland; aplasia of the thyroid gland; ineffective synthesis or utilization of thyroid hormones; transient hypothyroidism related to maternal antithyroid medications or fetal/neonatal exposure to high levels of thyroid hormone; congenital hypopituitarism
  - Iodine deficiency
- Secondary: lesions in pituitary gland (less common)
  - Pituitary adenoma
  - Certain drugs, such as lithium and para-aminosalicylic acid; previously treated hyperthyroidism, especially postpartum; coexisting autoimmune disorders (lupus, pernicious anemia, rheumatoid arthritis)
- Tertiary: thyrotropin-releasing hormone (TRH) deficiency from hypothalamus

Incidence and Demographics

- Predominant age older than 40; more frequent in women
- Hashimoto's thyroiditis can occur younger than age 3 years but usually older than age 6 years, with an increasing incidence in adolescence.
- Congenital hypothyroidism occurs in 1 in 3,700 live births in North America; more frequent in people of Asian and Hispanic descent

Risk Factors

- Previous hyperthyroidism treatment
- Autoimmune diseases; presence of thyroid antibodies
- Family history of thyroid or autoimmune disorders
- Pituitary disease; hypothalamic disease
- Postpartum women, maternal TSH-binding antibodies
- Lithium treatment
- Diabetes mellitus type 1 (10% will develop hypothyroidism)
- Infertility problems, repeated spontaneous abortions
- Fetal or newborn exposure to antithyroid drugs or excessive amounts of iodine
- Children with Down, Turner, Klinefelter, or Noonan syndromes

Prevention and Screening

- No official screening guidelines: however, periodic TSH screening for patients treated for hyperthyroidism or those who are symptomatic; expert groups recommend screening adult women older than 50 or 60
- Mandatory newborn screening at 2 to 6 days (5% to 10% false-negative rate); thyroid dysfunction must be confirmed with a venous sample
- People with diabetes may be at increased risk.
- Retest children with Down syndrome at age 3 months and periodically thereafter.
- Screen those with autoimmune diseases.

Assessment

History

- Adults: fatigue, dry skin, coarse dry hair, alopecia, receding hairline, constipation, cold intolerance, lethargy, increase in weight, irregular or heavy menses, memory loss, depression, muscle aches, paresthesias, medication history (especially lithium)
- Neonates: persistent jaundice, constipation, poor feeding, lethargy/somnolence, prolonged gestation, increased birth weight
- Children: family history, poor growth, learning disabilities or poor school performance, fatigue, constipation, weight gain, cold intolerance

Physical Exam

- Weight gain, short stature in pediatric patients, failure to grow, subnormal temperature, decreased level of consciousness
- Face: dull, blank expression, swollen; eyes: periorbital edema; ears: decreased auditory acuity
- Skin: dry skin; coarse, dry hair; brittle nails; hair loss; temporal thinning of eyebrows
- Mouth: swollen tongue, slow speech, hoarseness; thyroid: enlarged gland or atrophy, tender, nodules
- Cardiac: bradycardia, decrease heart tones, mild hypotension or diastolic hypertension, cardiomegaly
- Respiratory: dyspnea, pleural effusion; breasts; galactorrhea; electrolytes: hyponatremia
- Abdominal: hypoactive bowel sounds, ascites
- Extremities: swollen hands/feet, leg edema
- Neurological: dementia, paranoid ideation, slow/delayed reflexes, cerebellar ataxia, carpal tunnel syndrome
- Hematologic: anemia; hyperlipidemia, hypercholesterolemia
- Neonates: occasional large birth weight, jaundice, large fontanels, respiratory distress, hoarse cry, large abdomen, umbilical hernia (possibly), hypothermia, cool/ mottled extremities, bradycardia with murmurs and cardiomegaly, anemia

Diagnostic Studies

- TSH assay (use third-generation assay): elevated in primary hypothyroidism; TSH will be low in cases due to pituitary insufficiency
- Order free T4 when TSH elevated; low free T4 confirms diagnosis of hypothyroidism.
- Subclinical hypothyroidism: normal T4 and elevated TSH
- If secondary to pituitary or hypothalamic failure: normal TSH, low or mildly elevated T4
- Further tests when secondary hypothyroidism suspected, such as serum prolactin level, neuroradiologic studies, pituitary-adrenal and pituitary-gonadal function
- CBC, serum electrolytes, BUN, creatinine, glucose, calcium, phosphate, albumin levels, pregnancy test, urine protein, lipid studies as indicated
- Free thyroxine index (FTI) in most cases provides indirect estimate of T4.
- Children: bone age if short stature is suspected
- Neonates: thyroid scan

Differential Diagnosis

- Depression
- Obesity
- Dementia
- Ischemic heart disease
- Chronic heart failure (CHF)
- Kidney failure
- Cirrhosis
- Nephrotic syndrome
- Chronic renal disease
- Coexisting secondary cause
- Congenital hypothyroidism
- Transient hypothyroidism
    - Hypopituitarism
    - Euthyroid sick syndrome

- ◇ Iodine ingestion
- ◇ Thyroid hormone resistance

Management

Nonpharmacologic Treatment

- ♦ Education, high-fiber diet for constipation; diet and exercise for weight loss if obese
- ♦ Avoid drug interactions: cholestyramine (Questran); ferrous sulfate; aluminum hydroxide antacids; sucralfate; foods such as cabbage, turnips, kale, and soybeans that increase the loss of thyroid hormone, as they may interfere with levothyroxine absorption, should be spaced 4 hours from these medications
- ♦ Take medication in the morning on an empty stomach to increase absorption.
- ♦ For congenital hypothyroidism, monitor growth and development and be alert for signs of behavior changes.

Pharmacologic Treatment

- ♦ Primary hypothyroidism: Correct hormone deficiency with thyroxine replacement.
  - ◇ Levothyroxine (Synthroid) (T4) first-line therapy for primary hypothyroidism
  - ◇ Adults: starting dose 50–100 μg orally daily, increase 25 μg if TSH remains high after 6 weeks or may check T4 and TSH in 3 weeks based on patient's clinical condition; average dose 1.6 μg/kg body weight per day (112 μg in a 70 kg adult)
  - ◇ Older adults with coronary artery disease: Start levothyroxine at 25–50 μg orally daily with gradual increase every 4 to 6 weeks as tolerated, maximum dose of 75–150 μg.
- ♦ Children: Congenital hypothyroidism is a true endocrine emergency; goal is to begin therapy by 14 days of life.
  - ◇ Levothyroxine at 10–15 μg/kg/day; recheck T4 and TSH at 2 weeks and titrate to maintain normal levels.
- ♦ Subclinical hypothyroidism
  - ◇ Treat pharmacologically if TSH is higher than 10 mU/mL with presence of thyroid autoantibodies.
  - ◇ Just monitor the older adult, due to risk of coronary artery disease (CAD) with treatment.

- Transient, subacute hypothyroidism
  - Self-limited with symptoms resolving after 2 to 3 months
  - No therapy for minimal symptoms
- Congenital hypothyroidism
  - Initially, levothyroxine 10–15 µg/kg/day orally; recheck thyroid function tests within 2 to 3 weeks (goal: raise T4 and decrease TSH; TSH may not decrease to normal levels for several months, despite normal T4)
  - Management is usually with a pediatric endocrinologist.
  - May consider stopping levothyroxine at age 2 to 3 years in children with congenital hypothyroidism to reevaluate, if medication was started before a thyroid scan or if child had a normal gland on initial scan.
  - Hashimoto's thyroiditis may be self-limited in older children; reevaluate periodically throughout life.

Special Considerations

- Adults/geriatric patients: Concomitant use of CNS depressants, digoxin may decrease efficacy of thyroid replacement dosage; older adults are at risk for angina as thyroid levels increase.
- Patients with severe hypothyroidism are at risk for bacterial pneumonia or megacolon
- Pregnancy: If hypothyroidism is present during pregnancy, monitor TSH every trimester.
- Children: T4 may be normally low and TSH high in premature infants; soy-based formula may interfere with absorption of levothyroxine; untreated hypothyroidism in children leads to facial edema, hirsute forehead, growth delays, and intellectual disability or intellectual development disorder.
- Myxedema particularly affects older adults women and can occur spontaneously with prolonged exposure to the cold or administration of certain medications.

When to Consult, Refer, Hospitalize

- Refer developing myxedema coma, hypothermia, decreased mentation, respiratory acidosis, hypotension, hyponatremia, hypoglycemia, hypoventilation, significant cardiac disease, secondary hypothyroidism, or radically abnormal thyroid function tests to an endocrinologist.

- Consult or refer for co-management of congenital hypothyroidism.
- Refer pregnant and pediatric patients to an endocrinologist for ongoing management.
- Hospitalization is not usually required.

Follow-Up

- Adults: Measure TSH 4 to 6 weeks after initial dosage, then every 2 months until within normal limits, then every 6 to 12 months (TSH levels may remain elevated for several months despite effective treatment); if drug dosage changed, recheck TSH levels in 2 to 3 months.
- Annual lipid levels
- Confirm patient compliance if TSH is high

Expected Course

- Improvement within 1 month of starting medication; symptoms resolve within 3 to 6 months.
- Treatment usually lifelong; maintain medication at lowest dosage to maintain euthyroid state.
- Excellent prognosis with appropriate treatment

Complications

- Chronic heart failure
- Depression, psychoses
- Miscarriages during pregnancy
- Thyrotoxicity, myxedema coma (rare)
- Bone demineralization due to over-treatment
- Intellectual disability or intellectual developmental disorder in children

THYROID NODULE

Description

- Localized enlargements within thyroid gland; may function independently of hypothalamic/pituitary feedback
- Evaluation of thyroid nodule is important to detect thyroid cancer, which accounts for 4% to 6.5% of all thyroid nodules.

Etiology

- Unknown
- Autonomously functioning nodules (hot nodule on thyroid scan) are usually benign and may cause symptoms of hyperthyroidism.
- Nonfunctioning nodule (cold nodule) may be malignant carcinoma.

Incidence and Demographics

- Clinical exam uncovers 3–7% of thyroid nodules and ultrasound uncovers 20–76% of thyroid nodules. There has been an increase in thyroid cancer diagnosis related to better detection but at the same time, there is a trend towards overdiagnosis and overtreatment.
- 50–60% of people have thyroid nodules, and most are benign and asymptomatic.
- Most thyroid malignancies are low risk and do not impact survival.
  - Solitary nodules in 4% to 7% of U.S. population
  - More common with age, women, exposure to ionizing radiation, living in areas with iodine deficiency
  - Less than 10% of solitary nodules are malignant.
  - 10,000 to 20,000 new cases of thyroid cancer per year
  - Papillary carcinoma 75% of thyroid cancers; follicular carcinoma (aggressive) less than 10% of thyroid cancers
  - Papillary nodules twice as common in women than men; slow-growing
  - Cysts comprise 15% to 25% of thyroid nodules.
  - Uncommon in children; if they occur, usually asymptomatic and 25% to 75% malignant

Risk Factors

- For thyroid nodule
  - Female, increasing age, residing in area of endemic iodine deficiency
- For thyroid cancer
  - Family history of thyroid cancer or multiple endocrine metaplastic type II carcinoma
  - Family history of medullary thyroid cancer
  - Male gender, extremes in age (younger than 15 and older than 70)
  - Exposure of head, neck, or chest to radiation
  - Single nodule

Assessment

History

- Hoarseness, cough, dysphagia, obstruction, neck tenderness, neck swelling or enlargement
- History of hypo or hyperthyroidism; external radiation to head, neck, chest; or nuclear fallout
- Family history of thyroid disease
- Medication history
- Pregnancy status
- Benign or malignant nodules often asymptomatic but may have symptoms of hypo- or hyperthyroidism

Physical Exam

- Malignant: hoarseness; enlarged cervical lymph nodes; dyspnea; tumor palpable as fixed, painless, hard, irregular-shaped mass; does not move with swallowing
- Document thyroid dimensions, consistency, size, and number of nodules; tenderness or pain; cervical lymphadenopathy.
- Benign: multiple nodules palpable (nodular Hashimoto's thyroiditis or multinodular goiter)

Diagnostic Studies

- All palpable nodules should have ultrasound.
- Labs: OrderTSH and ifTSH is low, order FreeT4 and FreeT3; ifTSH is high, then order Thyroid Peroxidase antibodies. If non-medullary thyroid cancer is suspected based on fine needle aspiration, then order serum calcitonin.
- Use simplified US 3 class rating system to guide decisions for fine needle aspiration of thyroid nodules (FNA). Decision is based on balancing the risk between unnecessary procedures versus potential of harm due to delayed diagnosis.
  - Class 1 (low risk of malignancy): mostly cystic nodules (greater than 50%), spongiform (1% chance of malignancy)
  - Class 2 (Intermediate risk of malignancy): slightly hypoechoic or isoechoic, ovoid to round in shape, smooth margins, intramodular vascularization, continuous rim calcification (5–15% chance of malignancy)
  - Class 3 (High risk of malignancy with one of the following): hypoechogenicity, spiculated or microlobulated margins, microcalcifications, taller than wide in shape, extrathyroidal growth, pathologic lymphadenopathy (50–90% chance of malignancy)
- Size guides FNA according to the following:
  - less than 5 mm, monitor rather than biopsy
  - 5–10 mm monitor or do FNA based on setting and patient preference
  - FNA is specifically recommended for nodules associated with a suspicious lymph node, extrathyroid spread, + or personal family history of thyroid cancer, greater than 10 mm with suspicious findings and greater than 20 mm if isoechoic, slightly hypoechoic, ovoid shape, smooth or ill-defined borders. If nodule is cystic and spongiform and greater than 20 mm or growing, then do FNA.
- TheThyroid Nodule App (TNAPP) is being developed as an electronic tool to guide clinicians in deciding to order a FNA. It is based on the three-class system above. The tool and instructions are found atTNAPP is web-based (https://aace-thyroid.deontics.com) and features a tutorial on how to use it (https://deontics-external-publication.s3-eu-west-1.amazonaws.com/aace/ThyroidþnoduleþAppþvideos.pptx).
- Multinodular goiter is usually euthyroid
- Radionuclide scans to determine cytologic results; hot nodules are benign in 98% of cases; 5% to 10% cold nodules are malignant (meaning decreased amount of radionuclide uptake)
- Serum calcitonin with family history of medullary thyroid carcinoma
- Evaluate anithyroperoxidase antibodies and antithyroglobulin antibodies to rule out thyroiditis.

Differential Diagnosis

- Malignant nodules vs. benign nodules
- Cysts
- Thyroiditis

Management

Nonpharmacologic Treatment

- Adequate iodine intake
- Surgery for malignant or disfiguring tumors
- Carefully follow patients with benign nodules (see follow-up).
- Instruct patients to follow-up for size changes, lymphadenopathy, dysphasia, hoarseness, or new or worsening symptoms of hypo- or hyperthyroidism.

Pharmacologic Treatment

- *Levothyroxine suppressive therapy is not recommended for thyroid nodules in euthyroid patients*
- Treat abnormal thyroid hormone levels following guidelines for hypo- or hyperthyroidism.

Special Considerations

- Pregnancy and lactation: Avoid radionuclide scan.

When to Consult, Refer, Hospitalize

- Refer all patients with thyroid nodules to endocrinologist for evaluation to rule out malignancy.

Follow-Up

- Re-evaluate euthyroid patients with benign nodules annually to check size and TSH.
- Benign nodules with abnormal thyroid function require frequent monitoring according to hypothyroidism and hyperthyroidism guidelines.
- Patients with malignancy must be followed up by an endocrinologist and possibly an oncologist.

Expected Course

- Good survival rate with malignant nodules unless due to follicular carcinoma

Complications

- Tumor recurrence
- Hypo- or hyperthyroidism

Adrenal Disorders

CUSHING SYNDROME

Description

- Syndrome of clinical abnormalities resulting from exogenous glucocorticoid excess (mainly cortisol)
- Due to endogenous hypercortisolism related to adrenal or pituitary dysfunction

Etiology

- Excess glucocorticoid production caused by adrenocorticotrophic hormone (ACTH) secreting pituitary tumor (two-thirds of cases), ectopic production by a nonpituitary tumor (small cell carcinoma of lung), or ACTH-independent adrenal tumor
- Prolonged use of glucocorticoids

- Serum concentration of glucocorticoids is regulated by the negative-feedback loop of the hypothalamic-pituitary-adrenal (HPA) system. Corticotropin-releasing hormone (CRH) stimulates the production and release of ACTH by the anterior pituitary, which stimulates the adrenal cortex to produce cortisol. Cortisol levels increase in response to increased ACTH levels and will decrease in response to decreasing ACTH levels.

Incidence and Demographics

- Cushing disease and primary adrenal tumors are more common in women
- Pituitary tumors are five times more frequent in women than men
- Age of onset 20 to 40 years
- Rare in childhood and infancy; most cases in children younger than 8 years old are malignant adrenal tumor

Risk Factors

- Adrenal tumor
- Pituitary tumor
- Neuroendocrine tumor
- Long-term or frequent high-dose corticosteroid use

Prevention and Screening

- Limit corticosteroid use
- Screen for unprescribed steroid use

Assessment

History

- Acne, back pain, headache, emotional lability, depression, mental changes, muscle weakness, fatigue, poor wound healing, thin skin, menstrual disorders/amenorrhea, hyperglycemia, susceptibility to infections, weight gain, easy bruising, decreased libido, insomnia, hirsutism
- Therapeutic or factitious use of corticosteroids

Physical Exam

- High blood pressure
- Truncal obesity with thin extremities, dorsal fat pad ("buffalo hump"), moon face
- Skin: thin, atrophic, acne, hirsutism, ecchymosis, hyperpigmentation; purple striae around breasts, abdomen, thighs
- Eyes: increased intraocular pressure
- Musculoskeletal: weakness, atrophy of muscles, thinning bones

Diagnostic Studies

- Initial late night salivary cortisol and late-night serum cortisol
- Glycosuria and elevated urine cortisol (24-hour urine free cortisol)
- Plasma cortisol level elevated evenings (higher than 5–7.5 μg/dL)
- Serum glucose elevated, hypokalemia without hypernatremia
- Screening tests: Refer to endocrinologist.
    - Dexamethasone overnight suppression test: suppression cortisol level less than 5 μg/dL normal result. If abnormal, more reliable suppression test performed by giving dexamethasone 0.5 mg orally q6h for 2 days.
- CT scans, chest and abdomen, for adrenal tumors and MRI for pituitary tumors

Differential Diagnosis

- Alcoholism
- Obesity
- Depression
- Familial cortisol resistance
- DM
- PCOS
- Drugs such as phenytoin, phenobarbital, and primidone accelerate dexamethasone metabolism, causing "false-positive" dexamethasone suppression test.

Management

Nonpharmacologic Treatment

- High-protein diet
- Reduce pituitary ACTH by transsphenoidal resection or radiation.
- Reduce adrenal cortisol secretion by bilateral adrenalectomy.
- Surgically remove ectopic ACTH-secreting tumors.

Pharmacologic Treatment

- Refer to endocrinologist for ongoing management.
- Replacement glucocorticoid therapy up to 1 year post–adrenal surgery, lifelong if bilateral adrenalectomy
- If patient is taken off glucocorticoid therapy, may need to restart if becomes ill

Special Considerations

- Pregnancy can exacerbate symptoms.

When to Consult, Refer, Hospitalize

- Refer all cases to endocrinologist and coordinate their primary care.
- Refer to surgeon and oncologist for adrenal or pituitary tumor.

Follow-Up

- For recurrence symptoms, measure urine-free cortisol.

Expected Course

- Post-treatment for pituitary adenoma: normal ACTH suppressed and requires 6 to 36 months to recover to normal function; hydrocortisone replacement therapy necessary

- Normal HPA function within 3 to 24 months after surgery if one adrenal gland is left
- 10% to 20% failure rate with transsphenoidal surgery; those with complete remission will have 15% to 20% recurrence rate over next 10 years

Complications

- Hypertension, CAD
- Osteoporosis, compression fractures of spine, aseptic necrosis femur head
- Diabetes mellitus
- Overwhelming infection
- Nephrolithiasis
- Psychosis
- If untreated, morbidity and death

ADRENAL INSUFFICIENCY/ADDISON'S DISEASE

Description

- Primary adrenal insufficiency is a loss of all adrenal hormones, including mineralocorticoids, glucocorticoids, and adrenal androgens. It is an insidious, chronic disease of adrenal destruction, also known as Addison's disease or primary adrenal failure.
- Secondary adrenal insufficiency is a lack of glucocorticoids due to pituitary dysfunction.
- Tertiary adrenal insufficiency is lack of glucocorticoids caused by hypothalamic failure.

Etiology

- Autoimmune destruction of the adrenal gland accounts for 80% of Addison's disease, followed by tuberculosis as second leading cause.
- Rarer causes include AIDS and other infections, genetic disorder, carcinoma, amyloid disease, hemochromatosis, antineoplastic chemotherapy, and bilateral adrenal hemorrhage, or it may be idiopathic.
- Secondary and tertiary adrenal insufficiency result from suppression of HPA axis through glucocorticoid replacement or adrenalectomy; pituitary tumor, trauma, surgery, or infarction; or hypothalamic disease.

Incidence and Demographics

- Usually affects those aged 30 to 50, but may occur at any age, incidence higher in women than men
- Prevalence approximately 4/100,000

Risk Factors

- Autoimmune disease
- Family history of adrenal insufficiency
- Prolonged steroid use followed by infection, trauma, surgery
- Medications: ketoconazole, phenytoin, rifampin, opiates

Assessment

History

- Progressive weakness, fatigue, weight loss, lightheadedness, anorexia, possible nausea and vomiting, diarrhea, cold intolerance, abdominal pain (like peptic ulcer disease), salt craving, emotional changes

Physical Exam

- Postural hypotension
- 90% systolic blood pressure lower than 110 mm Hg and rarely higher than 130 mm Hg
- Skin: hyperpigmentation (especially hand creases, knuckles, elbows, buccal mucosa) in White people, multiple freckles, change in body hair distribution with scant axillary and pubic hair, areas of vitiligo
- Breasts: dark nipples and areola
- Cardiac: small heart
- Lymph: hyperplasia, lymphadenopathy
- Acute adrenal insufficiency or Addisonian crisis may present with profound fatigue, dehydration, severe abdominal pain, nausea and vomiting, hypotension, hypoglycemia, and shock with vascular collapse and renal shut-down, and is precipitated by surgery, infection, exacerbation of comorbid illness, sudden withdrawal of long-term glucocorticoid replacement.

Diagnostic Studies

- Diagnostic: low plasma cortisol less than 5μg/dL at 8:00 a.m.; low morning salivary cortisol concentration (less than 1.8ng/ml)
- Sodium, chloride, glucose, and bicarbonate levels low with high potassium level
- BUN, plasma renin, ACTH, calcium all elevated
- CBC, decreased hemoglobin, neutrophils, and eosinophils
- Serum anti-adrenal antibodies in 50% cases of autoimmune Addison's disease
- ECG: nonspecific changes
- EEG: generalized slowing
- Abdominal CT scan: small adrenals
- Chest X-ray: small heart size and adrenal calcification

Differential Diagnosis

- Hyperparathyroidism
- Depression
- Mild thyrotoxicosis in older adults
- Gastrointestinal malignancy
- Chronic infection
- Heavy metal poisoning
- Hemochromatosis, anemia
- Salt-wasting nephritis
- Myopathies
- ACTH-secreting tumors

Management

Nonpharmacologic Treatment

- Monitor fluid and electrolytes.
- Ensure adequate dietary intake of sodium.
- Treat all infections immediately and vigorously and raise cortisol dose.

Pharmacologic Treatment

- Chronic phase: management initiated by endocrinologist; replace deficient hormones
- Cortisol 10–20 mg orally every morning; 5–10 mg orally at 4:00 to 6:00 p.m. (total of 15–25 mg of hydrocortisone daily in two divided doses with two-thirds morning and one-third afternoon) or prednisone 3 mg orally every morning, 2 mg orally every evening
    - Dose will be increased in case of stress, trauma, surgery, stressful diagnostic procedures, postural hypotension, hyperkalemia, or weight loss.
- Fludrocortisone acetate 0.05–0.3 mg orally daily or q.o.d. for cases of primary adrenal insufficiency if insufficient sodium retention with cortisol alone
    - If edema, hypokalemia, or hypertensive crisis occurs, lower dose.
    - Salt additives for excess heat or humidity
- Acute adrenal insufficiency: Hospitalize for IV hydrocortisone, mineralocorticoid, and normal saline.

When to Consult, Refer, Hospitalize

- Refer all suspected cases to endocrinologist for management.
- Hospitalization with acute crisis, dehydration, severe stress

Follow-Up

- Periodic evaluations of blood pressure, weight, electrolytes and other labs, muscle strength, appetite, cardiac status
- Medic Alert or similar identification bracelet or necklace

Expected Course

- Excellent prognosis with lifelong steroid replacement therapy

Complications

- Acute adrenal crisis
- Complications of steroid therapy: osteoporosis, psychosis, hyperglycemia, Cushing syndrome

Pituitary Disorders

PITUITARY ADENOMA

Description

- Pituitary adenoma or tumor can manifest by disturbance of function (hyper- or hyposecretion of trophic hormones), anatomic invasion into surrounding structures (enlargement of tumors), or a combination.
- Microadenoma is less than 10 mm, and macroadenoma is 10 mm or larger in size.

Etiology

- Largely unknown
- Occasionally part of multiple endocrine neoplasia type 1 (MEN1) syndrome, autosomal dominant chromosomal mutation
- If adenoma is secretory, usually only one hormone is secreted (frequently growth hormone, ACTH, or prolactin), causing characteristic symptoms. Secretion of prolactin (common) causes syndrome of hyperprolactinemia.

Incidence and Demographics

- More frequent in women
- Growth hormone secretion with gigantism almost always occurs in males.
- Fairly common and may be asymptomatic; often found on autopsy

Assessment

History

- Headaches, visual field loss due to pituitary enlargement; rare: loss of consciousness, seizures, mental state changes, brainstem dysfunction
- Amenorrhea, infertility, galactorrhea, impotence due to hyperprolactinemia
- Symptoms of Cushing syndrome with ACTH secretion (acne, weight gain, depression)
- Symptoms of acromegaly with growth hormone secretion (enlargement of head and face, feet and hands)

Physical Exam

- Body habitus for signs of gigantism, acromegaly, Cushing syndrome
- Eyes: ocular motor dysfunctions, pupillary dysfunction, limited visual fields
- Breast exam: bilateral galactorrhea (milky discharge)

Diagnostic Studies

- Serum prolactin, growth hormone, adrenal steroids may be elevated
  - Prolactin should be considered for complaint of headache with visual changes, amenorrhea, or galactorrhea.
- MRI of brain preferred over CT scan for pituitary imaging; angiography, visual field testing
  - Imaging indicated for men or women with serum prolactin higher than 200 ng/mL.

Differential Diagnosis

- Pituitary inflammation
- Other causes of headache
- Other causes of amenorrhea and galactorrhea
- Aneurysm
- Cushing syndrome

Management

Nonpharmacologic Treatment

- Transsphenoidal surgery or stereotactic radiosurgery to remove pituitary adenoma
- Radiation to pituitary

Pharmacologic Treatment

- Dopamine agonist bromocriptine (Parlodel) for hyperprolactinemia; may shrink tumors by 50% in 40% of patients within 3 months; treatment may be long term. Withdrawal from drug may result in recurrent hyperprolactinemia.

- Octreotide (Sandostatin), a somatotropin for treatment of acromegaly
- Postoperative substitution, including adrenal steroids, thyroxin, and testosterone or estrogen may be given.

Special Considerations

- Stop bromocriptine treatment with pregnancy/lactation.

When to Consult, Refer, Hospitalize

- Refer all suspected cases to endocrinologist; neurologist if surgery indicated

Follow-Up

- MRI scans at 6 months, 12 months, and annually for those treated with bromocriptine
- Growth of tumor indicates need for surgery or radiation therapy.

Expected Course

- Recurrence can occur within 5 to 10 years.

Complications

- Hypopituitarism
- Pituitary hemorrhage, infarct
- Diabetes insipidus
- Surgical complications including menstruation ceases and infertility

SHORT STATURE

Description

- Genetic: height below the 2.3 percentile (or two standard deviations below the norm) with no known etiology with appropriate growth in relation to parents' heights; normal growth rate and bone age

- Constitutional delay in growth also a normal variant of short stature. Well child who is short, takes longer to get to his or her eventual height (which is usually average height), with a biologically slower maturation and delay in puberty; delayed bone age by about 2 years; often progresses to delayed puberty; parents' heights are normal; predicted final height is comparable to target height.
- Turner syndrome: short stature in women due to an absence or abnormality of an X chromosome

Etiology

- Genetic: usually normal variant; possible genetic tendency toward growth hormone (GH) deficiency or GH receptor defect; possible inherited pathologic condition (e.g., hypochondroplasia)
- Constitutional delay in growth: often no known cause; possible causes include decreased GH secretion, abnormal GH structure, GH receptor defect
- Turner syndrome: absence or defect of an X chromosome, usually 45,X (monosomy) or 46,XX (mosaicism)

Incidence and Demographics

- Genetic: 3% of all normal children are below the 3rd to 5th percentile in height; equal incidence in boys and girls
- Constitutional delay in growth: increased incidence in boys
- Turner syndrome: occurs in 1 in 2,000 live female births (no males)

Risk Factors

- Genetic: parents who are below the 3rd to 5th percentile in height or with a pathologic cause for short height (e.g., hypochondroplasia)
- Constitutional delay in growth: usually a positive family history of growth delay
- Turner syndrome: no known risk factors

Prevention and Screening

- No known prevention
- Assess parents' heights.
- Fetal ultrasound may detect abnormality associated with Turner syndrome (no known prevention).
- Amniocentesis or chorionic villus sampling may detect Turner syndrome, but also has the potential to over-diagnose an X-chromosome abnormality.

Assessment

History

- Genetic: normal birth size; no intrauterine growth retardation; short parents below the 3rd to 5th percentile with or without known pathologic reason
- Constitutional delay in growth: normal birth weight and size; gradual decrease in rate of growth in first 2 years of life, then maintains growth curve approximately two standard deviations (SDs) below normal
- Turner syndrome: no family history, slightly small birth size, puffy hands and feet in neonatal period; short stature with a marked deviation of a decreased height on the normal growth curve

Physical Exam

- Genetic: gradual decrease in growth rate within the first 2 years of life; normal growth rate after age 2 years; normal onset of puberty
- Constitutional delay: aside from short stature, healthy; reduced growth rate until about age 2 years secondary to delayed bone age; in early adolescence, rate of growth decreases secondary to delayed puberty but then resumes after onset of puberty with some catch-up growth noted (see Table 17–5)
- Turner syndrome: short stature, small jaw, short or webbed neck (20% to 30% cases), high arched palate; absence or delayed puberty with ovarian failure; skeletal abnormalities; possible cardiovascular and renal abnormalities; recurrent otitis media, hearing loss, Hashimoto's thyroiditis, usually normal intelligence
- Height should be assessed on a carefully calibrated scale with a built-in level for children and on measuring boards for infants.

TABLE 17–7.
COMPARISON OF NORMAL VARIANTS

	FAMILIAR SHORT STATURE	CONSTITUTIONAL DELAY
Parents	Short (or family history)	Average height
Birth history and early years	Normal; often born at 25th to 75th percentile followed by a deceleration period until age 2, at which point they are in 3rd to 5th percentile	Same growth shift as genetic short stature
Growth velocity	Steady after age 2 to adulthood; parallels growth curve	Steady until puberty and because pubertal growth spurt is delayed, begins to fall away further from growth chart
Puberty changes	Normal age	Boys: failure to achieve Tanner genital 2 by age 13.8 years, or Tanner pubic 2 by 15.6 years. Girls: failure to achieve Tanner breast 2 by age 13.3 years
Bone age	Normal	Delayed (usually 2 to 4 years)
Ultimate height	Short	Average (can be tall) Males more than163 cm (64 inches) Females more than150 cm (59 inches)
Diagnostic studies	All normal	All normal except delayed bone age; a more extensive workup likely will be done because of the delayed puberty
Treatment	Reassurance	Reassurance

Diagnostic Studies

- X-rays for bone age: normal in genetic, delayed in constitutional delay
- Check for decreased serum GH and GH receptor defect.
- Diagnostic tests for Turner syndrome should be directed by a pediatric endocrinologist and may include chromosomal karyotype, FSH and LH, thyroid function tests, glucose tolerance test, echocardiogram, and renal and pelvic ultrasound.

Differential Diagnoses

- Constitutional short stature
- Familial short stature
- Malnutrition
- Chronic renal failure
- GI malabsorption
- Skeletal defects
- Pulmonary disease
- Cardiac disease
- Failure to thrive
- Metabolic diseases
- DM type 1
- Anemia
- Hypothyroidism
- GH deficiency
- Turner syndrome
- IUGR
- Chromosomal abnormalities

Management

Nonpharmacologic Treatment

- Genetic: No treatment is necessary as this is usually a normal variant; occasional uses of subcutaneous injections of GH have not proven to significantly increase final height.
- Reassurance that child is healthy aside from short stature

Pharmacologic Treatment

- Constitutional delay: Treatment with injections of GH occasionally renders a brief increase in growth but it is unclear whether final height is truly affected; appropriate time to discontinue therapy is controversial.

- Adolescents with constitutional delay may be treated with low doses of androgen.
- Turner syndrome: Use hormone replacement at puberty, GH therapy, and anabolic steroid therapy managed by a pediatric endocrinologist.

Special Considerations

- Educate families that growth hormone treatment will not make their child tall but will restore the normal growth pattern.

When to Consult, Refer, Hospitalize

- Consult with pediatrician or pediatric endocrinologist for evaluation and diagnosis; no further referral needed for genetic short stature.
- Constitutional delay and Turner syndrome: refer to pediatric endocrinologist for management.

Follow-Up

- Continue to assess growth and development in routine physical exams.
- Follow-up with pediatric endocrinologist and other pediatric specialists as appropriate for clinical manifestations.
- Periodic monitoring of thyroid function in all ages and lipid levels in adults is indicated at 6-month intervals for patients treated with GH who have constitutional delay.
- Carefully monitor bone maturation and serum glucose levels in patients with Turner syndrome.

Pubertal Disorders

Normal onset of puberty is 8 to 13 years in girls and 9 to 14 years in boys.

PRECOCIOUS PUBERTY

Description

- Early onset of pubertal changes (secondary sexual development) before age 6
  - Girls less than 8 years of age
  - Boys less than 9 years of age
- Normal development sequence is thelarche followed closely by pubarche and menarche 2 to 3 years later.
- Normal variants of early onset puberty:
  - Premature thelarche: benign breast development (typicallyTanner 2) usually in toddlers (see next section)
  - Premature adrenarche: small amounts of pubic hair younger than age 8 in girls and younger than age 9 in boys (possibly axillary hair and body odor); no growth spurt, breast development, testicular enlargement (needs to be differentiated from true and pseudo precocious puberty)

Etiology

- True precocious puberty or gonadotropin-dependent precocious puberty (central precocious puberty [CPP]) results from premature activation of the hypothalamic pituitary-gonadal axis. Hypothalamic-pituitary (CNS) stimulation of gonads produces estrogen and testosterone, which induces the pubertal changes. May be:
  - Idiopathic: no identifiable cause (system turns on spontaneously at an earlier than expected age); 75% of precocious puberty in girls is idiopathic, approximately 33% in boys
  - Neurogenic: damage to areas of the CNS that affect the hypothalamic pituitary axis and may include CNS tumors, infections, trauma, radiation, cerebral malformations, hydrocephalus, seizure disorders, neurofibromatosis, and tuberous sclerosis
- Pseudo (or peripheral) precocious puberty or gonadotropin-independent precocious puberty
  - Cause is from a source outside the central hypothalamic-pituitary system, such as the ovaries or adrenals; hypothalamic-pituitary system is not activated and does not mature
  - Results in the same secretion of pubertal amounts of estrogen and testosterone
  - Can occur from ovarian or testicular tumors, liver tumors (hepatomas), congenital adrenal hyperplasia, exposure to exogenous sex steroids from food (e.g., soybeans), drugs (e.g., oral contraceptives or estrogen-containing creams), or familial trait (e.g., familial testotoxicosis)

Incidence and Demographics

- More common in girls than in boys
- Usually idiopathic in girls
- In boys, approximately 50% related to a tumor, congenital adrenal hyperplasia, or familial testotoxicosis

Risk Factors

- CNS insult
- Family history
- Obesity

Prevention and Screening

- No known prevention

Assessment

History

- Pubertal changes: age of onset, progression, and specific symptoms (e.g., breast budding, hair, menses)
- Symptoms of possible underlying etiology such as headaches, weight loss, fatigue, and constipation (hypothyroid)
- History of CNS insult (meningitis, radiation)
- Exogenous sources of hormones
- Family history of early-onset puberty

Physical Exam

- Assess all pubertal changes: breast development, testicular size, pubic hair staging, presence of adult body odor, acne, any growth spurt (plot on growth chart)
- Obtain blood pressure: increased blood pressure may be consistent with increased intracranial pressure or congenital adrenal hyperplasia.

- Thorough neurological exam, including funduscopic exam (papilledema), visual acuity, and visual fields
- Palpate scrotum/testicles for any masses; abdomen for possible hepatomegaly or enlarged ovary or uterus
- Assess skin for café-au-lait spots, myxedema
- Palpate thyroid

Diagnostic Studies

- Results of tests will vary depending on the etiology.
- Levels of FSH and LH are usually in the prepubertal ranges with true precocious puberty; therefore, to document the premature activation of the hypothalamic-pituitary axis, a gonadotropin-stimulating test must be obtained. If premature activation has occurred, an increase in LH in response to a GnRH stimulation (i.e., serum concentration higher than 10 IU/L 30 to 40 minutes after administering GnRH subcutaneous) will occur. A positive response indicates the presence of true precocious puberty (not the cause but the presence). If LH/FSH is high, follow with prolactin.
- In both true and pseudo precocious puberty, levels of testosterone or estradiol will be elevated. Levels are normal for normal variants such as premature adrenarche.
- Adrenal androgens, particularly dehydroepiandrosterone sulfate (DHEAS), are obtained to rule out congenital adrenal hyperplasia. Levels would be elevated.
- Thyroid function studies (free T4 and TSH) if hypothyroidism suspected
- Bone age should be obtained on all patients to assist with determining etiology (i.e., advanced with true precocious puberty, normal with normal variants), height potential, and whether treatment is warranted; may need to be repeated in the follow-up of patients.
- Pelvic and testicular ultrasounds may be obtained to rule out tumors.
- Cranial CT scan or MRI of the hypothalamic/pituitary regions can determine tumors or structural abnormalities.
- CT scan of the adrenals if adrenal tumor suspected

Differential Diagnosis

- Premature thelarche
- Premature adrenarche

- Ovarian tumors
- Ovarian cysts
- Adrenal tumors
- McCune-Albright syndrome
- Exogenous sex steroids
- Congenital adrenal hyperplasia
- Familial testotoxicosis (Leydig cell tumors)
- Cerebral lesions

Management

Nonpharmacologic Treatment

- Treatment directed at underlying cause
- Reassurance if pubescent and postpubescent if evaluation negative and lack of pathology
- Referral to surgeon if fibrous tissue present causing breast enlargement, or breast mass present
- Weight reduction

Pharmacologic Treatment

- Antiestrogens (tamoxifen, clomiphene), dehydrotestosterone, diethylstilbestrol in older adults
- Eliminate or decrease any medication that may have a side effect of gynecomastia.
- Treat specific hormone disorders.

Special Considerations

- None

When to Consult, Refer, Hospitalize

- Refer to endocrinologist when history and/or workup compatible with pathologic origin.
- Urologist if cryptorchidism, testicular neoplasm
- Surgeon for removal of mass if indicated

Follow-Up

- Pubescent males every 3 to 6 months
- Watch for signs of abnormal progression of puberty, chronic illness, or emotional/psychological disorders.
- Perform/repeat diagnostic workup if clinical picture changes.

Expected Course

- Pubescent males should normalize within a 2-year period.
- Usually, good prognosis

Complications

- Self-image problems
- Increased risk of breast cancer in patients with Klinefelter syndrome

OBESITY

Description

- Condition involving accumulation of excess adipose tissue more than 20% over ideal body weight or body mass index (BMI) higher than 30

Etiology

- May be secondary to disease processes or a primary result of overeating and inadequate exercise

- Genetic predisposition: 60% risk of obesity if one parent obese, 90% risk if both
- Multifactorial, including environmental and psychological factors
- Abdominal fat (visceral fat) is associated with metabolic disorders (diabetes mellitus, Cushing syndrome) and cardiovascular disease.
- Hip and thigh fat (subcutaneous fat) more common in women and pose less medical risk than abdominal fat.
- Waist measurements over 35 inches in women and over 40 inches in men pose significant health risk for cardiovascular disease; risk of death increases with BMI over 30.
- Secondary causes such as adrenal problems, hypothyroid, polycystic ovary disease cause less than 1% of cases.
- Many medications cause increased appetite and weight gain, including steroids, antidepressants, hormones, mood stabilizers, and antipsychotics.

Incidence and Demographics

- Most prevalent chronic medical disorder in world
- Incidence and prevalence increasing in all genders and ages
- One-third of U.S. population is obese.
- Prevalence rates higher in Hispanic and Black women, and people of Asian and Pacific Island, Native American, Native Hawaiian, and Alaskan Native descent.
- Childhood obesity has been rising over the past 30 years; approximately 17% (or 12.7 million) children and adolescents aged 2 to 19 years are obese. However, the prevalence of obesity among children aged 2 to 5 years decreased significantly from 13.9% in 2003–2004 to 8.4% in 2011–2012.
- New onset in older adults is rare, requires investigation.

Risk Factors

- Overeating or other poor dietary habits
- Sedentary lifestyle
- Genetic predisposition

Prevention and Screening

- Balanced dietary intake throughout life span
- Exercise regularly

Assessment

History

- Obtain weight history of life span.
- Collect comprehensive diet history, including food categories, number of servings, number of meals per day, fluid intake, snacks
- Exercise history
- Motivation to lose weight and prior attempts to lose weight
- Smoking and alcohol intake
- Occupational history
- Past medical history of diabetes mellitus, thyroid disease, cardiovascular disease, cerebral vascular disease, hypertension, orthopedic problems
- Medication use, with particular attention to laxatives, diuretics, hormones, nutritional supplements, OTC medications
- Family history of obesity, overeating, metabolic disorders, cardiovascular disease, cerebral vascular disease, hypertension, diabetes mellitus

Physical Exam

- Height and weight: Calculate BMI by using tables or formula (see Diagnostic Studies).
- Obtain waist and hip measurement; waist more than 35 inches in women and more than 40 inches in men is dangerous.
- Children: weight exceeds 120% of that expected for their height (95th percentile on weight-for-height plot)
- Complete physical exam to assess for conditions associated with obesity:
  - Skin: assess for changes of Cushing syndrome or intertrigo caused by obese skin folds, striae, dermatitis, poor wound healing
  - Respiratory: compromise due to restrictive lung disease, hypoventilation

- ◊ Cardiovascular: hypertension, coronary artery disease
- ◊ Peripheral vascular: venous insufficiency
- ◊ Musculoskeletal: arthritis

Diagnostic Studies

- Adults: calculate BMI: weight in kilograms divided by height in meters squared
  - Pounds divided by 2.2 equal kilograms: inches times 0.0254 equal meters
  - Also, can be calculated by (weight in pounds times 703) divided by (height in inches^2)
- BMI between 18.5 and 25 is healthy, normal weight.
- BMI 30 to 34.9 is class I obesity; 35 to 39.9 is class II obesity; higher than 40 is class III obesity.
  - Asian populations have lower BMI thresholds.
- 18.5 to 23.9 healthy weight range, 24 to 26.9 overweight, over 27 obese
- Waist–hip ratio: Estimate fat distribution using waist–hip ratio by measuring waist at navel and measure hips over buttocks, then divide waist measurement by hip measurement to get ratio.
  - Men: Low risk less than 0.85, moderate risk 0.85 to 0.95, high risk over 0.95
  - Women: Low risk less than 0.75, moderate risk 0.75 to 0.85, high risk over 0.85
  - Upper body obesity has more significant health consequences than lower body obesity; therefore, large abdominal circumference or increased waist-to-hip ratio suggests increased risk of diabetes or vascular disease.
- Calculate ideal body weight.
  - Men: height (cm) equals 64.19 minus (0.04 times age) plus (2.02 times knee height)
  - Women: height (cm) equals 84.88 minus (0.24 times age) plus (1.83 times knee height)
  - A rough estimate of ideal body weight can be obtained by starting with 100 lbs (women) or 106 lbs (men) and adding 5 lbs (women) or 6 lbs (men) for each inch over 5 feet.
- Instruments to quantify body adipose tissue: hydrostatic densitometry (gold standard), skin-fold thickness measurement (simplest, most common), dual energy X-ray absorptiometry (DEXA) scan (most reliable and accurate, especially in older adults)
- Lipid profile, fasting blood glucose, metabolic and chemistry panel, thyroid function, consider urine-free cortisol measures for workup of secondary cause of obesity, or complication of obesity

- Children: Calculate BMI (interpretation depends on the child's age) and plot the BMI for-age according to sex-specific charts through puberty.
  - ◊ BMI equals (weight in pounds divided by height in inches divided by height in inches) times 703
  - ◊ Fractions and ounces must be entered as decimal values.
- BMI-for-age less than 5th percentile equals underweight
- BMI-for-age 85th percentile or higher equals overweight
- BMI-for-age 95th percentile or higher equals obese

Differential Diagnosis

- Endocrine disorders presenting with obesity include hypothalamic disease, thyroid disease, pituitary dysfunction, Cushing syndrome, and polycystic ovary disease.

Management

Nonpharmacologic Treatment

- The U.S. Preventive Services Task Force suggests that a combination of diet, exercise, and behavioral modifications is essential to obtain and maintain weight reduction.
- Children: Develop an alliance with the family; treat parents also; use positive reinforcement; emphasize the importance of family involvement in physical activity program.
- Long-term lifestyle changes
- Comprehensive multidisciplinary approach to weight reduction includes dietary control, exercise, eating behavior modifications, and psychosocial modification.
- To lose 1 pound, 3,500 more calories must be expended than consumed (500 calories per day to lose 1 pound per week).
- Moderate calorie deficit or low-calorie diet for obese men and women attempting to lose weight:
  - ◊ 800 to 1,200 calories per day women; 800 to 1,500 calories per day men
- Follow U.S. Department of Agriculture (USDA) food pyramid; avoid controversial fad diets; high-fiber, low-fat diets have proven most successful.
- Exercise: For energy expenditure, exercise 5 to 7 times a week for minimum of 30 minutes of moderate-intensity activity (walking, jogging, cycling, ice/roller skating, swimming).
- May require cardiac stress test before initiating exercise plan

- Eating behavior modification: emphasize planning and record-keeping.
- Psychosocial modification: support for losing weight essential, whether form of close friend, peer, therapist, or formal organization of people (such as Overeaters Anonymous, TOPS, Weight Watchers)
- Surgical approach with morbid obesity includes gastric operations, such as vertical banded (Mason) gastroplasty and gastric bypass.
- Pediatric obesity is best managed by increasing the child's activity level and improving nutrition; avoid medication or hypocaloric approaches.

Pharmacologic Treatment

- Recommended for BMI higher than 30 in conjunction with diet modification and exercise regimen or BMI 27 to 29 with at least one major comorbidity
- Long-term use:
  - Serotinin-2C receptor agonist: lorcaserin 10 mg twice daily; avoid in patients with severe hepatic or renal insufficiency
  - Phentermine-topiramate 3.75 mg/23 mg once daily in the morning for 14 days, titrate up upon response to max 15 mg/92 mg
  - Pancreatic lipase inhibitor: orlistat (Xenical) 120 mg three times a day with meals (no systemic absorption); discuss GI side effects; consider fat-soluble vitamin supplementation
  - Bupropion-naltrexone 90 mg/8 mg once daily titrate to max two tablets in the morning and evening
  - Liraglutide 0.6 mg daily titrate up to 3 mg daily
- Short-term use:
  - Benzphetamine: initially 25 mg once daily and then titrate to max dose of 50 mg three times per day; high abuse potential
  - Diethylpropion: initially 25 mg three times per day or controlled release 75 mg daily; less than 12 weeks
  - Phentermine: 15–37.5 mg daily
  - Phendimetrazine: initially 17.5–35 mg two to three times per day, max dose of 70 mg three times per day

Special Considerations

- Encourage patient to set goal of 10% weight loss for improved health and repeat as necessary.

When to Consult, Refer, Hospitalize

- May consider registered dietician when designing a low-calorie diet after determination of caloric requirements based on daily energy intake, expenditure, and average weight-loss goal of 1 pound per week after the first month
- Counselor for behavior modification
- Refer adults and children with morbid obesity to specialists.

Follow-Up

- Frequently, at least initially, to evaluate progress
- Monthly to monitor blood pressure if taking sibutramine
- Regular monitoring and reinforcement of progress until goal weight reached

Expected Course

- Slow progress with expected loss from ½ lb to 2 to 3 lbs per week maximum
- Continue to monitor for obesity complications.
- Many regain if they do not maintain the lifestyle modifications

Complications

- Cardiovascular disease: hypertension, coronary artery disease, varicose veins, CVA
- Metabolic disorders: hyperinsulinemia, diabetes mellitus type 2, hyperlipidemia
- Pulmonary: sleep apnea syndrome, chronic respiratory infections, hypoventilation
- Cholelithiasis; nephrotic syndrome
- Depression, loss of self-esteem; psychosocial disability
- Degenerative joint disease, chronic orthopedic problems
- Structural disorders; skin disorders
- Cancers: colon, rectum, prostate, uterine, biliary tract, breast, ovary
- Surgery increases perioperative morbidity and mortality.

CASE STUDIES

CASE 1

A 52-year-old woman arrives at your clinic. She states she has been fatigued for 3 months, has gained weight since her last visit (6 months ago), and is urinating more frequently, but that she is consuming more water and relates the urination to increased intake of fluids.

PMH: Hypertension and obesity; medications benazepril (Lotensin) 10 mg daily and Prempro 0.625 mg/2.5 daily

1. What additional history would you ask for?

   Exam: Vital signs: BP 130/88, HR 72, RR 12, temperature 97.9° F, weight 196 lbs, height 5′4″, BMI 33.7; general appearance is alert without distress. HEENT exam is normal, lungs clear, and heart rate and rhythm regular without murmurs; abdomen is obese with waist circumference 39 inches; no masses or tenderness. Extremities' pulses are normal; skin is warm and dry, sensation intact without lesions. Neuro exam is within normal limits.

2. What diagnostic tests would you order?
3. If your suspicions were correct, what actions would be required?
4. What is your treatment plan and follow-up?

CASE 2

A mother arrives at your clinic with her 7-year-old daughter, stating that she is developing breasts early and has hair under her arms.

PMH: Normal growth and development at well child visits; current on immunizations.

1. What additional history would you ask for?

   Exam: Vital signs within normal limits, height 95th percentile on the growth curve, Tanner stage III; the rest of the exam is normal.

2. What diagnostic tests would you order?
3. What is your next course of action?

CASE 3

A couple brings their 11-year-old son to the community clinic, stating he has lost 15 pounds in 3 weeks and is urinating frequently. He is also "drinking a lot."

PMH: Recent recovery from chickenpox (4 weeks); otherwise normal growth and development; immunizations up to date

1. What additional history would you ask for?

   Exam: Alert and oriented but appears ill, thin; fruity odor to breath, vital signs stable; mucous membranes slightly dry

2. What are your differential diagnoses?
3. What diagnostic tests would you order?
4. The lab results return with a glucose of 420 mg/dL (fasting) and urine dip positive for ketones and glucose. What is your next course of action?

CASE STUDIES DISCUSSION

CASE 1

1. What additional history would you ask for?

   Allergies, sleeping pattern, appetite/weight change, level of activity/exercise, 24-hour diet recall, social history including ETOH and cigarette use, family history of DM, thyroid disorders, hypertension, cardiovascular disease. ROS questions should include a statement about how the patient feels in general; changes in skin integrity, nails, or hair; visual changes; problems with breathing; chest pain/palpitations; urinary symptoms such as incontinence, urgency, burning; vaginal dryness; frequent yeast infections; bowel habit changes such as constipation, diarrhea, bloating; frequent hunger or thirst.

2. What diagnostic tests would you order?

   Complete metabolic panel to check glucose level, renal and hepatic function due to the history of hypertension and exam findings; complete blood count to rule out anemia or other blood dyscrasias due to complaint of fatigue; thyroid panel to rule out hypothyroidism due to increased risk of age and gender and the complaint of fatigue and weight increase; lipid profile for risk of lipid abnormalities with the history of hypertension, obesity, and age; urinalysis to rule out infection as a result of the history of frequency; may consider ECG and CXR as baseline studies.

3. If your suspicions were correct, what actions would be required?

   Order fasting blood glucose on a separate day to confirm the diagnosis.

4. What is your treatment plan and follow-up?

   If her blood glucose was more than 250 mg/dL but less than 400 mg/dL, this would require immediate treatment with oral medications. If her blood glucose was less than 250 mg/dL, diet and exercise would be the initial therapy. Nonpharmacologic therapy to include patient education: basic pathophysiology, cause, general management, and long-term complications of type 2 diabetes; lifestyle modifications including diet and exercise counseling and plan, foot care, MedicAlert bracelet, self-glucose monitoring and log; pharmacotherapy would include initial monotherapy. The medication will be adjusted based on home glucose monitoring in 1 week. Referral to a diabetes educator and dietician should be considered.

CASE 2

1. What additional history would you ask for?

   Family history, medication use or medications in the home, history of chronic disease, onset of menses, recent increase in rate of growth, changes in behavior or mood, illness or head trauma

2. What diagnostic tests would you order?

   Consider hormone and GnRH testing, thyroid function test. May consider bone age, MRI of pituitary gland, and CT of adrenal glands.

3. What is your next course of action?

   Refer to a pediatric endocrinologist for management if precocity is confirmed.

CASE 3

1. What additional history would you ask for?

   Incidence of fatigue, abdominal pain, nausea, vomiting or diarrhea, headaches, medication use or drug ingestion; changes in behavior of school performance

2. What are your differential diagnoses?

   DM type 1, urinary tract infection, hypercalcemia, sepsis, acute abdomen, salicylate intoxication

3. What diagnostic tests would you order?

   Blood glucose (by monitor) and urine dip for glucose, ketones, and signs of infection; urgent comprehensive metabolic panel

4. The lab results return with a glucose of 420 mg/dL (fasting) and urine dip positive for ketones and glucose. What is your next course of action?

   Consult with pediatrician or endocrinologist for hospitalization and management; educate parents on cause/course of illness and need for hospitalization.

REFERENCES

Adeyinka A, Kondamudi NP. Hyperosmolar hyperglycemic syndrome. [Updated 2022 May 22]. In: StatPearls [Internet]. Treasure Island (FL): StatPearls Publishing; 2022 Jan-. Available from: https://www.ncbi.nlm.nih.gov/books/NBK482142/

American Association of Clinical Endocrinologists. (2016). *Medical guidelines for clinical practice for the diagnosis and management of thyroid nodules*. Endocrine Practice (22) Supplement 1: 2–57.

American Association of Clinical Endocrinologists. (2011a). *Hyperthyroidism and other causes of thyrotoxicosis: Management guidelines of the American thyroid.* Retrieved from https:// www.aace.com/files/hyperguidelinesapril2013.pdf

American Association of Clinical Endocrinologists. (2012). *Medical guidelines for clinical practice: Clinical practice guidelines for hypothyroidism in adults.* Retrieved from https://www.aace.com/files/final-file-hypo-guidelines.pdf

American Association of Clinical Endocrinologists. (2019). *Clinical Practice Guidelines.* Retrieved from; https://www.aace.com/publications/guidelines

American Diabetes Association. (2019). 2. Classification and diagnosis of diabetes: Standards of medical care in diabetes—2019. *Diabetes Care, 42,* (Supplement 1), S13–S28.

American Diabetes Association Professional Practice Committee. 14. Children and adolescents: Standards of Medical Care in Diabetes—2022. Diabetes Care 2022;45 (Suppl. 1):S208–S23

American Diabetes Association. (2018). Economic costs of diabetes in the US in 2017. *Diabetes care, 41*(5), 917–28.

American Diabetes Association Professional Practice Committee. 2. Classification and diagnosis of diabetes: Standards of Medical Care in Diabetes—2022. Diabetes Care 2022;45(Suppl. 1): S17–S38

American Diabetes Association (2019) Lifestyle management: Standards of Medical Care in Diabetes 2019. Diabetes Care 2019;42 (Suppl. 1): S46–S60

American Diabetes Association Professional Practice Committee. 15. Management of diabetes in pregnancy: Standards of Medical Care in Diabetes—2022. Diabetes Care 2022;45(Suppl. 1):S232–S243

American Diabetes Association Professional Practice Committee. 9. Pharmacologic approaches to glycemic treatment: Standards of Medical Care in Diabetes—2022.Diabetes Care 2022;45(Suppl. 1):S125–S143

American Diabetes Association Professional Practice Committee; 3. Prevention or delay of Type 2 Diabetes and associated comorbidities: *Standards of Medical Care in Diabetes—2022. Diabetes Care* 1 January 2022; 45 (Supplement_1): S39–S45. https://doi.org/10.2337/dc22-S003

Appel, S. J., & Jones, S. J. (2012). Latent autoimmune diabetes of adulthood: A case presentation. *Nurse Practitioner, 37*(10), 6–9. doi:10.1097/01.NPR.0000419302.54267.d8

Appel, S. J., Wadas, T. M., Rosenthal, R. S., & Ovalle, F. (2009). Latent autoimmune diabetes of adulthood (LADA): an often misdiagnosed type of diabetes mellitus. *Journal of the American Academy of Nurse Practitioners, 21*(3), 156–59.

Bingham, M. (2018). ADA and EASD Update guidance on the management of hyperglycemia in type 2 diabetes. *Diabetes, 41*, 2625–33.

Benoit, S. R., Zhang, Y., Geiss, L. S., Gregg, E. W., & Albright, A. (2018). Trends in diabetic ketoacidosis hospitalizations and in-hospital mortality—United States, 2000–2014. *Morbidity and Mortality Weekly Report, 67*(12), 362.

Bonora, B. M., Avogaro, A., & Fadini, G. P. (2018). Sodium-glucose co-transporter-2 inhibitors and diabetic ketoacidosis: an updated review of the literature. *Diabetes, Obesity and Metabolism, 20*(1), 25–33.

Care, D. (2019). Standards of medical care in diabetes 2019. *Diabetes Care, 42*, S81.

Centers for Disease Control and Prevention (2020). *National Diabetes Statistics Report, Estimates of diabetes and its burden on the United States.* Retrieved from https://www.cdc.gov/diabetes/pdfs/data/statistics/national-diabetes-statistics-report.pdf

Atlanta, GA: Centers for Disease Control and Prevention, US Dept of Health and Human Services; 2019. https://www.aace.com/files/growth-hormone-guidelines.pdf

Centers for Disease Control and Prevention. (2020). *Childhood obesity facts: Prevalence of childhood obesity in the United States.* Retrieved from https://www.cdc.gov/obesity/data/childhood.html

Centers for Disease Control and Prevention. (2020). *Overweight and obesity.* Retrieved from https://www.cdc.gov/obesity/data/index.html

Centers for Disease Control and Prevention (2022). *Diabetes Report Card 2021.* Retrieved from: https://www.cdc.gov/diabetes/library/reports/reportcard.html

Centers for Disease Control and Prevention. National Diabetes Statistics Report website. https://www.cdc.gov/diabetes/data/statistics-report/index.html. Accessed June 28, 2022.

Cook, D. M., Yuen, C. J., Biller, B. M., Kemp, S. F., & Vance, M. L. (2009). American Association of Clinical Endocrinologists medical guidelines for clinical practice for growth hormone use in growth hormone-deficient adults and transition patients—2009 update. *Endocrine Practice, 15*(Suppl. 2). Retrieved from https://www.aace.com/files/growth-hormone-guidelines.pdf

Davies, M. J., D'Alessio, D. A., Fradkin, J., Kernan, W. N., Mathieu, C., Mingrone, G., . . . & Buse, J. B. (2018). Management of hyperglycaemia in type 2 diabetes, 2018. A consensus report by the American Diabetes Association (ADA) and the European Association for the Study of Diabetes (EASD). *Diabetologia, 61*(12), 2461–98.

Davis, C. S., Fleming, J. W., Malinowski, S. S., Brown, M. A., & Fleming, L. W. (2018). Ultralong-acting insulins: A review of efficacy, safety, and implications for practice. *Journal of the American Association of Nurse Practitioners, 30*(7), 373–80.

J.R. Garber, E. Papini, A. Frasoldati et al., American Association of Clinical Endocrinology and Associazione Medici EndocrinologiThyroid Nodule AlgorithmicTool, Endocrine Practice, https://doi.org/10.1016/j.eprac.2021.04.007

Garber, A. J., Abrahamson, M. J., Barzilay, J. I., Blonde, L., Bloomgarden, Z. T., Bush, M. A., . . . Umpierrez, G. (2018). Consensus statement by the American Association of Clinical Endocrinologists and American College of Endocrinology on the comprehensive type 2 diabetes management algorithm—2018 executive summary. *Endocrine Practice, 24*(1), 91–120. doi:http://dx.doi.org/10.4158/CS-2017-0153

Gastaldelli, A., Balas, B., Ratner, R., Rosenstock, J., Charbonnel, B., Bolli, G. B., . . . Balena, R. (2014). A direct comparison of long and short-acting GLP-1 receptor agonists (taspoglutide once weekly and exenatide BID) on postprandial metabolism after 24 weeks of treatment. *Diabetes, Obesity and Metabolism, 16*(2), 170–78. doi:10.1111/dom.12192

Gosmanov, A. R., & Umpierrez, G. E. (2013). Management of hyperglycemia during enteral and parenteral nutrition therapy. *Current Diabetes Reports, 13*(1), 155–62. doi:10.1007/s11892-012-0335-y

Gray, A.Threlkeld, R.J. (2019) Nutrition recommendations for individuals with diabetes. n: Feingold KR, Anawalt B, Boyce A, et al., editors. Endotext [Internet]. South Dartmouth (MA): MDText.com, Inc.; 2000-. Available from: https://www.ncbi.nlm.nih.gov/books/NBK279012/

Joslin Diabetes Center. (2013). *Asian American Diabetes Initiative: BMI calculator.* Retrieved from https://aadi.joslin.org/en/am-i-at-risk/asian-bmi-calculator

Loscalzo, J., Fauci, A., Kasper, D., Hauser, S., Longo, D., Jameson, L. (2022) *Harrison's principles of internal medicine.* McGraw Hill.

Mompoint-Williams, D. F., Watts, P. I., & Appel, S. J. (2012). Detecting and treating hypoglycemia in patients with diabetes. *Nursing, 42*(8), 50–52. doi:10.1097/01. NURSE.0000414629.07884.7f

National Center for Chronic Disease Prevention and Health Promotion. (2012). *Body mass indexfor-age: BMI is used differently with children than it is with adults.* Retrieved from www.cdc. gov/healthyweight/assessing/bmi/adult_bmi/

National Institute of Health (2022). *Hyperosmolar Hyperglycemic Syndrome.* Retrieved from https://www.ncbi.nlm.nih.gov/books/NBK482142/

Novo Nordisk receives FDA approval for Xultophy 100/3.6 (insulin degludec and liraglutide injection) [news release]. Plainsboro, NJ: Novo Nordisk; November 21, 2016. press.novonordisk-us.com/2016-11-21-Novo-Nordisk-Receives-FDA-Approval-for-Xultophy-100-3-6-insulin-degludec-and-liraglutide-injection

Papadakis, M. A., McPhee, S. J., Rabow, M.W. & McQuaid, K.R. (2022). *Current medical diagnosis & treatment* (61st edition). McGraw Hill

Stiles, L. (2018) ADA releases updated guidelines for managing pediatricType 1 Diabetes. Endocrinology Advisor https://www.endocrinologyadvisor.com/home/topics/diabetes/type-1-diabetes/ada-releases-updated-guidelines-for-managing-pediatric-type-1-diabetes/3/

Radin M. S. (2013). Pitfalls in hemoglobin A1c measurement: when results may be misleading. *Journal of General Internal Medicine, 29*(2), 388–94. doi:10.1007/s11606-013-2595-x

Sanofi receives FDA approval of Soliqua 100/33 for the treatment of adults with type 2 diabetes. [news release]. Paris, France: Sanofi; November 21, 2016. http://news.sanofi.us/2016-11-21-Sanofi-Receives-FDA-Approval-of-Soliqua-100-33-for-the-Treatment-of-Adults-with-Type-2-Diabetes

Soliqua [prescribing information]. Bridgewater, NJ: Sanofi-Aventis U.S. LLC; 2016.

Sudhakaran, S., & Surani, S. R. (2015). Guidelines for perioperative management of the diabetic patient. *Surgery Research and Practice*, 2015, 284063. doi:10.1155/2015/284063

Tibaldi, J., Hadley-Brown, M., Liebl, A., Haldrup, S., Sandberg, V., Wolden, M. L., & Rodbard, H. W. (2019). A comparative effectiveness study of degludec and insulin glargine 300 U/mL in insulin-naïve patients with type 2 diabetes. *Diabetes, Obesity and Metabolism, 21*(4), 1001–09.

U.S. Preventive ServicesTaskforce (2015) Final recommendation statement: Thyroid dysfunction: Screening. https://www.uspreventiveservicestaskforce.org/uspstf/recommendation/thyroid-dysfunction-screening

U.S. Preventive ServicesTaskforce (2021) Screening for gestation diabetes: US Preventive ServicesTaskforce Recommendation Statement. *JAMA 326 (6), 531–538*

Vilsbøll, T., Blevins, T. C., Jodar, E., Poulter, N., Tentolouris, N., Ross Agner, B. F., . . . & Leiter, L. A. (2019). Fixed-ratio combination of insulin degludec and liraglutide (IDegLira) improves cardiovascular risk markers in patients with type 2 diabetes uncontrolled on basal insulin. *Diabetes, Obesity and Metabolism.*

Zheng SL, Roddick AJ, Aghar-Jaffar R, et al. Association between use of sodium-glucose cotransporter 2 inhibitors,glucagon-like peptide 1 agonists, and dipeptidyl peptidase 4 inhibitors with all-cause mortality in patients with type 2 diabetes: a systematic review and metaanalysis. *JAMA, 319*(15):1580–91.

CHAPTER 18

PSYCHIATRIC–MENTAL HEALTH DISORDERS

Rosita Rodriguez, DNP, PMHNP-BC, AGPCNP-BC, FNP-BC, WHNP-BC, CDCES, CNE

General Approach

DESCRIPTION

- Mental illnesses are common, serious brain disorders that affect thinking, motivation, emotions, and social interactions and the ability to perform one's roles at work and at home. An estimated one in four adults has a diagnosable mental disorder each year.
- Untreated mental illness increases the morbidity of other chronic illnesses and results in decreased life expectancy.
- Obtain a complete history, including past medical, family, social history, medications, and review of systems.
- Obtain a mental status exam, using specific screening tools as appropriate.
- Distinguish between a mental disorder and a medical condition or substance abuse.
- The U.S. standard psychiatric diagnostic system (*Diagnostic and Statistical Manual of Mental Disorders*, 5th Edition, Text Revision (DSM-5-TR)) uses a categorical approach in which each disorder has its own set of criteria.
- Concomitant disorders are common.
- Most mild (and some moderate) mental disorders can be treated effectively in the primary care setting.
- With the presence of a developmental delay of a child, the clinician should consider a psychiatric disorder.
- Approximately 20% to 25% of children visiting pediatric outpatient settings have psychiatric disorders, either diagnosed or undiagnosed.

RED FLAGS

- Persons with mental illness often self-medicate with alcohol or other substances.
- Consult, refer, or hospitalize when presenting symptoms are severe, chronic, or unresponsive.
- Suicidal ideation with a plan or attempt is always a psychiatric emergency.
- Persons who represent a clear and present danger to themselves or others should never be left alone and should be hospitalized immediately, even when it is contrary to their wishes.

Anxiety Disorders

DESCRIPTION

- Anxiety disorders are characterized by fear (an emotional response to a real or perceived threat) and anxiety or preoccupation with a future event. These emotions and cognitions are associated with physical symptoms, the autonomic arousal and fight or flight reaction in the case of fear, and increased muscle tension and vigilance in the case of anxiety. Anxiety disorders are more extreme than developmentally appropriate fears and persist for a longer period than stress-induced fears. The diagnosis of anxiety disorder is made when the symptoms cannot be attributed to other medical conditions, other psychiatric conditions, or a substance abuse disorder. Anxiety disorders result in significant difficulties in social, academic, occupational, or other types of functioning.

SUBTYPES

- Separation anxiety disorder (F93.0)
  - Developmentally inappropriate or excessive distress related to separation from parents or caretakers
  - Persistent and excessive worry about losing an attachment figure or fear of possible harm to them or fear of experiencing a harmful event, such as kidnapping or hospitalization, which would result in a separation from significant caretakers
  - Other symptoms include nightmares about separation, fear of being alone, physical symptoms (headaches, nausea, vomiting) that occur when separation is anticipated, inability to go to sleep when attachment figure is not physically nearby.
  - The fear and anxiety are persistent, lasting more than 4 weeks in children and several months in adults.

- Selective mutism (F95.0)
  - ◊ Consistent inability to speak or respond when spoken to in certain social situations while maintaining normal speech in certain environments such as the home or when with close family members
  - ◊ Duration of the disorder is at least 1 month.
- Panic disorder (F41.0)
  - ◊ Episodes of recurrent and intense fear or feeling of impending doom that occur without apparent warning and reach a peak within minutes
  - ◊ Physical symptoms including palpitations, shortness of breath, trembling or shaking, paresthesia, tachycardia, sweating, abdominal distress, dizziness, tightness in chest; fear of dying, a sense of unreality
  - ◊ At least one of the attacks must be accompanied by either persistent fear of having an additional attack and the consequences of it, or an avoidance of situations that they perceive as dangerous or threatening. Patients may prefer to be accompanied by a friend or family member in tunnels, elevators, crowded streets, subways, airplanes, etc. Some patients may refuse to leave their homes.
- Phobias
  - ◊ Social anxiety disorder (F40.10)
- Severe, persistent fear of social or performance situations in which the person will be observed by others. The fear or anxiety is related to fear of negative evaluation, judgment, humiliation, or embarrassment, provoking an immediate and intense anxiety response; extreme, irrational fear leads to avoidance of people or social situations.
  - ◊ Specific phobia (F40.8)
- Extreme, irrational fear of specific objects, such as animals (snakes or insects), specific situations (enclosed spaces, elevators), or aspects of the natural environment that leads to avoidant behavior of that object
- Fear or anxiety lasts 6 months or more.
  - ◊ Generalized anxiety disorder (GAD) (F41.1)
- Excessive worry, with person reporting little or no ability to control the worry, along with significant distress and impairment in social, occupational, and interpersonal areas. Anxiety may seem groundless or appear disproportionate to issue.
- Must have three or more of the following symptoms in adults, present at least 6 months, occurring more days than not. Only one item is required for children.
  - ◊ Restlessness or feeling on edge
  - ◊ Easily fatigued
  - ◊ Difficulty concentrating or mind going blank
  - ◊ Irritability

- ◊ Muscle tension
- ◊ Sleep issues

Sleep Disturbance Etiology

- Psychodynamic theory
  - ◊ Severe conflict between the id and superego
  - ◊ Irrational guilt and shame
- Behavioral theory
  - ◊ Conditioned behavioral response to earlier interpersonal or social experiences
- Biologic theory
  - ◊ Genetic predisposition
  - ◊ Overstimulated autonomic nervous system, stress response
  - ◊ Abnormalities of neurotransmitter receptors in the central nervous system (CNS), specifically γ-aminobutyric acid (GABA) receptors
- Existential theory
  - ◊ Response to an awareness of living in a world without purpose or meaning

Incidence and Demographics

- Anxiety disorders are one of the most common mental illnesses in the United States.
- Approximately 19% of adults are diagnosed with an anxiety disorder.
- Most anxiety disorders are more common in women than in men (approximately 2:1 ratio).
- Anxiety is a common concomitant disorder in patients with a history of early traumatic experiences such as abuse, separation, or loss of a parent.
- Phobias affect children and adults with a lifetime prevalence of 8% to 12%.
- Most common psychiatric disorder diagnosed in childhood and adolescence
- Anxiety disorders frequently co-occur with depressive disorders or substance abuse, occupational difficulties, and suicidal behaviors.
- Separation anxiety disorder occurs during preschool, although one-third to one-half of patients have onset in adulthood.
- Left untreated, anxiety disorders persist into adulthood.

Risk Factors

- Temperamental; tendency to experience negative emotions (neuroticism), behavioral inhibition, and anxiety sensitivity
- Family history; genetic predisposition; one-third of the risk of GAD is genetic.
- Environmental; exposure to traumatic events such as a disease or death in the family, childhood physical or sexual abuse, history of depression and/or substance abuse

Prevention and Screening

- Public and patient education and awareness
- Reduced exposure to real or potential trauma
- Strong social support systems and strategies to develop personal resilience

Assessment

History

General

- Determine onset, frequency, and duration of symptoms.
- Determine degree of distress and symptom interference with daily function.
- Elicit predisposing factors or stressors, such as divorce, financial difficulties, job loss, or victimization.
- Obtain complete medical history, including medications, over-the-counter (OTC) medications, and supplements taken.
- Obtain history and current patterns of use of caffeine, alcohol, nicotine, and other addictive substances.
- Ask about:
  - ◊ Feelings of loss of control, panic, impending doom or dread, depersonalization, difficulty concentrating
  - ◊ Excessive worry, irrational fear, concern over “losing one’s mind” or death, memory changes
  - ◊ Difficulty concentrating, making decisions, irritable, agitated mood, motor restlessness
  - ◊ Sleep disturbances (insomnia, frequent awakenings), fatigue, irritation, agitated mood

- ◇ Nausea, diarrhea, vomiting, frequent urination
- ◇ Feeling of lump in the throat, difficulty swallowing, dry mouth

For Children

- ◇ Failure to speak in specific situations but able to speak at home or with family
- ◇ Excessive distress related to separation from parents or caretakers
- ◇ Excessive worry about losing an attachment figure or fear of possible harm to them or fear of experiencing a harmful event, such as kidnapping or hospitalization, which would result in a separation from significant caretakers

Phobias

- Excessive, persistent fear and avoidance of specific objects or situations
- In children: avoidance of school; impaired social, family, and academic functioning
- In adults: avoidance of work, social activities

General Anxiety and Panic Attacks

- Palpitations, tachycardia, tightness in chest or chest pain
- Difficulty breathing, tachypnea, hyperventilation
- Lightheadedness, dizziness, diaphoresis
- Tingling, numbness in extremities
- Fear of losing control or going crazy
- Fear of dying

Physical Exam

- Perform general exam to rule out serious CNS, cardiopulmonary, or endocrine disorder.
- Focus on vital signs, cardiac, pulmonary, and neurological exam.

Diagnostic Studies

- Diagnostic labs such as electrocardiography (ECG), thyroid-stimulating hormone (TSH), complete blood count (CBC), chemistry panel to rule out medical conditions
- Minnesota Multiphasic Personality Inventory (MMPI-II), Hamilton Anxiety Rating Scale, Adult Manifest Anxiety Scale (AMAS), Revised Children's Manifest Anxiety Scale (RCMAS-2) may be done
- Potential screening instruments include Generalized Anxiety Disorder-7 (GAD-7) or GAD-2 two-question screener

Differential Diagnosis

- Any medical condition with CNS involvement
- Substance abuse, including acute withdrawal or intoxication

Metabolic Disorders

- Seizure disorders
- Mood disorders
- Caffeine, nicotine
- Delirium, especially in older adults

Cardiac Disorders

- Arrhythmias
- Myocardial infarction
- Cardiovascular disease
- Chronic heart failure (CHF)

Endocrine Disorders

- Cushing syndrome
- Hyperthyroidism
- Hypoglycemia

Pulmonary Disorders

- Chronic obstructive pulmonary disease (COPD)
- Asthma
- Pulmonary embolism
- Pneumothorax

Inflammatory Disorders

- Lupus erythematosus
- Rheumatoid arthritis

Substances That may Produce Anxiety

- Amphetamines (methylenedioxymethamphetamine [MDMA])
- Herbal substances such as ginseng
- Hallucinogens (marijuana, lysergic acid diethylamide [LSD])
- Inhalants
- Phencyclidine (PCP)

Medications That may Produce Anxiety as a Side Effect

- Antihistamines
- Corticosteroids
- Antihypertensives
- Antipsychotics
- Antidepressants
- Bronchodilators
- Anesthetics

Management

- Mild cases of anxiety disorder and GAD are responsive to treatment in primary care settings.
- Refer nonresponsive or moderate to moderately severe primary anxiety disorders that meet DSM-5 or DSM-5-TR criteria to a mental health provider.
- Provide patient education to ensure compliance and effective treatment.

Nonpharmacologic Treatment

- Cognitive behavioral therapy (CBT); supportive psychotherapy, insight-oriented psychotherapy, group therapy promoting healthy lifestyles
- Relaxation therapy
- Stress management education, courses, workshops; behavioral conditioning, biofeedback
- Community self-help and support groups
- Education of patient and family about the disorder and treatment
- Self-management and self-help

Pharmacologic Treatment

- Benzodiazepines are effective in the short-term management of some anxiety disorders; however, selective serotonin reuptake inhibitors (SSRIs) and serotonin and norepinephrine reuptake inhibitors (SNRIs) are the preferred first-line treatment (see Table 18–1).
  - ◊ Significant potential for dependence and abuse; limit use to when SSRI or SNRI becomes therapeutic, about 2 weeks

TABLE 18–1.
BENZODIAZEPINE THERAPY FOR ADULT ANXIETY DISORDERS

BENZODIAZEPINE	INITIAL DOSAGE	THERAPEUTIC DOSAGE
Alprazolam (Xanax)	0.25–0.5 mg three times a day	0.5–4 mg/day
Clonazepam (Klonopin)	0.25–1 mg twice a day	1–4 mg/day
Lorazepam (Ativan)	1–1.5 mg twice a day	2–6 mg/day
Diazepam (Valium)	2–10 mg twice a day	4–40 mg/day

    - ◊ Rapid onset of action with quick symptom relief
    - ◊ Alprazolam (Xanax), diazepam (Valium), and clonazepam (Klonopin) frequently used to treat panic disorders when there is marked anticipatory anxiety
    - ◊ Patients with substance abuse histories at risk for abuse should avoid these medications
- Other antianxiety medications
    - ◊ Buspirone (Buspar): 7.5 mg twice a day up to 20–30 mg a day, non-addictive
- Slower onset of action—may take up to 4 weeks for antianxiety effects
- Maximum therapeutic effect may not be reached for 4 to 8 weeks.
- Antidepressants are commonly the first-line drug of choice for anxiety disorders (see Table 18–2).
    - ◊ Potential for substance abuse and dependence is significantly less than with benzodiazepines.
    - ◊ Main therapeutic effect may take 2 to 4 weeks.
    - ◊ Educating patient on time required to reach main effect of drug is essential for compliance.
    - ◊ Pregabalin has been shown to be effective in the treatment of GAD and is approved for that indication in Europe but not in the United States, 50–300 mg per day (see Table 18–2). Side effects include sedation and dizziness. It is better tolerated than benzodiazepines but should be prescribed with caution to patients with substance abuse disorder.
- Maximum therapeutic effect may not be reached for 4 to 8 weeks.

TABLE 18–2. SSRI/SNRI THERAPY IN ANXIETY DISORDERS

SSRI/SNRI MEDICATION	INITIAL DOSAGE	THERAPEUTIC DOSAGE
Fluoxetine (Prozac)	20 mg daily	20–80 mg/day
Paroxetine (Paxil)	20 mg daily	20–60 mg/day
Sertraline (Zoloft)	25 mg daily	25–200 mg/day
Fluvoxamine (Luvox)	50 mg q.h.s.	100–300 mg/day
Venlafaxine (Effexor)	12.5–25 mg twice a day	150–375 mg/day
Escitalopram (Lexapro)	10 mg daily	20 mg/day

How Long to Treat

- Length varies according to individual response and symptom management.
- Mild and situational anxiety usually resolves within 2 months.
- Long-term use of antidepressants can be required.
- Chronic, disabling anxiety requires a psychiatric consultation and referral.

Special Considerations

- It is common for anxiety disorders to occur concomitantly with other disorders, such as depression, eating disorders, and substance abuse, or with attention-deficit/hyperactivity disorder (ADHD), obsessive-compulsive disorder (OCD), and Tourette syndrome in children.
- Anxiety disorders are seen commonly with medical disorders. Always rule out underlying medical causes and ensure appropriate treatment of any concomitant disorders.
- Patients with anxiety disorders need reassurance that their disorders can be treated effectively.
- Establishing a trusting, safe, therapeutic patient provider relationship is essential for compliance and effective treatment.

When to Consult, Refer, Hospitalize

- Severe panic attacks, intense posttraumatic stress disorder (PTSD), and disabling OCD always require a psychiatric consult or referral and usually require a combination of pharmacotherapy and CBT.
- SSRIs and SNRIs, particularly venlafaxine and sertraline, have been found to be effective for pediatric anxiety disorders and should be the first-line treatment in combination with CBT for severe pediatric anxiety disorders that are unresponsive to CBT. CBT should be the first-line treatment for mild to moderate anxiety disorders.
- There is a black box warning of increased suicidal ideation and behavior in children and young adults under the age of 25 taking antidepressants, which was issued by the U.S. Food and Drug Administration (FDA) in 2004. The evidence is inadequate to establish this connection and the consensus is that the benefits of treatment outweigh the risks.
- Referral to a psychiatrist or psychiatric nurse practitioner or other mental health professional is indicated for anxiety in children. If started on medication, children should be monitored weekly for the first 4 weeks when started on medication, and parents and children should be informed of the risks.

Follow-Up

- Patients should be seen weekly during the acute phase of treatment.
- Medications need to be monitored for effectiveness, appropriate dose, and potential abuse.

Complications

- Drug abuse or dependence, dysfunctional social or occupational performance
- Treatment resistance or undertreatment, side effects from medications

OBSESSIVE–COMPULSIVE DISORDER (OCD)

Description

- OCD is characterized by the presence of obsessions or compulsions. *Obsessions* are recurrent, repetitive, and intrusive thoughts that are extremely difficult or impossible to control, are unreasonable or excessive, and that interfere significantly with a person's ability to function. *Compulsions* are repetitive behaviors that a person feels driven to perform and according to rigid internalized rules.

Subtypes

- Obsessive–compulsive disorder (OCD) (F42.2)
  - Either recurrent and persistent unwanted thoughts that are difficult or impossible to control, and/or
  - Repetitive, uncontrollable behaviors such as excessive handwashing, counting
  - Behaviors consume more than 1 hour of time each day.
- Body dysmorphic disorder (F45.22)
  - Preoccupation with a perceived body flaw in appearance that is not observable or is inconsequential to others resulting in obsessive behaviors
- Hoarding disorder (F42.3)
  - Persistent distress related to discarding possessions even when they have little economic or sentimental value. The accumulated possessions severely clutter and compromise the safety of living areas.

- Trichotillomania (F63.3)
  - Recurrent pulling out of one's hair resulting in hair loss
- Excoriation (F42.4)
  - Recurrent skin picking that results in lesions

Etiology

- Cause unknown
- Evolutionary psychology
  - Evolutionary advantage to compulsive behaviors and hoarding
- Biologic theory
  - Genetic predisposition, OCD 45% to 65%, mutation in human serotonin transporter (*5-HTT*) gene identified in OCD
  - Abnormalities of neurotransmitter receptors in the CNS, specifically dysregulation of the serotonin system
  - Abnormal brain structure and function in caudate region, frontal lobe, and cingulate gyrus
  - Possible infectious trigger for OCD

Risk Factors

- Environmental stressors, adverse prenatal events such as preterm birth or maternal tobacco use during pregnancy
- Disturbances in childhood development during the anal phase

Incidence and Demographics

- OCD typically starts in childhood or adolescent years.
- OCD can occur but is rare in persons 35 years of age or older.
- In the United States, OCD affects approximately 1.2% of the population.
- Adult onset of OCD affects slightly more women than men; childhood onset is more common in boys.
- About 76% of persons with OCD have a comorbid anxiety disorder.
- Approximately 30% of persons diagnosed with OCD have a comorbid tiic disorder.

Assessment

History

General

- Assess content and characteristics of obsessions and/or compulsions (obsessions: contamination; need for symmetry; pathological doubt; sexual) (compulsions: checking, counting, hoarding).
- Distinguish between preoccupations and worries about real-life concerns vs. inappropriate obsessive thoughts.
- Determine onset, frequency, and duration of symptoms.
- Determine degree of distress and symptom interference with daily function.
- Determine onset or precipitating factors for obsessions/compulsions.
- Elicit predisposing factors or stressors, such as divorce, financial difficulties, job loss, or victimization.
- Obtain complete medical history, including prescription medications, OTC medications, and supplements taken, history and current patterns of use of caffeine, alcohol, nicotine, and other substances.
- Ask about:
  - Attempts to control or neutralize thoughts or behaviors
  - Insight into excessive irrational nature of thoughts and behaviors
  - Feelings of anxiety or fear that accompany obsession
  - Suicidal thoughts or behaviors

Physical Exam

- Perform general exam to rule out serious CNS, cardiopulmonary, or endocrine disorder.

Diagnostic Studies

- Diagnostic labs such as ECG,TSH, CBC, and chemistry panel to rule out medical conditions
- Yale-Brown Obsessive Compulsive Scale (Y-BOCS)

Differential Diagnosis

- Any medical condition with CNS involvement, particularly basal ganglia diseases
- Major depressive disorder
- Tics and stereotyped movements
- Tourette syndrome
- Psychotic disorders
- Other compulsive-like behaviors (gambling, paraphilias)
- Obsessive-compulsive personality disorder

Management

- Mild cases are responsive to treatment in primary care settings.
- Refer moderately severe or disabling OCD to a mental health provider.
- Provide patient education to ensure compliance and effective treatment.

Nonpharmacologic Treatment

- Behavior therapy (BT), exposure and response prevention (ERP). BT is as effective as pharmacological therapy and effects longer lasting.
- Family therapy
- Relaxation therapy
- Stress management education, courses, workshops
- Biofeedback
- Community self-help and support groups
- Education of patient and family about the disorder and treatment
- Self-management and self-help

Pharmacologic Treatment

- Tricyclic antidepressants, particularly clomipramine, SSRIs, and an atypical antipsychotic in conjunction with SSRI

Other Treatments

- Electroconvulsive therapy (ECT)
- Deep brain stimulation
- Vagus nerve stimulation
- Surgical lesion to cingulate cortex (cingulotomy)

TRAUMA AND STRESSOR-RELATED DISORDERS

Description

- Disorders precipitated by exposure to a traumatic event resulting in sustained fear or anxiety-based reactions

Subtypes

- Reactive attachment disorder (F94.1)
    - A childhood disorder characterized by a pattern of emotionally withdrawn behavior towards adult caregivers
    - The child rarely seeks comfort or responds to comfort from caregivers when distressed.
    - Results from extreme deprivation or social neglect and failure to meet basic needs for comfort, stimulation, and affection during the first few months of life
- Post-traumatic stress disorder (PTSD) (F43.10)
    - Exposure to an extreme traumatic stressor such as rape, sexual or physical abuse, natural disasters, war, or other perceived or actual threat to a person's physical being or self-concept
    - Response to event is intense fear, helplessness, or horror
    - Results in persistent symptoms, including nightmares, flashbacks, numbing of emotion, dissociative episodes, or inability to recall specific events
    - Hyper-arousal
    - Avoidance of stimuli associated with the event
    - Intense psychological distress at exposure to reminders of the original event
    - Symptoms must last more than 1 month after event.
    - Depression, anxiety, cognitive difficulties

- Acute stress disorder (ASD) (F43.0)
  - Exposure to a traumatic event that involved actual or threatened death or serious injury
  - Response to event is intense fear, helplessness, or horror
  - Results in same symptoms as PTSD, but occur within 4 weeks of the event
  - Dissociation maybe a predominant symptom in some individuals
  - Lasts for minimum of 3 days and maximum of 4 weeks
- Prolonged grief disorder (F43.8)
  - An abnormally persistent grief response to the death of a loved one
  - There is an intense yearning for the deceased individual or a preoccupation of the deceased person
  - Results in clinically significant identity disruption, disbelief about the death, avoidance of reminders of the dead person, emotional pain or numbness, loneliness, purposelessness, or difficulty in moving forward with life, exhibiting three of these symptoms lasting about 1 month
  - The death of a loved one occurred in the preceding 12 months, for adults
  - The death of a loved one occurred in the preceding 6 months, for children
  - New DSM-5-TR diagnosis

Etiology

- Exposure to stressor and response to stressor
- Biologic theory
  - Genetic predisposition to psychiatric illness
  - Abnormalities of neurotransmitter receptors in the CNS, specifically GABA receptors, increased catecholamines
  - Abnormalities in the opioid system
  - Hypothalamic-pituitary-adrenal (HPA)–axis dysfunction and low plasma and urinary free cortisol
- Psychodynamic theory
  - Subjective meaning of stressor may determine traumatic effect
  - Resonance with childhood traumas
  - Inability to regulate emotions
  - Use of defense mechanisms of repression, denial, reaction formation, and undoing
  - Alexithymia, which is an inability to identify and express feelings

- Behavioral model
  - The trauma is an unconditioned stimulus that produces a fear response that is paired with it through class conditioning. Reminders of the stimulus elicit the fear response through instrumental learning.

Incidence and Demographics

- The lifetime prevalence of PTSD in the United States is 6.8%,
- High-risk groups include combat veterans, survivors of rape and domestic violence, and workers in vocations that increase a person's likelihood of exposure to a trauma such as first responders
- Prevalence in women is twice as high as in men.
- Prevalence of prolonged grief disorder may be higher in populations with elevated exposure to trauma.

Risk Factors

- Severity, duration, and proximity to actual trauma
- Presence of childhood trauma
- Borderline, paranoid, dependent, or antisocial personality disorders
- Single, divorced, socially withdrawn, inadequate family or peer support system
- Female gender
- Low socioeconomic status
- Recent excessive alcohol intake
- External locus of control
- Risk of developing PTSD after exposure to trauma greater in first-degree relatives of persons who have history of depression

Assessment

History

General

- Determine onset, frequency, and duration of symptoms.
- Determine degree of distress and symptom interference with daily function.

- Elicit predisposing factors or stressors, such as divorce, financial difficulties, job loss, or victimization.
- Obtain complete medical history, including prescription medications, OTC medications, and supplements taken.
- Obtain history and current patterns of use of caffeine, alcohol, nicotine, and other substances.
- Assess for suicidal ideation or attempt.
- Ask about:
  - Feelings of loss of control, panic, impending doom or dread, depersonalization, difficulty concentrating
  - Flashbacks, reliving the event
  - Hypervigilance
  - Emotional numbness and avoidance
  - Difficulty concentrating, making decisions, irritable, agitated mood, motor restlessness
  - Sleep disturbances (insomnia, frequent awakenings), fatigue, irritation, agitated mood

Physical Exam

- Perform general exam to rule out serious CNS, cardiopulmonary, or endocrine disorder.
- Focus on vital signs, cardiac, pulmonary, and neurological exam.

Differential Diagnosis

- Adjustment disorders
- Traumatic brain injury
- Major depression
- Personality disorders
- Psychotic disorders, schizophrenia
- Alcohol and substance abuse
- Anxiety disorder
- Panic disorder
- Dissociative disorders

Management

Nonpharmacologic Treatment

- Behavior therapy and exposure therapy, cognitive behavioral therapy, and stress management, coping skills, psychodynamic psychotherapy, hypnosis
- Psychoeducation related to symptom management
- Offer reassurance to destigmatize experiences.
- Encourage participation in support groups, group therapy.

Pharmacologic Treatment

- SSRIs (sertraline and paroxetine)
- Other possible options: SNRI (venlafaxine), anticonvulsant (topiramate), antipsychotic (risperidone)
- Symptom management: Alpha-1 adrenergic antagonist (prazosin) for nightmares; trazodone for insomnia

Mood Disorders

DESCRIPTION

- Includes symptoms of depressed mood and includes depressive disorder, dysthymic disorder, and bipolar disorder

GRIEF/BEREAVEMENT

- A normal emotional and physiological reaction to loss; situational and time-limited
- May cause varying degrees of symptoms, such as feeling of profound sadness, crying spells, insomnia, loss of appetite, survivor guilt
- Distinguish between grief and major depressive episode (MDE). Grief decreases in intensity over days to weeks and comes in waves. It is not accompanied by self-criticism, feelings of worthlessness, self-loathing, and being undeserving of life.

RISK FACTORS

- All people, for uncomplicated grief
- Risk of developing more complicated mood disorders: poor coping skills, lack of support, history of previous mood disorder, alcohol, or substance abuse

MANAGEMENT

Nonpharmacologic Treatment

- Encourage the expression of grief and mourning over loss.
- Offer reassurance that grief is a normal, nonpathologic reaction to loss and is self-limited.
- Encourage participation in support groups.

Pharmacologic Treatment

- Mild antianxiety agents at the lowest effective dose may be used to treat symptoms, but do not treat symptoms of major depression.

When to Consult, Refer, Hospitalize

- Grief that lasts longer than 1 month should be evaluated for mood disorders or prolonged grief disorder and referred to a mental health specialist.
- Suicidal ideation is a psychiatric emergency; the patient should be referred immediately for psychiatric evaluation.

Follow-Up

- The duration of normal grief reaction varies among different persons and may vary among cultures, but usually begins to show marked improvement within 8 weeks.
- The diagnosis of major depressive disorder is not given unless symptoms are still present after 2 months and represent a significant change in function and impairment.

- Older adults and patients without adequate social/familial support are at high risk for developing major depression and suicidal ideation.
- Children may harbor feelings of guilt and responsibility and may require referral to psychiatrist or mental health specialist.

Depressive Disorders

DESCRIPTION

- Major depression is a complex mood disorder lasting at least 2 weeks, with sad, "blue" mood that may or may not be accompanied by the loss of interest or pleasure in nearly all activities, every day.
- In children, the mood may be irritable rather than sad.
- Depression is associated with abnormalities in neurotransmission, neurophysiology, and neuroendocrine function.
- Clinical manifestations of childhood depression vary according to the child's developmental age.

SUBTYPES

- Adjustment disorder with depressed mood (F43.21)
- Depressive disorders
- Major depressive disorder (F32.9): single or recurrent episodes of depression associated with other symptoms lasting at least 2 weeks but without mood elevation, elation, or mania
- Dysthymic disorder (Persistent depressive disorder; F34.1): chronic, sustained depressed mood ongoing for a minimum of 2 years, more days than not, symptoms less severe than in depressive disorder
- Premenstrual dysphoric disorder (F32.81)
- Mood disorders due to illness and drugs
- Bipolar disorder (mania, cyclothymic disorder): recurrent episodes of depression with episodes of mania characterized by lack of impulse control, excessive energy, grandiose or delusional thinking, elated mood, inappropriate behaviors, hyperactivity, pressured speech, decreased need for sleep

- Atypical depression: characterized by hypersomnia, fatigue, rejection sensitivity, overeating
- Melancholic depression: characterized by insomnia, early morning or frequent awakenings, anxiety, loss of appetite, difficulty concentrating, fatigue
- Postpartum: symptom onset within 2 weeks to 6 months postpartum
- Suicide: Suicide rates in the United States increased 37% between 2000 and 2018, decreased 5% between 2018 and 2020, rates increased to peak again in 2021, and increased by 2.5% in 2022. The highest rate of suicide is among middle-aged White men.

ETIOLOGY

- Genetic predisposition—30% to 40% hereditable
- Theoretical: Biological dysregulation of the hypopituitary axis (stress response). The core symptoms of depression—such as sleep, appetite, and mood disturbances—are related to the functions of the hypothalamus and the pituitary glands and associated hormones such as cortisol, leptin, and corticotropin-releasing hormone (CRH).
- Theoretical: Abnormalities in neurotransmitters in the brain are associated with serotonin, acetylcholine, dopamine, norepinephrine, epinephrine, and GABA; possible structural changes in the brain.
- Social-Ecological Model: theory of multiple influences, individual, interpersonal, institutional, community, societal, or policy level
- Additional environmental factors and learned behaviors may influence neurotransmitter function or exert independent influence.

INCIDENCE AND DEMOGRAPHICS

- Third most important cause of disease burden worldwide; first most important in high-income countries
- Depression is the most common mental illness seen in primary care practices.
- Depressive disorders often co-occur with anxiety and substance use disorders.
- The 12-month prevalence of a major depressive disorder for the U.S. adult population is about 7%.
- Depression is more common in women than men and in persons without close interpersonal relationships.

- Patients with depression have two to three times the normal death rate at any age (independent of suicide) and are more likely to incur long-term medical consequences, such as premature osteoporosis, coronary artery disease, dysfunction of inflammatory mediators and the immune system, and increased insulin resistance.
- The presence of a chronic illness increases the risk for a major depressive disorder.
- The peak onset of a bipolar I disorder ranges from 20 to 30 years of age and for bipolar II disorder is in the mid-20s.
- In the United States, the mean age for onset of major depressive disorder and for persistent depressive disorder is about 30 years of age.
- About 75% of suicide victims have a depressive or alcohol use disorder.

RISK FACTORS

- Recent stressful life events are the most powerful predictors of onset of a depressive disorder.
- Prior episodes of depression
- People without close interpersonal relationships
- Losing a parent before age 11
- Family history, especially having first-degree relative who is diagnosed
- Alcohol and substance abuse
- Postpartum period
- Significant psychosocial stressors such as poverty, homelessness, divorce, finances, job loss, political refugee, trauma, or abuse
- Chronic medical illness
- Risk factors for suicide:
    - Personal or family history of one or more mental or substance abuse disorders
    - Severe psychosocial stressors: divorce, unemployment, legal problems, perception of poor health
    - Anxiety
    - Depression in childhood or adolescence
    - Previous suicide attempt(s)
    - Family or domestic violence, including physical or sexual abuse
    - Firearms in the home

- ◊ Specific plan
- ◊ Family history of suicide
- ◊ Mental illness: anxiety, depression, bipolar disorder, and schizophrenia

PREVENTION AND SCREENING

- U.S. Preventive Services Task Force (USPSTF) recommendation: Screen adults for depression in clinical practices that have systems in place to assure accurate diagnosis, effective treatment, and follow-up. The benefits of screening are likely to outweigh any potential harms. There is little evidence to recommend one screening tool over another.
- Patient education/public awareness of signs, symptoms, and available treatment modalities: Patient Health Questionnaire-9 (PHQ-9) most widely used screening tool
- PHQ-2: two-question screening questionnaire is reliable when followed with clinical evaluation
- The American Academy of Pediatrics (AAP) recommendation: routine screening for postpartum depression (PPD) in mothers during well-child visits at 1, 2, 4, and 6 months of age.

ASSESSMENT

History

- Establish frequency, type, and duration of symptoms.
- Degree of disruption or impairment in daily activities
- Past medical history, including thyroid disease
- Prior personal psychiatric history
- Social history including alcohol and substance use
- Family psychiatric/psychosocial history
- Identify acute and chronic stressors.
- Ask about suicidal thoughts, impulses, and history of prior attempts or current plans.
- Inquire about homicidal ideations.
- Rule out a bipolar disorder.
- According to the DSM-5-TR, sad, blue, or depressed mood and/or absence of pleasure plus four or more of listed symptoms must be present for a minimum of 2 weeks and

represent a change from previous function to diagnose major depression. Classic symptoms of major depression (DSM-5-TR):

- ◊ Depressed mood most of the day, nearly every day; in children, can be irritable mood
- ◊ Significant weight loss when not dieting, or weight gain, or increase or decrease in appetite
- ◊ Markedly diminished interest or pleasure in all or almost all activities
- ◊ Psychomotor agitation or retardation
- ◊ Difficulty concentrating or making decisions
- ◊ Change in sleep patterns (insomnia or hypersomnia)
- ◊ Low self-esteem; feelings of worthlessness or excessive, inappropriate guilt
- ◊ Recurrent thoughts of death, suicidal ideation with or without a specific plan, prior suicide attempt
- ◊ Decreased energy and fatigue; increased somatic complaints such as headache
- ◊ Feelings of hopelessness
- ◊ Use a scale such as the PHQ-9, which has good test–retest reliability, internal consistency, and sensitivity to change in depression over time. It has been studied extensively as a screening measure for major depression in primary care settings.

- ♦ Use a scale such as the Geriatric Depression Scale (for older adults).
- ♦ Adjustment disorder
  - ◊ A less-severe form of depression in which symptoms occur within 3 months of an identifiable stressor; mild sadness, inability to concentrate, excess worry, somatic complaints
- ♦ Bipolar disorder
  - ◊ Extreme swings in mood, hyperactivity, flight of ideas, decreased need for sleep, grandiosity, impaired judgment, depression, aggressive behavior, sexual acting out, delusions, or ideation
- ♦ Depression in children
  - ◊ Sadness, crying, withdrawal, fatigue, anger, irritability or agitation, somatic complaints, separation anxiety, difficulty concentrating, feelings of guilt or worthlessness, weight change, change in sleep patterns, increased social isolation, substance abuse, or suicidal ideation
- ♦ Dysthymic disorder
  - ◊ Depressed mood most of the day, present almost continuously; complaint that has always been depressed

Physical Exam

- Complete physical exam with a mental status exam to rule out any underlying medical conditions
- Observation of personal appearance, grooming, hygiene, affect

Diagnostic Studies

- Primarily a clinical diagnosis; tests (CBC, TSH, sedimentation rate, chemistry profile, B12 and folate, rapid plasma regain [RPR], computed tomography [CT] scan) used to rule out suspected underlying medical causes
- ECG before initiation of tricyclic antidepressants (TCAs)
- Cortisol levels, EEG may be done by specialist.
- Psychometric tests include Minnesota Multiphasic Personality Inventory (MMPI-2).
- Self-report scales commonly used are Beck Depression Inventory, Hamilton Rating Scale for Depression, Zung Self-Rating Depression Scale, and Geriatric Depression Scale.
- Self-report scales commonly used include the Edinburgh Postpartum Depression Scale (EPDS).

Differential Diagnosis

- Electrolyte imbalances
- Chronic fatigue syndrome
- COPD
- Bereavement or grief reaction over recent loss
- Bipolar disorders
- Psychotic disorders, schizophrenia
- Alcohol and substance abuse
- Mononucleosis

Endocrine Disorders

- Hyperthyroidism
- Cushing syndrome

- Addison's disease
- Diabetes

Neurological Disorders

- Neoplasms
- Stroke
- Severe trauma
- Head injury
- Multiple sclerosis
- Seizure disorders
- Parkinson's disease
- Dementia
- Chronic pain

Cardiac Disorders

- Arrhythmia
- CHF
- MI
- Hypertension

Medications That Can Induce Depression

- Opioids
- Steroids
- Estrogen
- Antihypertensive agents
- Digoxin
- Anti-Parkinson's drugs

- Non-steroidal anti-inflammatory drugs (NSAIDs)
- Beta blockers
- Sedatives and hypnotics
- Antibacterial/antifungals
- Antineoplastic drugs
- Psychotropic drugs
- Analgesics
- Anti-inflammatories

Management

- Mild depression may be managed safely by a primary practitioner with frequent evaluation.
- Frequent follow-up is necessary to educate patients regarding their illness and to adequately treat.
- Any antidepressant may precipitate a manic episode in those patients prone to bipolar illness.
- Patient education concerning the nature of the illness, course of treatment, and expected outcome is essential.
- A complete diagnostic evaluation is essential, with evaluation of suicide risk.
- Treatment for adolescents with mental health specialist.

Nonpharmacologic Treatment

- Psychotherapy, alone or in combination with antidepressant medication, is an option for patients with mild to moderate major depression.
- CBT and dialectical behavior therapy with a focus on cognitive distortions and behaviors that exacerbate depressive illness
- Psychoanalysis or psychotherapy with a focus on interpersonal skills
- Consider transcranial magnetic stimulation (TMS) for treatment-resistant depression or for use during pregnancy.

- Suicidal ideation or behavior is a psychiatric emergency and should always be evaluated further and treated by a mental health practitioner immediately.
- ECT is indicated for severely depressed or suicidal patients who do not respond to pharmacological agents; the main side effect is temporary memory impairment that may last up to 2 weeks.
- Provide community resources, hotlines, and a list of local support groups.

Pharmacologic Treatment

See Table 18–3

- SSRIs are the first-line drug of choice because of their effectiveness and safety record in adults.
  - All antidepressants including SSRIs carry a black box warning of suicidal ideations in children, adolescents, and young adults up to the age of 24. Treatment of children should be initiated and managed by a mental health specialist.
  - Information from an increasing number of studies indicates an increase in suicidal and homicidal behavior with SSRI use in some children. An FDA advisory panel has recently recommended warnings on all antidepressants, indicating that suicide risk may be increased in children taking these products.
  - Other cautions include abrupt withdrawal of SSRIs and SNRIs, which may cause discontinuation syndrome including unpleasant symptoms such as fatigue, paresthesia, abnormal dreams, and/or irritability, so SSRIs should be tapered. During treatment, children may experience "behavior activation" (the underactive child may become agitated and impulsive).

TABLE 18–3. COMMON SSRI THERAPY FOR TREATMENT OF ADULT DEPRESSION

SSRI/SNRI MEDICATION	INITIAL DOSAGE	THERAPEUTIC DOSAGE
Fluoxetine (Prozac)	20 mg daily in a.m.	20–80 mg daily
Sertraline (Zoloft)	50 mg daily	50–200 mg daily
Paroxetine (Paxil)	20 mg daily in a.m.	20–50 mg daily
Citalopram (Celexa)	20 mg daily	20–40 mg daily
Escitalopram (Lexapro)	10 mg daily	10–20 mg daily
Duloxetine (Cymbalta)	40 mg daily	40–60 mg daily in divided dose
Venlafaxine (Effexor)	25–50 mg daily with food in 2–3 doses	75–375 mg daily divided

- Tricyclic antidepressants (or TCAs) (see Table 18–4) are also effective but are associated with a greater incidence of side effects.
    - ◊ Tricyclics block cholinergic muscarinic receptors, resulting in possible constipation, dry mouth, urinary retention, blurred vision, and sinus tachycardia; other side effects include sedation, postural hypotension, weight gain, potentiation of CNS medications, and dizziness.
    - ◊ Tricyclics are contraindicated in patients with cardiac conduction disorders, narrow angle glaucoma, and prostatic hypertrophy.
    - ◊ Tricyclics cause weight gain; monitor weight and body mass index (BMI).
- Monoamine oxidase inhibitors (MAOIs), such as phenelzine (Nardil) and tranylcypromine (Parnate), are used in the treatment of refractory or treatment-resistant depression. Potentially serious and lethal side effects, such as hypertensive crisis, may occur. These drugs should be initiated by a psychiatrist.
- Atypical antipsychotics may be used in refractory depression.
- Other antidepressants used in adults and children are listed in Table 18–5. Dose should be increased every 2 weeks in adults until a therapeutic dose is reached. Children and adolescents should be monitored more frequently upon starting an antidepressant.

How Long to Treat

- Duration and course of treatment is individualized, depends upon severity of illness and response to treatment.
- 33% of patients achieve full remission with one antidepressant.
- If the patient is nonresponsive to medication, increase to maximum dose slowly. If no response, change within the drug class (switch from one SSRI to another) or to another antidepressant drug class. Table 18–4 and 18–5 include treatment options. Start with SSRI, add another antidepressant (Wellbutrin, Effexor, Remeron); add next or switch to second-line tricyclics; and, finally, refer out for MAOIs.

TABLE 18–4.
COMMON TRICYCLIC ANTIDEPRESSANTS

MEDICATION	INITIAL DOSAGE	TARGET DOSAGE
Amitriptyline (Elavil)	25 mg q.h.s.	50–150 mg divided
Desipramine (Norpramin)	25 mg daily	75–300 mg daily
Imipramine (Tofranil)	25 mg q.h.s.	75–300 mg q.h.s.
Nortriptyline (Pamelor)	10–25 mg q.h.s.	75–150 mg daily or divided

TABLE 18–5. OTHER ANTIDEPRESSANTS COMMONLY USED IN TREATING ADULTS AND CHILDREN

MEDICATION	INITIAL DOSAGE	TARGET DOSAGE
Bupropion (Wellbutrin)	75 mg twice a day; avoid bedtime dosing	300–400 mg/day divided 3–4x daily
Mirtazapine (Remeron)	15 mg q.h.s.	15–45 mg q.h.s.
Nefazodone (Serzone)	200 mg/day divided 2x/day	300–600 mg/day divided 2x daily
Venlafaxine (Effexor)	25–50 mg daily with food in 2–3 doses	75–375 mg daily divided

- In March of 2019, the FDA approved esketamine (Spravato) nasal spray for patients who have treatment-resistant depression or have failed to improve on at least two other antidepressant medications. The drug is similar to the anesthetic ketamine. It is the first new depression treatment approved in decades and targets brain pathways different from those targeted by other antidepressants. Unlike SSRIs, which can take 4–6 weeks to take effect, Spravato's effect can occur within hours or days.
    - Serious adverse outcomes are contained in a boxed warning and include sedation and dissociation (difficulty with attention, judgment, and thinking) and the potential for abuse and misuse of the drug, as well as suicidal thoughts and behaviors. It is available only through a restricted distribution system, and it must be administered in a certified medical office under a Risk Evaluation and Mitigation Strategy (REMS). The patient cannot take the medication home and must be monitored for at least 2 hours after taking the medication in the office setting.
- Depression is a chronic illness with frequent episodes of recurrence.
- Antidepressants are most effective when taken for at least 1 year after remission of symptoms.
- If patient has had two or more episodes, consider remaining on antidepressants.
- If patient is unresponsive to treatment, consider combination treatment with psychotherapy and/or refer to a mental health specialist.
- Genetic testing is not recommended due to lack of standardization.

Special Considerations

- Patients treated for major depression in a general practice setting have more pain, physical illness, and social and interpersonal impairment than other patient populations.
- Sustained release (SR) or extended release (XR) versions are more easily tolerated.

- Tricyclic medications have a high potential for lethality in overdose.
- Depression in older adults may be difficult to diagnose because of the greater incidence of dementia and the number and types of medications taken for other medical conditions.
- Older adult patients require smaller starting doses but may require the same therapeutic dosage as younger adults and frequently require closer medical management.
- In clients age 60 or older, the maximum daily dose is 20 mg per day of citalopram because of the risk of QTc interval prolongation

When to Consult, Refer, Hospitalize

- All patients who present with suicidal ideation with plan or history of prior attempt should immediately be referred to an emergency department or psychiatrist for further evaluation and treatment.
- Symptoms of bipolar disorder (history of mania or hypomania, frequent depressive episodes, earlier age at onset, strong family history) should be referred to a mental health professional.
- All patients should be referred to the appropriate mental health practitioner for therapy.
- Consult for all women who are pregnant or plan to become pregnant before initiating medication.
- Patients who are severely impaired by their symptomology or present with comorbid disorders, such as OCD, substance abuse, eating disorders, or no social support, should be referred to a psychiatrist or other mental health specialist.
- Patients who represent a clear and present danger to themselves or others should be hospitalized immediately.
- Children should be referred to a child and adolescent psychiatrist or psychiatric nurse practitioner and, at minimum, consult with a mental health professional.
- *Antidepressant medication in children should be managed by a mental health professional.*
- Patients who prefer therapy to medication should be referred to a psychologist or other mental health specialist.

Follow-Up

- Patients should initially be seen weekly or least biweekly to titrate dosage and monitor symptom management and compliance.

- Medication compliance is a serious issue, with patients often discontinuing treatment before medication has time to work and symptoms subside.
- Educate patients concerning risks, benefits, and possible side effects of medications.
- Patients are at the highest risk for suicide 2–4 weeks after initiating antidepressants
- Educate patients about onset of effectiveness.

Expected Course

- Most patients respond to antidepressants within 2 to 3 weeks of treatment but should be educated that drug therapy may take months to reach full effect.
- Risk factors for recurrence are several prior episodes and early discontinuance of medication.
- To ensure the most effective response, antidepressants need to be taken at least 1 year after remission of symptoms, as depression is a chronic disease with frequent episodes of recurrence.

Complications

- Social isolation, impairment of vocation and interpersonal relationships, suicide

Somatic Symptom Disorders

DESCRIPTION

- Multiple and ongoing chronic physical complaints (somatic symptoms) occur over a period of years, causing significant functional impairment. Commonly presenting in primary care settings; less frequently in psychiatric settings

SUBTYPES

- Somatic symptom disorder—many physical complaints affecting many body systems for which the patient seeks treatment. Somatic symptoms are accompanied by abnormal thoughts, feelings, and behaviors related to the symptoms. (1) One or more somatic symptoms that cause distress or significant functional impairment. (2) Excessive cognitions, feelings, or behaviors about symptoms evidenced by one of the following:

persistent thoughts about seriousness of symptoms; high anxiety about symptoms; excessive time and energy devoted to health concerns. (3) Having symptoms is persistent and lasts longer than 6 months.

- Symptoms are more than known medical conditions or cannot be explained by a medical condition or substance abuse.
- Illness anxiety disorder (previously referred to as hypochondriasis): patient's belief that he or she has a specific disease
- Conversion disorder: one or more neurological complaints with the absence of substantiating physical and laboratory findings
- Factitious disorder: falsification of physical signs or symptoms or self-infliction of injury or disease associated with identified deception

ETIOLOGY

- Cause unknown
- Psychodynamic: symptoms substitute for repressed unacceptable instincts
- Psychosocial: secondary gains from symptoms to avoid work; symptoms are a form of communication, to unconsciously express beliefs and feelings
- Biological factors: faulty perception and interpretation of somatosensory input
- Temperamental: A personality trait of negative affectivity (neuroticism) is a potential risk factor for the development of somatic symptom disorder
- Environment: Adverse childhood experiences, stress, low socioeconomic status including limited education are all risk factors
- Theoretical: biological dysregulation of the cytokine system
- Additional environmental factors and learned behaviors may influence development of symptoms.

INCIDENCE AND DEMOGRAPHICS

- The lifetime prevalence of somatic symptom disorder in the adult population is estimated to be 4% to 6%; there is a higher prevalence in the primary care setting.
- Women are diagnosed more often with a somatic symptom disorder because they tend to report somatic symptoms more often than men.
- Begins before age 30, usually in adolescent years

RISK FACTORS

- Low education
- Low socioeconomic status
- Other psychiatric disorders
- Personality disorders (avoidant, OCD, paranoid)
- Depression
- Anxiety
- Childhood physical or sexual abuse
- Negative affectivity (neuroticism)
- Recent stressful events

ASSESSMENT

History

- Establish frequency, type, and duration of symptoms.
- Degree of disruption or impairment in daily activities
- Past medical history, including thyroid disease
- Prior personal psychiatric history
- Social history including alcohol and substance use
- Family psychiatric/psychosocial history
- Identify acute and chronic stressors.
- Ask about prior diagnostic tests, laboratory studies, experiences with other providers.

Physical Exam

- Complete physical exam with a mental status exam to rule out any underlying medical conditions

Diagnostic Studies

- Primarily a clinical diagnosis; tests (CBC, TSH, sedimentation rate, chemistry profile, B12 and folate, RPR, CT scan) used to rule out suspected underlying medical causes

DIFFERENTIAL DIAGNOSIS

Other Medical Conditions

- Chronic fatigue syndrome
- Mononucleosis
- Multiple sclerosis

Psychiatric Disorders

- Psychotic disorders, schizophrenia
- Alcohol and substance abuse
- Grief and bereavement with physical symptoms
- Mood disorders
- Anxiety disorders
- Malingering
- Delusional disorder

Endocrine Disorders

- Hyperthyroidism
- Hyperparathyroidism
- Intermittent porphyria

Management

- Respond to physical complaints as emotional expressions of need rather than medical complaints
- Conduct brief visit, with episodic physical exam in response to new physical complaints.
- Avoid extensive laboratory and diagnostic studies.
- Increase patient's awareness that physical symptoms may have psychological factors.

Nonpharmacologic Treatment

- Psychotherapy, individual and group

Pharmacologic Treatment

See Table 18–3

- SSRIs only if underlying mood disorder is present
- Monitor for adherence

Substance Use Disorders

TOBACCO DEPENDENCE

Description

- Tobacco is smoked, chewed, and snuffed. Electronic cigarettes or e-cigarettes use a liquid nicotine cartridge, rather than tobacco. Nicotine is the main source of dependence.

Incidence and Demographics

- An average of 10% to 12% of adults in the U.S. are tobacco smokers.
- The most used nicotine product is tobacco from cigarettes in adults; among middle and high school students the most used route is via e-cigarettes.
- Greater incidence of smoking in men than women
- Almost every adult who smokes started by the age of 18.

Risks of Tobacco Use

- More than 400,000 people die each year of tobacco-related illnesses.
- Deaths from use include cardiovascular disease, cancer, and COPD.
- Direct and indirect health costs each year are estimated at more than $300 billion.
- Tobacco usage is established in adolescence. In 2018, 7.2% of middle school students and 27% of high school students were currently using some form of tobacco. Although

cigarette use has declined, e-cigarette use has increased, accounting for 21% of all tobacco use among high school students.

- In 2019, about 25% of U.S. middle and high school students were exposed to environmental tobacco smoke in their own home; another 23% in vehicles

Prevention and Screening

- Discuss the effects of tobacco use at all health care visits with children, adolescents, and adults.
- Screen persons for exposure to secondhand smoke.
    - Inquire at adolescent health visits if an adolescent's friends are smokers. If an adolescent's friends smoke, the adolescent is more likely to smoke.
    - Take a complete smoking history at all health care visits and encourage attempts to quit.

Assessment

- Use 5As algorithm:
    - **Ask** about their smoking status.
    - **Advise** smokers to quit.
    - **Assess** their readiness to quit.
    - **Assist** them with smoking cessation effort.
    - **Arrange** for follow-up visits or contact.

Management

Smoking Cessation

- Combination of education, support, behavioral strategies, pharmacotherapy (with nicotine replacement, bupropion, or varenicline) is more effective than any method alone.
- Encourage patient to quit and offer therapy at every visit.
- Brief tobacco dependence treatment is effective. Clinicians should offer at least brief treatments to every patient who uses tobacco.
- Individual, group, and telephone counseling are effective, and their effectiveness increases with treatment intensity. Two components of counseling are especially

effective; clinicians should use practical counseling (problem-solving/skills training) and social support delivered as part of treatment.

- Numerous effective medications are available for tobacco dependence; clinicians should encourage their use by all patients attempting to quit smoking—except when medically contraindicated or with specific populations for which there is insufficient evidence of effectiveness (i.e., pregnant women, smokeless tobacco users, light smokers, and adolescents).
- Seven first-line medications (five nicotine and two non-nicotine) reliably increase long-term smoking abstinence rates:
  - Bupropion SR (Wellbutrin SR): 150 mg twice a day for 7 to 12 weeks.
  - Nicotine gum (Nicorette): 2–4 mg orally every 1 to 2 hours. Taper use after 6 weeks. Max 24 pieces/24 hours.
  - Nicotine inhaler (Nicotrol): 4 mg per cartridge. Taper use. Maximum 16 cartridges/24 hours.
  - Nicotine lozenge (Nicorette): 2–4 mg orally every 1 to 2 hours. Taper use after 6 weeks.
  - Nicotine nasal spray (Nicotrol NS): 10 mg/mL (0.5 mg/spray). One spray each nostril every 1 to 5 hours for 8 weeks. Then taper. Maximum 80 sprays (40 mg)/24 hours.
  - Nicotine transdermal patch: Dose based on cigarette consumption. 7 mg, 14 mg, 21 mg patches. Tapered dosing.
  - Varenicline (Chantix): Start drug 1 week before planned quit date. Increase dose first week, then 1 mg orally twice a day for 11 weeks. May continue for an additional 12 weeks if initial treatment is unsuccessful.
- Consider combination therapies.
- Nicotine-replacement product adverse reactions include local irritation of skin or mucous membranes, withdrawal symptoms, gastrointestinal (GI) upset, tachycardia, and spontaneous abortion. Avoid use immediately post-MI, accelerated hypertension, severe angina, chronic nasal disorders (spray), hepatic and renal dysfunction, hyperthyroidism, and other disorders.
- Counseling and medication are effective when used by themselves for treating tobacco dependence. The combination of counseling and medication, however, is more effective than either alone. Thus clinicians should encourage all persons making a quit attempt to use both counseling and medication.
- Telephone quit-line counseling is effective with diverse populations and has a broad reach, so clinicians should promote quit-line use.

Follow-Up

- Patient must stop smoking before nicotine preparation is used.
- Pregnant women should be encouraged to stop smoking without pharmacologic support.
- Relapse is common and occurs frequently within the first 1 to 2 weeks during withdrawal.
- Provide weekly visits during attempts to quit.
- Long-term success is greater with multiple attempts.

ALCOHOL DEPENDENCE

Description

- Alcohol dependence is defined as a maladaptive pattern of use associated with three or more of the following:
  - Tolerance
  - Withdrawal
  - Taking in more than intended
  - Persistent desire to cut down/control use
  - Time spent obtaining, using, or recovering from the substance
  - Social/occupational/recreational tasks sacrificed
  - Uses despite physical and psychological problems

Etiology

- Alcohol is absorbed rapidly from the GI tract and acts as a CNS depressant.
  - Excessive quantity will cause stupor, coma, and death (from respiratory depression or toxicity to neurons).
  - Physical and psychological dependence vary; there may be genetic predisposition to alcoholism, as well as social and cultural conditioning to its use.

Incidence and Demographics

- Alcohol dependence and abuse are prevalent worldwide.
- The first episode of alcohol intoxication is likely to occur in adolescence.

- Alcohol is the most frequently used depressant in the world.
- Greater incidence of alcohol use disorder in men than women
- Middle-aged adults are at the highest risk of abuse; abuse and dependence are prevalent across the age spectrum but decline with age.

Risk Factors

- Genetics: Tends to run in families, 40% to 60% of cases with a genetic influence
- Environment: Poverty, discrimination, low educational levels, stress, unemployment, access to alcohol, and cultural attitudes about alcohol consumption

Prevention and Screening

- Screen using a brief, simple questionnaire, such as the single-item screening, Cutdown, Annoyed, Guilty, and Eye opener (CAGE) Questionnaire, or Alcohol Use Disorders Identification Test Concise (AUDIT-C):
    - ◊ How often do you have a drink containing alcohol?
    - ◊ How many drinks containing alcohol do you have on a typical day that you are drinking?
    - ◊ How often do you have six or more drinks on one occasion?
- Early public education as to the nature, course, and consequences of alcohol
- Primary intervention programs in the community and schools
- Increased social and public awareness through educational mass media campaigns
- Community groups such as Mothers Against Drunk Driving (MADD)

Assessment

History

- Inquire about patterns of use; however, denial is a common coping mechanism.
- History of prior substance abuse treatment
- Psychiatric history and mental status exam
- Current use of prescribed and OTC medications

Physical Exam

- Clinical manifestations of alcoholism and alcohol abuse include:
  - Withdrawal symptoms such as tremors, confusion, hallucinations, disorientation, seizures
  - Neurological: memory impairment, forgetfulness, loss of time or blackouts, hyperreflexia, ataxia, confabulation
  - Cardiovascular: cardiomyopathy, hypertension, and arrhythmias
  - Compromised immune system, frequent infections
  - Gastrointestinal: peptic ulcer; diarrhea; nausea; gastric distention; ascites; enlarged liver; hepatitis; cirrhosis; pancreatitis; malnutrition; thiamin, folic acid, and vitamin B deficiency
  - Musculoskeletal: muscle wasting, frequent fractures
  - Generally unkempt appearance, poor personal hygiene
  - Integumentary: Cushing appearance, flushed face, spider nevi, ecchymosis
  - HEENT: nystagmus, angiomas, smell of alcohol on breath, blurred vision
  - Impotence, sexual dysfunction
  - Generalized edema
  - Higher incidence of sexually transmitted diseases (STDs), HIV infections
- Acute intoxication: ataxia, drowsiness, disinhibition, delayed responses, nystagmus, psychomotor dysfunction
- Overdosing: coma, respiratory depression, seizures, stupor
- Chronic indicators of alcoholism: flushed face, frequent accidents, positive response to CAGE questionnaire, scleral injection, unexplained work/school absences

Diagnostic Studies

- Blood alcohol levels; CBC: decreased white blood cell (WBC) count, platelets, hematocrit; increased mean corpuscular volume (MCV)
- Chemistry profile for liver function studies (aspartate aminotransferase [AST], alanine aminotransferase [ALT], γ-glutamyl transpeptidase [GGT], lactate dehydrogenase [LDH], alkaline phosphatase, total bilirubin), cholesterol, triglycerides, uric acid, amylase all increased (AST higher than ALT by factor of 2)
- Consider HIV, thyroid function tests, glucose, electrolytes to clarify the diagnosis.
- Prothrombin time, partial thromboplastin time (PTT) if liver disease suspected
- Urinalysis, ECG, chest X-ray to fully evaluate health

Differential Diagnosis

- Major depressive mood disorders
- Anxiety disorders
- Bipolar disorder
- Personality disorders
- Polysubstance abuse disorder
- Endocrine disorders such as Cushing syndrome
- Neurological disorders, seizure disorders
- Cardiovascular disease

Management

Nonpharmacologic Treatment

- Substance abuse counseling; treatment program such as Alcoholics Anonymous, employee-assistance programs
- CBT, psychoanalysis

Pharmacologic Treatment

- Detoxification for symptoms of withdrawal. Commonly used agents include the benzodiazepines lorazepam (Ativan), chlordiazepoxide (Librium), and oxazepam (Serax). Use of atenolol (Tenormin) to reduce the need for benzodiazepines; clonidine, carbamazepine when benzodiazepines are not a good choice.
- Maintenance therapy includes disulfiram (Antabuse), naltrexone (ReVia), thiamine, folic acid, and B complex.
- Pharmacologic and medical management of underlying medical disorders as appropriate

How Long to Treat

- Physical withdrawal can be treated in 1 week; however, psychological dependence is long term.
- Treatment for maintenance can be 2 to 6 months of medication with an additional 6 months of follow-up.

Special Considerations

- Alcohol abuse during pregnancy can lead to severe birth defects or fetal alcohol syndrome.
- Alcoholism and alcohol abuse have long-term medical, social, and legal consequences.
- Severe intoxication is a medical emergency and may lead to coma, respiratory depression, aspiration, and death.

When to Consult, Refer, Hospitalize

- Refer patients who are diagnosed with or suspected of alcoholism to a substance abuse specialist.
- Hospitalize for acute intoxication and withdrawal.
- Refer social issues to a mental health specialist for long-term management.
- Refer all legal issues to the appropriate legal authority.

Follow-Up

Expected Course

- Treatment and outcome are variable for each person, with recovery as a lifelong commitment.

Complications

- Peak at 65 to 74 years of age, depending on length of exposure, frequency, and quantity of consumption
- See Assessment for list of medical complications, fetal alcohol syndrome

SUBSTANCE USE DISORDERS (SUDS)

Description

- A maladaptive pattern of substance use manifested by recurrent and significant adverse medical, psychosocial, and legal consequences related to the repeated use of the substance

- Drug dependence manifests as substance-seeking behaviors, physical dependence, tolerance—requiring increasingly higher doses to achieve the desired effect—and withdrawal.

Etiology

- Acquired brain disease; not well-understood, underlying change in brain circuits that persists beyond detoxification
- Neurons in the locus coeruleus are thought to adapt to chronic opiate exposure and fire at a higher-than-normal rate when withdrawal occurs and are responsible for producing the physical symptoms of withdrawal.
- Contributing factors to individual vulnerability:
  - Genetic predisposition
  - Neurotransmitter abnormalities
  - Environmental stressors
  - Psychodynamic factors, such as unstable childhood, impaired developmental stages, personality disorders
  - Social cultural factors, such as increased availability and prevalence, cultural acceptance and peer pressure, impaired family and peer relations, stress, lack of valued alternatives

Incidence and Demographics

- SUDs are more common in men than in women.
- The average onset age of substance use is 12 to 14 years of age. Early use of substances predicts later drug addiction, psychopathology, and social and occupational impairments.
- There is a link between substance use and suicide in adolescents.
- Usage crosses all cultural and socioeconomic barriers.
- Marijuana is the most used substance, excluding alcohol and tobacco.
- Strong links occur among alcohol, substances, and nicotine use.
- In the United States approximately 20.3 million people have an SUD
- In 2020, 75% of drug overdose deaths were related to an opioid (illicit or prescribed)

Risk Factors

- Genetic vulnerability
- Personal or family history
- Social, cultural, peer acceptance, and frequent use
- Psychiatric diagnosis, history of previous addiction
- Chronic pain

Prevention and Screening

- National and local public education and awareness through mass media educational campaigns
- Early prevention and education programs in school systems
- All patients interviewed for possible SUD
- CBT to enhance coping skills
- Substance Abuse and Mental Health Services Administration (SAMHSA) behavioral health treatment locator for substance abuse treatment referrals
- Screening tools for SUD: National Institute on Drug Abuse (NIDA) Quick Screen, NIDA Modified (NM), Alcohol, Smoking and Substance Involvement Screening Test (ASSIST), CAGE Adapted to Include Drugs (CAGE-AID), AUDIT, Drug Abuse Screening Test (DAST)

Assessment

History

- Personal, family history of abuse
- Patterns of use, substances of choice
- History of accidents, traumas, overdoses; legal difficulties
- Effects in Table 18–6

TABLE 18–6.
EFFECTS OF DRUG ABUSE

NAME OF DRUG	EFFECT	METHOD OF USE	CHARACTERISTICS	EFFECTS ON USER
Tobacco	No alterations in mood or effect	Smoked, chewed	Addicting	Frequent respiratory symptoms, infections. Lowered high-density lipoprotein (HDL) cholesterol, increased heart disease. Smokeless tobacco increases incidence of oral cancer, periodontal disease
Alcohol	Initial euphoria, impaired judgment, long-term depressant effects	Swallowed	Withdrawal symptoms with frequent, prolonged use	Gastritis, vomiting, anorexia Blackouts with heavy use
Marijuana	Relaxation, depressant; may have mild hallucinogenic effects	Smoked, swallowed	Referred to as "gateway" drug, may lead to use of other products; tolerance with regular use	Chronic users develop apathy, decreased motivation, flat affect, global cognitive impairment (memory, problem-solving), chronic cough
Cocaine	Stimulant, produces euphoria, increased physical activity, may lead to aggression, paranoia	Smoked, snorted, sniffed	Highly addictive, tolerance develops	Hypertensive crisis, coronary artery vasospasm, arrhythmias may occur

Methamphetamine Stimulant, similar to cocaine	Snorted, smoked, ingested	Withdrawal symptoms with	Similar to cocaine, cessation	Tachycardia
Hallucinogens (LSD, PCP, MDMA "Ecstasy")	Visual, auditory hallucinations, altered mood and dream-like state	Ingested	MDMA commonly abused at raves, music clubs, and festivals to produce euphoria	Hallucinations may occur weeks after use. Renal damage may occur with ecstasy.
Inhalants (glue, paint thinner, gasoline, Freon)	Euphoria, dream-like state, often with hallucinations; some products may have aphrodisiac properties	Directly inhaled or inhaled by huffing (putting a substance-soaked cloth in a bag and inhaling)	Commonly used by younger adolescents because of easy access	Most are CNS toxins, possible permanent sequelae such as peripheral neuropathy, ataxia, cognitive loss, language difficulty, loss of coordination. Lung, kidney damage may occur.
Heroin	Sedation, soothing and numbing effect with euphoria	Snorted, sniffed, subcutaneous (skin popping), and IV use	Sniffing most common method of use with adolescents	Chronic symptoms include constipation, chronic pruritus, bronchospasm
Prescription medications (opioids, benzodiazepines, stimulants)	Concurrent with drug of use	Ingested	Often manifests as patients presenting with pain complaints	Necessary to treat patient for pain; however, recognize addiction can present this way

Physical Exam

- Stimulants
    - Anxiety, agitation, panic, restlessness, irritability, aggression
    - Mood swings, grandiose, elated mood, hallucinations
    - Tachycardia, arrhythmias, chest pain, hypertension; hypothermia, hyperthermia
    - Abdominal pain, nausea, vomiting, insomnia, mydriasis
    - Hypersexuality, frequent urination
- Depressants
    - Dysphoria, depressed affect, apathy, psychomotor retardation, slurred speech, drowsiness
    - Diaphoresis, hypotension, miosis, rhinorrhea, sneezing, headache, nausea, vomiting
    - Myalgia, muscle pain, ataxia, tremors, impaired coordination, impotence
    - Mood swings, aggression, combativeness, lack of impulse control, disinhibition
    - Impaired attention, memory and judgment, hallucinations, paranoia
- Hallucinogens
    - Mydriasis, nystagmus, tachycardia, hypertension, ataxia, tremors
    - Severe anxiety, panic, mood swings, aggression, hallucinations, paranoia, flashbacks
    - Impaired concentration, memory, judgment, ability to make decisions
- Cannabis
    - Paranoia, confusion, hallucinations, distortion of time and spatial orientation
- Inhalants/solvents
    - Odor on breath, ataxia, slurred speech, euphoria, agitation, tachycardia, arrhythmias
    - Delirium, confusion, stupor, hallucinations, organic brain damage

Diagnostic Studies

- Urine and serum toxicology screens
- CBC, chemistry profiles, liver, kidney, cardiac, thyroid functions to rule out other disorders
- Venereal Disease Research Laboratory (VDRL), HIV because of high rate of STDs and blood-borne disease in this population
- CT, magnetic resonance imaging (MRI) scans, X-rays as indicated by history and physical to rule out other conditions

Differential Diagnosis

- Polysubstance abuse
- Psychiatric disorders
- Hypothyroidism, hyperthyroidism
- Hypoglycemia, hyperglycemia
- Head trauma
- Stroke, dementia, delirium, seizure disorder

Management

- Treatment and management depend on patient motivation, characteristics, and ability to engage in a therapeutic relationship. Nonjudgmental support by provider facilitates recovery.
- Before treatment, identify type and amount of substance ingested and route taken.
- Minimization and denial are hallmark characteristics and interfere with recovery.
- Motivational Interviewing (MI): evidenced-based approach to improve treatment engagement and retention.

Nonpharmacologic Treatment

- Multiple treatment modalities and interventions
  - CBT: strongest evidence for efficacy in adolescents; may be useful for comorbid ADHD and mood disorders
  - Family therapy for adolescents
  - Behavioral therapy: contingency management (CM)—positive reinforcement for negative drug screens and prosocial behavior
  - Narcotics Anonymous, Cocaine Anonymous, Marijuana Anonymous
  - Long-term residential treatment programs
  - Adolescent Community Reinforcement Approach (A-CRA): community-based approach for adolescents that helps youth and families improve access to alternatives and positive approaches to reduce substance use
  - Multisystemic therapy: intensive home-based therapy including multidisciplinary treatment teams

Pharmacologic Treatment

- Methadone hydrochloride levo-alpha-acetylmethadol (LAAM) used to treat heroin addiction, to block effects of heroin, and yield stable, non-euphoric state free from drug craving
- Buprenorphine/naloxone (Suboxone), an opioid (narcotic) partial agonist-antagonist, prevents withdrawal symptoms in opioid addiction. First dose: 2–4 mg sublingual (SL). Monitor in office for 1+ hours after first dose. Aim for dose of 8–12 mg in the first 24 hours
  - Comprehensive Addiction and Recovery Act (CARA) of 2016 and buprenorphine (Suboxone). The Drug Abuse Treatment Act of 2000 is an amendment to the 1970 Controlled Substances Act (CSA). The Act allows nurse practitioners to prescribe FDA-approved buprenorphine, a schedule III medication, upon completing 24 hours of certification from an approved provider and receipt of approval from The U.S. Department of Health and Human Services (HHS). May treat up to 30 patients in outpatient setting during the first year.
- *N*-Acetylcysteine, an amino acid supplement, 1,200 mg twice a day for cannabis SUD
- Stimulant abuse
  - Amphetamine withdrawal: Treatment in an inpatient setting; diazepam (Valium) to reduce agitation and hyperactivity if no psychosis is present
  - Cocaine withdrawal: Treatment in an inpatient setting—especially with severe depression with suicidal ideations; no reliable drug treatment; however, an anxiolytic such as diazepam (Valium)
  - Monitor cardiac rate and rhythm.
- Depressant abuse
  - Phenobarbital for withdrawal
  - Haloperidol commonly used to treat assaultive and psychotic behaviors

How Long to Treat

- Varies according to individual response
- Substance abuse commonly occurs with psychiatric disorders, requiring treatment of other disorder.
- Prognosis and recovery are highly dependent on personal motivation and social support.
- Residential treatment needs to exceed 90 days to be effective.
- Methadone maintenance is 12 months minimum.
- Opiate treatment is a minimum of 2 years.

Special Considerations

- Legal issues are common with substance abuse disorders.
- Abuse of substances during pregnancy increases the risk of spontaneous abortion, premature birth, preeclampsia and eclampsia, low birth weight, and birth defects.
- DSM-5-TR criteria apply to the adult population and may not be applicable to adolescents and children.

When to Consult, Refer, Hospitalize

- The role of the primary provider is diagnosis, referral to a substance abuse specialist, and co-management of medical consequences.
- Hospitalize for severe intoxication and medical compromise.

Follow-Up

- Frequency dictated by substance abuse specialist

Expected Course

- Substance abuse is a chronic disorder characterized by periods of relapse and remission.
- Outcomes are contingent on adequate length of time in treatment and support systems.

Complications

- Long-term use results in significant changes in brain function, as well as severe impairment in social, vocational, and interpersonal relations.
- High-risk behavior places substance abusers at risk for infections such as HIV, STDs, and hepatitis.
- Poor nutritional status, dental problems, poor personal hygiene

Care for Survivors of Abuse Domestic Violence and Abuse

DOMESTIC VIOLENCE WITH AN EMPHASIS INTIMATE PARTNER VIOLENCE (IPV)

Description

- Domestic or family violence generally involves physical, emotional, economic, or sexual pain and injury inflicted deliberately upon a family member or partner with the aim of controlling, manipulating, or intimidating that person within the relationship.
- Intimate partner violence (IPV) refers to abuse within a relationship between a spouse or romantic partner, including same-sex partnerships. In addition to previously mentioned acts of violence, other acts of abuse include, but are not limited to, gaslighting, humiliating, restricting movement or access to resources, and stalking.

Etiology

- Social learning theory—aggression as a learned behavior
- Genetic predisposition toward aggression
- Personality disorders (antisocial disorder, narcissistic disorder, borderline personality disorder)
- Environmental stressors (unemployment, poverty, crime, teenage pregnancy, social isolation)
  - Developmental traumatology: Exposure to violence at an early developmental age produces physiological changes in the developing brain that can result in impulsivity and antisocial behavior.
  - Feminist sociopolitical theory: Violence is the outgrowth of a patriarchal society, unequal power distribution, and male privilege.

Incidence and Demographics

- Domestic violence is the leading cause of injury to women ages 15 to 44.
- More women than men experience IPV and stalking.
- Women between the ages of 18 and 34 years of age have the highest rate of IPV

- In adolescence, about 1 in 11 females vs. 1 in 15 males experience teen dating violence (TDV)
- About half of female homicides are due to IPV.
- The indirect and direct cost of IPV is estimated to be about $3.6 trillion.
- 7% to 17% of pregnant women experience domestic violence.
- About 35% of all women sustain physical injury as a result of domestic violence.
- Profile of known, reported abusers: male under age 25, lower socioeconomic status, inner-city resident.
- IPV survivors experience short- and long-term mental and physical health consequences, including injury and death; PTSD, chronic pain, asthma, diabetes, and irritable bowel syndrome; unintended pregnancy; pelvic inflammatory disease and STDs.

Risk Factors

- Female gender
- Physical, emotional, financial dependence
- Poverty, housing problems, lack of education, lack of vocational skills
- Divorced and single-parent families
- Psychiatric diagnosis
- Alcohol and substance abuse
- Pregnancy
- Physical and emotional disabilities
- Family or personal history of physical or sexual abuse; long-term exposure to violence
- Social isolation, lack of support systems
- Undocumented immigrant status

Prevention and Screening

- The USPSTF recommends routine screening for IPV among women of childbearing age: 18 to 46.
- Inform your patient that you routinely screen everyone.
- Public education and awareness campaigns

- Educated primary providers
- Provide community resources, support
- Community emergency shelters, hotlines, and safe houses
- Organizations such as the National Coalition Against Domestic Violence (NCADV)

Assessment

History

- Interview persons alone.
- Include questions concerning domestic violence in medical history.
- Appropriate documentation
- Trouble expressing anger
- Passive role in the relationship

Physical Exam

- Withdrawn, fearful, evasive
- Poor personal hygiene, neglect; bruises, burns, fractures, injuries to abdomen, breasts, torso, pelvic region; injuries inconsistent with explanation offered
- Significant delay between time of injury and treatment
- Substance abuse; depression, anxiety; suicidal or homicidal ideation; PTSD; somatization of symptoms

Diagnostic Studies

- As injuries warrant:
    - X-ray
    - CT, MRI
    - CBC, chemistry profiles, electrolytes, STD testing, VDRL, HIV

Differential Diagnosis

- Accidental injuries
- Depression or anxiety
- Hypochondriasis
- Substance abuse
- Borderline personality disorder

Management

Nonpharmacologic Treatment

- Establishment of safe, supportive environment, including counseling to develop a safety plan
- Development of plan of action regarding safety and escape
- Provide community resources, shelters, and hotlines.
- CBT

Pharmacologic Treatment

- Varies according to individual injuries
- Antidepressants
- Antianxiety agents

Special Considerations

- Persons who are victims of domestic violence have a greater incidence of substance abuse.
- Persons with a history of being a victim of domestic violence are more likely to commit violent acts.
- Persons who are feeling trapped or hopeless have a greater incidence of suicidal ideation and depression.
- It is mandatory by law to report all acts of violence or abuse against children or older adults. Check state laws for reporting domestic violence.

When to Consult, Refer, Hospitalize

- Refer all cases to a mental health specialist for counseling.
- Refer patients with injuries to an emergency department.

Follow-Up

- Long-term with mental health specialist often needed, or return to therapy at a later time

OLDER ADULT AND DISABLED ADULT ABUSE AND NEGLECT

Description

- Emotional or physical injury deliberately inflicted upon an older adult partner or family member with the goal of control and intimidation by a person who has control or a position of trust. Goal is manipulation, intimidation, or control of the dependent person.

Etiology

- Physical, emotional, sexual, and financial dependency due to disability or age; unreasonable physical restraint; deprivation of food, water, shelter, or medical treatment; and physical abandonment
- Limited economic and financial resources

Incidence and Demographics

- One of 10 adults 60 years of age or older who live at home are victims of abuse; often underreported
- Persons older than 84 years of age are more likely to be abused.
- Women are more likely to be victimized than men.
- There is a greater incidence of abuse by family members than by paid providers.
- More than 50% of victims are cognitively impaired.

Risk Factors

- Over age 84
- Social isolation, lack of support
- Cognitively impaired
- Physical, financial dependency

Prevention and Screening

- Public education and awareness
- Social programs such as Adult Protective Services
- Caregiver support/respite
- Assess caregivers for depression.

Assessment

History

- Interview patient alone.
- Mental status exam
- Determine primary caregivers, living arrangements, legal custodian, and power of attorney.
- History of medical treatment, accidents, fractures, physical injuries, trauma, overdose of medications
- Determine environmental, psychosocial, and financial stressors.

Physical Exam

- Monitor nutritional status for dehydration and malnutrition.
- Lacerations, bruises, wounds, burns, fractures
- Poor skin and personal hygiene
- Evidence of sexual abuse: pain or soreness in anogenital area, venereal diseases, vaginal/rectal bruises, or bleeding
- Fearful, evasive, guarded, depressed

Other

- Unusual or inappropriate activity in bank accounts
- Numerous unpaid bills
- Lack of amenities
- Missing belongings
- Missed medical appointments

Diagnostic Studies

- Specific to presenting symptomology
- Signs of poor nutritional status

Differential Diagnosis

- Accidental injury
- Depression
- Self-neglect due to cognitive status or physical impairment

Management

Nonpharmacologic Treatment

- Goal is to maintain independence of the patient and caregiver. If patient needs care beyond ability of caregiver, consider institutionalization, home care services, respite for caregiver, adult day care program, etc.
- Potential removal from the home for care and safety
- Monitor nutritional status and vital signs, cognitive status, medical status as symptomology presents.
- Counseling for the perpetrator and the abused may be indicated; consider need for psychiatric or alcohol abuse treatment.

Pharmacologic Treatment

- Antidepressants may be indicated.

Special Considerations

- Report all older and disabled adult abuse and neglect to Adult Protective Services.
- Depending on the state, health care workers may be mandatory reporters of elder abuse. Under the Elder Justice Act (2010), any abuse occurring in long-term care facilities must be reported to Adult Protective Services.

When to Consult, Refer, Hospitalize

- Hospitalization or institutionalization when in the best interest of the person

Follow-Up

- Routine medical follow-up for signs of further abuse

Complications

- Wide variety of medical and emotional consequences is possible

CHILD ABUSE AND NEGLECT

Description

- Physical or emotional pain and injury inflicted upon a child or failure to provide a child with adequate food, clothing, shelter, supervision, or care
- Includes physical abuse; sexual assault; unreasonable physical restraint; deprivation of food, water, shelter, or medical treatment; emotional deprivation; and physical abandonment

Etiology

- No single set of factors produces abusive and/or neglectful persons
- Often abuser was a victim of abuse

Incidence and Demographics

- About 1 in 7 children experience abuse or neglect in the United States each year.
- Neglect is the most common form of child abuse, followed by physical abuse.
- About 16% of victims suffer from more than one type of abuse.
- Youngest children are most vulnerable to child abuse.

Risk Factors

- History of abuse in a family is common.
- Nonbiologic primary caregiver, live-in girlfriend/boyfriend of child's parent
- Increased family stress and social isolation are linked to abuse.
- Low socioeconomic level and financial stress are correlated with increased rates of neglect and abuse.
- Some psychiatric conditions in parents or guardians are associated with abuse and neglect.
- Alcohol and drug abuse are related to high rates of neglect and abuse.
- Characteristics of the child, including dependency, being a fussy baby, slow growth, developmental delay, disability, and male gender increase rates of abuse and neglect.

Prevention and Screening

- Public education and awareness
- Government social agencies such as Child Protective Services

Assessment

History

- Interview child and parents separately. Start with open-ended questions.
- Interview by persons with specialized training in the history process is preferred.
- If physical injury is present, ask specific questions eliciting detailed answers, including when and how it occurred.

- Inconsistencies, contradictions, and failure to adequately explain should arouse suspicion of abuse.
- Take a complete social history, including information about parents, caretakers, and family functioning; determine environmental, psychosocial, or financial stressors.
- Explore child's past and present history of medical treatment, including accidents, fractures, physical injuries, traumas, ingestions, and illnesses.
- Explore child's developmental and behavioral history, including the perinatal period, labor and delivery, neonatal period, feeding difficulties, sleeping problems, toilet training, encopresis, or enuresis.

Physical Exam

- Measure height and weight, using growth chart, and compare findings to norms and child's own growth curve; note nutritional status and hydration.
- Findings on physical exam suggestive of abuse include:
  - Bruising: in unexpected areas (abdomen, lower back, inner thighs, neck, around the mouth, pinna, inner aspects of arms—as child raises arms to protect face), in infants younger than 6 months of age; multiple bruises in various stages
  - Marks with characteristic shapes: belt buckles, looped cords, palm of hand, human bite marks; marks around the wrists or ankles may indicate tying the child down
  - Burns: cigarette marks, specific objects (curling iron), immersion burn from hot bathtub (discrete water level marks are around buttocks, feet, and hands); scalds from tap water are the most common type of intentional burn
  - Hair: patchy areas of alopecia from pulling out hair
  - Mouth: torn frenula, petechial lesions, lacerations or bruising to the palate
  - Neurological signs (signs of increased intracranial pressure [ICP] from bleeding into the head): bulging anterior fontanel, palpable split in suture lines, increasing head circumference, papilledema, behavior changes and/or decreased level of consciousness, vomiting. Most subdural hematomas are due to abuse. Head trauma accounts for approximately 50% of deaths due to physical abuse.
  - Eyes (fundus): retinal hemorrhages (from shaking), papilledema (from increased ICP)
  - Abdomen: vomiting, abdominal distention, tenderness, decreased or absent bowel sounds may indicate trauma; bruising on the abdomen may not always be present. Abdominal trauma is the second leading cause of death from physical abuse.
  - Genitalia and buttocks: Most sexual abuse leaves no visible scars; injuries that occur heal quickly.
    - In girls: unusually enlarged hymenal opening (requires expert evaluation because of wide range of normal in sizes and shapes), extensive vaginal adhesions, purulent vaginal discharge.

- In boys: penile and/or scrotal injuries are uncommon; most findings are in the rectal area and may include abrasions, perirectal skin tags outside the midline (these develop as small areas of bleeding heal), hemorrhoids (normally very uncommon in children), poor rectal tone (dilation greater than 15 mm), penile erection during entire exam in prepubertal boys (may be a normal variant).
- In both genders: any sexually transmitted skin lesion such as warts is highly suggestive of abuse.

Diagnostic Studies

- Bony injuries are most common in children younger than 3 years.
- Fractures highly suggestive of abuse include metaphyseal (or buckle fracture), rib, scapular, vertebral, spiral fractures of the humerus or femur in the young infant, and/or fractures of the hands or feet in children younger than 2 years of age.
- Metaphyseal injuries are fractures through newly forming bone that occur when limbs are forcefully moved (usually rotated), such as commonly seen in the distal humerus and femur or proximal tibia. They are highly suggestive of abuse. Changes may not be seen on X-ray for days to weeks.
- Skull fractures suggestive of abuse are wide (greater than 3 mm), complex (branching, involvement of suture lines), occurring outside the parietal area, and/or multiple.
- Simple skull fractures may or may not be associated with abuse. Falls of less than 2½ feet do not usually result in skull fractures.
- Multiple fractures in various stages of healing are almost pathognomonic of abuse once osteogenesis imperfecta is ruled out.
- Fractures not highly suggestive of abuse are those of the distal radius and ulna (from falling on outstretched hands), simple linear fracture of a long bone, midclavicular fractures, and nondisplaced spiral fracture of the tibia in a toddler.
- Blunt trauma to a bone can cause subperiosteal hemorrhage, with subsequent periosteal thickening and elevation visible on X-ray.
- Full skeletal surveys are recommended in children younger than 3 years of age who are suspected of being abused.
- New, nondisplaced fractures may not be evident on X-ray for 1 to 2 weeks, and a repeat X-ray or a bone scan is recommended.
- Sexual abuse requires a specialized exam and collection of laboratory and forensic evidence.

Differential Diagnosis

- Unintended injury
- Poverty resulting in poor hygiene, clothing, or nutrition
- Osteogenesis imperfecta

Management

- Suspicion of neglect or abuse mandates reporting to local (or state, depending on region) child protection authority. Consider reporting to local law enforcement.
- Inform parent/guardian that you are required by law to report suspected abuse.

Special Considerations

- The child protection agency is responsible for investigating the case and assisting the family and child to obtain or access support services.
- Documentation is critical and should be done carefully, as it may be part of a court case.

When to Consult, Refer, Hospitalize

- If injuries are severe or involve suspected sexual abuse, child should be referred to the hospital for evaluation and treatment with child abuse team.

Follow-Up

- The family nurse practitioner (FNP) has the responsibility to follow-up closely and advocate for the safety and medical well-being of the child.

Complications

- Victims are at risk for depression; other psychological, educational, and behavioral problems; and repeating the cycle of violence.

SEXUAL ASSAULT AND ABUSE

Description

- Any sexual act or penetration committed through coercion or physical force, including rape, incest, sodomy, oral and anal acts, or use of a foreign object

Etiology

- Character disorders
- Behavioral: act of violence is reinforcing; once done, likely to do again
- Social: exposure to violence in culture, media, and home

Incidence and Demographics

- Women have a greater incidence of being assaulted; men are more frequently perpetrators.
- Every year in the United States, nearly 1.5 million women and 834,700 men are victims of sexual violence
- The most common perpetrators of abuse are fathers, stepfathers, uncles, older siblings, and dates.
- Incestuous behavior is reported more frequently among families of low socioeconomic status.
- Most victims of rape (79%) report first rape before the age of 25 and about 40% report first rape before age 18.
- Sexual violence is the costliest crime in the United States at an estimated $127 billion per year between legal and medical fees.

Risk Factors

In the abuser

- Substance abuse disorders, psychiatric disorders
- Divorce, pregnancy
- Family or personal history of physical or sexual abuse

- Long-term exposure to violence
- Lower socioeconomic status
- Social isolation, lack of support systems
- Factors such as unemployment, financial difficulty, housing problems, overcrowding

In the abused

- Vulnerable, dependent, young
- Opportunity for abuser to be alone with them

Prevention and Screening

- Public education and awareness campaigns
- Providing community resources, support
- Community emergency shelters, hotlines, and safe houses
- Organizations such as the NCADV
- Assertiveness and self-defense training

Assessment

- The FNP is required to know and follow specific rape-evaluation protocols regarding history, physical, and collection of specimens, or information/findings may not be admissible in court.
- If FNP is not educated in rape evaluation, refer to a specially trained provider.

History

- Social history, living environment, relationships
- Inclusion of questions concerning domestic violence in medical history
- Interview persons alone when possible.

Physical Exam

- Withdrawn, frightened appearance; depressive symptoms
- Dislocations and fractures
- Unexplained bruises, abrasions, cuts, laceration, burns, soft tissue swellings, hematomas
- STDs, genital rash, discharge
- Rectal tissue swelling, discharge

Diagnostic Studies

- Forensic specimens and extensive STD testing per protocol, including HIV screening
- Pregnancy test now and 2–4 weeks later
- X-rays, CT scans, MRI as indicated

Differential Diagnosis

- Consenting sex among adults
- Accidental injury to pelvic and groin area
- PTSD

Management

- Ensure safety, well-being, confidentiality.
- Accurate documentation
- Be aware of depressive symptoms and potential for suicide.
- Offer option for empiric and prophylactic STD treatment instead of STD testing

Nonpharmacologic Treatment

- CBT
- Psychoanalysis

- Support groups and community resources
- Legal intervention

Pharmacologic Treatment

- Emergency contraception (rule out pregnancy with urine or serum human chorionic gonadotropin [hCG] first)
  - Yuzpe regimen (100 µg of ethinyl estradiol and 0.5 mg levonorgestrel: two doses 12 hours apart as soon as possible)
  - Levonorgestrel 0.75 mg (Plan B). Two doses 12 hours apart as soon as possible, or 1.5 mg orally single dose (Plan B One-Step). Effective up to 72 hours; less effective in overweight women.
  - Ulipristal acetate (Ella) 30 mg oral single dose, effective up to 120 hours. It is preferred in overweight women.
  - Copper IUD 313.4 mg intrauterine single device (Paragard) is effective up to 120 hours after intercourse. This method is considered the most effective emergency contraceptive.
  - Antiemetic may be necessary with oral emergency contraception.

How Long to Treat

- Varies with individual medical and emotional needs

Special Considerations

- Persons with other mental disorders at higher risk of abusing others
- Nature of relationship between abuser and the person affects recovery.
- Persons with developmental delays are at risk of being abused.

When to Consult, Refer, Hospitalize

- All injuries and all cases of recent rape should be referred to an emergency department (with rape protocol).
- Refer all patients with recent or past sexual abuse to mental health professional with experience in sexual abuse for treatment of psychosocial issues and possible PTSD.

Follow-Up

- Depends on individual coping strategies and support system

Complications

- PTSD, injuries to external genitalia, STDs

Eating Disorders

DESCRIPTION

- Disorders that are characterized by severe disturbances in eating behavior. The two major types are anorexia nervosa and bulimia nervosa. Binge eating and avoidant restrictive food intake are also disorders that exist by themselves.

SUBTYPES

- Anorexia nervosa (see the following section) (F50.00)
- Binge eating disorder (F50.81): eating more than what a normal person would eat in a specific time frame with a lack of control; overeating: eating when not physically hungry
- Bulimia nervosa (see upcoming section) (F50.2)
- Avoidant restrictive food intake disorder (ARFID) (F50.82): failure to meet appropriate nutritional needs based on an aversion to food, lack of interest in food, or dislike of the sensory characteristics of food, with absence of a disturbance of body image

ANOREXIA NERVOSA

Description

- Eating behavior characterized by a person's refusal to maintain a normal body weight (and body weight is less than 85% of expected), severe restriction of caloric intake, intense fear of gaining weight and a severely distorted perception of one's body, and absence of menses; weight loss to more than 15% below expected weight for height
- Types: restricting, binge eating and purging

Etiology

- Biological
  - Genetic vulnerability and predisposition, neurotransmitter abnormalities
  - Biological: altered brain function in corticolimbal regions controlling appetite
- Psychodynamic
  - Reaction to the demand of adolescence; perfectionist personality with obsessive, rigid characteristics
  - Lacking self-confidence; close, troubled relations with parents; influence of family dynamics; parents may be overbearing/demanding; father may be distant while mother is overprotective and intrusive; disordered attachment
- Social/cultural
  - Peer pressure to be thin; media and cultural emphasis on thinness, youth, body image
- Pathophysiology of starvation: lack of energy and nutrients causes fat and protein store breakdown

Incidence and Demographics

- The lifetime prevalence in the United States is up to 0.08% in women and 0.01% in men
- Anorexia begins in adolescence and is more common in females
- Anorexia nervosa is associated with depressive disorder, bipolar disorder, substance use, OCD, and anxiety disorder.

Risk Factors

- Family histories of mood disorders, alcoholism, or eating disorders
- Perfectionistic, compulsive, high expectations of self
- Caucasian, middle-class females; adolescence
- Dancers, athletes, gymnasts

Prevention and Screening

- Public education and awareness
- Early intervention

Assessment

History

- Weight history, onset of weight loss
- Symptoms such as constipation, cold hands and feet, fatigue
- Dietary habits, patterns of eating, food rituals, weight loss, binge eating or purging
- Menstrual history: amenorrhea
- Perception of body weight and shape, fears of gaining weight
- Exercise history, frequency, and duration—may be excessive
- Use of medication for weight control
- Psychiatric history, including comorbidity and previous eating disorders
- Family history of eating or psychiatric disorders
- Previous psychiatric treatments

Physical Exam

- Weigh patient without clothes. Weight is often 15% below ideal body weight with significantly low BMI.
- Amenorrhea, lanugo, delayed growth, sexual maturation
- Altered vital signs: hypothermia, hypotension, bradycardia
- Muscular atrophy, ridges in fingernails, erosion of enamel of teeth from stomach acid

Diagnostic Studies

- A multitude of endocrine and medical problems can occur secondary to the starvation that occurs with this disorder. There are no definite laboratory tests to diagnosis anorexia.
- ECG (look for flattening or inversion of T waves, ST-segment depression, lengthening of QT interval), CBC (anemia, leukopenia), chemistry panel with electrolytes (low potassium and magnesium levels), luteinizing hormone (LH) and follicle-stimulating hormone (FSH) diminished; TSH, triiodothyronine (T3), thyroxine (T4), glucose levels may be diminished.

Differential Diagnosis

- Bulimia nervosa
- Mood disorders
- Medical disorders such as cancer, diabetes mellitus, Crohn's disease, endocrine disorders
- Substance abuse

Management (Should Be Based on the Severity of the Disorder)

- Requires multidisciplinary approach
- Recovery-oriented, maximizing self-determination and self-management
- Least-intrusive and least-restrictive environment
- First consideration in treatment is to restore the person's nutritional state.

Nonpharmacologic Treatment

- Nutritional and medical management
  - Establish appropriate eating habits.
  - Rehydrate and correct electrolyte balance.
  - Restore weight; stop exercising.
  - Assess for excessive exercise as weight-loss mechanism.
- Psychotherapy
  - Psychotherapy is standard treatment, but there is no evidence that one type of therapy is more effective than another type.
  - Involvement of family, family therapy
  - Nutritional and dietary education and weekly monitoring
  - No research evidence for Internet-based CBT efficacy

Pharmacologic Treatment

- Lack of evidence for routine use of pharmacotherapy

How Long to Treat

- Varies according to individual characteristics, severity of symptoms, and motivation
- Inpatient stays may last 4 to 8 weeks, followed by day-treatment program of 4 to 6 weeks

Special Considerations

- Denial is a classic characteristic of this disorder.
- People resist medical treatment.
- Symptoms of bulimia occur in 30% to 50% of persons with anorexia.
- In a pregnant patient, poor nutritional status may endanger fetus and status of the pregnancy.

When to Consult, Refer, Hospitalize

- A psychiatric consult should always be obtained.
- Mandatory hospitalization should occur when the risk of death from complications of malnutrition is high, postural hypotension or electrolyte imbalances are present.
- Inpatient treatment required when BMI is 14 kg/m2 or less, weight loss more than 1 kg/week, nutritional intake of less than 100 kcal a day, continued weight loss despite treatment

Follow-Up

- The role of the primary care provider is to monitor the medical component, including weekly weight and nutritional status, periodic lab tests, and collaboration with involved professionals.

Expected Course

- 40% can make full recovery with appropriate treatment for 5 years.
- Short-term response to hospitalization is good but relapse is common.
- Food rituals, low self-esteem, and distorted body image commonly persist after treatment.

- Indicators of a favorable outcome are decreased denial, admission of hunger, and improved self-esteem and perceptions of body image and self.

Complications

- Cardiac arrhythmias if purging, heart failure, convulsions, osteoporosis, infertility, death

BULIMIA NERVOSA

Description

- Recurrent episodes of overeating followed by purging behavior (episodes occur at least twice a week for 3 months). Feeling of self-worth unduly influenced by weight
- Eating a larger amount of food than most in a discrete period
- Sense of lack of control over eating during episode
- Recurrent compensatory behavior to prevent weight gain with use of laxative, diuretic, enema, induced vomiting (purging type); or fasting or excessive exercise (nonpurging type)

Etiology

- Neurotransmitter abnormalities: poor serotonergic function; depression
- Poor impulse control disorder as high prevalence of alcoholism and drug abuse in this population
- Genetic predisposition
- Social, cultural, and peer pressure to be thin
- Demands of adolescence
- Family dynamics, particularly family disorganization and lack of interest

Incidence and Demographics

- More common in females than in males
- More common than anorexia, but may occur with it

- Occurs in late adolescence
- About 30% with bulimia nervosa have a comorbid substance use disorder with alcohol or stimulant.

Risk Factors

- Approximately 90% to 95% of persons with bulimia nervosa are female; adolescents and young adults; family history of obesity, family conflict
- Poor impulse control, low self-esteem; high expectations of self-performance
- Normal weight or overweight; history of dieting, obesity, fluctuating weight
- Substance abuse, mood disorders

Prevention and Screening

- Public education and awareness
- Early intervention

Assessment

History

- Onset of symptoms such as constipation, muscle cramps; menstrual history
- Dietary habits, patterns of eating, food rituals, and purging behaviors
- Use of medication, especially for weight control; use of laxatives
- Weight history, exercise history
- Psychiatric history, body perception

Physical Exam

- Complete physical exam to rule out medical causes.
- Weight measurement without clothes (weight fluctuations—typically remain within 20% normal)
- Dental carries, dental erosions, gum disease, parotid swelling

- Abdominal distress (from putting pressure on the abdomen to vomit), esophagitis, irritation of the pharynx
- Ridges in fingernails, calluses, or abrasions on knuckles (Russell's sign)

Diagnostic Studies

- CBC, chemistry panel with electrolytes (low potassium and magnesium levels), ECG, TSH, T3, T4
- Amylase levels elevated with vomiting; return to normal in 72 hours after vomiting stops

Differential Diagnosis

- Anorexia nervosa
- GI disorders
- Endocrine disorders
- Neurological disorders
- Mood disorders
- Anxiety disorders
- Personality disorders

Management (Should Be Based on the Severity of the Disorder)

Nonpharmacologic Treatment

- CBT, including individual and family therapy
- Nutritional counseling: goal is to restore appropriate eating patterns
- Community support groups and resources

Pharmacologic Treatment

- Antidepressant medications—SSRIs and TCAs—are considered effective in reducing binge eating and purging behaviors. Use doses given in the treatment of depressive disorders.

- Avoid MAOIs due to the potential for severe food interactions and hypertensive crisis.
- Avoid bupropion because of risk for seizure
- Topiramate can promote weight loss and alleviate bulimia symptoms.
- Medication is used as adjunct therapy, combined with psychological and nutritional counseling.

How Long to Treat

- Duration varies, often months to years

Special Considerations

- Patients will try to hide behaviors associated with the disorder; family may see patient make frequent trips to bathroom after eating, excessive exercise, up during night binging

When to Consult, Refer, Hospitalize

- Refer every case to a mental health professional who is an eating disorder specialist.
- Treatment may be managed on an outpatient basis in consultation with a nutritionist and psychotherapist.
- Hospitalization is indicated when outpatient treatment is unsuccessful, or if cardiac complications, hemodynamic instability, or hypovolemia is present.

Follow-Up

- Role of primary care provider is to monitor medical aspects, including nutritional status (weekly weight) and periodic lab testing, and coordinate care with other involved professionals

Expected Course

- Frequent relapses
- 50% achieve full remission
- Prognosis depends on severity, electrolyte imbalances, and other medical complications.

Complications

- Chronic induced emesis results in volume depletion, renal compensation, cardiac arrhythmia, esophagitis, dental decay

Other Disorders

ATTENTION-DEFICIT/HYPERACTIVITY DISORDER (ADHD)

Description

- A neurobiological disorder affecting attention, impulse control, and level of activity
- One of the most common psychiatric disorders of childhood and adolescence; also recognized in adults
- Pervasiveness or evidence of symptoms in two or more settings. Symptoms may be reduced in highly supervised situations, one-on-one encounters, and/or when an activity is new or enjoyable. Symptoms may worsen when the activity is nonpreferred, difficult, or unstructured.
- Onset of symptoms is usually before age 12.
- Main behavioral aspects: inattentiveness, impulsivity, and hyperactivity, more frequent and severe than what would be expected for child's developmental level. Symptoms vary from person to person and may include:
  - Easily distracted
  - Daydreams
  - Appears to be in another world
  - Fidgety, restless
  - Inappropriate or excessive activity
  - Seems to be "driven by a motor"; always on the go
  - Talks constantly
  - Interrupts others
  - Has difficulty getting along with others
  - Forgetful: fails to turn in work or complete assignments ("forgets")
  - Poor sustained attention
  - Poor self-esteem

- Symptoms may vary with the type of setting. Often minimized in highly supervised situations, one-on-one encounters, and/or when an activity is new or enjoyable. Symptoms may worsen when the activity is non-preferred, difficult, or unstructured.
- Age at onset of symptoms is usually before age 7. (Diagnosis may be made later.)

Subtypes (DSM-5-TR)

- Attention-deficit/hyperactivity disorder, combined type
- Attention-deficit/hyperactivity disorder, predominantly inattentive type
- Attention-deficit/hyperactivity disorder, predominantly hyperactive-impulsive type

Etiology

- No single known cause; may be multiple etiologies. Possible causes:
  - Genetic factors: Up to 75% of children may have inherited this disorder.
  - Adoption: adopted children five times more likely to have ADHD than non-adopted children; may be related to poor prenatal care, malnutrition, or lack of stimulation
  - Neurochemical differences: possible dopamine or norepinephrine deficiencies
  - Brain structure differences: possible frontal lobe and striatum alterations
  - Pregnancy and delivery complication
  - Prenatal substance abuse
  - Prenatal exposure to smoking
  - Low birth weight
  - Traumatic brain injury

Incidence and Demographics

- Approximately 7.2% of all school-age children have ADHD worldwide
- Ratio of boys to girls with ADHD approximately 2:1; however, girls may be underdiagnosed because, although they are inattentive, their behavior tends to be less aggressive than boys.
- Most common psychiatric disorder in school-age children; less recognized in adults
- Symptoms may be present as early as age 3 years.
- One of the most common referrals to mental health care providers

Risk Factors

- See Etiology.

Prevention and Screening

- Public education and awareness
- Early screening and evaluation
- Patient and family education

Assessment

History

- Specific symptoms, age at onset (younger than 7 years), duration of symptoms (older than 6 months), presence in more than one setting
- Has a negative impact on child's quality of life
- CNS insult/injury such as fetal alcohol syndrome, prematurity, CNS infection/injury, lead poisoning, neurodegenerative disorders, and seizures
- Family/child history of medical conditions such as anemia, thyroid dysfunction, fragile X syndrome
- Interpersonal dynamics: interactions between the child and each family member and peer relationships
- Past or present stressors such as divorce or loss of a parent
- School history: grades (past and present), school problems, absenteeism
- Family history of psychiatric illnesses, ADHD, or "school problems" (diagnosed or undiagnosed)
- History should be obtained from multiple sources, including parents, child, teachers, or other people involved with the child, such as mental health care providers.

Physical Exam

- Usually no findings on physical exam. There may be an increased incidence of neurological "soft signs," which can aid with diagnosis.

- Perform a complete physical exam to rule out possible medical etiologies.
- Obtain vision and hearing tests.

Diagnostic Studies

- No laboratory tests diagnose ADHD.
- Parent and teacher rating scales, such as Conners, Vanderbilt, Achenbach, and Barkley, should be used in addition to the clinical history.
- Psychological, educational, and language evaluations may be performed if learning disabilities are suspected. Psychoeducational testing may be obtained through the child's school or a psychologist.
- If indicated, obtain a CBC, lead level, and/or thyroid studies.
- EEG recordings may be obtained to rule out seizure disorders; MRI studies are indicated only for children with neurological findings.

Differential Diagnosis

- Anxiety
- Depression
- Learning disabilities
- Pervasive developmental disorder
- Substance abuse
- Medical disorders—absence seizures, hypothyroidism, anemia, lead poisoning
- Hearing and vision impairment
- Disorganized and chaotic family

Possible Comorbid or Coexisting Conditions

- Depression
- Dysthymia
- Learning disabilities
- Oppositional defiant disorder

- Conduct disorder
- Bipolar disorder
- Tourette syndrome
- Drug or alcohol abuse
- Adjustment disorder
- PTSD

Management

Nonpharmacologic Treatment

- Education of child and family
  - Assess their understanding of ADHD and provide information as needed.
  - Discuss the treatment plan with the child and family, including behavioral and educational plans and medication use.
  - Often find that one of the parents has symptoms and may need to provide support and assistance for them. Adults often have a history of problems in school or jobs and require assistance with organization and social skills.
- Social skills training
  - Children with ADHD often have problems with peer relationships because of their inability to read social cues and impulsive, hyperactive, or aggressive behaviors; tend to be immature
  - Training facilitates the child in recognizing problem areas in relationships and teaches strategies to help improve social skills.
- Psychotherapy
  - Often helpful in understanding ADHD and its impact on the child and family
  - May include CBT for the child and family, and group therapy
  - Behavioral and educational interventions (see Table 18–7)

Pharmacologic Treatment

- Approximately 80% of children with ADHD respond positively to medication; adults may also respond (see Table 18–8).
- Some positive effects of medication include improvement in attention, concentration, and academic achievement; decrease in hyperactive behaviors, disruptive and aggressive behaviors, and emotional lability (emotional ups and downs).

TABLE 18–7.
SELECTED BEHAVIORAL AND EDUCATIONAL INTERVENTIONS FOR CHILDREN WITH ADHD

BEHAVIORAL INTERVENTIONS AT HOME	ACCOMMODATIVE INTERVENTIONS AT SCHOOL
Establish a list of appropriate behaviors (a targeted small number but consistently reinforced)	Assess for possible learning disorders
Provide a structured environment (predictable routines)	Tutoring
Give only 1–3 shortly stated instructions at a time	Untimed testing
Use chart for reminders	Preferential seating in the classroom
Use timers or bells for transitions	Note-taking services
Reward positive behaviors	Modified textbooks
Ignore minor misbehaviors or give nonverbal cues	Tailoring of homework assignments
Consistently discipline targeted behaviors	Organizational aids
	Use visual cues
	Use peer helper

TABLE 18–8.
PHARMACOLOGIC MANAGEMENT OF ADHD

MEDICATION	DAILY DOSE RANGE	MAXIMUM DOSE
Methylphenidate HCl		
(Ritalin, Ritalin LA, Ritalin SR)	5–60 mg	60 mg
(Metadate CD, Metadate ER)	10–60 mg	60 mg
(Concerta)	18–54 mg	54 mg
(Aptensio XR)	10–40 mg	60 mg
(Daytrana)	10/15/20 mg patch on 9 hours, off 15 hours	30 mg patch on 9 hours,
(Quillivant XR)	10–20 mg	30 mg
Dextroamphetamine sulfate (Dexedrine, Dexedrine Spansule)	5–30 mg	40 mg
Dextroamphetamine/amphetamine (Adderall, Adderall XR)	5–30 mg	40 mg 30 mg (XR)
Dexmethylphenidate HCl (Focalin)	2.5–10 mg	20 mg
Atomoxetine HCl (Strattera)	10–60 mg	100 mg
Pemoline (Cylert) (not used as first-line therapy because of liver toxicity)	18.75–75 mg	112.5 mg

- Psychostimulants are the first-line choice for the treatment of ADHD.
- Side effects of the psychostimulants include
  - Decreased appetite, anorexia, insomnia, headache, stomachache, irritability, dysphoria, nausea, and vomiting
  - Rebound effect (increased hyperactive or impulsive behavior or marked irritability as medication wears off)
  - Most side effects dissipate after several days; however, if they persist, medication change should be considered.
  - Less-common side effects seen, particularly with methylphenidate, are tics in susceptible children (5% to 10%) and possible growth suppression at high doses.
  - Nonstimulant medication may be used to treat ADHD if the child does not respond to or tolerate stimulants. These may include atomoxetine HCl (Strattera), clonidine (Catapres), imipramine (Tofranil), venlafaxine (Effexor), and/or bupropion (Wellbutrin).
  - Unlike psychostimulants, nonstimulants may not treat all behaviors associated with ADHD. A combination of stimulants and nonstimulants may be needed.

How Long to Treat

- ADHD treatment in adolescents should be reassessed when they enter adulthood to establish the need for continuing treatment.

Special Considerations

- Diagnosis of ADHD before the age of 4 years should be done cautiously.
- Girls may often be underdiagnosed, particularly if child is inattentive but does not exhibit impulsive or hyperactive behavior.
- Adolescents typically are not hyperactive, but restless.
  - Hyperactive children often exhibit quiet behavior while in an office setting.
  - If hyperactive behavior appears suddenly, this is often due to a stressor in the child's life, not ADHD.
  - Inattention or lack of motivation may be easily confused with ADHD and needs to be examined further.
  - Children with ADHD are at an increased risk for developing other conditions, such as substance abuse, depression, conduct and anxiety disorders, and driving violations.

When to Consult, Refer, Hospitalize

- If the child has an atypical ADHD presentation or has a complicated comorbid condition
- When the child does not respond to treatment
- If the child exhibits severe antisocial or aggressive behavior
- If the child is threatening or attempting suicide

Follow-Up

- Medications should be monitored closely to determine effectiveness and possible side effects.
- Behavioral rating scales are useful to establish the effectiveness of medication during school.
- Initially frequent telephone follow-up with an office visit 1 month after starting medication
- Frequent follow-up when titrating medication dosage and every 3 to 6 months when stabilized
- Monitor height, weight, and blood pressure at every visit.
- Provide close monitoring of the child's functioning in school and at home, and make appropriate adjustments and recommendations as needed.

AUTISM SPECTRUM DISORDER (ASD; F84.0)

Description

- A neurodevelopmental disorder characterized by impairments in three major domains: social interactions, communication, and behavior that is repetitive and restricted

Etiology

- No single known etiology. Multiple genetic and environmental factors are suspected to play a role.

Incidence and Demographics

- Affects 1% to 2% of U.S. population
- Three to four times more common in boys than girls
- Average age at diagnosis is 3 years of age

Risk Factors

- Genetic (multi-genomic) factors lead to altered brain development, resulting in neurobehavioral phenotype
- Little evidence to link any single environmental factor to autism
- Overwhelming evidence of lack of an association between immunizations and autism

Prevention and Screening

- Commonly recognized symptoms of autism are most often recognized in the second year of life
- Screening is not diagnostic but helps determine whether additional diagnostic evaluation by a specialist is warranted.
- Developmental-behavioral assessments should be done for all infants and young children routinely; an autism-specific screening tool should be used in children with delayed language/communication milestones, regression in milestones, a sibling with autism, and parents who raise concern.

Assessment

History

- Impaired social interaction, including a baby who resists cuddling, avoids eye contact, or fails to spread arms in anticipation of being picked up; older children have persistent routines
- Failure to develop peer relationships, prefers solitary play, older children lack understanding of social conventions or needs of others, responds inappropriately in conversation
- Language development: expressive and receptive delayed
- Pregnancy, neonatal development: toxic exposures, illness

- Sleep, feeding patterns
- Coordination and physical milestones delayed
- Use valid screening tools such as Checklist for Autism in Toddlers (CHAT), Infant-Toddler Checklist (ITC), Autism Spectrum Screening Questionnaire (ASSQ), and Autism Diagnostic Observation Schedule (ADOS-G).
- Stereotyped repetitive or obsessive-compulsive–like behaviors
- Aggression, impulsivity, cognitive disorganization, inattention, and hyperactivity
- Assess comorbid conditions, including seizure disorders, lead poisoning, genetic disorders, mental health disorders, sleep problems, gastrointestinal problems, nutrition problems, delays in acquisition of self-help skills.

Physical Exam

- Refer for a comprehensive diagnostic evaluation by a team that has expertise in the diagnosis and management of ASD.
- Complete a developmental and neurological exam.
- Evaluate for medical causes (uncommon).

Diagnostic Studies

- Genetic testing
- Metabolic testing
- Neuroimaging not recommended unless microcephaly or macrocephaly is present; consider MRI

Differential Diagnosis

- Phenylketonuria
- Fetal alcohol syndrome
- Tuberous sclerosis complex
- Fragile X
- Rett syndrome
- 15q chromosome disorders

- Smith-Lemli-Opitz syndrome
- Other chromosomal disorders

Management

Nonpharmacologic Treatment

- Main role of the primary care provider is to coordinate referrals to specialists for evaluation and management; routine health maintenance; and provision of support, guidance, and advocacy.
- Social skills training
- Behavioral therapy
- Speech and language therapy
- Parental education
- Early intensive behavioral and educational interventions that target the core symptoms are key due to neuroplasticity, which optimizes early intervention and developmental disruption present prior to age 3.
- 20 hours per week of year-round treatment results in the best outcomes.

Pharmacologic Treatment

- Medications helpful for management of symptoms may target hyperactivity, aggression, anxiety, obsessive-compulsive behaviors, depressive symptoms, and sleep dysfunction.
- Psychopharmacologic interventions do not treat the underlying symptoms but can improve the child's functioning and ability to participate in behavioral interventions.

How Long to Treat

- Individualized; management goal is to maximize functioning, improve quality of life, and move child toward independence

When to Consult, Refer, Hospitalize

- All suspected cases should be referred to a specialized team for comprehensive evaluation and management.

Follow-Up

- Close monitoring of support and treatment to child and family as needed

Expected Course

- Outcome is variable and difficult to predict. Some children will retain diagnosis despite improvement and others with milder symptoms may no longer meet diagnostic criteria for autism yet will still have delays or other mental health disorders.
- Early identification and early intervention are associated with better outcomes.

DISRUPTIVE, IMPULSE CONTROL, AND CONDUCT DISORDERS

Description

- Disorders involving difficulties in the self-control of emotions and behaviors. Persistent antisocial behavior, violating others' rights, conflict with authority figures, and typically aggressive behavior, inconsistent with societal norms. Conduct-disordered persons exhibit at least one of these symptom clusters:
    - Aggressive, bullying behavior toward people or animals
    - Vandalism, fire-setting, and property destruction
    - Lying, "conning," or theft
    - Serious violation of rules (truancy) or running away from home overnight
    - No sign of remorse for misconduct

Subtypes

- Oppositional defiant disorder: enduring patterns of disobedient and hostile behavior toward authority figures and an unwillingness to take responsibility for one's own actions or blaming others for actions
- Intermittent explosive disorder: recurrent behavioral outbursts such as verbal aggression, temper tantrums, physical aggression. Outbursts occur twice weekly for a period of at least 3 months. Episodes last 30 minutes or less and in contrast to conduct disorder, do not result in injury to self or others.
- Conduct disorder: severe repeated acts of aggression that cause physical harm to themselves and others

- Antisocial personality disorder: pervasive disregard for other people's rights starting at age 15, failure to conform to societal norms, lying, deceitful behavior, lack of remorse

Etiology

- No single known etiology. Multiple biological, psychological (cognitive and personality), and environmental factors are suspected to play a role.
  - Parental inconsistency, chaotic home environment, harsh and punitive parenting
  - Parental depression, parental antisocial personality disorder
  - Children who lack permanent family or absent father
  - Peer influences
- New evidence suggests neurotransmitters such as serotonin and abnormalities in catecholaminergic and peptidergic systems are linked to aggressive conduct disorder.

Incidence and Demographics

- More common in boys
- Lifetime prevalence in the United States is 7%.
- Conduct disorder is more common in children previously diagnosed with oppositional defiant disorder.
- Associated with ADHD, learning disorders, and depression

Risk Factors

- Dysfunctional family
- Socioeconomically deprived
- Family history of antisocial personality
- Substance abuse
- Learning disorders or ADHD

Prevention and Screening

- Early management of associated disorders decreases the likelihood that antisocial behaviors will develop.
- Parent education about child development and parenting techniques
- Social skills training

Assessment

History

- Specific behaviors of the person and effects on self and others
- Comorbid conditions such as depression, anxiety, substance abuse, learning disabilities, ADHD
- Academic history, past and present
- Family history of sociopathic and/or psychiatric illnesses
- Family functioning
- CNS insults/injuries, disorders, or symptoms

Physical Exam

- Evaluate for trauma or abuse
- Evaluate for medical causes (uncommon)

Diagnostic Studies

- Neuropsychiatric assessment
- Psychoeducational testing to rule out learning disabilities

Differential Diagnosis

- Depression
- ADHD

- Specific developmental disorders
- Substance abuse
- Bipolar disorder
- Psychotic disorders
- Dissociative disorder
- PTSD

Management

Nonpharmacologic Treatment

- Psychotherapy and anger management; individual and family therapy
- Parent training
- Treat comorbid conditions if present (depression, personality disorders, anxiety).

Pharmacologic Treatment

- Medications helpful for management of aggressive and antisocial behavior include lithium, risperidone (Risperdal), olanzapine (Zyprexa); atypical antipsychotics (diminish aggression); stimulants (with coexisting ADHD); clonidine (Catapres); and SSRIs (with coexisting depression or anxiety).

How Long to Treat

- Variable

Special Considerations

- Early age at onset and higher number of behaviors correlate with poorer prognosis.
- Referral to a pediatric psychiatrist who is a specialist in these disorders for evaluation and treatment.

When to Consult, Refer, Hospitalize

- All cases should be referred to a mental health professional.
- Emergency referral or hospitalization for aggressive, threatening behavior that jeopardizes the safety of others or the patient; homicidal or suicidal ideation

Follow-Up

- Close monitoring of medications and support to child and family as needed

Expected Course

- Course is variable and dependent on multiple factors, including patient's receptivity to treatment, stability of family, and access to resources; early intervention has a more favorable outcome.

Complications

- Treatment failure may result in criminalization and placement in a correctional facility.

SLEEP DISORDER—INSOMNIA

Description

Chronic (Persistent) Insomnia

- Difficulty initiating or maintaining sleep of a restorative nature that lasts for over 3 months and causes significant distress or social, educational, or occupational impairment

Transient Insomnia

- Lasts less than 30 days and is induced by substances, medications, jet lag, medical illness, stressful events

Etiology

- Normal sleep has two basic phases: rapid eye movement (REM; time of physical and mental activation) and non-REM (NREM; deep rest), which cycle in 90 minutes and repeat four to five times a night; with insomnia, the typical pattern is lost because of
  - Substance or medication effects
  - Situational stressors
  - Medical disorders
  - Sleep apnea conditions
  - Disturbance in circadian rhythms from jet lag, shift work
  - Psychiatric disorders such as anxiety, major depressive disorders
  - Primary sleep disorders with unknown etiology

Incidence and Demographics

- It is estimated that 5% to 35% of the population has had insomnia at any given time.
- About 40% to 50% of persons with insomnia have a comorbid mental health disorder
- Most common and widely recognized sleep disorder
- More prevalent with increasing age
- More common in women than men

Risk Factors

- Older adults
- Persons under severe situational stress, such as divorce, job loss, financial distress
- Occupations that require shift work, frequent travel through time zones
- Alcohol and substance abuse

Prevention and Screening

- Regular bedtime routines
- Normalized work hours
- Reduced daily stress; avoidance of stimulants late in the day

Assessment

History

- Inquire about onset, frequency, and duration of insomnia.
- Elicit present and past history of sleep patterns, routines, and naps.
- Inquire about patterns of use of caffeine, nicotine, alcohol, or other substances.
- Review current medications, including OTC and herbal products.
- Obtain psychiatric and medical history.

Physical Exam

- Physical exam should be tailored to the presenting symptomology, as primary insomnia is an illness of exclusion of other underlying medical conditions.

Diagnostic Studies

- CBC, chemistry profile, electrolytes, ECG
- EEG if warranted by abnormal exam or associated symptoms

Differential Diagnosis

- Alcohol or substance abuse
- Medication side effects
- Acute reaction to stressful life events

Psychiatric Disorders

- Anxiety disorder
- Major depressive disorder
- Grief reactions
- Bipolar disorder

Medical Conditions

- Cardiac disease
- GI disease
- Respiratory problems
  - COPD
  - Sleep apnea
  - CNS lesions
  - Endocrine disorders

Management

Nonpharmacologic Treatment

- Primary treatment consists of treating underlying cause.
- Eliminate or restrict use of caffeine, nicotine, and other CNS stimulants; alcohol may cause rebound stimulation.
- Establish routine:
  - Maintain a consistent bedtime.
  - Only go to bed when tired.
  - Do not use the bedroom for any activity other than sleeping and sexual activity.
  - Rise from bed at the same time every day, regardless of hours slept.
  - Do not nap during the day.
- Provide person with literature and community resources.

Pharmacologic Treatment

- Medications commonly prescribed for the treatment of insomnia include benzodiazepines, zolpidem (Ambien), and trazodone (Desyrel). Most medications (see Table 18–9) have some adverse effects, such as hangover, loss of effectiveness (tolerance), dependence, or constipation. Trazodone has TCA adverse reactions. Benzodiazepines are addictive; zolpidem may cause psychological dependence.
- Melatonin is not approved by the FDA but has shown some effectiveness in self-treatment of insomnia.

TABLE 18–9. INSOMNIA MEDICATIONS

MEDICATION	DOSAGE
BENZODIAZEPINE RECEPTOR AGONISTS	
Zolpidem (Ambien)	5–10 mg h.s.
Zolpidem CR	6.25 mg for women and 6.25 or 12.5 mg for men h.s.
Zaleplon (Sonata)	10–20 mg h.s.
TRICYCLIC ANTIDEPRESSANT	
Doxepin (Silenor)	6 mg h.s.
SEROTONIN ANTAGONIST AND REUPTAKE INHIBITOR	
Trazodone (Desyrel)	25–100 mg h.s.
MELATONIN RECEPTOR AGONIST	
Ramelteon (Rozerem)	8 mg h.s.
BENZODIAZEPINES	
Triazolam (Halcion)	0.125–0.25 mg h.s.
Temazepam (Restoril)	15–30 mg h.s.
Flurazepam (Dalmane)	15–30 mg h.s.
Estazolam (ProSom)	1–2 mg h.s.
Quazepam (Doral)	15–30 mg h.s.
OREXIN RECEPTOR AGONIST	
Suvorexant (Belsomra)	10–20 mg h.s.

How Long to Treat

- Non-benzodiazepines: Prescribe for short term (1 month), except Rozerem—can be used long term.
- Benzodiazepines: Prescribe for 7 to 10 days.
- Use lowest effective dose and discontinue gradually.
- Rebound insomnia may occur when medications are discontinued.
- Be aware of potential for drug tolerance, dependence, and withdrawal with benzodiazepines.
- Trazodone is effective only in insomnia associated with depression.

Special Considerations

- Do not prescribe for pregnant or lactating women or people with sleep apnea or renal or hepatic disease.
- Dose in older adults is usually lower, and short-acting agents are generally safer.
- Benzodiazepines have a potential for abuse; do not prescribe if history of substance abuse or mental illness.

When to Consult, Refer, Hospitalize

- Refer to mental health specialist when symptoms are secondary to anxiety disorder or mood disorder.
- When symptoms continue for longer than 1 month, refer to a sleep disorder specialist, neurologist, psychiatrist, or other qualified mental health practitioner.

Follow-Up

- Weekly monitoring of effectiveness of treatment, compliance, and potential abuse

Expected Course

- Most cases of primary insomnia will resolve with short-term management.

Complications

- Medication dependence

Websites with Important Information

Centers for Disease Control and Prevention: http://www.cdc.gov

National Institutes of Health: http://www.nih.gov

National Institute of Mental Health: http://www.nimh.nih.gov

Substance Abuse and Mental Health Services Administration (SAMSHA) https://www.samhsa.gov/

CASE STUDIES

CASE 1

A 32-year-old man presents to the FNP office for a routine wellness check. The client's PHQ-9 screening score is 9, indicating mild depressive symptoms. He states that he has been feeling sad for the last 2 months. He states he no longer enjoys golfing with friends and has preferred to stay home during his last two golf outings. The client denies suicidal ideations or behaviors. The client does not have a personal or family history of suicide. He denies symptoms consistent with a diagnosis of mania.

PMH: Smokes cigarettes regularly since age 15 years of age. Depression in early 20s treated with fluoxetine for 2 years. No hospitalizations or surgeries. No drug allergies or intolerance. Denies history of seizures.

Exam: Appeared well groomed. Speech slow. Affect congruent with mood. Physical exam otherwise unremarkable.

1. What additional history would you ask for?
2. What is the most likely mental health diagnosis?
3. What diagnostic tests would you offer?
4. What is your treatment plan?

CASE 2

A 52-year-old woman presents for a follow-up blood pressure check. The client reports issues with sleeping. She reports trouble falling asleep and getting about 5 hours of sleep. She denies nightmares. She works as a supervisor full time on the day shift in a merchant warehouse. She states during seasonal holidays "it can get hectic" at work. She states her husband is supportive of her career.

Past Medical History (PMH): Well-controlled hypertension with losartan (Avapro) 75 mg by mouth daily.

Exam: BP 124/70, HR 80, weight 145 pounds, height 5 feet 2 inches. PHQ-9 screen is negative for depression. Last menstrual period was 2 years ago. Skin intact with no apparent injuries. Remainder of physical examination was otherwise unremarkable

1. What additional history would you ask for?
2. What is the most likely mental health diagnosis?
3. What diagnostic tests would you offer?
4. What is your treatment plan?

CASE 3

A 30-year-old woman presents as a walk-in visit to the FNP led clinic for evaluation. The client shares witnessing a traumatic event at work over a month ago. The client states that since the incident she is experiencing intrusive thoughts, flashbacks, and nightmares of the traumatic event; difficulty sleeping; diminished interest in usual activities; feeling on edge like something terrible is going to happen; negative mood; and poor concentration.

PMH: Last menstrual period 2 weeks ago. She is currently taking daily oral contraceptives with good adherence and tolerance.

Exam: She appears alert, oriented, well-groomed, cooperative, and mildly anxious. She is breathing easy and regular, with oxygen saturation at 99% on room air. Her vital signs are within normal range.

1. What additional history would you ask for?
2. What is the most likely mental health diagnosis?
3. What diagnostic tests would you offer?
4. What is your treatment plan?

CASE STUDIES DISCUSSION

CASE 1

1. What additional history would you ask?

   Ask about onset, duration, and severity of symptoms and to what extent daily functioning is impaired. Identify any precipitating events or recent life changes such as divorce, financial difficulties, job loss, or victimization. Obtain complete medication history; caffeine intake; alcohol or drug use; and prescription and OTC medication, and alternative medication or treatments, including herbal supplements. Assess for alcohol and substance use. Calculate smoking pack-years. Obtain complete past medical history, any current medical problems, psychiatric history, social history, and family medical and psychiatric history. Inquire about a history of bipolar or symptoms of mania, as antidepressant medications may induce a manic episode. Assess for suicidal ideation or attempt. Inquire about homicidal thoughts or plans. Question the client about the symptoms of depression such as the following:

   - Depressed mood
   - Appetite changes
   - Anhedonia
   - Psychomotor agitation or retardation
   - Difficulty concentrating or making decisions
   - Change in sleep patterns
   - Low self-esteem; feelings of worthlessness or excessive, inappropriate guilt
   - Recurrent thoughts of death, suicidal ideation with or without a specific plan, prior suicide attempt
   - Decreased energy and fatigue; increased somatic complaints
   - Feelings of hopelessness

2. What is the most likely mental health diagnosis?

   The presumptive diagnosis for this client is major depressive disorder.

3. What diagnostic tests would you offer?

   Diagnostic labs depend on physical findings. Consider chemistry panel, TSH, CBC, sedimentation rate, chemistry profile, B12 and folate, and RPR; Consider the following screening tools other than PHQ-9: Beck Depression Inventory, Hamilton Rating Scale for Depression, Zung Self-Rating Depression Scale, and Adverse Childhood Experience (ACE) Questionnaire, as the higher score of adverse childhood experience increases the risk of a medical or mental condition.

4. What is your treatment plan?
   - Counsel regarding the benefits of quitting vs. the risks of smoking
   - Referral to psychotherapy
   - Pharmacologically the client is a good candidate for treatment with bupropion (Wellbutrin) as it is helpful for depression and smoking cessation. However, any other SSRI is also appropriate.

CASE 2

1. What additional history would you ask?

   Ask about onset, frequency, and duration of insomnia. Elicit present and past history of sleep patterns, routines, and naps. Inquire about patterns of use of caffeine, nicotine, alcohol, or other substances. Review current medications, including prescription, OTC, and herbal products. Obtain psychiatric and medical history.
2. What is the most likely mental health diagnosis?

   Presumptive diagnosis for this client is persistent insomnia.
3. What diagnostic tests would you offer?

   Diagnostic labs depend on physical findings. Consider chemistry panel, TSH, and CBC to rule out other medical conditions.
4. What is your treatment plan?
   - Psychoeducation regarding sleep hygiene
   - Ambien 5 mg as needed for insomnia, a 7-day supply. Counsel client regarding potential for addiction

CASE 3

1. What additional history would you ask?

   Ask about onset, duration, and severity of symptoms and to what extent daily functioning is impaired. Identify any precipitating events or recent life changes such as divorce, financial difficulties, job loss, or victimization. Obtain complete medication history, caffeine intake, alcohol or drug use, prescription and OTC medication, and alternative medication or treatments, including herbal supplements. Assess for nicotine or substance use. Obtain complete past medical history, any current medical problems, psychiatric history, social history, and family medical and psychiatric history. Assess for suicidal ideation or attempt. Question the client about the symptoms of PTSD such as the following:

   - Feelings of loss of control, panic, impending doom or dread, depersonalization, difficulty concentrating
   - Flashbacks, reliving the event
   - Hypervigilance
   - Emotional numbness and avoidance
   - Difficulty concentrating, making decisions, irritable, agitated mood, motor restlessness
   - Sleep disturbances (insomnia, frequent awakenings), fatigue, irritation, agitated mood

2. What is the most likely mental health diagnosis?

   Presumptive diagnosis is PTSD. The client is experiencing symptoms of both PTSD and ASD. However, the critical difference is the duration of the symptoms. ASD lasts for 3 days and a maximum of 4 weeks. This client has had symptoms for only over a month.

3. What diagnostic tests would you offer?

   Diagnostic labs depend on physical findings. Consider chemistry panel, TSH, and CBC to rule out other medical conditions. Consider the following screening tools: Primary Care PTSD Screen for DSM-5, PTSD Checklist (PCL-5), and ACE Questionnaire, as the higher score of adverse childhood experience increases the risk of a medical or mental condition.

4. What is your treatment plan?

   Referral for psychotherapy. Pharmacologic treatment with SSRI. Both sertraline and paroxetine are approved by the FDA for PTSD. However, sertraline has fewer drug interactions and a better side-effect profile. If nightmares persist would consider adding prazosin to treatment regimen. Provide psychoeducation on stress, stress reduction techniques, and psychotropic.

REFERENCES

Aiken, C., Feder, J. D., & Carlat, D. J. (2022). *Prescribing psychotropics: From drug interactions to genetics* (4th ed.). Newburyport, MA: Carlat Publishing

American Psychiatric Association. (2022). *Diagnostic and statistical manual of mental disorders* (5th ed., text rev.). Washington, DC: American Psychiatric Association.

Boland, R., Verduin, M. L., & Ruiz, P. (2022). *Kaplan & Sadock's synopsis of psychiatry* (12th ed.). Philadelphia, PA: Wolters Kluwer.

Centers for Disease Control and Prevention. (2019). *Tobacco and youth.* https://www.cdc.gov/tobacco/data_statistics/fact_sheets/youth_data/tobacco_use/index.htm

Centers for Disease Control and Prevention. (2021). *Preventing intimate partner violence.* https://www.cdc.gov/violenceprevention/intimatepartnerviolence/fastfact.html

Centers for Disease Control and Prevention. (2022a). *Smoking & tobacco use.* https://www.cdc.gov/tobacco/index.htm

Centers for Disease Control and Prevention. (2022b). *Opioids.* https://www.cdc.gov/opioids/index.html

Corrigan, J. D., Wolfe, M., Mysiw, W. J., Jackson, R. D., & Bogner, J. A. (2003). Early identification of mild traumatic brain injury in female victims of domestic violence. *American Journal of Obstetrics and Gynecology,* 188, S71–S76.

Davenport, L. (2015). New evidence-based guidelines for eating disorders issued. *Medscape Briefs,* 2015. https://www.medscape.org

Earls, F., Yogman, M. W., Mattson, G., Rafferty, J., & Committee on Psychosocial Aspects of Child and Family Health. (2019). Incorporating recognition and management of perinatal depression into pediatric practice. *Pediatrics, 143*(1), e20183259. https://publications.aap.org/pediatrics/article/143/1/e20183259/37241/Incorporating-Recognition-and-Management-of?autologincheck=redirected DOI: 10.1542/peds.2018-3259

Forman, S. F. (2018). Eating disorders: Overview of epidemiology, clinical features, and diagnosis. In J. A. Melin (Ed.). *UpToDate.* https://www-uptodate-com. proxy.libraries.rutgers.edu/contents/eating-disorders-overview-of-epidemiology-clinical-features-and-diagnosis

Gentzke A, S., Creamer, M., Cullen, K. A., Ambrose, B. K., Willis, G., Jamal, A., & King, B. A. (2019). Vital signs: Tobacco product use among middle and high school students—United States, 2011–2018. *MMWR Morbidity and Mortality Weekly Report, 68*(6), 157–64. http://dx.doi.org/10.15585/mmwr.mm6806e1

Glazier Leonte, K., Puliafico, A. Na, P., & Rynn, M. A. (2017). Pharmacotherapy for anxiety disorders in children and adolescents. In J. A. Melin (Ed.). *UpToDate.* https://www.uptodate.com/contents/pharmacotherapy-for-anxiety-disorders-in-children-and-adolescents

Halter, M. (2022). *Varcarolis' foundations of psychiatric-mental health nursing* (9th Ed.). St. Louis, Missouri: Elsevier.

Hasin, D. S., Sarvet, A. L., Meyers, J. L., Saha, T. D., Ruan, W. J., Stohl, M., & Grant, B. F. (2018). Epidemiology of adult DSM-5 major depressive disorder and its specifiers in the United States. *Journal of the American Medical Association Psychiatry, 75*(4), 336–346. https://doi.org/10.1001/jamapsychiatry.2017.4602

Moreland, C. S., & Bonin, L. (2018). Effect of antidepressants on suicide risk in children and adolescents. In J. A. Melin (Ed.). *UpToDate.* https://www.uptodate.com/contents/effect-of-antidepressants-on-suicide-risk-in-children-and-adolescents?topicRef=15928

National Vital Statistics System. (2018). QuickStats: *Age-adjusted suicide rates, by race/ethnicity—National Vital Statistics System, United States, 2015–2016. MMWR Morbidity and Mortality Weekly Report, 67*(14), 433. DOI: 10.15585/mmwr.mm6714a6

Puzantian, T., & Carlat, D. J. (2020). *Medication fact book for psychiatric practice* (5th ed.). Newburyport, MA: Carlat Publishing.

Tomko, R. L., Jones, J. L., Gilmore, A. K., Brady, K. T., Back, S. E., & Gray, K. M. (2018). N-acetylcysteine: A potential treatment for substance use disorders. *Current Psychiatry, 17*(6), 30–55.

United States Food and Drug Administration. (2019). *FDA approves new nasal spray medication for treatment-resistant depression; available only at a certified doctor's office or clinic.* https://www.fda.gov/NewsEvents/Newsroom/PressAnnouncements/ucm632761.htm

WebMD. (2019). *FDA panel backs ketamine-like drug for depression.* https://www.webmd.com/depression/news/20190213/fda-panel-backs-ketamine-like-drug-for-depression 5 Minute Clinical Consult. (2021). *Rape crisis syndrome.* https://5minuteconsult.com/collectioncontent/1-152038/diseases-and-conditions/rape-crisis-syndrome

APPENDIX A

REVIEW QUESTIONS

1. According to the Consensus Model for Advanced Practice Registered Nurses, which of the following may call themselves advanced practice registered nurses (APRNs)?

    a. Nurse administrators

    b. Nurse practitioners

    c. Nurse educators

    d. Clinical nurse leaders

2. Which of the following standards for quality nurse practitioner education does the National Organization of Nurse Practitioner Faculties (NONPF) National Task Force (NTF) consensus-based standards recommend?

    a. Site visits for accreditation

    b. Program quality

    c. Annual reports

    d. Program planning

3. Legislative authority for nurse practitioner practice is regulated by which of the following?

    a. The professional certifying organization, with a vote of the membership

    b. The board of medicine in each state jurisdiction, with the consent of the board of nursing

    c. The federal government's Bureau of Health Professions

    d. A legally designated authority that implements regulations, such as state boards of nursing

4. A nurse practitioner (NP) is planning to interview for a job with a physician practice that has not hired NPs previously. The NP is asked, "How can we bill for the services you provide?" Which response would be best?

    a. In most states, nurse practitioners (NPs) take direct payments from patients, so the patients pay NPs for services.

    b. Medicare will reimburse for an NP's services at 85% of the customary physician rate.

    c. Medicaid is the only insurance plan that does not reimburse NPs.

    d. Reimbursement is available from Medicare at the full physician rate, even if the physician is not in the office.

5. You are completing a quality improvement project involving Health Insurance Portability and Accountability Act (HIPAA) compliance at your primary care practice. For this project, you are following several colleagues throughout the day and observing their activities. Based on your knowledge of the HIPAA Act of 1996, which of the following demonstrates compliance with HIPAA?

   a. The nurse practitioner (NP) is unable to reach a patient so she calls and leaves a message on the patient's home phone asking the patient to call the practice.

   b. A patient's intake notes with vital signs and chief complaint are on a clipboard that is inserted face-down on the door rack.

   c. The clerk calls the patient in the waiting room up to registration by their first and last names and asks for their health insurance.

   d. The NP leaves the computer logged on to the practice web site with the screen on upon leaving for lunch.

6. Which of the following statements about Duvall's theory of the stages in family development is true?

   a. The stages cannot overlap.

   b. The stages are based on the age and school placement of the firstborn child.

   c. There are four stages.

   d. Marriage is strongest during the fourth stage.

7. Which of the following is true regarding the role of the family nurse practitioner (FNP) and evidence-based practice?

   a. The family nurse practitioner (FNP) must rely on tradition, intuition, and personal preference to deal with clinical problems.

   b. The FNP should accept and use clinical practice guidelines as valid and credible, regardless of the source of the recommendations.

   c. Cultural influences rarely influence health behaviors and should not be included in developing a treatment plan.

   d. It is prudent for the FNP to identify evidence-based practices and to critically evaluate and participate in outcome studies.

8. You have just graduated from your nurse practitioner (NP) program and are investigating malpractice insurance. You are aware that there are several different types of coverage. You select a policy that covers any claim that results from an incident that occurs during the term of the policy, regardless of how long it takes before the claim is made. This is referred to as a:

   a. Claims-made policy

   b. Tail policy

   c. Occurrence policy

   d. Nurse practitioner policy

9. Which of the following statements regarding health disparities is correct?
   a. Bias does not impact health outcomes.
   b. Bias does not influence health disparities.
   c. Health disparities are preventable, inequitable differences in disease burden and opportunities to achieve optimal health that are experienced by socially disadvantaged populations.
   d. Health disparities are a direct result of an individual's failure to care about their health and well-being.

10. Which of the following individuals would be the best candidate for palliative care?
    a. A 56-year-old man with diabetes
    b. An 18-year-old woman with a terminal brain tumor
    c. An 87-year-old patient with Alzheimer's disease
    d. A 47-year-old woman with chronic heart failure

11. You are seeing a 36-year-old patient with type 2 diabetes for a new patient visit. She tells you that she is starting a new job and is concerned about getting insurance coverage, as she has been told in the past that she could not get insurance because of her preexisting medical condition. You tell her:
    a. She may want to consider getting a second individual insurance policy outside work.
    b. She should not have any issues getting insurance because the Affordable Care Act ended preexisting conditions exclusions.
    c. She should see if she could remain on her old insurance.
    d. She should save extra funds to pay for services associated with her type 2 diabetes care.

12. You are treating a 52-year-old White woman who has no chronic health conditions and usually sees you only for minor acute problems. She was seen at a health fair and was told that she must begin getting mammogram screenings for breast cancer. You recommend the following:
    a. Begin doing self-breast exams at home.
    b. Refer her to an oncologist for further care.
    c. Order a screening bilateral mammogram to be performed every 2 years.
    d. Discuss that there is not current evidence supporting this test.

13. You are seeing a newborn for his 1-month well-child exam. His mother asks you why the nurses in the hospital drew blood from his heel before he was discharged home. You explain that this blood test was to detect any genetic abnormalities he may have. This is an example of:

    a. Primary prevention
    b. Secondary prevention
    c. Tertiary prevention
    d. Quaternary prevention

14. You are discussing the importance of exercising with a 68-year-old patient you are seeing for routine follow up. She tells you she does not feel safe walking outside in her neighborhood because of all the gang members that "hang out" on her street. This patient is experiencing which social determinant of health?

    a. Economic stability
    b. Education access and quality
    c. Health care access and quality
    d. Social and community context

15. Your 68-year-old patient reports that she has a new grandchild that she will be visiting about 2 months later during the summer. The baby's mother told the patient that she must receive a "booster shot" before she visits but does not remember which one. What is the most likely vaccine needed for this patient?

    a. MMR
    b. DTaP
    c. Zoster
    d. HPV

16. You are doing a routine wellness visit for an 8-year-old girl. Her mother reports she has already had two menstrual cycles this year. On your exam you note that she has developed breast tissue as well as pubertal hair. What is your next action?

    a. Nothing at this time
    b. Schedule back in 6 months for re-evaluation
    c. Order an MRI
    d. Refer the child to a specialist

17. Mrs. Smith is a 75-year-old woman who has questions about taking calcium dietary supplements. You have conducted a focused history and physical examination including all recommended screening exams. What do you recommend for her to take?

    a. Take 1000–1500 mg of calcium daily.
    b. Increase exercise until just unable to talk while exercising.
    c. Take in more dietary calcium in the form of dairy products.
    d. She does not need to take any calcium supplements.

18. Ms. Tsong is a 75-year-old woman who takes multiple over-the-counter vitamin and herbal supplements along with nine prescribed medications. She asks you if taking all these medications and vitamins is okay. What is your advice to her?

    a. Continue taking all the medications as well as the vitamins and supplements.
    b. Discontinue taking all the vitamins and supplements; take only the prescribed medications.
    c. Review all her medications, including vitamins and supplements, and decide which are safe and necessary for her to continue.
    d. Do not say anything.

19. J. Martinez is a 35-year-old woman whose grandmother had a history of osteoporosis. She asks for your advice about things she can do to help decrease her risk of developing this condition. Which of the following is recommended to decrease her risk of developing osteoporosis?

    a. Follow her bone density with annual measurements.
    b. Drink at least one glass of red wine per week.
    c. Ensure adequate dietary intake of vitamin C.
    d. Regularly engage in weight-bearing exercise.

20. Mr. King is a 78-year-old Black man who wants some advice about getting a colonoscopy. He has had one every 10 years since he was 50 and never had an abnormal one. He wants to know if he should continue to get one every 10 years. How do you advise Mr. King?

    a. Go ahead and get one if he wants to. That is his choice.
    b. Patient should be advised to ask his gastroenterologist for his recommendation.
    c. Colonoscopies are recommended only for ages 50 to 75, so he does not need another one.
    d. Recommend he get fecal occult blood test (FOBT) instead.

21. A 16-year-old adolescent presents to the clinic 30 days following her return from summer camp. She complains of fever, sore throat, and right upper quadrant abdominal pain. On exam the patient is noted to have exudative pharyngitis, lymphadenopathy, and splenomegaly. The FNP suspects which etiology?

    a. Coxsackievirus
    b. Hepatitis B
    c. Mononucleosis
    d. *Streptococcus*

22. What are the characteristic findings in a patient with suspected inhalation anthrax infection?

    a. Diffuse rash with erythema and pleuritic pain
    b. Elevated liver enzymes and leukopenia
    c. Fever, malaise, and thrombocytopenia
    d. Mediastinal widening and pleural effusion

23. An adolescent boy presents with fever and malaise for 24 hours, and now has developed orchitis. Which is a likely cause for these symptoms?

    a. Measles
    b. Mumps
    c. Rubella
    d. Rubeola

24. Which minor may consent for his or her own care?

    a. A 16-year-old visiting with relatives for the summer in another state
    b. A legally emancipated minor
    c. A 15-year-old who goes to the school nurse because of a headache
    d. A 14-year-old in the foster care system

25. Sally is 15 weeks pregnant. She is requesting a flu vaccine today. You tell her:

    a. You must wait until the pregnancy is over to receive the flu vaccine
    b. You must wait until the third trimester to receive the flu vaccine
    c. We will administer your flu vaccine today.
    d. You must wait until the pregnancy is over and you have finished breastfeeding to receive the vaccine

26. Jane is 19 weeks pregnant. Her titer for measles is negative; she has never had the disease or the immunization. What is your best course of action?

    a. Give measles, mumps, and rubella vaccine (MMR) #1 today and MMR #2 in one month.

    b. Give measles, mumps, and rubella vaccine (MMR) #1 today but wait until the pregnancy is over before giving MMR #2.

    c. Wait until the third trimester and give measles, mumps, and rubella vaccine (MMR) #1 and MMR #2 at the appropriate intervals.

    d. Do not give measles, mumps, and rubella vaccine (MMR) during the pregnancy.

27. Which is the best method for preventing spread of varicella zoster virus?

    a. Avoid touching lesions.

    b. Keep the patient in isolation.

    c. Keep lesions covered.

    d. Practice good handwashing.

28. A 6-year-old child is bitten by a dog. Her mother asks the nurse practitioner (NP) if the child needs anti-rabies treatment. You tell her:

    a. If the dog is a domestic pet that was vaccinated, the wound should be cleaned and irrigated.

    b. Anti-rabies treatment must be started immediately.

    c. Rabies can be contracted only through the bites of wild animals.

    d. Wait until you have observed the animal for 2 weeks to determine whether it is rabid.

29. What is the most effective way to prevent SARS-CoV-2 infection?

    a. Zinc/vitamin C

    b. Masking

    c. Vaccines

    d. Paxlovid

30. When a patient asks how she was infected with herpes simplex virus (HSV), the family nurse practitioner advises which of the following?

    a. Contact with a toilet seat

    b. Unprotected intercourse with an infected partner

    c. Swimming pool

    d. From catching the flu

31. Which of the following patients is at the greatest risk for basal cell carcinoma?

    a. 32-year-old African American male farmer

    b. 26-year-old Hispanic female teacher

    c. 67-year-old Caucasian male soybean farmer

    d. 41-year-old African American female nurse

32. A patient presents to an urgent care office with small, raised, bright red lesions on his legs and belt line. The family nurse practitioner is concerned about which of the following bites?

    a. Chiggers

    b. Mosquitoes

    c. Fleas

    d. Spiders

33. The family nurse practitioner is seeing a patient for follow-up of a herpes zoster infection and subsequent diagnosis of postherpetic neuralgia. Which of the following medications would be most appropriate to treat postherpetic neuralgia?

    a. Cymbalta (duloxetine)

    b. Neurontin (gabapentin)

    c. Ultram (tramadol)

    d. Celebrex (celecoxib)

34. When treating a patient following a human bite, the family nurse practitioner appropriately prescribes which medication?

    a. Erythromycin

    b. Cephalexin (Keflex)

    c. Dicloxacillin (Dycil)

    d. Amoxicillin/clavulanate (Augmentin)

35. After diagnosing a patient with extensive hidradenitis suppurativa, the family nurse practitioner understands that which of the following options is the top priority?

    a. Recommend local heat.

    b. Prescribe a prednisone taper.

    c. Refer to a general surgeon.

    d. Recommend avoiding antiperspirants.

36. When educating a patient about urticaria, the family nurse practitioner describes spontaneous urticaria as?

    a. Hives or wheals that have no identifiable causative factor
    b. Hives or wheals that have a specific identifiable causative factor
    c. Hives or wheals that last longer than 6 weeks
    d. Hives or wheals that last 24 to 36 hours

37. The family nurse practitioner understands the etiology of atopic dermatitis as?

    a. Idiopathic
    b. IgM-mediated
    c. IgE-mediated
    d. IgG-mediated

38. A 65-year-old man is diagnosed with rhinophyma. The family nurse practitioner would expect to see which of the following diagnoses in his medical history?

    a. Acne vulgaris
    b. Systemic lupus erythematosus (SLE)
    c. Nodulocystic acne
    d. Acne rosacea

39. The family nurse practitioner recognizes a herald patch as pathognomonic for this of the following dermatologic conditions?

    a. Dermatophytosis
    b. Pityriasis rosea
    c. Atopic dermatitis
    d. Alopecia

40. An 8-week-old boy presents to the clinic with his mother and older sister for a well-child exam. Both are concerned because the patient looks at them with crossed eyes. They state that the right eye fixates inward more than the left eye and this occurs more when he is tired. On examination, his eyes are crossed. When either eye is covered, he fixes and follows with the contralateral eye and appears to have normal motility. What is the most likely diagnosis in this patient?

    a. Sixth nerve palsy
    b. Monocular diplopia
    c. Congenital esotropia
    d. Accommodative dystropia

41. A 52-year-old African American man presents to the clinic for an annual well exam. He has a history of hypertension controlled with lifestyle modifications. He has been feeling well other than decreasing eyesight. His mother had a history of glaucoma. He denies nausea, vomiting, or eye pain. On examination, his visual acuity is OU (both eyes) 20/40 and his PERRLA with no injection. Intraocular pressure is elevated at 22 mmHg. Which of the following is a risk factor for open-angle glaucoma?

    a. African American
    b. Depression
    c. Hyperthyroidism
    d. Age 40–50 years

42. A 62-year-old Native American woman presents to the clinic with blood in her right eye. She states that she noticed it this morning. She denies eye pain, blurred vision, double vision, or decreased visual acuity. She denies any trauma and states that she was seen by her ophthalmologist 3 weeks ago with normal intraocular pressure. Her past medical history includes diabetes mellitus and generalized arthritic pain. Her current medications include metformin and ibuprofen. Exam findings: visual acuity 20/20 OU; no deformities of eyelids, lashes, lacrimal ducts, or cornea. EOMs intact with normal direct, consensual papillary response, and the visual fields are intact to confrontation. Blood is present in the right anterior chamber with partial filling. Which of the following is the most appropriate treatment for this patient?

    a. Hospital admission for IV corticosteroids and IV antibiotics
    b. Prednisolone acetate 1% one gtt OD twice daily
    c. Immediate referral to ophthalmology
    d. Send patient home with instructions to avoid vigorous activities and to keep her head elevated

43. A 32-year-old African American man presents to the clinic with red eyes, sensitivity to bright lights, tearing, gritty sensation, mild discharge, and swollen eyelids. He states he was seen and treated for conjunctivitis 10 days ago and has used the prescribed erythromycin ophthalmic ointment as directed. Although he has been feeling well otherwise, his symptoms have not improved. He denies any contact lens use or eye injury. He has no allergies or other medication use. He reports sexual activity with multiple female and male partners as well as marijuana use with alcohol every weekend. On exam: visual acuity 20/25 OU; PERRLA, EOMs intact, eyelid edema with matted eyelashes, and bilateral conjunctival injection. Preauricular lymphadenopathy is also present. Which of the following is appropriate for the treatment of gonococcal conjunctivitis?

    a. Penicillin VK orally
    b. Ceftriaxone IM/IV
    c. Latanoprost ophthalmic drops
    d. Timolol maleate

44. A 65-year-old White man presents to the clinic for a preoperative history and physical examination. He is scheduled to have cataract surgery in 2 weeks. He has a history of hypertension, non–insulin-dependent diabetes mellitus, benign prostatic hyperplasia, and generalized osteoarthritis. His current medications include lisinopril (Prinivil), furosemide (Lasix), metformin (Glucophage), exenatide (Byetta), tamsulosin (Flomax), meloxicam (Mobic), and multivitamin and garlic tablets. Which of the following medications can cause intraoperative floppy iris syndrome in patients undergoing cataract surgery?

a. Fur osemide

b. Tamsulosin

c. Meloxicam

d. Garlic

45. An 18-month-old boy presents to the clinic with his father who reports he has been "tugging" at his right ear. Father states that the pain started late yesterday afternoon and the child developed a fever (temperature of 102°F) last evening. The child has been less active, fussy, and more fatigued. No known drug allergies. On exam, the child is alert, lying in his father's arms, but interactive. Eyes unremarkable. Ears: left ear canal patent with Tympanic Membrane™ dull, intact. Right ear canal patent with air-fluid level behind TM with marked redness of TM and poor movement with pneumatic otoscopy. Nose: clear sinus drainage without congestion. Lungs: clear bilaterally. Heart: Regular rate and rhythm without murmurs. What is the most appropriate treatment for this patient?

a. Observation with pain management because symptoms just started yesterday

b. Ofloxacin (Floxin) otic drops

c. Azithromycin 10 mg/kg for 1 day then 5 mg/kg for days 2–5

d. Amoxicillin 80–90 mg/kg/day twice a day

46. An 18-month-old girl presents to the clinic with her mother with complaints of fever and poor appetite for the past 3 days. Her mother states that the patient is not her normal self because she is less active and more irritable. Her fluid intake has decreased from normal, although she has good urine output. There is no reported vomiting, diarrhea, sinus drainage, or tugging at her ears. Her immunizations are up to date, although another child in daycare had similar symptoms last week. On exam, she had a 103°F temperature and is alert, underweight for age, and nontoxic appearing. She appears fatigued and is drooling. Her ears and nose are unremarkable. There are small gray ulcers on the distal tongue and lips. Posterior pharynx is nonerythematous and without tonsillar enlargement. Neck is supple with enlarged anterior cervical adenopathy. Lungs are clear bilaterally and heart is regular sinus rhythm without murmurs. Skin is warm, dry, and intact. What is your most likely diagnosis?

a. Varicella

b. Herpetic gingivostomatitis

c. Hand, foot, and mouth disease

d. Aphthous ulcers

47. Which of the following is considered first-line treatment for otitis externa?

    a. Oral ciprofloxacin

    b. Carbamide peroxide otic solution

    c. Neomycin/polymyxin B/hydrocortisone otic solution

    d. Ceftriaxone 1 g IM

48. A 72-year-old woman presents to the office today for ringing in her ears. She is accompanied by her son who states he has had to speak louder around his mother over the last 2 months. Her symptoms have been constant and unchanged throughout the day. She has a history of congestive heart failure, hypertension, and coronary artery disease. Her medications include furosemide (Lasix), lisinopril (Prinivil), rosuvastatin (Crestor), metoprolol (Toprol XL), and aspirin. Physical examination is unremarkable except for decreased bilateral auditory acuity. Which of the following is the mainstay of therapy for her condition?

    a. Hypnosis

    b. Cognitive behavioral therapy

    c. Avoid exposure to loud noises

    d. Supportive care

49. A 23-year-old woman without any significant past medical history presents to your office for left eye pain. She is not allergic to any medications and does not take any medications. She has worn contacts for the last 6 years and describes her left eye pain as excruciating with a foreign body sensation. She reports photophobia and excessive tearing. Examination of the left eye reveals conjunctival injection, increased lacrimation, and an abrasion via fluorescein stain. Visual acuity of the left eye is 20/80 without refraction. No foreign body was identified via upper or lower eyelid inversion. Which of the following treatments is most appropriate for this patient?

    a. Ganciclovir ophthalmic gtt

    b. Natamycin ophthalmic gtt

    c. Ciprofloxacin ophthalmic gtt

    d. Patanol ophthalmic gtt

50. The nurse practitioner is evaluating a 70-year-old woman who presented to the primary care office with complaints of sudden onset of fever with temperature of 102.0°F (38.3°C), a productive cough with rust-colored sputum, and sharp pain in the back and chest with coughing. Physical examination reveals tachycardia, tachypnea, dullness on percussion, and rales. The chest X-ray reveals lobar opacities. Which diagnosis is most likely?

    a. Atypical pneumonia

    b. Acute bronchitis

    c. Bacterial pneumonia

    d. Influenza

51. A 30-year-old client presents to the clinic with complaints of a nonproductive cough for 8 days. Breath sounds are clear to auscultation and there is no sign of fever. The client is diagnosed with acute bronchitis. Which of the following is an appropriate initial therapy?

    a. Antibiotics
    b. Antihistamines
    c. Inhaled beta agonist
    d. OTC cough suppressant

52. A 25-year-old client presents to the clinic for a physical and requests a tuberculin skin test as a requirement for an upcoming job in a correctional facility. The client has a negative medical history and is in good health. The client denies coming into contact with anyone with a history of tuberculosis. Which finding would indicate a positive tuberculin skin test (TST) finding in this patient?

    a. Erythema 10 mm in diameter
    b. Induration 10 mm in diameter
    c. Erythema 15 mm in diameter
    d. Induration 15 mm in diameter

53. Which is the initial therapy for a child diagnosed with uncomplicated bronchiolitis for the first time?

    a. Nebulized albuterol
    b. Dexamethasone
    c. Guaifenesin DM
    d. Frequent suctioning

54. Which is the preferred first-line treatment for community-acquired pneumonia in a 50-year-old patient with no comorbidities?

    a. Amoxicillin
    b. Amoxicillin/clavulanate
    c. Amoxicillin-clavulanate plus clarithromycin
    d. Levofloxacin

55. Which of the following pulmonary function test results are seen in a 17-year-old patient with mild asthma?

    a. FEV1 70% of predicted with FEV1/FVC ratio greater than85%
    b. FEV1 85% of predicted with FEV1/FVC ratio 75%
    c. Forced vital capacity (FVC) 50% of predicted
    d. FEV1 88% of predicted with FEV1/FVC ratio greater than85%

56. A 10-year-old girl presents to the clinic with complaints of wheezing for the past 2 weeks. She has a history of asthma and has been using her albuterol inhaler 4 times a day with some relief. She has awakened during the night once with symptoms. What is the next step in treatment for the client?

    a. Add low-dose fluticasone-salmeterol, 1 inhalation twice daily; continue albuterol as needed
    b. Add mometasone-formoterol, 2 inhalations twice daily
    c. Add formoterol, 1 inhalation twice daily
    d. Continue albuterol as needed

57. Which of the following medications may lead to increased risk of asthma-related adverse outcomes when used alone as maintenance therapy in the treatment of asthma?

    a. Oral prednisone
    b. Oral montelukast
    c. Inhaled fluticasone
    d. Inhaled formoterol

58. The goal of chronic obstructive pulmonary disease (COPD) management is to:

    a. Prevent lung cancer
    b. Prevent disease progression
    c. Prevent hemoptysis
    d. Prevent tuberculosis

59. A 65-year-old man presented to the clinic with complaints of a productive cough with bloody sputum for the past month. He denies fever, chills, or shortness of breath. He is former smoker and is retired. The family nurse practitioner should suspect?

    a. Bronchitis
    b. Lung cancer
    c. Chronic obstructive pulmonary disease (COPD)
    d. Asthma

60. A 55-year-old man with a history of hypertension, hyperlipidemia, type 2 diabetes, status post mechanical mitral valve replacement surgery 2 years ago, presents with complaint of shortness of breath, palpitations. ECG shows new-onset atrial fibrillation. His comprehensive metabolic panel, complete blood count (CBC), prothrombin time (PT), partial thromboplastin time (PTT), and international normalized ratio (INR) are all within the normal range. Which of the following medications may be started for anticoagulation?

    a. Warfarin (Coumadin)

    b. Apixaban (Eliquis)

    c. Dabigatran (Pradaxa)

    d. Rivaroxaban (Xarelto)

61. Murmurs loudest at the 5th intercostal space (ICS), midclavicular line (MCL), are likely which of the following?

    a. Aortic

    b. Tricuspid

    c. Mitral

    d. Pulmonic

62. A 75-year-old woman presents for a third follow-up visit for repeat blood pressure evaluation. On prior visits her blood pressure was 132/84 and 136/85. Today her blood pressure is 138/86. Atherosclerotic cardiovascular disease (ASCVD) or 10-year cardiovascular disease (CVD) risk is greater than 10%. In addition to lifestyle recommendations, what would the FNP do next?

    a. Start hydrocholorthiazide (HCTZ)25 mg orally daily.

    b. No medications at this time; continue lifestyle modification and reassess in 3 months.

    c. Reassess blood pressure in 1 month; if elevated then start an ACE inhibitor.

    d. Start furosemide 20 mg orally daily.

63. 45-year-old man with a history of myocardial infarction 2 weeks ago presents for follow-up. He has normal left ventricle function. Which of the following medications should he be taking?

    a. Acetaminophen (Tylenol)

    b. Fluoxetine (Prozac)

    c. Atorvastatin (Lipitor)

    d. Famotidine (Pepcid)

64. A 59-year-old man patient with Stage 1 hypertension who is at high risk (Atherosclerotic cardiovascular disease [ASCVD] 10-year risk is greater than 10%) is started on hydrocholorthiazide 25 mg orally daily in addition to lifestyle modification recommendations. When will you have the patient follow-up with repeat blood pressure after initial diagnosis?

    a. 3 months
    b. 1 month
    c. 2 weeks
    d. 6 months

65. A 29-year-old pregnant woman presents to the emergency department with left calf pain. Deep vein thrombosis (DVT) is confirmed on ultrasound. She has no other medical history. What would you do next?

    a. Insert an inferior vena cava filter
    b. Start Low-molecular-weight heparin (LMWH)
    c. Observe
    d. Start thrrombolytic

66. A 35-year-old woman with hypertension, taking lisinopril 10 mg orally daily, tells you she would like to have a baby. What will you tell her about her hypertension medication?

    a. You can continue lisinopril at 10 mg orally daily throughout pregnancy
    b. We may need to increase the dose of lisinopril later in pregnancy
    c. We will stop lisinopril and transition to labetalol
    d. You will not be able to take any blood pressure medications while you are pregnant

67. What is the recommended target for LDL level in a 30-year-old adult with no risk factors?

    a. Under 100
    b. Under 70
    c. Under 130
    d. Under 200

68. A 69-year-old man with a history of myocardial infarction who is status post stent to LAD 6 months ago, with hypertension, hyperlipidemia, 10-year risk greater than 20%, with an LDL of 150 on a high-dose statin, Lipitor 80 mg p. o. daily. What medication would you add?

    a. PCSK9 inhibitor
    b. Increase Lipitor dose
    c. Ezetimibe
    d. No change in medication; enhance lifestyle modification

69. What medication would you prescribe initially for a 68-year-old woman with Stage B chronic heart failure and no other past medical history? All labs (basic metabolic pane [BMP], complete blood count [CBC], coagulation times) are within normal limits.

    a. ACEI

    b. statin

    c. verapamil

    d. warfarin

70. Which of the following is true regarding dysphagia?

    a. Patients describe oropharyngeal dysphagia as a feeling of food getting stuck.

    b. Dysphagia may present as chest pain.

    c. Dysphagia may be a structural or neuromuscular problem.

    d. All of the above

71. In evaluation of a patient with elevated AST, which of the following is correct?

    a. Elevated AST should be fractionated to determine if it is predominantly from the liver.

    b. If a patient has normal liver function tests, hepatitis studies should not be ordered.

    c. AST is found in liver, cardiac, skeletal, kidney, and brain tissue; elevated levels alone may indicate tissue damage in any of those organ systems.

    d. Liver biopsy should be performed for definitive diagnosis prior to serological workup.

72. Which of the following is a risk factor for developing constipation?

    a. Excessive dietary intake of fiber and fluids

    b. Overactive lifestyle

    c. Use of anticholinergics

    d. Eating from animal sources (meat, dairy, eggs) that are pasteurized

73. When is it appropriate to use pharmacological treatment for AGE (acute gastroenteritis)?

    a. If vomiting continues despite slow intake of fluids, consider use of an antiemetic.

    b. If a patient has a fever and blood in the stool can use antidiarrheal agents.

    c. Antibiotics can be used prior to an organism causing the diarrhea being isolated.

    d. Initiate antihistamines for acute vomiting.

74. In caring for a child with gastroesophageal reflux, which of the following is most important for a clinician to remember?

    a. Infants outgrow gastroesophageal reflux at 2 years of age.

    b. Respiratory disorders can be caused by gastroesophageal reflux.

    c. Infants with gastroesophageal reflux gain weight at an increased rate compared to other infants.

    d. Forty-seven percent of infants younger than 2 months of age have gastroesophageal reflux with multiple daily symptoms.

75. What is the standard diagnostic definition of inflammatory bowel disease?

    a. A combination of chronic and recurrent GI symptoms not explained by structural or biochemical abnormalities

    b. Two or more weeks in the last 6 months of abdominal pain

    c. Discomfort that is relieved by urination

    d. Onset associated with consistent form of stool

76. When assessing a hernia, which of the following is a correct description?

    a. Herniated (contents are partially able to be pushed back into abdominal cavity)

    b. Strangulated (a non-reducible hernia in which the flow of intestinal contents is obstructed)

    c. Incarcerated (hernia in which the blood supply of the hernia contents is compromised)

    d. Reducible (contents can be pushed back into the abdominal cavity)

77. Risk factors for colorectal cancer include which of the following?

    a. Age over 30 years

    b. Cachexia

    c. History of inflammatory bowel disease

    d. History of brain cancer

78. In evaluating a child for acute intussusception, which of the following diagnosis should be included in the differential diagnoses?

    a. Reducible inguinal hernia

    b. Hirschsprung's disease

    c. Jejunal atresia

    d. AGE

79. Which of the following is true of viral hepatitis?

    a. ALT and AST are rarely elevated.

    b. If the patient has jaundice, it will be noted on clinical exam with a serum bilirubin level 2.5 mg/dL.

    c. Alkaline phosphatase level may be abnormal.

    d. Prolonged prothrombin time (PT) is an indicator of resolving disease.

80. What is the prime effect of antidiuretic hormone on kidneys?

    a. Increase collecting duct permeability

    b. Increase medullary blood flow

    c. Decrease cortical blood flow

    d. Decrease potassium secretion

81. An 11-month old girl presents for fever and fussiness. A urinalysis indicates she has a urinary tract infection. You treat with an appropriate antibiotic. What is your next step?

    a. IV pyelogram

    b. Cystoscopy

    c. Renal ultrasound and voiding cystourethrography (VCUG)

    d. Observation with no further testing

82. Which of the following statements about enuresis in childhood is true?

    a. Primary enuresis is defined as the onset of bed-wetting after a 6-month period of dryness.

    b. Bed-wetting usually occurs in Stage 1 of NREM sleep.

    c. Most outgrow the condition before 12 years of age.

    d. Diagnosis should include cystoscopy to rule out structural causes.

83. Which of the following tests is indicated in the initial workup of urinary incontinence in an older adult patient?

    a. Renal ultrasound

    b. Urodynamic studies

    c. Postvoid residual

    d. Urine cytology

84. Which of the following does asymptomatic hematuria workup include?
    a. Cystoscopy
    b. CT urography
    c. Urine cytology
    d. All the above

85. What is the most common cause of microscopic hematuria in men 60 years of age and over?
    a. Kidney stones
    b. Glomerulonephritis
    c. BPH
    d. Bladder cancer

86. What is false concerning fosfomycin antibiotic?
    a. Has a limited cross-resistance with most common antibacterial agents
    b. Causes injection site reactions
    c. Is active against most uropathogens
    d. Is effective as a single-dose agent

87. What is false concerning asymptomatic bacteriuria during pregnancy?
    a. It could lead to pyelonephritis, low birth weight, premature labor.
    b. Pregnant women are at higher risk of UTI in weeks 6 through 24.
    c. Antibiotics should be culture-based and given, preferably, intravenous in a single shot.
    d. Screening for asymptomatic bacteriuria should begin at the first antenatal visit.

88. What is (are) the prominent clinical finding(s) in the diagnosis of acute pyelonephritis?
    a. Fever, chills, abdominal pain
    b. Costovertebral angle tenderness
    c. Hypogastric and loin pain
    d. Flank pain, dysuria

89. What is false concerning stress incontinence pathophysiology?

   a. Physiologically, during sneezing, the intra-abdominal pressure increases over the bladder and the abdominal part of the urethra, ending in no leakage.

   b. While leaking, bladder pressure exceeds the urethral resistance.

   c. During episodes of stress incontinence, leakage ceases when bladder pressure falls below urethral pressure.

   d. The major cause of stress incontinence is intrinsic sphincter deficiency

90. Which of the following statements regarding asymptomatic bacteriuria in women is TRUE?

   a. Risk is increased with sexual intercourse.

   b. Risk is not increased in women who use diaphragms.

   c. It has been shown to lead to renal damage in all patients.

   d. Prevalence in older adult women may be as high as 75%.

91. Which of the following best describes the abnormal uterine bleeding (AUB) pattern termed menometrorrhagia?

   a. Menstrual periods occurring at irregular intervals of varying flow and duration

   b. Regular menstrual periods but with reduced amount or duration

   c. Irregular menstrual periods of increased amount or duration

   d. Regular menstrual periods but at intervals of less than 21 days

92. Which of the following describes a suitable candidate for a diaphragm contraceptive device?

   a. A postpartum patient who had a vaginal birth 3 weeks ago

   b. A 10-week status post-cesarean section, postpartum patient who is breastfeeding

   c. A female patient with a history of frequent urinary tract infections

   d. A female patient with a history of toxic shock syndrome

93. Which of the following is the most effective form of emergency contraceptive method that can be used up to 120 hours after an unprotected sexual encounter?

   a. Ulipristal acetate (UPA) progesterone receptor modulator

   b. Estrogen and progestin combined pill

   c. Copper T IUD

   d. Progestin-only pill

94. Which of the following medication combinations is appropriate for a client with pelvic inflammatory disease (PID)?

    a. Ceftriaxone (Rocephin), doxycycline, plus metronidazole (Flagyl)

    b. Ceftriaxone (Rocephin), doxycycline, plus a quinolone agent

    c. Oral cephalosporins and a quinolone agent

    d. Metronidazole (Flagyl) and doxycycline

95. Women with polycystic ovary syndrome are at high risk for developing which of the following conditions?

    a. Hypoglycemia

    b. Hypoinsulinemia

    c. Weight loss

    d. HAIR-AN syndrome

96. A piece of rusty metal cuts a 30-year-old woman who is 12 weeks pregnant. She does not remember the last time she received a tetanus toxoid booster. She should be advised that:

    a. it is safe to receive a booster now.

    b. she must wait until after the delivery.

    c. she should receive the booster in her third trimester.

    d. childhood immunizations will give her immunity now.

97. Which of the following vaccines is contraindicated in pregnancy?

    a. Mumps, Measles, Rubella (MMR)

    b. COVID-19

    c. Hepatitis B

    d. Polio

98. During a 6-week postpartum exam, an abdominal diastasis recti measuring 3 cm in diameter is noted in a multigravida patient. Which of the following is the best recommendation?

    a. Refer the patient for surgical repair.

    b. Perform daily abdominal crunch exercises.

    c. Bed rest

    d. Wear an abdominal binder.

99. A postpartum woman who chooses not to breastfeed should be advised to do which of the following relief measures for breast engorgement:

    a. Apply ice bags to breasts.
    b. Avoid analgesics.
    c. Apply warm compresses to breasts.
    d. Do not wear a bra.

100. Which of the following is the most common causative organism of mastitis?

    a. *Escherichia coli*
    b. *Klebsiella*
    c. *Mycoplasma*
    d. *Staphylococcus aureus*

101. A 16-year-old boy presents for his annual physical exam. On exam the nurse practitioner identifies the patient's pubertal development at Tanner I: he has small testes, no pubic hair development, no elongation of penis, and no facial hair. Your assessment is:

    a. Patient has normal pubertal development for a 16-year-old boy.
    b. Patient's pubertal development is slower than usual but still within the lower range of normal for his age.
    c. Patient's pubertal development is delayed and needs evaluation by a pediatric Endocrinologist.
    d. Patient should be reassessed in 3 months; if he still does not have secondary sexual characteristics a hormonal workup will be started.

102. Upon physical exam, the nurse practitioner assesses a 12-year-old boy patient to be at Tanner stage II in his pubertal development. Select the pubertal characteristics expected of Tanner stage II:

    a. Testicle and penile width and length are both developing quickly.
    b. Testicles are growing larger; skin of the scrotum is becoming darker with straight, fine, sparse hairs on the genitals and axilla.
    c. Penis is growing larger in width than in length with darker scrotal skin and dense. Pubic hairs are darker, curly, and coarse.
    d. Penis is growing larger in length than in width; testicles are becoming larger with darker scrotal skin and a moderate amount of pubic hair starting to curl.

103. Among cancer death rates for American men, prostate cancer is ranked as:

   a. First

   b. Second

   c. Third

   d. Fourth

104. The American Cancer Society recommends routine, annual, digital rectal examination and annual prostate specific antigen (PSA) measurement in asymptomatic African American men starting at which age?

   a. 30

   b. 35

   c. 40

   d. 45

105. Which age group would comprise the most realistic target for screening for testicular cancer?

   a. 10–15 years of age

   b. 15–35 years of age

   c. 35–55 years of age

   d. 55–75 years of age

106. In patients with testicular tumors, the most common presentation is:

   a. A dull ache in the scrotum and lower abdomen

   b. Gynecomastia

   c. Symptoms of epididymitis

   d. Absence of symptoms

107. On examination of a 9-year old boy, the testis is not palpable in the right scrotal sac, and a 1 cm, slightly firm testis is palpable in the left scrotal sac. Regarding this patient's risk for development of testicular carcinoma, which of the following statements is correct?

   a. The malignancy that most commonly develops in a patient such as this case is a seminoma.

   b. Placement of the right testis into the scrotal sac by surgical correction greatly reduces this patient's risk.

   c. Most testicular carcinomas occur in patients with undescended testicles.

   d. The risk is higher if the missing testicle is in the inguinal canal than if it is in the intra-abdominal area.

108. The mother of a 10-year old boy with sickle cell anemia calls the office stating that her son woke up this morning with a painful penile erection that will not go away. The nurse practitioner's appropriate intervention is:

a. Recommend an increase in the child's fluid intake
b. Instruct mother to apply an ice pack to her son's penis and scrotal area and monitor for the next 24 hours
c. Recommend immediate referral to the emergency department
d. Insert a Foley catheter to obtain a specimen for a urinalysis and urine for culture and sensitivity

109. A 70-year-old man patient presents to the office for his annual urologic exam. He has a history of benign prostatic hyperplasia (BPH). Which of the following clinical findings is expected during the prostatic exam for this patient?

a. Prostate feels rubbery and uniformly enlarged.
b. Prostate feels boggy and warm.
c. Prostate feels hard and indurated.
d. Presence of tender nodules on the lateral edge of the gland

110. Which of the following actions is contraindicated in patients with acute prostatitis?

a. Serial urine samples
b. Rectal exams
c. Massaging the infected prostate
d. Palpation of the epididymis

111. Spermatogenesis initiates in the following area of the male anatomy?

a. Epididymis
b. Seminal vesicles
c. Vas deferens
d. Testes

112. A 25-year-old sexually active man presents with a 3-day history of fever and pain over the right scrotum. He also reports frequency and dysuria. The scrotum is edematous and tender to touch. He denies flank pain, nausea, and vomiting. He states the pain is lessened when he uses a scrotal support. The urinalysis shows 2+ blood and a large number of leukocytes. What is the most likely diagnosis?

a. Urinary tract infection
b. Acute pyelonephritis
c. Acute orchitis
d. Acute epididymitis

113. A 55-year-old man complains of a 3-year history of progressively worsening nocturia 3–4 times per night, increased hesitancy upon initiation of urinary stream, and decreasing stream size. The nurse practitioner's next step is to do the following:

   a. Order an alkaline phosphatase test
   b. Order a bone scan
   c. Perform a digital rectal examination
   d. Order a PSA test

114. How long does sperm remain viable after ejaculation into the vagina?

   a. 24 hours
   b. 48 hours
   c. 3 days
   d. 6 days

115. A man who undergoes a semen analysis during an infertility workup has the following results:

Volume	1.0 mL
Sperm concentration	6 million/mL
Motility	55%
Morphology	50%

   These findings indicate:

   a. Poor velocity
   b. Abnormal sperm shape
   c. Slow-moving sperm
   d. Low sperm count

116. The first sign of puberty in a boy is:

   a. Testicular enlargement
   b. Appearance of pubic hair
   c. Appearance of axillary hair
   d. Growth

117. A testicular volume of 6–12 mL is which Tanner stage?

a. Stage II

b. Stage III

c. Stage IV

d. Stage V

118. A full triangle of adult-type coarse, curly pubic hair with no extension down the lateral thigh is which Tanner stage?

a. StageII

b. Stage III

c. Stage IV

d. Stage V

119. A physiologic protective mechanism to prevent urinary tract infections in men and boys is:

a. Alkaline urine pH

b. Adherent mucin lining of the bladder

c. Descending flow of seminal fluid

d. Acidic urine pH

120. As you are examining a newborn boy in the nursery, you notice that his testicles are not in the scrotum, and you are unable to palpate them in the inguinal canal. You tell his parents that you will be following this closely because of the risk of infertility and malignancy, and that medical or surgical correction may be necessary if the testicles do not descend into the scrotum. Of the following, the *most* appropriate age at which medical or surgical correction should take place if the testicles do not descend is:

a. Immediately at birth

b. 6 months to 1 year of age

c. At the onset of puberty

d. After puberty is fully completed

121. The most common cause of priapism in childhood is:

a. Sickle cell disease

b. Idiopathic

c. Medication side effect

d. Trauma

122. Which classification of medications is associated with erectile dysfunction:

   a. Antipyretics
   b. Antibiotics
   c. Anti-inflammatories
   d. Antihypertensives

123. Several patients in an outpatient clinic have requested prescriptions for sildenafil (Viagra). Sildenafil would be contraindicated for use in which of the following patients?

   a. A patient diagnosed with type 2 diabetes
   b. A patient with benign prostatic hypertrophy (BPH) who is being managed medically
   c. A patient taking medication for angina pectoris
   d. A patient who has chronic sinusitis with flare-ups in the spring

124. According to CDC recommendations, Expedited PartnerTherapy (EPT) should not be considered for use in which situation?

   a. Female client with gonorrhea and her male partner
   b. Male client with gonorrhea and his female partner
   c. Teenage female with gonorrhea and her teen male partner
   d. Male client with gonorrhea and his male partner

125. What time interval should be considered for repeat testing for repeat infection with *Chlamydia*?

   a. 2 weeks
   b. 1 month
   c. 3 months
   d. Repeat testing for repeat infection is not recommended for *Chlamydia*

126. What is the CDC 2020 preferred treatment for gonorrhea infections (for patient under 300 pounds) with a negative *Chlamydia* co-test of the cervix, urethra, and rectum?

   a. Doxycycline 100 mg twice daily for 7 days
   b. Fluoroquinolone single-dose therapy
   c. Ceftriaxone 250 mg IM and doxycycline 100 mg twice daily for 7 days
   d. Ceftriaxone 500 mg IM

127. A 23-year-old sexually active woman with no general medical concerns presents for exam in your office. She has no history of prior STD or abnormal Pap tests. Her visit last year included a Pap test with normal results, negative *Chlamydia*, and negative gonorrhea testing. She denies at-risk behaviors. Which of the following testing should be offered at the visit today?

a. No Pap or GC/CT testing is indicated at this visit.

b. No Pap test is indicated but GC/CT testing should be completed.

c. Both a Pap test and GC/CT testing should be completed.

d. A Pap test and CT testing only should be completed.

128. The most common cause of nongonococcal urethritis (NGU) is which of the following organisms?

a. *Trichomonas vaginalis*

b. *Neisseria gonorrhoeae*

c. Herpes simplex virus

d. *Chlamydia trachomatis*

129. A 22-year-old woman who has had unprotected intercourse presents for evaluation of an irritating vaginal discharge. Visual exam reveals a frothy discharge. Wet-mount exam is negative for all findings except a few white blood cells on high power. Which combination of testing should be considered?

a. Only gonorrhea

b. Both gonorrhea and *Chlamydia*

c. Gonorrhea, *Chlamydia,* and *Trichomonas* testing

d. None of the above. If wet mount is negative, this is sufficient testing.

130. A 16-year-old boy presents with questions regarding the human papillomavirus (HPV) vaccine, of which they have not received any doses. The patient was recently told they have genital warts. What are current recommendations for the HPV vaccine?

a. Males are not recommended for HPV vaccine at any age.

b. Advice should include consideration for vaccine for this patient.

c. The patient should be advised that it is too late to obtain the vaccine because he is already infected with HPV.

d. The patient should be told that he should defer vaccine until a later age because he is only an adolescent.

131. Syphilis is considered most contagious during what stage?
    a. Primary
    b. Secondary
    c. Tertiary
    d. All stages are equally contagious.

132. Which of the following people should have trichomoniasis screening annually?
    a. Adolescent boys, because they are at high risk for infection without complaints
    b. A 30-year-old man with prior diagnosis of syphilis without complaints
    c. A 40-year-old woman presenting for an annual pelvic exam without complaints
    d. A 23-year-old HIV-positive woman presenting for an annual pelvic exam without complaints

133. Routine bloodwork screening for STDs should include the following?
    a. Hepatitis B surface antibody, hepatitis C antibody with confirmatory quantitative viral level, HIV
    b. Hepatitis B surface antigen, hepatitis C antibody with confirmatory quantitative viral level, HIV
    c. Hepatitis B surface antigen, hepatitis C antibody with confirmatory quantitative viral level, HIV, syphilis testing
    d. Hepatitis B surface antigen, hepatitis C antibody with confirmatory quantitative viral level, HIV, syphilis testing, herpes IgG screening

134. Which of the following is a risk factor for developing osteoarthritis?
    a. Obesity
    b. History of athletic overuse
    c. Joint trauma
    d. All the above

135. Which of the following is recommended for management of rheumatoid arthritis?
    a. Care by an expert in rheumatic disease
    b. Shared decision-making
    c. Early use of disease-modifying antirheumatic drugs (DMARDs) to limit disease activity
    d. All the above

136. Which of the following is a special considering in women of childbearing age being treated with disease-modifying antirheumatic drugs (DMARDs)?

a. Pause treatment with methotrexate, hydroxychloroquine before conception to prevent fetal injury.

b. Increase doses of methotrexate in pregnancy.

c. Avoid folic acid supplementation.

d. Advise exclusive breastfeeding for 1 year.

137. Which of the following statements is true regarding the incidence of gout?

a. Women are affected 18 times more often than men.

b. Men are affected nine times as often as women.

c. Peak onset of new cases occurs in adolescent boys.

d. There is no gender difference in prevalence.

138. Which of the following is the goal for the management of developmental hip dysplasia?

a. Prevent long-term complications and pathologic changes through early diagnosis and treatment in infancy

b. Prompt referral to an orthopedist

c. Proper skin care while wearing harness

d. All the above

139. Which of the following symptoms is considered uncommon in adolescents with idiopathic scoliosis and requires further evaluation?

a. Back pain

b. Loss of height

c. Dysuria

d. Degenerative disk disease

140. Which of the following populations is most affected by osteoporosis?

a. Pregnant women

b. Postmenopausal women aged 50 years and older

c. Men aged 50 years and older

d. None of the above

141. Which of the following is considered first-line therapy for osteoporosis?

   a. Vitamin D and calcium supplementation
   b. Proton pump inhibitors
   c. Miacalcin nasal spray
   d. Oral bisphosphonates

142. Which of the following describes the etiology of slipped capital femoral epiphysis (SCFE)?

   a. Multiple factors contribute to weaking of the physis and the femoral head slipping off the femoral neck.
   b. The etiology is clear and distinct.
   c. Growth hormones are responsible for SCFE.
   d. Prevention is necessary.

143. Which of the following is considered a risk factor for the development of Osgood-Schlatter's disease?

   a. Sports that require running, jumping (e.g., soccer, basketball)
   b. Sedentary lifestyle in school-age children
   c. Secondary smoke exposure
   d. All the above

144. Risks for Tourette syndrome include:

   a. Folic acid deficiency, poor prenatal care, and a previous sibling with a neural tube defect
   b. Folic acid deficiency accompanied by a sibling with a history of seizures
   c. Low birth weight, maternal stress during pregnancy, and folic acid deficiency
   d. Obstetrical complications, maternal stress during pregnancy, and genetic disposition

145. A red flag for immediate referral to or consultation with a neurologist includes:

   a. Inability to walk by age 9 months
   b. Retention of normal newborn reflexes past the sixth month of life
   c. Persistent Moro reflex after age 4 months
   d. Open anterior fontanelle at age 10 months

146. Common findings in patients diagnosed with Down syndrome include:

  a. Intellectual disability, infant hypertonia, hearing loss, and hyperthyroidism.
  b. Intellectual disability, infant hypotonia, hearing loss, and visual refractive errors.
  c. Obesity, normal developmental milestone achievement, and hearing loss.
  d. Failure to thrive, infant hypertonia, and congenital heart disease.

147. During a physical exam of a 19-year-old patient, you notice pale blue irises, probable mitral valve prolapse through auscultation, and macroorchidism. What disorder do you suspect?

  a. Down syndrome
  b. Cerebral palsy
  c. Fragile X syndrome
  d. Multiple sclerosis

148. Sarah, age 34, presents to your clinic with a complaint of headaches that began in the last few months and have gradually worsened. The pain is always in the occipital region and may last for several hours. She mentions she gets visual disturbances (scintillation) in both eyes about 30 minutes before the headache begins. Sarah denies congestion. Which of the following is the most likely diagnosis for this patient?

  a. Migraine headache
  b. Sinus headache
  c. Cluster headache
  d. Tension headache

149. An abortive medication for migraine symptoms is:

  a. Sumatriptan (Imitrex)
  b. Butalbital (Fiorinal and Fioricet)
  c. Hydrocodone/acetaminophen (Lortab)
  d. Fentanyl (Sublimaze)

150. Gina, age 46, presents to your clinic accompanied by her partner. Gina's partner has noticed that she has had some memory changes, difficulty with spatial awareness and judging distances, loss of coordination including hand–eye coordination, and trouble speaking. You suspect a brain lesion. Given these symptoms, where is the lesion most likely located?

  a. Temporal region
  b. Frontal
  c. Parietal
  d. Occipital

151. Pain triggers for trigeminal neuralgia may be touch, cold, or chewing. Which cranial nerve is involved?

   a. First cranial nerve
   b. Fifth cranial nerve
   c. Eighth cranial nerve
   d. Tenth cranial nerve

152. A patient presents with Bell's palsy and is curious about what may have caused this condition. Which of the following statements about Bell's palsy is true?

   a. Reactivation of the herpes simplex virus is suspected in most cases.
   b. Surgical decompression leads to an improved outcome.
   c. All cases resolve in 1 month when treated with an antiviral medication.
   d. Use of high doses of glucocorticoids is indicated for a minimum of 6 months.

153. Aneurysms associated with a subarachnoid hemorrhage are typically caused by bleeding in what area of the brain:

   a. The parietal area
   b. The frontal area
   c. Interpeduncular cistern area
   d. Temporal area

154. Azi returns for a 1-month follow-up for iron-deficiency anemia. Lab work reveals no improvement in hemoglobin. Present treatment is ferrous sulfate 325 mg orally three times a day. Your response to this finding is:

   a. Begin parental iron administration
   b. Confirm adequate adherence
   c. Repeat blood work
   d. Refer to hematology

155. You receive Hulu's lab report, which identifies Bence-Jones protein in the urine. This confirms your suspected diagnosis of:

   a. Multiple myeloma
   b. Sickle cell anemia
   c. Urinary tract infection
   d. Renal failure

156. Smith presents to your sickle cell clinic requesting another prescription for oxycodone. The patient lost the prescription obtained 2 weeks ago. This is the third time over the past 6 months that this has occurred. After completing your ROS and exam, which are normal for the patient, your best response to this request is to:

a. Give another and clearly explain that you will not be able to do this again.

b. Establish a pain management contract.

c. Refer to social work.

d. Call the pharmacy to verify that the prescription was not filled.

157. Harry, 19 years old, presents for a well visit. PAST MEDICAL HISTORY: positive sickle cell trait, up to date on immuni zations, denies illicit drug use, no alcohol use, no tobacco use. Patient is concerned that sickle cell anemia will develop. Your best response to this concern is:

a. Tell the patient that you will order appropriate tests if signs or symptoms develop.

b. Tell the patient this would have developed already.

c. Say that this information is important if Harry considers having children.

d. Refer the patient to hematology for further evaluation.

158. Sarah, your 22-year-old patient, presents for an ill visit complaining of dysuria and hematuria. No fever, no abdominal pain, or back pain. PAST MEDICAL HISTORY: G6PD deficiency. The urine dipstick confirms a UTI. Which drug would you avoid prescribing?

a. Ciprofloxacin

b. Sulfamethoxazole/trimethoprim

c. Amoxicillin

d. Cephalexin

159. Mary, a 29-year-old woman, presents for an annual well visit. PAST MEDICAL HISTORY: none. PSH: tonsillectomy. Denies tobacco or illicit drug use. She admits to drinking alcohol socially, two to three glasses per week. She admits to trying to get pregnant. In response, you recommend the following:

a. Take 400 μg of folic acid when the patient gets pregnant.

b. Take 400 μg of folic acid daily beginning today.

c. Increase daily calcium intake.

d. Increase daily protein intake.

160. Jeremy, a 3-year-old, presents with mom who verbalizes concern that Jeremy bruises easy and bleeds more than usual after a small cut. Your exam is normal other than the large bruises on patient's lower leg. You order CBC with differential and PT and PTT. The lab contacts you because his PTT is prolonged. All other data are normal. Your response to this is:

    a. Repeat the test to confirm.
    b. Order factor VII and factor IX levels.
    c. Refer to hematology.
    d. Refer to the ED.

161. Seller, a 78-year-old patient, presents with a past medical history: hypertension, diabetes mellitus, chronic kidney disease. Was recently diagnosed with normocytic normochromic anemia. The most likely etiology for his anemia is:

    a. Pernicious
    b. Iron deficiency
    c. Folic acid deficiency
    d. Anemia of chronic disease

162. Erb's laboratory results were returned today. The abnormal results are Hgb 11 g/dL, Hct 34%, and MCV 110 f/L. What type of anemia does the patient have?

    a. Thalassemia
    b. Aplastic
    c. Iron deficiency
    d. Vitamin B12 deficiency

163. The presence of Reed-Sternberg cells on a peripheral smear is consistent with which disease?

    a. Hemophilia
    b. Hodgkin's lymphoma
    c. Sickle cell disease
    d. Hemochromatosis

164. You are evaluating the care of patients with diabetes at your clinic to see whether these patients have appropriate diabetes management. Which of the following metrics indicate that the patients with diabetes are being appropriately managed:

    a. All patients have an HbA1c test every 3 months.
    b. All patients with diabetes have a yearly retinopathy screen.
    c. All patients with diabetes have blood pressure less than 120/80.
    d. All patients have urine screened every 6 months for the presence of microalbumin.

165. You are seeing your 12-year-old patient for the first time after she was newly diagnosed with type 1 diabetes. You note that there are many gaps in the knowledge of both the patient and her parents and that she is next scheduled to see the endocrinologist in 3 months. Your next action is to:

   a. Schedule a follow-up visit with you in 3 months to see how they are managing.

   b. Call the patient's endocrinologist in an attempt to schedule the patient sooner.

   c. Make an appointment with a certified diabetes educator in the next week.

   d. No action needs to be taken; change is difficult and both the patient and parents need time to adjust to the new diagnosis.

166. Janet, a 32-year-old patient, asks you if you would consider her diabetes type 2 to be under control at the present time. You answer that presently you do consider her diabetes under control. A thorough explanation to her response would include which of the following:

   a. She has not had a vaginal yeast infection in over 1 year.

   b. Her HbA1c is currently 7.2 and her blood pressure is 128/80.

   c. Her HbA1c is less than 6.9 and according to her blood glucose logs, her blood glucose is between 70 mg/dL and 180 mg/dL about 80% of the time and below 70 mg/dL only twice in the past 6 months.

   d. Her HbA1c is 6.5 and she is not reporting symptoms of polyuria.

167. In your clinic you are evaluating a 30-year-old Black woman with a BMI of 29, a history of rapid weight loss, fatigue, abdominal pain, and polyuria, and you note a finger-stick blood glucose of 352 mg/dL. The most prudent decision is to:

   a. Send the patient to the lab to obtain necessary blood work and start the patient on lifestyle modifications.

   b. Send the patient to the lab to obtain necessary blood work and start the patient on metformin in addition to lifestyle behavioral modifications, because she likely has type 2 diabetes. Follow up in 2 weeks.

   c. Send the patient to the lab to obtain an HbA1c; start the patient on glipizide in addition to lifestyle behavioral modifications, because she likely has type 2 diabetes. Follow-up in 2 weeks.

   d. Send the patient to the emergency department for evaluation because you suspect diabetic ketoacidosis.

168. A 56-year-old Black man presents to your clinic for a well check-up. Upon review of his labs, you note that 3 months ago his HbA1c was 6.7% and today it is 7.2%. All his other lab values are within normal range. You tell him he has a diagnosis of type 2 diabetes and you:

    a. Start him on lifestyle modifications such as weight loss, low carbohydrate diet, exercise
    b. Tell him he likely has diabetes and repeat the test in 3 months
    c. Start him on lifestyle modifications such as weight loss, low carbohydrate diet, exercise, and glargine insulin 10 units q.h.s.
    d. Start him on lifestyle modifications such as weight loss, low carbohydrate diet, exercise, and metformin 500 mg orally twice a day

169. A 60-year-old white woman (74 kg) presents for follow-up care after you recently diagnosed her with hypothyroid disease. She reports to you that she feels well and has no complaints. You started her on levothyroxine 50 µg daily, and the repeat TSH 6 weeks later is 5.49 mU/L. Your next step is to:

    a. No changes to levothyroxine dose and repeat TSH in 6 weeks
    b. Increase levothyroxine dose to 75 µg daily and repeat TSH in 3 weeks
    c. Increase levothyroxine dose to 75 µg daily and repeat TSH in 6 weeks
    d. Increase levothyroxine dose to 75 µg daily and repeat TSH in 12 weeks

170. Denise, a 38-year-old woman, presents with weakness, hirsutism, fatigue, high blood pressure, late period, and complaints that her body is changing, and she does not understand why. You notice that her face appears round, and she has what looks like a "buffalo hump" on her back. You are considering a series of labs to aid in diagnosis. Which of the following is the best plan?

    a. Could we go over your medication list again? Are you taking any medications that contain steroids? If the answer is "no" then order a pregnancy test, TSH, HbA1c, a 24-hour urine free cortisol test, dexamethasone salivary test, and midnight salivary cortisol.
    b. I will order a pregnancy test and TSH and if they are negative, then I will ask you to return to the clinic to discuss some dietary changes.
    c. Could we go over your medication list again? Are you taking any medications that contain steroids? If yes, order a pregnancy test, TSH, HbA1c, a 24-hour urine free cortisol test, dexamethasone salivary test, and midnight salivary cortisol.
    d. I would like to do a complete work up to check you for polycystic ovarian syndrome. If that is negative, then I would like to schedule a follow-up to discuss dietary changes.

171. A 68-year-old Black male patient of yours has been admitted three times this year for heart failure. Upon reviewing his list of medications, which should be discontinued?

a. Metoprolol

b. Metformin

c. Lisinopril

d. Sitagliptin

172. Which of these symptoms may be absent in a patient with type 1 diabetes:

a. Abdominal pain

b. Lower-extremity edema

c. Polyuria

d. Fruity odor

173. You diagnose a patient with hyperthyroidism. The first intervention you chose to start is:

a. A beta-blocker

b. A thioamide

c. Thyroidectomy

d. Radioactive iodine

174. A 30-year-old patient presents with weakness, hypotension, severe abdominal pain, vomiting, weight loss, painful joints, darkening skin in the creases of her palms. She reports craving salt. These symptoms began a few months ago but were not very bad until this week after the patient was treated for a kidney infection. You plan to order labs and suspect the patient may have:

a. Latent autoimmune diabetes of adulthood (LADA)

b. Cushing syndrome

c. Addison's disease

d. Gastritis

175. A 22-year-old junior college student presents to the University Health Center for evaluation of sad mood. She shares feelings of sadness, poor appetite, difficulty falling asleep, and fatigue with low energy. She has been feeling down for about the past month. She states that because of her sadness she has trouble concentrating on academic studies; however, she is still maintaining a passing grade. She says her friends have noticed that she moves slower than usual, taking longer to get things done. She denies suicidal ideations, panic attacks, or the recent loss of a loved one. The most likely diagnosis is which of the following?

    a. Anxiety disorder
    b. Substance use disorder
    c. Major depressive disorder
    d. Post-traumatic stress disorder

176. Which of the following is an appropriate dose of citalopram for a client 60 years of age or older with depression?

    a. 20 mg by mouth once daily
    b. 20 mg by mouth twice daily
    c. 40 mg by mouth once daily
    d. 60 mg by mouth once daily

177. Which of the following case scenarios is the best example of integrated behavioral health care?

    a. The FNP screens every client for depression with a validated screening instrument.
    b. The FNP prescribes paroxetine to a patient with generalized anxiety disorder in consultation with an on-site psychologist who is treating the patient with psychotherapy.
    c. A client with schizophrenia presents for an annual physical exam; the FNP renews psychotropics the client is taking to manage psychotic symptoms.
    d. A client with obsessive compulsive disorder is referred to a community mental health center.

178. Which of the following is the best first-line treatment option for a person diagnosed with a mild to moderate major depressive disorder?

    a. Escitalopram 5 mg by mouth daily with a referral to psychotherapy
    b. Desipramine (Norpramin) 300 mg daily with a referral to psychotherapy
    c. Alprazolam (Xanax) 0.5 mg three times as day as needed when feeling down
    d. A monoamine oxidase inhibitor

179. Which of the following psychotropic medications is an appropriate treatment for a 25-year-old woman diagnosed with bulimia nervosa and a depressive disorder?

   a. Wellbutrin (Bupropion)

   b. Clonazepam (Klonopin)

   c. Fluoxetine (Prozac)

   d. Alprazolam (Xanax)

180. The FNP, in collaboration with the consulting child psychiatry specialist, starts an adolescent client on a selective serotonin reuptake inhibitor (SSRI) for depression. When initiating an SSRI, which health education needs to be imparted to the client and caregivers?

   a. Monitor for suicidal behavior.

   b. Monitor for the development of a tic disorder.

   c. Instruct to take the medication on an as-needed basis.

   d. Instruct that serum levels will be monitored every 3 months.

181. A 38-year-old client with a major depressive disorder is started on a selective serotonin reuptake inhibitor (SSRI). When initiating an SSRI, which education needs to be discussed with the client?

   a. Sexual side effects

   b. Urine discoloration

   c. Dehydration

   d. Sleep-driving

182. A 12-year-old client presents with parents for a routine wellness visit. The client has a mental health diagnosis of conduct disorder. Which of the following is a risk factor for this mental health disorder?

   a. History of oppositional defiant disorder

   b. History of obsessive compulsive disorder

   c. History of a tic disorder

   d. History of seizures

183. Which of the following is considered a first-line psychotropic treatment for children with attention-deficit/hyperactivity disorder (ADHD)?

   a. A selective serotonin reuptake inhibitor

   b. A serotonin and norepinephrine reuptake inhibitor

   c. A psychostimulant

   d. An antipsychotic

184. A client with an alcohol use disorder is on maintenance treatment with disulfiram (Antabuse) and a 12-step program. What education does the FNP provide in each health care–related encounter?

   a. Instruct the client to use a backup contraceptive method while taking this medication.

   b. Instruct to take the medication on an as-needed basis when having an alcohol craving.

   c. Instruct the client to take medication every other day.

   d. Instruct the client not to consume or use personal hygiene products containing alcohol.

APPENDIX B

REVIEW QUESTION ANSWERS

1. Correct Answer: B. According to the Consensus Model for Advanced Practice Registered Nurses (APRNs), nurse practitioners, nurse anesthetists, nurse midwives, and clinical nurse specialists are all APRNs. Nurse educators are not APRNs.
2. Correct Answer: B. The National Organization of Nurse Practitioner Faculties (NONPF) National Task Force (NTF) consensus-based standards facilitate program quality.
3. Correct Answer: D. Authority for nurse practitioner (NP) practice is found in state legislative statutes and in rules and regulations.
4. Correct Answer: B. Provided that the nurse practitioner (NP) has a Medicare provider number, Medicare will reimburse for services at 85% of the customary physician rate.
5. Correct Answer: A. Leaving a message without specific medical details on the patients' home phone does not violate HIPAA as there is no disclosure of medical information. Had the NP left a detailed message about the ~~patients'~~ patient's condition or medical care on the answering machine without the ~~patients'~~ patient's consent to do so, a HIPAA violation would have occurred.
6. Correct Answer: B. In Duvall's theory of the stages in family development, the stages are based on the age and school placement of the firstborn child.
7. Correct Answer: D. Family nurse practitioners (FNPs) must be able to identify and critically evaluate evidence-based research. This means evaluating current research in the context of the study parameters as well as evaluating the potential efficacy in specific patient populations. Participation in outcome studies is also a critical role for the FNP.
8. Correct Answer: C. An occurrence policy covers any claim that results from an incident that occurs during the term of the policy, regardless of how long it takes before the claim is made.
9. Correct Answer: C. According to the Centers for Disease Control and Prevention (CDC), health disparities are preventable, inequitable differences in disease burden and opportunities to achieve optimal health that are experienced by socially disadvantaged populations.
10. Correct Answer: D. Palliative care is comprehensive care for short- or long-term illnesses, including incurable conditions. The goal is to manage symptoms and improve quality of life. Unlike hospice care, palliative care allows for life-saving measures and does not

require a terminal illness diagnosis. It is a multidisciplinary approach that addresses social, psychological, and spiritual needs, as well as physical needs.

11. Correct answer: B. The Affordable Care Act allows adults younger than 26 years old to remain on their parent's policy, ended pre-existing condition exclusions, and covers preventive care with no copayment.
12. Correct answer: C. Agency for Healthcare Research and Quality recommends that women ages 50 to 74 years get a screening mammography every 2 years and get a diagnostic exam if positive or a mass is present. Self-breast exams at home are not a substitute for recommended screenings. An oncologist is not necessary for routine screenings.
13. Correct answer: B. This is an example of a genetic screening test that allows for early detection of an illness to reduce the progress or severity of the disease.
14. Correct answer: D. If you live in a neighborhood where you do not feel safe, this is identified as a social determinant of health under the Social and Community Context.
15. Correct answer: B. DTaP Many older adults may have had boosters of tetanus but not pertussis. Yet, pertussis can be present in older adults with a subclinical presentation. This can be harmful to the baby.
16. Correct answer: D. Refer the child to a specialist. This child will need to have a workup to determine the cause and potential treatments for precocious puberty.
17. Correct answer: A. Postmenopausal women should take 1000–1500 mg of calcium daily to reduce the risk of osteoporosis.
18. Correct answer: C. Polypharmacy of five or more drugs at one time is a common problem with potential drug interactions. Drug toxicities are more common and more serious in the older adults.
19. Correct answer: D. Bone density measurements are not recommended for women younger than age 65 and optimal intervals have not been established. Regular weight-bearing exercise is the only evidence-based recommendation to maintain optimal bone density.
20. Correct answer: C. Agency for Healthcare Research and Quality (AHRQ) recommends colonoscopies for adults ages 50 to 75 years. Since Mr. King is 78 years old, he does not need another colonoscopy.
21. Correct Answer: C. Mononucleosis is suspected because of the patient's age, the length of incubation, and the triad involving the pharynx, lymph nodes, and liver.
22. Correct Answer: D. Inhalation anthrax is evidenced by pulmonary complications, as opposed to cutaneous anthrax, which is evidenced by a skin abscess; there is no rash and there are no hematologic changes.
23. Correct Answer: B. Mumps is associated with parotitis (swelling of the salivary glands) and orchitis (inflammation of the testes) in males.

24. Correct Answer: B. Children under the age of 18 may not consent for their own medical care in most circumstances unless they have been deemed in charge of themselves (emancipated) by the court system.
25. Correct Answer: C. Influenza vaccination is a universal recommendation for all pregnant women.
26. Correct Answer: D. Measles, mumps, and rubella (MMR) vaccine is a live vaccine and is contraindicated in pregnancy because of potentially harmful or unknown effects to the fetus.
27. Correct Answer: B. Varicella zoster is spread by respiratory contagion and not through contact.
28. Correct Answer: A. In the United States, vaccinated, domesticated dogs do not carry rabies; all wounds should be cleaned and irrigated.
29. Correct Answer: C. Vaccination remains the most effective way to prevent SAR-CoV-2 infection and should be considered first line in prevention.
30. Correct Answer: B. HSV is a recurrent mucocutaneous infection spread by contact with HSV lesions on mucosal surfaces, in genital secretions or oral mucosa.
31. Correct Answer: C. Basal cell carcinoma tumors are slow growing and are the most common skin cancer. Patients most at risk are those with excess sun exposure, particularly fair-skinned individuals. Men and individuals over the age of 40 are most commonly affected.
32. Correct Answer: A. Chiggers present with discrete bright red papules on the legs and belt line. Flea bites present as irregularly grouped or linear urticarial wheals or papules with central puncta. Spider bites present as swelling or erythema at the site. Mosquito bites are scattered erythematous pruritic wheals with central puncta.
33. Correct Answer: B. Gabapentin and pregabalin are effective systemic agents to treat postherpetic neuralgia. Cymbalta (duloxetine) is an appropriate treatment for diabetic peripheral neuropathy, while Ultram (tramadol) and Celebrex (celecoxib) are not indicated for postherpetic neuralgia.
34. Correct Answer: D. Amoxicillin/clavulanate (Augmentin) is the most appropriate prophylactic antibiotic for human bites to cover for *Staphylococcus aureus*, alpha-hemolytic streptococci, and *Eikenella corrodens*.
35. Correct Answer: C. Referral to a general surgeon for extensive and chronic hidradenitis is the top priority for definitive treatment. Local heat and avoiding antiperspirants are appropriate non-pharmacologic treatments but are not the top priority as they will not treat the infection. Steroids, such as prednisone, may be indicated for episodic flares of chronic disease in conjunction with oral antibiotics.

36. Correct Answer: A. acute urticaria lasts 24 to 36 hours, chronic urticaria lasts longer than 6 weeks, spontaneous urticaria has no identifiable causative factor, and inducible urticaria has an identifiable causative factor.
37. Correct Answer: C. Atopic dermatitis is an IgE-mediated hypersensitivity reaction.
38. Correct Answer: D. Acne rosacea is a chronic acneiform inflammation of the central third of the face. Chronic inflammation can cause irreversible hypertrophy of the nose, known as rhinophyma, and is most commonly seen in men 40 and older.
39. Correct Answer: B. Pityriasis rosea is a benign self-limited skin eruption that presents with a sentinel herald patch. Herald patches are 2 to 6 cm in diameter scaly plaques commonly located on the trunk, followed by general exanthem in 1 to 2 weeks. The other conditions listed do not present with a herald patch.
40. Correct Answer: C. Congenital esotropia is generally found in children younger than 6 months. Monocular diplopia is double vision in one eye. Accommodative esotropia is the most common cause of esotropia in childhood and develops between the ages of 6 months and 7 years. It is rare for accommodative esotropia to develop before 4 months or after 8 years of age. There are no other CNS symptoms to suspect sixth nerve palsy.
41. Correct Answer: A. African American patients are much more likely than White patients to develop open-angle glaucoma and are also more likely to have vision loss from glaucoma. Depression and hyperthyroidism are not risk factors for open-angle glaucoma. Open-angle glaucoma affects the older adult. Angle-closure glaucoma can be seen in patients as young as 40–50 years of age.
42. Correct Answer: D. Patient has no history of trauma or infection. This is a spontaneous hyphema. In the past, accepted practice included hospital admission, but sending a patient home with instructions to avoid further trauma and vigorous activities is sufficient in reliable patients with limited disease. Outpatient referral to ophthalmology should be considered but does not need to be done emergently. Steroids ophthalmic groups are not clinically indicated with hyphemas.
43. Correct Answer: B. The hallmark of acute gonococcal conjunctivitis is severe purulent discharge, which occurs within 12–24 hours of infection. Preauricular adenopathy may also be seen. Management consists of Gram stain of purulent material to document gonococcus, culture, ceftriaxone IM/IV plus azithromycin (or spectinomycin if cephalosporin allergic), eye irrigation, and treatment for possible concurrent chlamydial infection. Penicillin is not an appropriate treatment for gonococcal infections. Latanoprost (Xalatan) and timolol maleate (Timoptic) ophthalmic drops are indicated for the treatment of glaucoma.
44. Correct Answer: B. Intraoperative floppy iris syndrome is a well-known risk factor for complications during cataract extraction in patients who are on or who have previously used tamsulosin (Flomax). Tamsulosin is the most commonly prescribed α-1 adrenergic blocker for the treatment of benign prostatic hyperplasia. It is important that the surgeon is aware of this prior to surgery.

45. Correct Answer: D. Amoxicillin is the first-line treatment of acute otitis media (AOM). The dose is 80–90 mg/kg/day via two doses in all patients, whether antibiotic naïve or not. Broad-spectrum (and expensive) drugs such as ceftriaxone, azithromycin, and amoxicillin/clavulanate should be reserved for patients who fail initial therapy with a first-line drug or have a penicillin allergy. All children under 6 months of age with otitis media should be treated with antibiotics. Patients from 6 months to 2 years should receive antibiotics if the diagnosis is certain or the diagnosis is suspected and the patient meets high-risk criteria (moderate-to-severe ear pain, fever of 102.2°F or higher, immunosuppressed). In patients 6 months to 2 years, observation is an option if the diagnosis is uncertain or they meet low-risk criteria (fever lower than 102.2°F, mild otalgia, immunocompetent, and follow-up assured within 48–72 hours). Patients with proven AOM who are older than 2 years may be observed rather than treated with antibiotics as long as they meet low-risk criteria. Analgesics should be given to all patients.

46. Correct Answer: B. Primary oral herpes (herpetic gingivostomatitis) is associated with a relatively high fever and anteriorly placed ulcerations and vesicles (gums, tongue, and lips). Symptoms tend to start relatively abruptly with pain, salivation, refusal to eat, and fever. Herpes gingivostomatitis may recur during life in the form of "cold sores." The patient does not have hand and foot lesions; therefore, C is incorrect. Varicella can occur in the oral pharynx but would have lesions elsewhere in various stages and respiratory symptoms as well. Aphthous ulcers are usually seen in older children/young adults, usually do not occur on the lips, and are not contagious.

47. Correct Answer: C. Otitis externa can be treated with a wide array of topical agents. One option is to acidify the external ear canal. Neither *Pseudomonas* nor *Staphylococcus* species can thrive at an acidic pH. Thus, acetic acid drops (VosoL) can be used: they are inexpensive and effective. Another approach is to use a topical antibiotic. Polymyxin/neomycin combinations are safe and effective. A number of other antibiotic preparations are available as well. Alcohol-based solutions are another alternative. Oral treatment is not indicated for simple otitis externa unless there is associated OM or cellulitis of the outer ear present. However, topical ciprofloxacin may be used. Carbamide peroxide otic solution is for earwax removal and has no role in the treatment of OE.

48. Correct Answer: D. Tinnitus is the perception of sound without external auditory stimulus. The examination is most commonly normal, and audiometry is the gold standard diagnostic study. Cognitive behavioral therapy, avoiding loud noises, and hypnosis are all adjuvant therapies. Supportive care and reassurance are mainstays of tinnitus therapy.

49. Correct Answer: C. This patient has a corneal abrasion from contact lens use. Corneal abrasions from contact lens use are commonly colonized with *Pseudomonas aeruginosa* and the best option would be a fluroquinolone such as ciprofloxacin (Ciloxan) or ofloxacin (Ocuflox). Patanol is appropriate for allergic conjunctivitis, whereas ganciclovir is used for viral infections. Natamycin is used for fungal infections.

50. Correct Answer: C. Patients with bacterial pneumonia normally present with sudden onset of high fevers, green- to rust-colored sputum, and pleuritic chest pain. Atypical pneumonia normally presents as a low-grade fever and headache; symptoms are more gradual. Acute bronchitis normally presents initially as an upper respiratory tract infection followed by a prolonged cough; abnormal vital signs are unlikely. Upper respiratory tract infection commonly presents as fever and cough; however, signs of consolidation are not seen on chest auscultation.

51. Correct Answer: D. Acute bronchitis is a self-limiting condition that usually resolves in 1 to 3 weeks. It is most commonly caused by a viral infection. Nonpharmacologic options for cough are usually recommended. OTC cough suppressants or other nonpharmacologic options are usually recommended for clients desiring something for the cough. Antibiotics are not routinely prescribed. Antihistamines dry out secretions and should not be used in patients with acute bronchitis. Inhaled beta agonists are used for patients with wheezing or other underlying pulmonary disease.

52. Correct Answer: D. The goal screening for TB infection is to identify individuals at risk for the development of active TB disease. Routine screening is not recommended for low-risk patients (e.g., community-dwelling individuals from a low-risk country). The client does not currently have risk factors for the new TB infection. The induration should be measured, not the erythema. An induration of ≥15 mm in individuals with no known factors for TB is considered positive. An induration of ≥10 mm is considered positive in recent immigrants, IV drug users, residents and employees of high-congregate settings, laboratory employees, individuals with preexisting health conditions, and children younger than 5 years of age. An induration of 5 mm or larger is positive in individuals with an old TB infection or in individuals who are HIV positive, immunosuppressed, or a recent contact of a person with TB disease. If the client had already been working in the correctional facility or had risk factors for new TB infection prior to testing, an induration of 10 mm or larger would have been the correct answer.

53. Correct Answer: D. Supportive care and anticipatory guidance are recommended for uncomplicated bronchiolitis. Glucocorticoids and bronchodilators are not routinely used for the management of a first episode of bronchiolitis or uncomplicated bronchiolitis. Cold preparations are not recommended in children younger than 6 years of age.

54. Correct Answer: A. The American Thoracic Society and Infectious Diseases Society of America (ATS/IDSA) recommends monotherapy with amoxicillin as a first-line therapy in healthy adults, younger than 65 years of age, and with no recent antibiotic use; monotherapy with doxycycline or a macrolide are suggested alternatives. Combination therapy with amoxicillin/clavulanate, amoxicillin-clavulanate plus clarithromycin, or levofloxacin is recommended for adults 65 years old or older, or with comorbidities, or recent antibiotic use.

55. Correct Answer: D. Patients greater than 12 years of age with mild asthma will have FEV1 greater than 80% predicted and FEV1/FVC ratio 85%, which is the same for intermittent disease.

56. Correct Answer: A. According to the 2022 GINA guidelines, the client should be moved to a Step 3 treatment: a low dose ICS-LABA (fluticasone-salmeterol) or medium-dose ICS should be added controller (maintenance) therapy. The patient should continue the short-acting beta adrenergic (albuterol) for acute symptom treatment. Formoterol is not indicated in children under 12 years of age. A short-acting beta adrenergic is only indicated as reliever therapy and is not controlling symptoms; better coverage with a controller therapy is needed.

57. Correct Answer: D. Inhaled formoterol, is a LABA and when used alone as a controller agent for asthma has been associated with a 2- to 4-fold increased risk of death related to asthma or other respiratory conditions. LABAs should always be used as combination therapy, such as ICS-LABA or ICS-LAMA-LABA, for safer use.

58. Correct Answer: B. The goal in management of COPD is to relieve symptoms, improve exercise tolerance and health status, prevent disease progression, prevent and treat exacerbations, and reduce mortality.

59. Correct Answer: B. Lung cancer should always be suspected in a current or former smoker with new onset cough or hemoptysis.

60. Correct Answer: A. Warfarin is the only anticoagulant approved for mechanical valve replacements

61. Correct Answer: C. Mitral stenosis is a diastolic murmur, best heard at the left 5th intercostal space (ICS), midclavicular line (MCL). It is associated with infective endocarditis and chronic rheumatic heart disease. Mitral regurgitation is a systolic murmur, best heard at the left 5th MCL with possible radiation to the left axilla. It is commonly associated with infective endocarditis, rheumatic heart disease, congenital anomalies, and inferior wall myocardial infarctions.

62. Correct Answer: A. This client has Stage 1 hypertension because her systolic blood pressure is between130–139 and diastolic blood pressure is between 80–89. Because she is considered high risk (with atherosclerotic cardiovascular disease [ASCVD] or 10-year cardiovascular disease [CVD] risk greater than 10%), the appropriate treatment is to initiate drug therapy immediately. For most clients, the FNP should start with a thiazide-type diuretic . The FNP will need to reassess blood pressure in 1 month and if at goal, reassess again in 3 to 6 months. If blood pressure is not at goal at 1 month reassessment, the FNP will consider adding another blood pressure-lowering medications.

63. Correct Answer: C. Postinfarction according to the American College of Cardiology (ACC), a person with a recent history of myocardial infarction should be on aspirin, an antiplatelet such as clopidogrel, (or prasugrel, ticagrelor), high-dose statin atorvastatin 80 mg once daily, and a beta-blocker. There is no recommendation for the patient to be on acetaminophen (Tylenol), fluoxetine (Prozsac), or famotidine (Pepcid) for cardiovascular concerns.

64. Correct Answer: B. According to American College of Cardiology (ACC), for adults with Stage 1 hypertension who are at high risk (Atherosclerotic cardiovascular disease [ASCVD]

10-year risk is greater than 10%) lifestyle modification plus medication treatment is recommended with repeat blood pressure assessment 1 month after initial diagnosis.

65. Correct Answer: B. Low-molecular-weight heparin (LMWH) is the recommended anticoagulation therapy for a pregnant client with deep vein thrombosis (DVT). Most other anticoagulants are not appropriate for a pregnant client because they have the potential to cross the placenta.

66. Correct Answer: C. During pregnancy the client can continue drug(s) used before pregnancy, except ACE inhibitors (like lisinopril), Angiotensin II Receptor Blockers (ARBs), and direct renin inhibitors; beta-blockers may cause growth retardation in early pregnancy; if hypertension develops during pregnancy (after the first 20 weeks of pregnancy), use or transition to labetalol, nifedipine, or methyldopa (Whelton, 2017).

67. Correct Answer: C. According to the American College of Cardiology (ACC)/American Heart Association (AHA) an LDL below 130 is recommended for adults who are low risk: fewer than 2 risk factors.

68. Correct Answer: C. For very high-risk adults: If LDL-C level remains ≥70 mg/dL (≥1.8 mmol/L) on high-intensity statin may add ezetimibe to maximally dosed (tolerated) statin therapy. If after adding ezetimibe to statin, LDL is greater than 70 may add a PCSK9 inhibitor

69. Correct Answer: A. A client with Stage B (pre-HF) (class I recommendations):

- ♦ Left ventricular ejection fraction (LVEF) ≤ 40%:
  - ◊ use an ACEI (decreases mortality, prevents symptomatic HF) or
  - ◊ BB (prevents symptomatic HF)
- ♦ LVEF ≤ 40% and recent or remote history of ACS/MI:
  - ◊ statins to prevent adverse CV events and prevent symptomatic HF,
  - ◊ use evidence-based BB to decrease mortality
- ♦ LVEF ≤ 40% and recent ACS/MI and unable to tolerate ACEI, use an ARB
- ♦ LVEF < 30% with minimum of 40 days post-MI with NYHA class I symptoms while on GDMT and with life expectancy greater than1 year, ACC/AHA recommends implantable cardioverter-defibrillator (ICD) as primary prevention of sudden death

70. Correct Answer: D. Patients describe oropharyngeal dysphagia as a feeling of food getting stuck, indicative of upper esophageal or pharyngeal disease; may present as difficulty swallowing solids or liquids, described as trouble initiating a swallow; coughing; choking; nasal regurgitation (oropharyngeal dysplasia); sensation of food "sticking" after it is swallowed (esophageal dysphasia). May be a structural or neuromuscular problem and can present as chest pain.

71. Correct Answer: C. AST is found in liver, cardiac, skeletal, kidney, and brain tissue; elevated levels alone may indicate tissue damage in any of those organ systems. AST cannot be fractionated. Liver biopsy should not be done prior to serological workup.

72. Correct Answer: C. Most common cause: functional—poor dietary intake of fiber and fluids, behavioral habits such as change in environment with travel or schedule, sedentary life-style; occurs in children most often when cereal is first introduced to diet, during toilet training, or entry to school. Commonly reported peripheral side effects of anticholinergic medicines include dry mouth, dry eyes, constipation, urinary retention, blurred vision, and increased heart rate

73. Correct Answer: A. If vomiting continues despite slow intake of fluids, consider use of an antiemetic.

    Antidiarrheal agents are controversial in AGE because the causative pathogen needs to be eliminated from the body. In mild to moderate diarrheal illness, antidiarrheal medications can be used with caution (but not if fever and blood in stool). Chemoreceptor trigger zone suppressors will suppress vomiting; antihistamines are more effective for nausea than for acute vomiting; antimotility agents to suppress diarrhea prolong absorption time of water in the gut but also may cause retention of bacteria.

    Antibiotics are used only when an organism is isolated, and symptoms are not resolved.

74. Correct Answer: B. Symptomatic condition characterized by reflux or retrograde passage of low pH gastroduodenal contents into the esophagus, larynx, or lungs causing in children poor weight gain, respiratory disorders. In infants, regurgitation of some of a feeding; 47% of all infants under 2 months of age display normal physiologic gastro-esophageal reflux without associated symptoms at least two times daily and outgrow by 10 months to 1 year.

    May cause damage to esophageal mucosa with or without failure to thrive, occult blood loss, anemia, and possibly aspiration pneumonia with or without wheezing

75. Correct Answer: A. American Gastroenterological Association: combination of chronic and recurrent GI symptoms not explained by structural or biochemical abnormalities. Rome III criteria for diagnosis: 12 or more weeks in the last 12 months of abdominal pain or dis-comfort that has two of three features; relieved by defecation, onset associated in change of frequency of stool, onset associated with change in form of stool.

76. Correct Answer: D. Clinically, hernias can be described as reducible (contents can be pushed back into the abdominal cavity), nonreducible (contents cannot be pushed back into the abdominal cavity), incarcerated (a nonreducible hernia in which the flow of intesti-nal contents is obstructed), or strangulated (an incarcerated hernia in which the blood supply of the hernia contents is compromised).

77. Correct Answer: C. Risk factors include incidence increases at and after age 40, with 90% of new cases occurring in adults age 50 and older. Previous history or family history of adenomatous polyps. Family history of colorectal cancer, especially in a first-degree relative diagnosed before age 55. Familial polyposis. Inflammatory bowel disease. History of breast or gynecological cancer. Barrett's esophagus. Obesity. Cigarette smoking

78. Correct Answer: B. Differential Diagnosis. Gastroenteritis. Tumor. Constipation/impaction. Meckel's diverticulum. Incarcerated inguinal hernia. Malrotation/volvulus. Hirschsprung's disease

79. Correct Answer: B. ALT and AST may be elevated; levels peak (400 to several thousand U/L) during the icteric phase, and then decrease progressively during the convalescent phase. Serum bilirubin is normal to markedly elevated; clinical jaundice evident at levels higher than 2.5 mg/dL. Alkaline phosphatase may be normal or mildly elevated. Prothrombin time, if prolonged, may indicate serious disease.

80. Correct Answer: A. The primary effect of antidiuretic hormone (ADH) is to increase water retention through the collecting ducts.

81. Correct Answer: C. All children 2 months to 2 years of age with a documented first UTI should have VCUG to exclude anatomic abnormality.

82. Correct answer: C . Nocturnal enuresis beyond 5 years of age in girls and 6 years in boys is a relatively common problem. Primary enuresis is defined as a patient who has never had an extended period of dryness since birth. Secondary enuresis is the onset of bed-wetting after a 6-month period of dryness. Bed-wetting usually occurs during the first REM sleep cycle, when sleep is relatively light. It may also occur in other stages, except for Stage 1. Diagnostic testing is typically limited to UA to rule out infection.

83. Correct answer: C. In most cases the evaluation of urinary incontinence requires only a history, pulmonary embolism, urinalysis, and measurement of postvoid residual. This initial evaluation is to identify conditions requiring referral or a specialized workup to detect and treat reversible causes, which may include infection, atrophic urethritis, pelvic floor weakness, medications, change in mental status, or overflow urinary incontinence related to obstruction (constipation vs. benign prostatic hyperplasia [BPH]).

84. Correct answer: D. All potential causes of hematuria must be considered, and all individual risk factors considered, so that an underlying disease requiring treatment can be identified or ruled out. Approximately 80%–90% of patients with bladder cancer present with painless gross hematuria.

85. Correct Answer: C. BPH is the most common cause of microscopic hematuria in men over 60; however, gross hematuria demands further evaluation to rule out etiology, which includes cancer.

86. Correct Answer: B. Fosfomycin is an oral, not injectable, antimicrobial agent.

87. Correct Answer: C. Antibiotics should be prescribed, first broad spectrum then based on culture for 7 days.

88. Correct Answer B: Costovertebral angle (CVA) tenderness on fist percussion is diagnostic for acute pyelonephritis in addition to pertinent subjective symptoms.

89. Correct Answer D: The major cause of stress incontinence is urethral hypermobility due to impaired support from pelvic floor.

90. Correct answer: A . Asymptomatic bacteriuria has never been shown to lead to renal dam age in women without anatomic abnormality or obstruction. Intercourse and diaphragm use have both been shown to increase risk for asymptomatic as well as symptomatic UTI. Prevalence in older adult women is 20%–50%. *Treatment is indicated only in pregnancy.*

91. Correct Answer: C. Menometrorrhagia is described as an irregular pattern of menstrual periods of increased amount or duration. Metrorrhagia is the term used for menstrual periods occurring at irregular intervals of varying flow and duration. Hypomenorrhea involves regular menstrual periods with a reduced amount of time and reduced volume about less than 60 mL . Polymenorrhea is a term used to characterize regular menstrual periods but at intervals of less than 21 days.

92. Correct Answer: B. The diaphragm birth control method is best used after about 6 to 8 weeks postpartum when uterine involution is complete, and the vagina has regained its tone following childbirth. Patients with a history of urinary tract infections, toxic shock syndrome, or a vaginal delivery within 6 weeks are unsuitable candidates for the diaphragm birth control method.

93. Correct Answer: C. The Copper T IUD may be inserted within 5 days (120 hours) after unprotected intercourse to reduce the risk of pregnancy by 99.9%. This form of emergency contraception prevents fertilization of the ovum and may prevent the implantation of a fertilized egg.

94. Correct Answer: A. The first-line outpatient treatment for PID is a multiple-drug regimen that covers several pathogens, including gonorrhea and chlamydia. This includes ceftriaxone (Rocephin), doxycycline, and metronidazole. Both oral cephalosporins and quinolone agents are no longer recommended treatments for gonococcal infections because of resistance.

95. Correct Answer: D. Acanthosis nigricans, hirsutism, and obesity occur with PCOS, as well as hyperinsulinemia and insulin resistance. HAIR-AN syndrome = hyperandrogenism, insulin resistance, acanthosis nigricans.

96. Correct Answer: A. It is safe to administer tetanus toxoid (Td) in pregnancy. The Td booster protection is considered active for 10 years. However, suppose the patient does not remember when she received the last booster or have documentation. In that case, it is safe to revaccinate with Td because the benefit outweighs the risk of the disease. Note that the Tdap vaccine is preferred in pregnant patients at over 20 weeks of gestation and is recommended in each pregnancy, regardless of tetanus vaccination history.

97. Correct Answer: A. Mumps, Measles, Rubella (MMR) contains a live vaccine and is thereby not safe to use in pregnancy. According to CDC guidelines, the COVID-19 vaccine is recommended for pregnant patients and Hepatitis B and Polio vaccines may be administered to pregnant patients in some circumstances.

98. Correct Answer: B. It is a normal pregnancy change for the rectus abdominis muscles to stretch apart with the growth of the uterus. Teaching the postpartum patient to perform daily abdominal crunch exercises (sit-ups) will promote closure of the rectus abdominis musculature and strengthen the abdominal muscle wall.

99. Correct Answer: A. Breast engorgement is an inflammatory process. Applying ice, taking analgesics, and wearing a supportive bra will help reduce breast engorgement; applying heat is not recommended to reduce inflammation and will promote milk ejection.

100. Correct Answer: D. Most cases of mastitis are caused by *Staphylococcus aureus,* an organism found commonly on the skin and in normal oral flora.

101. Correct Answer C. At 16 years of age without any signs of secondary sexual characteristics being present, this patient's pubertal development is markedly delayed. If there is no testicular development noted by age 14, a referral to an endocrinologist is indicated. There is a normal range of pubertal development and some boys develop secondary sexual characteristics sooner than others, but still within the normal range. Those who start pubertal development at a later age are monitored and considered to have constitutional delay providing secondary sexual characteristics are noted before or by age 14. Pubertal development can also be delayed in patients due to malnutrition, systemic disease, and defects of the reproductive system such as hypogonadism.

102. Correct Answer B. Tanner stage II is when the testicles start to grow. The scrotal skin becomes thicker and starts to get darker. The pubic hair is of a fine texture and straight and there are a few countable hairs on the genitals and the axilla.

103. Correct Answer B. Lung cancer is rated as the number 1 leading cause of death among men and prostate cancer is the second highest cause of death.

104. Correct Answer: C. The American Cancer Society recommends age 40 to begin routine, annual digital rectal examination and prostate-specific antigen (PSA) testing in asymptomatic African American men. This population has a higher incidence of prostate cancer and is more likely to have aggressive tumors than men of other races. In asymptomatic Caucasian men, age 40 is recommended for the start of digital rectal examinations, and age 50 to start PSA testing.

105. Correct Answer: B. The age group of 15–35 years is the one in which testicular cancer is most prevalent. Because of the common occurrence of testicular cancer in this age group, testicular self-examination should be taught to young men in early puberty. Approximately 35% of testicular tumors are seminomas, which are malignant neoplasms. These tumor types are highly radiosensitive where if the tumor stage is low, radiation alone is used after transinguinal radical orchiectomy is performed.

106. Correct Answer: D. Testicular tumors most commonly present with no symptoms. They are usually picked up incidentally on palpation or self-examination when the patient finds a painless mass in the testicle.

107. Correct Answer: A. The testicular malignancy that develops most commonly in a patient with an undescended testicle (cryptorchidism) is a seminoma. Cryptorchidism is slightly more common on the right side than the left. About 10% of all testicular carcinomas (not majority) develop in patients with a history of cryptorchidism, and 5%–10%of these develop in the contralateral (normally descended) testicle. The risk of malignancy is greater if the undescended testicle is in the intra-abdominal area than if it is in the inguinal canal. Surgical placement of the undescended testicle into the scrotal sac offers no decrease in the risk but helps earlier detection of malignancy.

108. Correct Answer: C. Priapism (painful penile erections not caused by sexual activity) is an urgent urological emergency that if left untreated could result in permanent erectile dysfunction and penile necrosis.

109. Correct Answer: A. The prostate should feel rubbery and uniformly enlarged with benign prostatic hyperplasia (BPH). A boggy and warm prostate with tenderness is consistent with acute prostatitis. Hard nodules and indurated areas are highly suggestive of prostate cancer.

110. Correct Answer: C. Massaging the infected prostate is contraindicated for acute prostatitis because the massage can spread the bacteria from the prostate into the bloodstream and lead to sepsis.

111. Correct Answer: D. Initial stages of spermatogenesis occurs within the testes and progress onto the epididymis where the developing gametes mature and are stored until ejaculation.

112. Correct Answer: D. Acute epididymitis is the infection noted in this case. Scrotal edema and pain with palpation do not occur with urinary tract infection or pyelonephritis. Acute orchitis symptoms include testicular pain and edema and do not have frequency and dysuria. Acute orchitis is usually associated with mumps.

113. Correct Answer: C. The digital rectal examination is the first evaluative step to be done for this patient who has prostatism. Prostatism (enlarged prostate gland) is commonly caused by either benign prostatic hypertrophy/hyperplasia (most common), prostatitis, or prostatic carcinoma. A combination of more than one of these conditions can also occur simultaneously.

114. Correct Answer: C. Sperm are viable for 3 days, or 72 hours.

115. Correct Answer: D. A normal sperm count is greater than 39 million/mL. All other findings in this semen analysis are within the normal, expected range. The volume of 1.0 mL is below average. A very low volume indicates that the seminal vesicles may not be making enough fluid or that these ducts may be blocked. It may also indicate a problem with the prostate gland. The sperm count of greater than 39 million is the normal range for the number of sperm per milliliter. Counts below 10 million are considered poor; counts of 20 million or more may be fine if motility and morphology are normal. Two aspects of motility are evaluated: the number of active cells as a percentage of the total number of cells (rated from 0–100%, at least 50% should be active) and the quality of the movement of the sperm (rated from 0–4; a score of 2 or more is satisfactory). At least 30% of cells should be of normal shape according to the World Health Organization. The Kruger (strict) morphology test examines the shape and size of the sperm head. Normal results are when 14% or more of the sperm have normal-shaped heads. Men with less than 4% normal-shaped sperm may have a significant infertility problem.

116. Correct Answer: A. Testicular enlargement is the hallmark sign of puberty in a boy.

117. Correct Answer: B. When using Prader beads to assess testicular volume, a volume of 6–12 mL is consistent with Tanner stage 3 for boys.

118. Correct Answer: C. A full triangle of adult-type coarse, curly pubic hair without extension onto the thighs is consistent with Tanner stage 4 in boys and girls.

119. Correct Answer: D. Acidic urine pH, anti-adherent mucin lining the walls of the urinary bladder, and descending flow of urine from the urethra all serve as protective physiologic mechanisms to prevent urinary tract infection in men and boys. Descending flow of seminal fluid serves no role in preventing UTIs in men and boys.

120. Correct Answer: B. Observation is not recommended beyond 1 year of age because it delays treatment, lowers the rate of surgical success, and may impair spermatogenesis. By 6 months of age, patients with undescended testicles should be evaluated by a pediatric urologist or other qualified subspecialist who can assist with diagnosis and treatment. Earlier referral may be warranted for bilateral nonpalpable testes in the newborn or for any child with both hypospadias and an undescended testis. Therapy for an undescended testicle should begin between 6 months and 1 year of age and may consist of hormone or surgical treatment.

121. Correct Answer: A. Sickle cell disease (SCD) is the most common cause of priapism in childhood being responsible for 65% of cases. Leukemia, trauma, and idiopathic causes are the causes in 10% of patients. Priapism in childhood commonly presents as a common symptom of SCD, especially after puberty, mainly as low flow or as a complication of penile trauma (normally high-flow, nonischemic episodes). This phenotypic manifestation of SCD can cause persistent impotence, erectile dysfunction, and behavioral problems in the sexual realm, as affected individuals fear the induction of an episode of painful erection in the course of normal sexual activity, which is the most common cause of priapism episodes after puberty.

122. Correct Answer: D. Beta blockers such as propranolol and ACE inhibitors such as captopril, furosemide, and digoxin have all been implicated in inhibiting erectile function.

123. Correct Answer: C. Nitrates are the most common drugs used in the management of angina. Current evidence indicates that patients taking nitrates should not ingest sildenafil at the same time because a sudden drop in blood pressure could occur that could lead to sudden death. A diagnosis of diabetes would not be a contraindication for use of sildenafil. Finasteride used to treat BPH may cause impotence and may decrease the effectiveness of sildenafil, but these effects are not as significant as the risk of cardiac arrest. Sildenafil may worsen chronic sinusitis, but the effect is not as significant as cardiac arrest.

124. Correct Answer: D. Evidence has been shown supporting EPT in clinical trials involving heterosexual men and women with chlamydia or gonorrhea. In addition, teens can consent for STD treatment. Data on use of EPT for men who have sex with men (MSM) is limited and is not currently recommended by Centers for Disease Control and Prevention for routine practice.

125. Correct Answer: C. Any person who tests positive for chlamydia or gonorrhea, along with women who test positive for *Trichomonas,* should be rescreened once 3 months of treatment is completed. This recommendation is related to high rates of repeat infection and should not be confused with the recommended interval for test of cure.

126. Correct Answer: D. Current recommendations are for treatment with only ceftriaxone 500 mg IM. Doxycycline alone will not cover gonorrhea infection. Because of concerns about emerging gonococcal resistance to cephalosporins, the CDC discontinued recommendations for oral cephalosporins for treatment of gonococcal infection. Single treatment for gonorrhea was made the new treatment recommendation in 2020 if negative *Chlamydia* testing is obtained.

127. Correct Answer: B. Pap test intervals for female patients ages 21–29 with no abnormal Pap history is every 3 years. CDC guidelines recommend both gonorrhea and *Chlamydia* testing annually for sexually active women and girls younger than 25 years of age.

128. Correct Answer: D. *C. trachomatis* is the major cause of NGU (23%–55%).

129. Correct Answer: C. If a 22-year-old woman presents for evaluation with vaginal discharge and history of unprotected intercourse, testing for both gonorrhea and *Chlamydia* should be ordered. *Trichomonas* testing is also recommended if wet mount is negative, because office studies detect only 51%–65% of infections.

130. Answer: B. All genders are now recommended for vaccine between the ages of 9 and 26 regardless of prior or current known HPV infection. Possible consideration for dosing up through age 45.

131. Correct Answer: B. Secondary syphilis, which occurs 6 weeks to 6 months after infection, is considered the most contagious.

132. Correct Answer: D. Trichomoniasis testing is recommended annually for female HIV-positive patients. Up to 53% of HIV-positive women are coinfected with *Trichomonas vaginalis. If results are positive, repeat testing is advised within 3 months after treatment is completed.*

133. Correct Answer: C. STD blood labs should include hepatitis B, hepatitis C, syphilis, and HIV testing. Hepatitis B surface antigen is done to check for infection, whereas hepatitis B surface antibody is used to check immune status. Herpes IgG by blood is not advised for routine screening for herpes. Herpes testing should occur via swab when lesion is present.

134. Correct Answer: D. obesity, overuse, and history of trauma are all risk factors for developing OA. Additional factors include occupation, heredity, and endocrine disorders.

135. Correct Answer: D. Management goals of rheumatoid arthritis include early diagnosis, care by an expert in rheumatology, shared decision making, disease-modifying antirheumatic drugs (DMARDs), preventing irreversible joint damage, maximizing mobility, and limiting pain.

136. Correct Answer: A. Women being treated with disease-modifying antirheumatic drugs (DMARDs) require preconceptual counseling, as it is necessary to pause DMARD treatment to prevent fetal harm. Doses of methotrexate are not increased. Folic acid would be advised as per usual treatment of pregnant women. Breastfeeding is not advised because DMARDs are secreted in breast milk.

137. Correct Answer: B. Men are affected nine times as often as women. Gout rarely affects men before adolescence or women before menopause. Peak incidence for men is the fourth to fifth decades and women the sixth to seventh decades of life.

138. Correct Answer: D. All are goals of management of developmental hip dysplasia. The goal is to prevent long-term complications and pathologic changes through early diagnosis and treatment in infancy. Prompt referral to an orthopedist. Pavlik harness, worn 24 hours per day, is the treatment of choice with a success rate of 80%–97%. Weekly follow-ups are needed. Proper skin care while wearing harness. Surgery recommended if harness treatment is unsuccessful.

139. Correct Answer: A. Back pain is uncommon in adolescents with idiopathic scoliosis, so further examination warranted if pain present. Loss of height, dysuria, and degenerative disk disease are not associated with scoliosis of adolescents.

140. Correct Answer: B. Osteoporosis primarily affects postmenopausal women 50 years of age and older. Pregnant women and men 50 years of age and older are not the groups typically diagnosed with osteoporosis.

141. Correct Answer: D. First-line therapy for osteoporosis is oral bisphosphonates: alendronate or risedronate. The other options are not considered first-line therapy. Proton pump inhibitors are not indicated in the treatment of osteoporosis.

142. Correct Answer: A. Multiple factors contribute to the slipping of the femoral head from the femoral neck. None of the other options is true.

143. Correct Answer: A. Sports that require running, jumping—soccer, basketball, football, ballet, figure skating, and gymnastics—are considered risk factors for OSD. Symptoms often present after a growth spurt in adolescents.

144. Correct Answer: D. Folic acid deficiency not recognized as a risk factor for Tourette syndrome.

145. Correct Answer: B. The inability to walk by 9 months, Moro reflex after 4 months, and an open anterior fontanelle at 10 months are considered normal findings. Retention of normal newborn reflexes past the sixth month of life may indicate neurological developmental concern and requires immediate intervention.

146. Correct Answer: B. Intellectual disability, infant hypotonia, hearing loss, and visual refractive errors are all associated with Down syndrome making B the correct answer. Infant hypertonia, hyperthyroidism, failure to thrive, and normal developmental milestone achievement are not associated with Down syndrome.

147. Correct Answer: C. Fragile X syndrome is a genetic defect that may result in pale blue irises, mitral valve prolapse, and macroorchidism (greater than 18 years of age). Persons with Down syndrome, cerebral palsy, and multiple sclerosis do not typically present with these symptoms.

148. Correct Answer: A. Migraine headache pain may present in various areas of the head and are commonly associated with auras (sensory disturbances) and typically last for minutes to hours. Sinus headaches typically present with fever and/or congestion, and cluster headaches usually present with several episodes per day. Tension headaches are usually described as squeezing, band-like pain that gradually increases over days to years.

149. Correct Answer: A. Sumatriptan in a migraine abortive agent that is effective in most people. Barbiturates and opioids are not recommended treatment for migraine.

150. Correct Answer: C. Brain lesions with spatial awareness changes and loss of hand–eye coordination are typically found in the parietal lesion of the brain.

151. Correct Answer: B. Trigeminal neuralgia involves the fifth cranial nerve.

152. Correct Answer: A. Reactivation of herpes simplex virus is suspected in most cases. Surgical intervention is not indicated for Bell's palsy. Use of antiviral medications and steroids as a treatment for Bell's palsy remains controversial and is typically reserved for a severe presentation. Antivirals are given for no more than 7 days and normal dosing of glucocorticoid doses for treatment would be for no more than 14 days.

153. Correct Answer: C. Aneurysms that cause subarachnoid bleeding are typically associated with bleeding in the circle of Willis located in the interpeduncular cistern area of the brain.

154. Correct answer: B. The most likely reason for no improvement in anemia is adherence to the regimen. If adequate adherence is confirmed, re-evaluate the etiology of anemia. Refer to hematology for cases that are unresponsive to treatment. Parenteral iron is used in resistant cases.

155. Correct answer: A . Bence-Jones protein in urine is indicative of multiple myeloma. It is not associated with sickle cell anemia, renal failure, or a UTI.

156. Correct answer: B. Using a pain contract establishes a mutually beneficial agreement in a positive manner. Consulting the social worker is not appropriate for this situation. Providing another prescription perpetuates the situation. Verifying the prescription is time consuming and can lead to a confrontation.

157. Correct answer: C . Sickle cell disease is an autosomal recessive genetic disorder requiring the gene from each parent. To have sickle cell disease, a person has to have both recessive alleles . No need for hematology referral for sickle cell trait.

158. Correct answer: B. Sulfa drugs are contraindicated in persons with G6PD deficiency because of the likelihood of hemolysis. Fluoroquinolones, cephalosporins, and penicillin are feasible options for patients with G6PD.

159. Correct answer: B. Neural tube defects are related to folic acid deficiencies; preconception increase of folic acid is recommended. No preconception recommendations for increased calcium or protein intake.

160. Correct answer: C. Referral to hematology as this situation requires specialty evaluation; not life-threatening for an ED referral. Not appropriate to repeat test as it correlates with the clinical picture.

161. Correct answer: D. Anemia of chronic disease is normocytic normochromic. Folic acid and pernicious anemia are macrocytic. Iron deficiency is microcytic.

162. Correct answer: D. MCV greater than100 in vitamin B12 deficiency, MCV normal in aplastic anemia and thalassemia, MCV decreased in iron-deficiency anemia.

163. Correct answer: B. Reed-Sternberg cells are associated with Hodgkin's lymphoma. Sickle-cell disease have sickled cells on peripheral smear. No specific cells are identified on peripheral smear with hemophilia or hemochromatosis.

164. Correct Answer: B: All patients with diabetes should have a comprehensive annual eye exam to evaluate for retinopathy. Biannual HbA1c is appropriate for well-controlled patients, making A incorrect.

165. Correct Answer: C: People with diabetes (and their families) should receive diabetes self-management education when they are diagnosed and as needed thereafter.

166. Correct Answer C: The common treatment plan is a goal for non-pregnant adults to maximize the time in glucose range (70–180 mg/dL) for 70% or more of the time, based on continuous glucose monitoring (CGM) or self-monitoring, HbA1c less than 7.0, and minimizing hypoglycemia to a goal of 4% or less of the time. Glycemic goals should be individualized and based on ASCVD, CHF, and renal status.

167. Correct Answer: D: Given the acute presentation of rapid weight loss, fatigue, elevated glucose, and abdominal pain, it is likely that patient has type 1 diabetes and may be in diabetic ketoacidosis, so she should be evaluated immediately.

168. Correct Answer: D: Weight loss, low carbohydrate diet, and exercise along with metformin are first-line interventions in someone with a new diagnosis of diabetes, so long as metformin is not contraindicated. Although glargine insulin theoretically could be started, its cost, risk of hypoglycemia, and weight gain makes it less favorable than metformin.

169. Correct Answer: C: Therapeutic TSH concentrations are not achieved for at least 6 weeks. Serum thyroid hormone concentrations increase first, and then TSH secretion begins to fall because of the negative feedback action of T4 on the pituitary and hypothalamus. Thus, after adjustment of T4 therapy, given that the patient is asymptomatic, the patient should be reevaluated and serum TSH measured again in 6 weeks.

170. Correct Answer A: This patient presents with classic symptoms of Cushing disease, but it would be important to screen for pregnancy, diabetes, and elevated TSH as well. Always screen for prescribed or unprescribed steroid use because long-term use of glucocorticoids could precipitate iatrogenic Cushing disease. If positive for steroid use, to avoid misdiagnosis, discontinue use and re-evaluate symptoms. Be sure not to discontinue too suddenly, however.

171. Correct Answer: B: Metformin should not be used in patients with unstable heart failure because of the risk of poor kidney perfusion leading to an increased risk of lactic acidosis.

172. Correct Answer: B. Lower-extremity edema is not a common symptom of type 1 diabetes, whereas the other answers are classic symptoms.

173. Correct Answer: A: A beta-blocker should be started (assuming there are no contraindications to its use) in most patients as soon as the diagnosis of hyperthyroidism is made. Beta-blockers ameliorate the symptoms of hyperthyroidism that are caused by increased beta-adrenergic tone while the workup of the cause of hyperthyroidism is done.

174. Correct Answer: C: Symptoms of Addison's disease may come on gradually or suddenly, especially if precipitated by infection or crisis. Common symptoms include weakness, fatigue, weight loss, nausea and vomiting, abdominal pain, craving salt, and feeling lightheaded or dizzy when standing. Patients may also report losing hair from armpits and pubic region. Patients may present with an adrenal crisis, in which case they are usually also confused and passing out.

175. Correct Answer: C. This client meets the criteria for a DSM-5 or DSM-5-TR diagnosis of major depressive disorder.

176. Correct Answer: A. 20 mg by mouth once daily. In clients age 60 years or older, the maximum daily dose is 20 mg/per day of citalopram because of the risk of QTc-interval prolongation.

177. Correct Answer: B. The FNP prescribes paroxetine to a patient with generalized anxiety disorder in consultation with an on-site psychologist who is treating the patient with psychotherapy. There are many models of integrated behavioral health care, but all involve a collaborative, multidisciplinary approach and systems for follow-up and monitoring of patient response to treatment. Answer B is the best example of this collaborative treatment approach.

178. Correct Answer: A. Escitalopram 5 mg by mouth daily with a referral to psychotherapy. Selective serotonin reuptake inhibitors with or without psychotherapy are considered first-line treatment for depression. In addition, escitalopram has minimal drug interactions.

179. Correct Answer: C. Fluoxetine (Prozac) has FDA approval for the treatment of bulimia nervosa and major depressive disorder. Wellbutrin (Bupropion) should be avoided in clients with an eating disorder because of the potential for a seizure, particularly in clients who induce vomiting.

180. Correct Answer: A. Monitor for suicidal behavior. There is a black box warning of increased suicidal ideation and behavior in children and young adults under 25 taking antidepressants. All the other options are not true.

181. Correct Answer: A. Sexual side effects. It is important to discuss with any client, whether male or female, the potential sexual side effects associated with SSRIs (especially paroxetine) and serotonin and norepinephrine reuptake inhibitors.

182. Correct Answer: A. History of oppositional defiant disorder. Conduct disorder is more common in children previously diagnosed with oppositional defiant disorder.

183. Correct Answer: C. A psychostimulants are the first-line choice for the treatment of ADHD.

184. Correct Answer: D. Instruct the client not to consume or use personal hygiene products containing alcohol. The ingestion of alcohol while on disulfiram (Antabuse) will bring on a disulfiram–alcohol reaction in which the person may get mildly to severely ill.

INDEX

Note: This index includes both volumes. Pages i–825 are in volume 1 and pages 829–1672 are in volume 2.

C

G

L

M

N

O

P

R

S

T